CLINICIAN'S HANDBOOK
OF
PRESCRIPTION DRUGS

D1272678

Notice

Medicine is an ever-changing science. As new research and clinical experience broaden our knowledge, changes in treatment and drug therapy are required. The authors and the publisher of this work have checked with sources believed to be reliable in their efforts to provide information that is complete and generally in accord with the standards accepted at the time of publication. However, in view of the possibility of human error or changes in medical sciences, neither the authors nor the publisher nor any other party who has been involved in the preparation or publication of this work warrants that the information contained herein is in every respect accurate or complete, and they disclaim all responsibility for any errors or omissions or for the results obtained from use of the information contained in this work. Readers are encouraged to confirm the information contained herein with other sources. For example and in particular, readers are advised to check the product information sheet included in the package of each drug they plan to administer to be certain that the information contained in this work is accurate and that changes have not been made in the recommended dose or in the contraindications for administration. This recommendation is of particular importance in connection with new or infrequently used drugs.

CLINICIAN'S HANDBOOK
OF
PRESCRIPTION DRUGS

Seymour Ehrenpreis, PhD

Former Chairman and Professor Emeritus of Pharmacology
Chicago Medical School
Chicago, IL

Eli D. Ehrenpreis, MD

Department of Gastroenterology
University of Chicago
Chicago, IL

McGRAW-HILL
Medical Publishing Division

New York Chicago San Francisco Lisbon London
Madrid Mexico City Milan New Delhi San Juan
Seoul Singapore Sydney Toronto

McGraw-Hill
*A Division of The **McGraw-Hill** Companies*

Clinician's Handbook of Prescription Drugs

Copyright © 2001 by The **McGraw-Hill Companies**, Inc. All rights reserved. Printed in the United States of America. Except as permitted under the United States Copyright Act of 1976, no part of this publication may be reproduced or distributed in any form or by any means, or stored in a data base or retrieval system, without the prior written permission of the publisher.

1 2 3 4 5 6 7 8 9 0   DOC/DOC   0 9 8 7 6 5 4 3 2 1

ISBN 0-07-134385-7

This book was set in QuarkXPress by Software Services.
The editors were Andrea Seils and Barbara Holton.
The production manager was Clare Stanley.
The cover designer was Elizabeth Schmitz.
R. R. Donnelley & Sons was printer and binder.

This book is printed on acid-free paper.

Library of Congress Cataloging-in-Publication Data

Ehrenpreis, Seymour.
    Clinician's handbook of prescription drugs/Seymour Ehrenpreis, Eli Ehrenpreis.
        p.; cm.
    Includes bibliographical references and index.
    ISBN 0-07-134385-7
        1. Drugs—Handbooks, manuals, etc. I. Ehrenpreis, Eli. II. Title.
    [DNLM: 1. Pharmaceutical Preparations—Handbooks. QV 39 E33c 2001]
RM301.12.E37 2001
615'.1—dc21   2001030501

TABLE OF CONTENTS

ADVISORY BOARD

PREFACE

A recent article published in the *New York Times* quoted the astounding statistic that as many as 7,000–10,000 deaths in the United States can be attributed on an annual basis to prescription errors. Countless hospital days, loss of productivity, and an atmosphere of distrust of modern medicine all result from such errors. Many causes can be found for these mistakes; drugs with completely different properties, uses, and toxicity profiles may have similar names. Polypharmacy, a common phenomenon in the elderly, places patients at risk for complex drug–drug interactions. Difficulty with high-volume record keeping and the loss of personal interaction with the "family pharmacist" certainly result in more patients receiving the wrong medication or dosage when a prescription is filled. Finally, the rapid pace of modern medical practices coupled with the ever–bewildering numbers of medications on the market result in a situation in which the busy practitioner may have difficulty keeping abreast of important aspects of the drugs they are prescribing. It was with these concerns in mind that we undertook the task of writing a manual of drug prescription for the practicing clinician. No one can be expected to commit to memory everything important about all the drugs available on the market. It can be quite time consuming and frustrating to search for important information on individual entries in a large comprehensive volume such as the *Physician's Desk Reference*. Thus, our main objective in creating this book was to provide the most essential information on all commonly prescribed drugs in a concise, accurate and easy-to-read manner.

In producing this book, it is our hope that we can help clinicians give the best care possible to patients taking prescription drugs. We believe this book will benefit you in looking up drugs that are not frequently prescribed. In addition, you will have an opportunity to reacquaint yourself with details about familiar drugs when using this book "at the bedside."

The book does not have complete entries for all prescription drugs. Some have been left out simply because of lack of sufficient available information or because of very limited use. In addition, we have not included many drug combinations because of space considerations. Furthermore, we have restricted our discussion in the case of drugs that are members of the same drug class. Most if not all of the drugs in a particular pharmacologic class have similar if not identical characteristics, for example, side effects, drug–drug interactions, contraindications. Accordingly, we have selected one or more drugs to serve as prototypes and these have been given a complete entry (as described below). For other members of the particular class, we have presented only essential information, referring the reader in each case to the prototype for additional details.

On the other hand, we have discussed in full a number of widely used drugs that for one reason or another are not listed in the *Physician's Drug Reference 2000* or for which only the drug name is stated without any details. In other instances, we provide even more complete information than offered by the manufacturer. For example, no drug–drug interactions are listed by the manufacturers for benzodiazepines in the *Physician's Desk Reference,* whereas we list a number of these interactions that are clinically important. The reader should note that some information provided may differ from that contained in the manufacturer's package insert. The decision to include or exclude information is based on our best judgment or on the advice of our Advisory Board after reviewing all available data.

A handbook such as this, with its emphasis on conciseness, can present only a relatively small fraction of the total knowledge available about any particular drug. Thus, it is our considered opinion that the clinician attempt to review available product information sheets as approved by the Food and Drug Administration should the need arise to expand on the information presented herein. We strongly believe that accessing the information provided with the easy-to-follow format we have created for this manual will make this book an important reference for clinicians in a wide variety of settings. If, overall, we are able to assist the health care provider to administer medications to their patients safely and effectively and thereby to treat their ailments as well as prevent complications of drug therapy, we will have achieved our desired goals.

The following format is used for all drugs:

Brand name: For drugs that have multiple brand names, we have listed those drugs that are widely prescribed.

Mechanism of action: This is stated succinctly, using at most one or two lines.

Indications/dosage/route: All approved indications are listed; occasionally, widely used unapproved indications are mentioned. For the most part, dosages recommended by the manufacturer are listed. Dosages are mainly the usual adult dose (persons <60 or 65 years). The following specific information about dosing is included wherever possible: initial dose, follow-up dose, maintenance and maximum doses, duration of drug administration, details for parenteral (in particular IV) administration. Wherever available, doses for children and the elderly are included.

Adjustment of dosage: Related primarily to kidney and liver disease. Guidelines are presented for adjusting dosage in relation to creatinine clearance or creatinine blood levels. We indicate if there is no need to adjust dosage for kidney or liver disease or for elderly or pediatric patients. Also stated are age limits for prescribing the drug for children or if the drug should be prescribed for this age group at all.

Onset of action, peak effect, and duration: Wherever available, time of onset of action, peak effect, and duration are listed. This information is considered most important for the proper spacing of drug administration. Other aspects of pharmacokinetics—peak serum levels, bioavailability, protein binding, half-life—as included in many sources, are not considered of utmost importance in pharmacotherapy per se and are not included.

Food: Wherever possible, mention is made of those foods to be avoided and whether or not the drug should be taken with food.

Pregnancy: The pregnancy category as proposed by the Food and Drug Administration is indicated for each drug. See Table 1 on page 958 for the definition of these categories.

Lactation: Available information regarding the presence of the drug in breast milk is given. Guidelines as set forth by the

American Academy of Pediatrics, if available, are presented. A general guideline provided in a brief statement (such as "avoid breastfeeding") is provided.

Warnings/precautions: All warnings provided by the manufacturer have been set forth as succinctly as possible. Other statements are made to alert the health provider to potential problems with the drug and how to avoid them.

Advice to patients: This represents our opinions regarding what the treating clinician needs to tell the patient to attempt to avoid or minimize problems with the drug. Included are the following "tips": when to avoid alcohol or other CNS depressants because of adverse interactions; how to protect oneself if the drug causes photosensitivity reactions; when to anticipate and minimize orthostatic hypotension; when to avoid driving; which appropriate contraceptive measures to use; when to avoid heat, cold, extreme exertion; how to cope with anticholinergic drug side effects; when and how to stop taking the drug.

Adverse reactions: These are defined as common (occurring in ≥ 10% of the patients taking the drug in pre- or postmarketing testing) and serious (potentially life threatening or with the risk of causing organ damage). **Side effects that are serious as well as common are listed as serious but in boldface type**.

Clinically important drug interactions: All too frequently, drug compendia list too many such interactions and/or fail to indicate which of these enhance or diminish the actions of a particular drug. Our list of drug interactions includes only those that, by consensus, are clinically relevant and include a statement regarding the actual effect of the interaction.

Parameters to monitor: We consider it to be of great importance that the treating clinician follow up on how a drug is acting on the patient by monitoring various vital functions. If these suggestions are followed, we believe many serious adverse reactions may be avoided or minimized. The following are some of the suggested parameters to be monitored: blood testing, hemodynamics, blood pressure, ECG, liver and kidney function, drug levels and efficacy of the drug in achieving its intended result. Judgment regarding actual monitoring in individual patients must ultimately be made by the treating clinician.

Editorial comments: Finally, the editors and their advisors have presented information in the form of editorial comments regarding certain aspects of many of the drugs included in this manual that are not covered by the preceding.

All drugs are listed by generic name in alphabetical order. A cross referenced list of brand name drugs is supplied in the front matter. With respect to the actual use of this book, the authors state the following:

1. Despite our best efforts to provide accurate information and opinions about each drug considered, the authors, members of the Advisory Board, and publisher do not guarantee that all of the material presented is completely accurate. The authors, reviewers, and publishers are not responsible for any errors, either those of omission or commission, that may arise in applying the enclosed information. Furthermore, not all authorities will agree with all our facts and/or evaluations. Accordingly, we can consider the material presented only as guidelines for drug administration, not the final word. The clinician or other health care provider must use his or her personal, independent judgment in applying the information in actual practice. In this regard, it is suggested that if the clinician disagrees with something in our drug monograph, he or she should check with the manufacturer's label for the particular drug before using it.

2. The authors, reviewers, and publisher disclaim any liability for any claim for losses or alleged losses that may have resulted from the use of the information contained herein whether directly or indirectly applied.

3. The authors, reviewers, and publisher have no connection with any pharmaceutical company or federal agency. They have not received compensation from any such organization. This book was commissioned solely by McGraw–Hill Company and the authors have written it without endorsement from any pharmaceutical company or federal agency. Any opinions expressed herein are solely those of the authors and members of their Advisory Board.

4. The authors, Advisory Board, and publisher will not be held liable if the material presented is misused or not applied appropriately by the clinician.

5. In many instances, a particular drug may have several brand names. We have included those that in our opinion are commonly used. Inclusion of one or more brand names should not be construed as an endorsement of the product just as its exclusion does not imply that we have rejected the product or consider it inferior to another. The publisher does not endorse or reject any of the products described and has no opinion regarding any of the products. The publisher has not engaged in or provided any kind of financial support for any of the products described herein.

ACKNOWLEDGEMENTS

We acknowledge the invaluable advice of our Advisory Board. Their knowledge and hands-on experience in specialty patient care has added greatly to the depth of information provided by the book. We also acknowledge Catherine Will and Cheryl Serdar for their excellent assistance with manuscript preparation. Special thanks go to Lynn Kaczmarz for administrative assistance with the book and to the editors of McGraw–Hill for their support and encouragement.

Seymour Ehrenpreis: My heartfelt thanks to my wife, Bella, for her forbearance throughout the time devoted to the task of writing this book. Never once did she complain! It is to her that I gratefully dedicate this book.

Eli Ehrenpreis: I would like to dedicate this book to my wife, Ana, for her encouragement and enthusiasm during the writing of the book and to my children, Benjamin, Jamie, and Joseph, for being so understanding and for sacrificing time that could have been spent with their father. Finally, I dedicate this book to my grandfather, the late Joseph Goodman, a man of great wisdom, energy, and humor who inspired me to achieve these qualities in my personal and professional life.

BRAND NAMES

Abelcet see Amphotericin B
Accolate see Zafirlukast
Accupril see Quinapril
Accurbron see Theophylline
Accutane see Isotretinoin
Achromycin see Tetracycline
Acticort see Hydrocortisone
Actic see Fentanyl
Actinin see Permethrin
Activase see Alteplase
Actonel see Riseronate
Acular see Ketorolac
Adalat see Nifedipine
Adapin see Doxepin
Adapryl see Selegiline
Adenocard see Adenosine
Adrenalin see Epinephrine
Adrucil see Fluorouracil
Aerobid see Flunisolide
Aerolate see Theophylline
Airet see Albuterol
AK-Chlor see Chloramphenicol
AK-Cide see Prednisolone
AK-Dex see Dexamethasone
Albenza see Albendazole
Aldactone see Spironolactone
Aldomet see Methyldopa
Aldoril see Methyldopa Hydrochlorothiazide
Alesse see Estrogen-Progestin
Aleve see Naproxen

Alfenta see Alfentanil
Alkeran see Melphalan
Allegra see Fexofenadine
Aloprim see Allopurinol
Aloprin see Allopurinol
Alphatrex see Betamethasone
Altace see Ramipril
Alupent see Metaproterenol
Amaryl see Glimepiride
Ambien see Zolpidem
Ambisome see Amphotericin B
Ambophen see Diphenhydramine
Amcort see Triamcinolone
Amen see Medroxyprogesterone
Amethopterin see Methotrexate
Amfebutamone see Bupropion
Amikin see Amikacin
Aminophylline see Theophylline
Amoxil see Amoxicillin
Amphocin see Amphotericin B
Amphotec see Amphotericin B
Anafranil see Clomipramine
Anaprox see Naproxyn
Ancef see Cefazolin
Ancobon see Flucytosine
Android see Methyltestosterone
Anectine see Succinylcholine

Anergan see Promethazine
Ansaid see Flurbiprofen
Antabuse see Disulfiram
Antigout see Colchicine
Antilirium see Physostigmine
Antinaus see Promethazine
Antivert see Meclizine
Anucort-HC see Hydrocortisone
Anx see Hydroxyzine
Anzemet see Dolasetron
Apresazide see Hydralazine
Apresoline see Hydralazine
AquaMephyton see Phytonadione
Aquaphylline see Theophylline
Aquatensen see Methyclothiazide
Aralen see Chloroquine
Arava see Leflunomide
Aristocort see Triamcinolone
Artane see Trihexyphenidyl
Asacol see Mesalamine
Asendin see Amoxapine
Asmalix see Theophylline
Atamet see Carbidopa/Levodopa/Carbidopa
Atarax see Hydroyzine
Ativan see Lorazepam
Atretol see Carbamazepine
Atromid-S see Clofibrate
Atropine see Atropine
Atropisol see Atropine
Augmentin see Amoxicillin, Clavulanate
Aureomycin see Tetracycline

Avandia see Rosiglitazone
Aventyl see Nortriptyline
Axid see Nizatidine
Aygestin see Norethindrone
Azamacort see Triamcimolone
Azifidine see Sulfasalazine
Azmacort see Triamcinolone
AZT see Zidovudine
Azulfidine see Sulfasalazine

Baciguent see Bacitracin
Bactocil see Oxacillin
Bactramycin see Lincomycin
Bactrim see Trimethoprin-Sulfamethoxazole
Baycol see Cerivastatin
Beclovent see Beclomethasone
Beconase see Beclomethasone
Benadryl see Diphenhydramine
Benemid see Probenecid
Bentylol see Dicyclomine
Benzamycin see Erythromycin
Betapace see Sotalol
Betaseron see Beta Interferon
Betatrex see Betamethasone
Betoptic see Betaxolol
Biaxin see Clarithromycin
Bicillin see Penicillin G
BICNU see Carmustine
Blenoxane see Bleomycin
Blocadren see Timolol
Bonine see Meclizine
Brethaire see Terbutaline
Brethine see Terbutaline

Bretylol see Bretylium
Brevibloc see Esmolol
Brevicon see Estrogen-Progesterone
Bromaline see Brompheniramine
Bromfed see Brompheniramine
Bronkaid see Epinephrine
Bronkodyl see Theophylline
Bumex see Bumetanide
Buprenex see Buprenorphine
BuSpar see Buspirone
Butalan see Butabarbital
Butisol see Butabarbital

Calan see Verapamil
Calcijex see Calcitriol
Calcimar see Calcitonin
Capastat see Capreomycin
Capoten see Captopril
Carbex see Seligine
Carbitrol see Carbamazepine
Carbocaine see Mepivacaine
Cardene see Nicardipine
Cardioquin see Quinidine
Cardizem see Diltiazem
Cardura see Doxazosin
Cartrol see Carteolol
Cataflam see Diclofenac
Catapres see Clonidine
Caverject see Alprostadil
CCNU see Lomustine
Ceclor see Cefaclor
Cedax see Ceftibuten
CeeNU see Lomustine

Cefizox see Ceftizoxime
Cefobid see Cefoperazone
Cefotan see Cefotetan
Ceftin see Cefuroxime
Cefzil see Cefprozil
Celebrex see Celecoxib
Celestone see Betamethasone
Celexa see Citalopram
CellCept see Mycophenolate
Ceptaz see Ceftazidime
Cerubidine see Daunorubicin
Chibroxin see Norfloxacin
Chloromycetin see Chloramphenicol
Chloroptic see Chloramphenicol
Chlor-Trimeton see Chlorpheniramine
Cibacalcin see Calcitonin
Cibalith-S see Lithium
Cibroxin see Norfloxacin
Ciloxan see Ciprofloxacin
Cinalone see Triamcinolone
Cipro see Ciprofloxacin
Claforan see Cefotaxime
Claritin see Loratadine
Clavulanate see Amoxicillin/Clavulanate
Clinoril see Sulindac
Clomid see Clomiphene
Cloxapen see Cloxacillin
Cogentin see Benztropine
Cognex see Tacrine
ColBENEMID see Probenecid
Colestid see Colestipol

Dilaudid see Hydromorphone

Dimetane see Brompheniramine

Diprolene see Betamethasone

Diprosone see Betamethasone

Ditropan see Oxybutinin

Diucardin see Hydroflumethiazide

Diuril see Chlorothiazide

Dizac see Diazepam

Dobutrex see Dobutamine

Dolene see Propoxyphene

Dolophine see Methadone

Dopar see Levadopa/Carbidopa

Dopastate see Dopamine

Doryx see Doxyclycline

Doxil see Doxorubicin

Droxia see Hydroxyurea

DTIC-Dome see Dacarbazine

Duraclon see Clonidine

Duragesic see Fentanyl

Duramorph see Morphine

Duranest see Etidocaine

Duricef see Cafadroxil

Duvoid see Bethanechol

D-Vert see Meclizine

Dyazide see Hydrochlorothiazide Trimterene

Dycill see Dicloxacillin

Dymelor see Acetohexamide

Dynacin see Minocycline

Dynapen see Dicloxacillin

Dyphylline see Theophylline

Dyrenium see Triamterane

Econopred see Prednisolone

Edecrin see Ethacrynic Acid

EES see qErythromycin

Effexor see Venlafaxine

Efudex see Fluorouracil

Elavil see Amitriptyline

Eldepryl see Selegiline

Elimite see Permethrin

Elixophyllin see Theophylline

Endodan see Methyclothiazide

Enduron see Methylclothiazide

Ephedrine see Ephedrine

Epifrin see Epinephrine

Epinal see Epinephrine

Epipen see Epinephrine

Epitol see Carbamazepine

Epivir see Lamivudine

Equanil see Meprobamate

Ergamisol see Levamisole

Ergostat see Ergotamine

Erycette see Erythromycin

Erythrocin see Erythromycin

Eserine see Physostigmine

Esgic see Butabarbital

Esidrix see Hydrochlorothiazide

Eskalith see Lithium

Estratest see Methyltestosterone

Ethmozine see Moricizine

Etopophos see Etoposide

Etrafon see Amitriptyline, Perphenazine

Eulexin see Flutamide

Everone see Testosterone

Famvir see Famciclovir
Feldene see Piroxicam
Feosol see Ferrous Sulfate
Flagyl see Metronidazole
Flexeril see Cyclobenzaprine
Flomax see Tamsulosin
Flonase see Fluticasone
Florinef see Fludrocortisone
Flovent see Fluticasone
Floxin see Ofloxacin
Flubenisolon see Betametha-
sone
Fludara see Fludarabine Phos-
phate
Flumadine see Rimantadine
Fluoroplex see Fluorouracil
Flutex see Triamcinolone
Folex see Methotrexate
Fortaz see Ceftazidime
Fosamax see Alendronate
Foscavir see Foscarnet
FUDR see Floxuridine
Fulvicin see Griseofulvin
Fungizone see Amphotericin B
Furacin see Nitrofurazone
Furadantin see Nitrofurantoin

Ganite see Gallium Nitrate
Garamycin see Gentamycin
Gastrocrom see Cromolyn
Genoptic see Gentamicin
Genora see Estrogen-Proges-
tin
Genotropin see Somatropin
Geocillin see Carbenicillin

Glaucon see Epinephrine
Glucagon see Glucagon
Glucotrol see Glipizide
Glynase see Glyburide
Grifulvin see Griseofulvin
Gynecort see Hydrocortisone

Haldol see Haloperidol
Halodrin see Fluoxymeste-
rone
Halotestin see Fluoxymeste-
rone
Hemabate see Carboprost
Herplex see Idoxuridine
Histalet see Chlorpheniramine
Hivid see Zalcitabine
Humalog see Insulin
Humatin see Paromomycin
Humatrope see Somatropin
Hycodan see Hydrocodone
Hydramine see Diphenhy-
dramine
Hydrea see Hydroxyurea
Hydrocortone see Hydrocorti-
sone
Hydro-Diuril see Hydrochloro-
thiazide
Hydroxacen see Hydroxyzine
Hygroton see Chlorthalidone
Hylutin see Hydroxyproges-
terone
Hyoscine see Scopolamine
Hyoscyamine
Hyperstat see Diazoxide
Hytrin see Terazosin

Hyzaar see Losartan
Hyzine see Hydroxyzine

Ifex see Ifosamide
Imdur see Isosorbide Mono-nitrate
Immitrex see Sumatriptan
Imuran see Azathioprine
Inapsine see Droperidol
Inderal see Propranolol
Indocin see Indomethacin
Inflamase see Prednisolone
Infumorph see Morphine
Innovar see Droperidol, Fentanyl
Inocor see Amrinone
Intal see Cromolyn
Integrilin see Eptifibatide
Intropin see Dopamine
Ismo see Isosorbide Mononit-rate
Isoproterenol see Isoprote-renol
Isoptin see Verapardl
Isopto see Atropine
Isopto-Hyoscine see Scopola-mine
Isordil see Isosorbide, Dini-trate
Isuprel see Isoproterenol

Kayexalate see Sodium Polystyrene Sulfonate
K-Dur see Potassium Chloride
Keflet see Cephalexin
Keflex see Cephalexin
Keflin see Cephalothin

Keftab see Cephalexin
Kefurox see Cefuroxime
Kefzol see Cefazolin
Kenalog see Triamcinolone
Kerlone see Betaxolol
Ketalor see Ketamine
K-Lor see Potassium Chloride
Klor-Con see Potassium Chloride
Konakion see Phytonadione
Kwell see Lindane
Kwildane see Lindane

Lamictal see Lamotrigine
Lanacort see Hydrocortisone
Lanoxicaps see Digoxin
Lanoxin see Digoxin
Laradopa see Levodopa/Carbidopa
Lasix see Furosemide
Ledercillin VK see Penicillin V
Lelvan see Estrogen/Progestin
Lescol see Fluvastatin
Leucovorin see Leucovorin
Leukeran see Chlorambucil
Leustatin see Cladribine
Levaquin see Levofloxicin
Levbid see Hyoscyamine
Levo-Dromoran see Levor-phanol
Levora see Estrogen-Proges-terone
Levothroid see Levothyroxine
Levoxyl see Levothroxine
Levsin see Hyoscyamine
Lexxel see Enalapril
Librium see Chlordiazepoxide

Lidex see Fluocinonide
Lioresal see Baclofen
Lipitor see Atorvastatin
Lithobid see Lithium
Lithonate see Lithium
LoCholest see Cholestyramine
Locoid see Hydrocortisone
Lodine see Etodolac
Lodosyn see Levodopa/Carbidopa
Lodrane see Brompheniramine
Loestrin see Estrogen-Progestin
Lopressor see Metoprolol
Lorabid see Loracarbef
Lotensin see Benazepril
Loxitane see Loxapine
Lozol see Indapamide
Luminal see Phenobarbital
Lupron see Leuprolide
Luvox see Fluvoxamine
Lyphocin see Vancomycin
Lysodren see Mitotane

Macrobid see Nitrofurantoin
Mandol see Cefamandole
Marax see Theophylline
Marinol see Dronabinol
Matulane see Procarbazine
Maxaquin see Lomefloxacin
Maxidex see Dexamethasone
Maxipeme see Cefepime
Maxivate see Betamethasone
Mebural see Mephobarbital
Medihaler see Isoproterenol

Medihaler-Iso see Isoproterenol
Medrol see Methylprednisolone
Mefoxin see Cefoxitin
Megase see Megestrol
Mellaril see Thioridazine
Menadol see Ibuprofen
Menest see Estrogen
Meni-D see Meclizine
Meperidine see Demerol
Mephyton see Phytonadione
Meprospan see Meprobamate
Mesnex see Mesna
Mestinon see Pyridostigmine
Methadose see Methadone
Methylin see Methylphenidate
Meticorten see Prednisone
Metric see Metronidazole
Mevacor see Lovastatin
Mevinolin see Lovastatin
Mexate see Methotrexate
Mexith see Mexiletine
Mezlin see Mezlocillin
Miacalcin see Calcitonin
Micatin see Miconzaole
Micro-K see Potassium Chloride
Micronase see Glyburide
Micronor see Estrogen/Progestin
Midamor see Amiloride
Milophene see Clomiphene
Milprem see Meprobamate
Miltown see Meprobamate
Minipress see Prazosin

Minitran see Nitroglycerin

Minitran see Nitroglycerin (Transdermel)

Minocin see Minocycline

Mintezole see Thiabendazole

Mithracin see Plicamycin

Mivacron see Mivacurium

Moban see Molindone

Modicon see Estrogen-Progestin

Monacolin see Lovastatin

Monistate see Miconazole

Monodox see Doxycycline

Monoket see Isosorbide Mononitrate

Monopril see Fosinopril

8-MOP see Methoxsalen

MTX see Methotrexate

Mucomyst see Acetyleysteine

Muse see Alprostadil

Mutamycin see Mitomycin

Myambutol see Ethambutol

Myambutol see Mitomycin

Mycostatin see Nystatin

Myidone see Primidone

Mykrox see Metolazone

Myleran see Busulfan

Myotrol see Orphenadrine

Mysoline see Primidone

Nalfon see Fenoprofen

Nallpen see Nafcillin

Naprosyn see Naproxen

Narcan see Naloxone

Nardil see Phenelzine

Nasalcrom see Cromolyn

Nasalide see Flunisolide

Nasocort see Triamcinolone

Naturectin see Bendroflumethiazide

Navane see Thiothixene

Nebcin see Tobramycin

NebuPent see Pentamidine

Necon see Estrogen-Protestin

Nembutal see Pentobarbital

Neoral see Cyclosporine

Neosar see Cyclophosphamide

Neo-Synephrine see Phenylephrine

Netromycin see Netilmicin

Neucalm see Hydroxyzine

Neuromax see Doxacurium

Neurontin see Gabapentin

Neutrexin see Cabapantin

Nexate see Methotrexate

Nilstat see Nystatin

Nimotop see Nimodipine

Nipride see Nitroprusside

Nitro-Bid see Nitroglycerin IV

Nitro-Derm see Nitroglycerin (Transdermal)

Nitroglyn see Nitroglycerine (Sustained Release)

Nitrol see Nitroglycerin (Topical)

Nitrong see Nitroglycerine (Sustained Release)

Nitropress see Nitroprusside

Nitrostat see Nitroglycerin (sublingual)

Nix see Permethrin
Nizoral see Ketoconazole
Nolvadex see Tamoxifen
Nordette see Estrogen-Progestin
Norditropin see Somatropin
Norgestrel see Levonorgestrel
Normgdyne see Labetolol
Norpace see Disopyramide
Norpath see Propanthaline
Norplant see Levonorgestrel
Norpromin see Desipramine
Norvasc see Amlodipine
Novantrone see Mitoxantrone
Novocaine see Procaine
NubuPent see Pentamidine
Numorphan see Oxymorphone
Nuprin see Ibuprofen
Nuromax see Doxacurium
Nutracort see Hydrocortisone
Nutropin see Somatropin
Nydrazid see Isoniazid
Nystex see Nystatin

Ocuflox see Ofloxacin
Omnicef see Cefdinir
Omnipen see Ampicillin
OMS see Morphine
Opticrom see Cromolyn
Oramorph see Morphine
Orasone see Prednisone
Oretic see Hydrochlorothiazide
Orinase see Tolbutamide
Orlaam see Levomethadyl

Ortho-Cept see Estrogen/Progestin
Orudis see Ketoprofen
Ovcon see Estrogen/Progestin
Oxitriptan see Levodopa/Carbidopa
Oxsoralen see Methoxsalen
Oxycontin see Oxycodene

Panaldine see Ticlopidine
Paraflex see Chlorzoxazone
Paraplatin see Carboplatin
Parlodel see Bromocriptine
Parnate see Tranylcypromine
PAS Sodium see Para-Aminosalicylic acid
Pavulon see Pancuronium
Paxil see Paroxetine
Pediazole see Erythromycin
Penetrex see Enoxacin
Pentam-300 see Pentamidine
Pentasa see Mesalamine
Pen-Vee see Penicillin
Pepsid see Famotidine
Percocet see Oxycodone
Percodan see Oxycodone
Periactin see Cyproheptadine
Permapen see Penicillin G, Benzathine
Permax see Pergolide
Permitil see Fluphenazine
Persantin see Dipyridamole
Pertofrane see Desipramine
Pfizerpen see Penicillin G
Phenergan see Promethazine
Phrenilin see Butabarbital

Pipracil see Piperacillin
Pitocin see Oxytocin
Pitressin see Vasopressin
Platinol see Cisplatin
Plendil see Felodipine
Ponstel see Mefenamic Acid
Prandin see Repaglinide
Pravachol see Pravastatin
Prevalite see Cholestyramine
Prilosec see Omeprazole
Primacor see Milrinone
Principen see Ampicillin
Prinivil see Lisinopril
Probalan see Probenecid
Pro-Banthine see Propantheline
Procanbid see Procainamide
Procardia see Nifedipine
Proglycem see Diazoxide
Prograf see Tacrolimus
Proleukin see Aldesleukin
Prolixin see Fluphenazine
Promet see Promethazine
Promethegan see Promethazine
Prometrium see Progesterone
Promine see Procainamide
Pronestyl see Procainamide
Propanthel see Propantheline
Propecia see Finasteride
Propocet see Propoxyphene
Propulsid see Cisapride
Propyl-Thyracil see Propylthiouracil
Proscar see Finasteride
Prostaphlin see Oxacillin
Prostat see Metronidazole

Prostigmin see Neostigmine
Prostin VR see Alprostadil
Prostin VR Pediatric see Alprostadil
Protamine see Protamine
Protopam see Pralidoxime
Proventil see Albuterol
Provera see Medroxyprogesterone
Prozac see Fluoxetine
Pulmicort see Budesonide
Purinethol see Mercaptopurine
Pyrazinamide see Pyrazinamide

Quelicin see Succinylcholine
Questran see Cholestyramine
Quibron see Theophylline
Quinaglute see Quinidine
Quinidex see Quinidine
Quinora see Quinidine

Regitine see Phentolamine
Reglan see Metoclopramide
Regonol see Pyridostigmine Bromide
Relafen see Nabumetone
Rescon see Chlorpheniramine
Respbid see Theophylline
Restoril see Temazepam
Retrovir see Zidovudine
Reversol see Edrophonium
ReVia see Naltrexone
Rheumatrex see Methotrexate
Rhinocort see Budesonide
Ridaira see Auranofin

Rifadin see Rifampin

Rifamate see Isoniazid, Rifampin

Rifampicin see Rifampin

Rifater see Isoniazid, Pyrazinamide, Rifampin

Rimactane see Rifampin

Risperdal see Risperidone

Ritalin see Methylphenidate

Rocaltrol see Calcitriol

Rocephin see Ceftriaxone

Roferon-A see Interferon Alfa 2_a

Rogaine see Minoxidil

Romazicon see Flumazenil

Rowasa see Mesalamine

Roxanol see Morphine

Roxicodone see Oxycodone

Ru-Vert-M see Meclizine

Ryna-C see Codeine

Rynatan see Azatadine

Rythmol see Propafanone

Saizem see Somatropin

Sandimmune see Cyclosporine

Sansert see Methysergide

Sarisol see Butabarbital

Scabene see Lindane

Scalpicin see Hydrocortisone

Sectral see Acebutolol

Selestoject see Betamethasone

Septra see Trimethoprim-Sulfamethoxazole

Serax see Oxazepam

Sereen see Chlordiazepoxide

Serentil see Mesoridazine

Serevent see Salmeterol

Seromycin see Cycloserine

Serophene see Clomiphene

Sertan see Primidone

Silvadene see Silver Sulfadiazine

Sinemet see Levadopa/Carbidopa

Sinequan see Doxepin

Slo-Phylline see Theophylline

Solfoton see Phenobarbital

Solu-Cortef see Hydrocortisone

Solu-Medrol see Methylprednisolone

Solurex see Dexamethasone

Soma see Carisoprodol

Sorbitrate see Isosorbide Dinitrate

Sparine see Promazine

Spectrobid see Bacampicillin

Sporanox see Itraconazole

SSKI see Potassium Iodide

Stadol see Butophanol

Staphicillin see Methicillin

Staticin see Erythromycin

Stelazine see Trifluoperazine

Sterapred see Prednisone

Streptase see Streptokinase

Streptomycin see Streptomycin

Sublimaze see Fentanyl

Sucostrin see Succinylcholine

Sufenta see Sufentanil

Sumycin see Tetracycline

Suprax see Cefixime

Surmontil see Trimipramine

Sus-Phrine see Epinephrine

Sustiva see Efavirenz
Symmetrel see Amantadine
Synalar see Fluocinolone
Synemol see Fluocinolone
Synthroid see Levothyroxine
Syntocinon see Oxytocin
Synvinolin see Simvastatin

Tacrium see Atracurium Acracurium
Tagemet see Cimetidine
Talacen see Pentazocine
Talwin see Pentazocine
Tambocor see Flecainide
TAO see Troleandomycin
Tapazole see Methimazole
Tavist see Clemastine
Tazicef see Ceftazidime
Tazicel see Ceftazidime
Tazidime see Ceftazidime
Tegretol see Carbamazepine
Teldrin see Chlorpheniramine
Tenormin see Atenolol
Tensilon see Edrophonium
Testoderm see Testosterone
Testopel see Testosterone
Testred see Methyltestosterone
Tetracycline see Tetracycline
Thalitone see Chlorthalidone
THC see Dronabinol
Theo-Dur see Theophylline
Theolair see Theophylline
Thioplex see Thiotepa
Thorazine see Chlorpromazine
Thysin see Levothyroxine

Tiazel see Dilitiazem
Ticar see Ticarcillin
Tigan see Trimethobenzamide
Timoptic see Timolol
Tobrex see Tobramycin
Tofranil see Imipramine
Togepen see Cloxacillin
Tolectin see Tolmetin
Tonocard see Tocainide
Toposar see Etoposide
Toprol see Metoprolol
Toradol see Ketorolac
Tornalate see Bitolterol
Totacillin see Ampicillin
Trandate see Lebetolol
Transderm-Nitro see Nitroglycerin (Transdermal)
Transderm-Scop see Scopolamine
Tranxene see Clorazepate
Tridil see Nitroglycerin
Trilafon see Perphenazine
Trimox see Amoxicillin
Trimpex see Trimethoprim
Trinalin see Azatadine
Tri-Norinyl see Estrogen-Progestin
Triostat see Liothyronine
Triphasil see Estrogen-Progestin
Tristoject see Triamcinolone
Tritec see Ranitidine
Tropol see Metoprolol
T-Stat see Erythromycin
Tubocurarine see Tubocurarine
Tussar see Codeine

Ultram see Tramadol
Unasyn see Ampicillin, Sulbactam
Unipen see Nafcillin
Univasc see Moexipril
Urecholine see Bethanechol
Uticort see Betamethasone

Valergen see Estradiol
Valisone see Betamethasone
Valium see Diazepan
Valrelease see Diazepam
Valtrex see Valacyclovir
Vancenase see Beclomethasone
Vanceril see Beclomethasone
Vancocin see Vancomycin
Vancoled see Vancomycin
Vantin see Cefpodoxime
Vascor see Bepridil
Vasotec see Enalapril
V-Cillin see Penicillin V
Veetids see Penicillin V
Velban see Vinblastine
Ventolin see Albuterol
Vepesid see Etoposide
Verelan see Verapamil
Vermox see Mebendazole
Versed see Midazolam
Vesprin see Triflupromazine
Vexol see Rimexolone
V-Gan see Promethazine
Viagra see Sildenafil
Vibramycin see Doxycycline
Vioxx see Rofecoxib
Vira-A see Vidarabine

Virilon IM see Testosterone
Visken see Pindolol
Vistacon see Hydroxyzine
Vistaril see Hydroxyzine
Vivactil see Protriptyline
Volina see Albuterol
Voltaren see Diclofenac

Wellbutrin see Bupropion
Wellcovorin see Leucovorin
Westcort see Hydrocortisone
Wigraine see Ergotamine
Wycillin see Penicillin G Procaine
Wydase see Hyaluronidase
Wygesic see Propxythphene
Wymox see Amoxicillin

Xanax see Alprazolam
Xanthotoxin see Methoxsalen
Xenical see Orlistat
Xylocaine see Lidocaine

Yutopar see Ritodrine

Zagam see Sparfloxacin
Zantac see Ranitidine
Zaroxolyn see Metolazone
Zeasorb-AF see Miconazole
Zebutal see Butabarbital
Zemuron see Rocuronium
Zerit see Stavudine
Zestril see Lisinopril
Zetran see Diazepam
Zinacef see Cefuroxime
Zithromax see Azithromycin

Zocor see Simvastatin
Zofran see Ondansetron
Zoloft see Sertraline
Zomig see Zolmitriptan

Zovirax see Acyclovir
Zyban see Bupropion
Zyloprim see Allopurinol
Zyrtec see Cetirizine

Acebutolol

Brand name: Sectral.
Class of drug: β-Adrenergic receptor blocker.
Mechanism of action: Competitive blocker of β adrenergic receptors in heart and blood vessels.
Indications/dosage/route: Oral only.
• Hypertension
  – Adults: Initial: 400 mg/d. Maintenance: 200–1200 mg/d.
• Premature ventricular contractions
  – Adults: Initial: 200 mg b.i.d. Maintenance: 600–1200 mg/d.
Adjustment of dosage
• Kidney disease: Creatinine clearance 25–50 mL/min: decrease dose by 50%; creatinine clearance <25 mL/min: decrease dose by 75%.
• Liver disease: None.
• Elderly: Avoid doses >800 mg/d.
• Pediatric: Safety and efficacy have not been established in children.
Food: No restriction.
Pregnancy: Category B.
Lactation: Appears in breast milk. Potentially toxic to infant. Considered compatible by the American Academy of Pediatrics. Observe infant for hypotension, bradycardia.
Contraindications: Cardiogenic shock, CHF unless it is secondary to tachyarrhythmia treated with a β blocker, sinus bradycardia and AV block greater than first degree, severe COPD.
Warnings/precautions
• Use with caution in patients with the following conditions: diabetes, kidney disease, liver disease, COPD, peripheral vascular disease.
• Do not stop drug abruptly as this may precipitate arrhythmias, angina, MI or cause rebound hypertension. If necessary to discontinue, taper as follows: reduce dose and reassess after 1–2 weeks; if status is unchanged, reduce by another 50% and reassess after 1–2 weeks.

- Drug may mask the symptoms of hyperthyroidism, mainly tachycardia.
- Drug may exacerbate symptoms of arterial insufficiency in patients with peripheral or mesenteric vascular disease.

Advice to patient

- Avoid driving and other activities requiring mental alertness or that are potentially dangerous until response to drug is known.
- Dress warmly in winter and avoid prolonged exposure to cold as drug may cause increased sensitivity to cold.
- Avoid drinks that contain xanthines (caffeine, theophylline, theobromine) including colas, tea, and chocolate because they may counteract the effect of the drug.
- Restrict dietary sodium to avoid volume expansion.
- Drug may blunt response to usual rise in blood pressure and chest pain under stressful conditions such as vigorous exercise and fever.

Adverse reactions

- Common: fatigue.
- Serious: symptomatic bradycardia, CHF, worsened AV block, hypotension, depression, bone marrow depression, SLE-like condition, bronchospasm, Peyronie's disease, hepatitis.

Clinically important drug interactions

- Drugs that increase effects/toxicity of beta blockers: reserpine, bretylium, calcium channel blockers.
- Drugs that decrease effects/toxicity of beta blockers: aluminum salts, calcium salts, cholestyramine, barbiturates, NSAIDs, rifampin.

Parameters to monitor

- Liver enzymes, serum BUN and creatinine, CBC with differential and platelets.
- Patient's pulse rate near end of dosing interval or before next dose is taken. A reasonable target is 60–80 bpm for resting apical ventricular rate. If severe bradycardia develops, consider treatment with glucagon, isoproterenol, IV atropine (1–3 mg in divided doses). If hypotension occurs despite correction of

bradycardia, administer vasopressor (norephinephrine, dopamine, or dobutamine).

- Symptoms of CHF. Digitalize patient and administer a diuretic or glucagon.
- Efficacy of treatment: decreased blood pressure, decreased number and severity of anginal attacks, improvement in exercise tolerance. Confirm control of arrhythmias by ECG, apical pulse, BP, circulation in extremities, and respiration. Monitor closely when changing dose.
- Central nervous system effects. If patient experiences mental depression reduce dosage by 50%. The elderly are particularly sensitive to adverse CNS effects.
- Signs of bronchospasm. Stop therapy and administer large doses of β-adrenergic bronchodilator, eg, albuterol, terbutaline, or aminophylline.
- Signs of cold extremities. If severe, stop drug. Consider β blocker with sympathomimetic property.

Editorial comments

- Stopping a β blocker before surgery is controversial. Some advocate discontinuing the drug 48 hours before surgery; others recommend withdrawal for a considerably longer time. Notify anesthesiologist that patient has been on β blocker.
- β Blockers are first-line treatments for hypertension, particularly in patients with the following conditions: previous MI, ischemic heart disease, aneurysm, atrioventricular arrhythmias, migraine. These are drugs of first choice for chronic stable angina, used in conjunction with nitroglycerin.
- Many studies indicate benefit from administration of a β blocker following an MI.
- β Blockers are considered to be first-line drugs for prophylaxis of migraine headache in patients who have two or more attacks per month.
- Note that this drug is pregnancy category B (most β blockers are category C).

Acetohexamide

Brand name: Dymelor.
Class of drug: Oral hypoglycemic agent, second generation.
Mechanism of action: Stimulates release of insulin from pancreatic beta cells; decreases glucose production in liver; increases sensitivity of receptors for insulin, thereby promoting effectiveness of insulin.
Indications/dosage/route: Oral only.
• Diabetes
 – Adults: Initial: 250–1500 mg/d. Adjust dosage until optimum control is achieved. Maximum: 1500 mg/d.
 – Elderly: Initial, 125–250 mg/d. Adjust dosage gradually until optimum control is achieved.
Adjustment of dosage
• Kidney disease: None.
• Liver disease: None.
• Elderly: See above.
• Pediatric: Not recommended.
Food: No restriction. Patient should be told to eat regularly and not to skip meals. Sugar supply should be kept handy at all times. If stomach is upset Tums should be taken with meal. Dose is best administered before breakfast or, if taken twice a day, before the evening meal.
Pregnancy: Category C.
Lactation: No data available. Potentially toxic to infant. Avoid breastfeeding.
Contraindications: Hypersensitivity to the drug; diabetes complicated by ketoacidosis.
Editorial comments
• This drug is not listed in *Physician's Desk Reference*, 54th edition, 2000.
• For additional information, see *glyburide*, p. 409.

Acetylcysteine

Brand name: Mucomyst.
Class of drug: Mucolytic agent; antidote for acetaminophen toxicity.
Mechanism of action: As mucolytic agent: disrupts disulfide bonds in mucoproteins thereby lowering viscosity of mucus. As antidote for acetaminophen poisoning: complexes with hepatotoxic free radial metabolite of acetaminophen and inactivates it.
Indications/dosage/route: Oral, inhalation, IV.
- Bronchial disorders, chronic bronchitis, asthma, emphysema, pulmonary complications of surgery
  - Adults: 6–10 mL of 10% solution, q2–3 hours by nebulizer.
  - Children: 3–5 mL of 10% solution, q2–3 hours by nebulizer.
  - Infants: 2–4 mL of 10% solution, t.i.d. to q.i.d., IV.
  - Alternate: 20% solution may be given in half of above volumes.
- Antidote for acetaminophen poisoning
  - Quaterdoze with Bronchical
  - Adults, children: Initial: PO 140 mg/kg, then 70 mg/kg q4h. Total of 17 doses. Complete therapy despite acetaminophen level. If patient has emesis with 1 hour of dose, repeat dose immediately.

Adjustment of dosage
- Kidney disease: None.
- Liver disease: None.
- Elderly: None.
- Pediatric: See above.

Onset of Action	Duration
5–10 min	>1 h

Food: Given before meals and just before bedtime for asthma.
Pregnancy: Category B.
Lactation: No data available. Best to avoid.

Contraindications: As mucolytic agent: hypersensitivity to acetylcysteine.

Warnings/precautions

• As antidote for acetaminophen poisoning: Administer as quickly as possible. Most useful if given within 12 hours of ingestion of acetaminophen.

• As inhaled drug: may induce bronchospasm. If this occurs, administer bronchodilator; suction bronchial secretions if they develop after inhalation.

• Elderly: May have reduced cough reflex and therefore reduced ability to clear airway of liquefied mucus. May need concomitant suction.

• For patient with asthma or hyperactive airway disease, a bronchodilator should be administered before acetylcysteine.

Advice to patient: Rinse mouth out and wash face after treatment to remove adhering drug.

Adverse reactions

• Common: vomiting, olfactory disturbance.

• Serious: bronchospasm (especially in asthmatics), hypotension.

Clinically important drug interactions: None.

Parameters to monitor

• As antidote for acetaminophen poisoning: Monitor acetaminophen plasma levels, liver enzymes, bilirubin. Monitor for nausea, vomiting, skin rash. Acetaminophen levels: Determine at least 4 hours after acetaminophen ingestion. Administer acetylcysteine if acetaminophen level is >150 mg/mL 12 hours after ingestion. Hepatotoxicity occurs if peak level is >200 mg/mL. Monitor cardiac function, renal function, prothrombin time. Administer fresh-frozen plasma or vitamin K if prothrombin time >3 seconds compared with control.

• As mucolytic agent: Monitor respiratory function for respiratory fluid increases, amount and consistency of secretions before and after treatment. Apply suction or endotrachial aspiration if necessary. Signs and symptoms of bronchospasm: if this occurs, administer bronchodilator or discontinue if necessary.

Acyclovir

Brand name: Zovirax.
Class of drug: Antiviral agent.
Mechanism of action: Nucleotide analog; inhibits viral replication by termination of viral DNA chain and inhibition and inactivation of viral DNA polymerase.
Indications/dosage/route: Oral, IV.

- Herpes simplex (HSV-1 and HSV-2) infections (immunocompromised host)
  - Adults, children >12 years: IV 5 mg/kg (infuse at constant rate over 1 hour), q8h for 7 days.
  - Children <12 years: IV 250 mg/m^2 (infuse at constant rate for 1 hour), q8h.
- Genital herpes
  - Adults, children >12 years: PO 200 mg q4h, five doses/day; 10 days for initial therapy. Dose for 5 days for intermittent recurrent disease. Administer up to 12 months for chronic disease (suppressive therapy).
  - Children <12 years: IV 250 mg/m^2, t.i.d. for 10 days.
- Herpes simplex encephalitis
  - Adults, children >12 years: IV 10 mg/kg (infuse at constant rate over 1 hour), q8h for 10 days.
  - Children, 6 months to 12 years: IV 500 mg/m^2 (infuse at constant rate over 1 hour), q8h for 10 days.
- Herpes zoster
  - Adults, children >12 years: PO 80 mg, q4h, five doses/day, 7–10 days.
  - Children <12 years: PO 250–600 mg/m^2, 4–5 times/day, 7–10 days.
- Chickenpox
  - Adults, children >40 kg: PO 800 mg, q.i.d. 5 days.
  - Children >2 years: PO 20 mg/kg q.i.d. (maximum 800 mg), 5 days.

Adjustment of dosage

- Kidney disease: Creatinine clearance 25–50 mL/min: dose q12h; creatinine clearance 10–25 mL/min: dose q24h; creatinine clearance <10 mL/min: half dose q24h (IV doses).
- Liver disease: None.
- Elderly: None.
- Pediatric: Safety has not been established in children <2 years old.

Food: No restrictions.

Pregnancy: Category C.

Lactation: Appears in breast milk; considered compatible by American Academy of Pediatrics.

Contraindications: Hypersensitivity to acyclovir.

Warnings/precautions

- Use with caution in patients with the following conditions: kidney disease, neurologic disease.
- Beware of renal dysfunction especially if patient is taking other nephrotoxic drugs.
- Women with genital herpes should have annual Pap smears.
- Rapid bolus administration may cause crystalline precipitation in renal tubules and renal insufficiency.
- Patients receiving acyclovir IV must remain well hydrated during treatment and for 24 hours after treatment.
- Cases of thrombotic thrombocytopenic purpura/hemolytic uremia syndrome have been reported with high-dose acyclovir in immunocompromised patients.

Advice to patient

- Drink 2–3 L of fluid per day. This is particularly important following IV infusion.
- Avoid sexual intercourse when lesions are present; otherwise use condoms.
- Avoid contact of the drug with or around the eyes.
- Resume treatment at first indication of recurrence of infection.

Adverse reactions

- Common: headache, phlebitis (IV only).

- Serious: seizures, renal failure, anaphylaxis, encephalopathy (confusion, hallucinations), coma, leukopenia, renal crystalline precipitant, elevated liver enzymes, Stevens–Johnson syndrome, urticaria.

Clinically important drug interactions

- Drugs that increase effects/toxicity of acyclovir: MAO inhibitors, probenecid, ziduvine, CNS depressants.
- Drugs that decrease effects/toxicity of acyclovir: β blockers, guanethidine.

Parameters to monitor

- Serum BUN and creatinine, CBC with differential and platelets, liver enzymes.
- Signs and symptoms of ocular herpetic infection as this may cause blindness.
- Serum creatinine level: If this increases during therapy, adjust dose, increase hydration or discontinue drug.
- Signs and symptoms of hepatotoxicity.
- Signs and symptoms of renal toxicity.
- Signs and symptoms of drug-induced psychologic disturbances: Changes in mood, behavior or orientation of patient, agitation, hallucinations, suicidal tendencies, sleep disturbances, lethargy.
- Intake of fluids and urinary and other fluids. Closely monitor electrolyte levels.

Adenosine

Brand name: Adenocard.
Class of drug: Antiarrhythmic.
Mechanism of action: Vagolytic effect: Slows conduction through AV node; prevents reentry through AV node. Restores normal sinus rhythm in patients with paroxysmal supraventricular tachycardia including Wolff–Parkinson–White syndrome.
Indications/dosage/route: IV only.

- Paroxysmal supraventricular tachycardia
  - Adults: bolus of 6 mg. If no effect after 1–2 min, 12-mg bolus. May repeat 12-mg dose × 2.
  - Child: bolus of 0.05 mg/kg; repeat dosage every 2 min. Maximum 0.25 mg/kg (not approved).

Adjustment of dosage
- Kidney disease: None.
- Liver disease: None.
- Elderly: None.
- Pediatric: See above.

Onset of Action	Peak Effect	Duration
10 s	No data	10–20 s

Pregnancy: Category C.

Lactation: Unlikely to be problematic.

Contraindications: Second- or third-degree AV block (without pacemaker), sick sinus syndrome, symptomatic bradycardia.

Warnings/precautions
- Use with caution in patients with the following condition: stroke, asthma, unstable angina (higher risk of arrythmias, MI).
- Cardiac arrest (including fatalities), ventricular tachycardia, and MI have been reported coincident with use.
- May produce transient first-, second-, third-degree AV block.
- Asystole has been reported in atrial flutter when given with carbamazepine.
- Use cautiously in patients receiving digoxin and/or verapamil.
- May cause ventricular fibrillation.
- Resuscitative equipment should be readily available when adenosine is administered.
- May produce hypotension or hypertension as side effects.
- May cause bronchoconstriction in patients with asthma or COPD.

Adverse reactions
- Common: facial flushing (18%), nausea, hyperventilation, thoracic constriction, palpitations.

• Serious: **hypotension, dyspnea** (12%), heart block, ventricular fibrillation, asystole, hypertension.

Clinically important drug interactions

• Drugs that increase effects/toxicity of adenosine: carbamazepine, digoxin, verapamil, dipyridamole.

Parameters to monitor: ECG for signs and symptoms of AV block and increased arrhythmias when converting to normal sinus rhythm.

Editorial comments

• Adenosine is highly useful as an acute antiarrhythmic agent.

• In narrow complex supraventricular tachycardia, it can be used simultaneously to diagnose the mechanism and to terminate it.

• Because it can terminate some catecholamine-requiring ventricular tachycardias, it can be safely used in wide complex tachycardia as well.

• It is necessary to inject adenosine rapidly by peripheral IV route followed by saline bolus because of its short half-life. Solution should be checked for presence of crystals; if present, warm solution. Do not inject if crystals are present.

Albendazole

Brand name: Albenza.
Class of drug: Anthelmintic.
Mechanism of action: Inhibits uptake of glucose and other nutrients by parasitic helminths.
Indications/dosage/route: Oral only.

• Hydatid disease
  – Adults ≥ 60 kg: 400 mg b.i.d. with meals, 28-hour cycle followed by 14-day drug-free interval for total of 3 cycles.
  – Adults <60 kg: 15 mg/kg/d in divided doses b.i.d. with meals. Maximum total daily dose: 800 mg.

• Neurocysticercosis

– Adults ≥ 60 kg: 400 mg b.i.d. with meals, 8–30 days.
– Adults < 60 kg: 50 mg/kg/d in divided doses b.i.d. with meals. Maximum total daily dose: 800 mg.

Food: Take with food.
Pregnancy: Category C.
Lactation: Probably present in breast milk. Best to avoid.
Contraindications: Hypersensitivity to mabendazole.
Editorial comments: For additional information, see *mebendazole*, p. 550.

Albuterol

Brand names: Proventil, Ventolin.
Class of drug: β-adrenergic agonist, bronchodilator.
Mechanism of action: Relaxes smooth muscles of the bronchioles by stimulating β_2-adrenergic receptors.
Indications/dosage/route: Oral, inhalation

• Bronchodilation
  – Adults, children >12 years: 2 inhalations q4–6h.
• Prophylaxis of exercise-induced bronchospasm
  – Adults, children >12 years: 2.5 mg t.i.d. to q.i.d. by nebulization.
• Bronchodilation: Capsule for inhalation
  – Adults, children >12 years: 200 μg q4–6h.
• Prophylaxis of exercise-induced bronchospasm
  – Adults, children >12 years: 200 μg 15 minutes before exercise.
• Bronchodilation: syrup
  – Adults, children >14 years: 2–4 mg t.i.d. to q.i.d.
  – Children 2–6 years: Initial: 2–4 mg, Maximum: 8 mg t.i.d. to q.i.d.
  – Children 6–12 years: 4 mg q12h. Maximum: 12 mg q12h.
  – Elderly: Initial: 2 mg t.i.d. to q.i.d. Increase dose if needed to maximum of 8 mg t.i.d. to q.i.d.
• Bronchodilation: extended-release tablets

– Adults, children >12 years: 4–8 mg q12h. Maximum: 32 mg/d.

Adjustment of dosage
- Kidney disease: None.
- Liver disease: None.
- Elderly: See above.
- Pediatric: See above.

Onset of Action		Duration
<30 min	Inhalation	4–8 h
<5 min	oral	3–8 h

Food: Not applicable.

Pregnancy: Category C.

Lactation: No data available. Other drugs in the same class such as terbutaline are considered compatible with breastfeeding.

Contraindications: Hypersensitivity to adrenergic compounds.

Warnings/precautions
- Use with caution in patients with the following conditions: hyperthyroidism, diabetes, coronary insufficiency, ischemic heart disease, history of stroke, CHF, hypertension.
- Some preparations contain bisulfite, which may cause an allergic reaction in sensitive individuals.
- Instruct patient in proper technique for using nebulizer and/or inhaler.

Advice to patient
- Avoid OTC products without consulting treating physician.
- Do not use solutions that contain a precipitate or are discolored.
- Contact treating physician if more than 3 inhalations are required within a 24-hour period to obtain relief.
- Wait at least 1 minute after 1 or 2 inhalations before taking a third dose.
- Keep spray away from eyes.
- Maintain adequate fluid intake (2000–3000 mL/d) to facilitate clearing of secretions.

- Rinse mouth with water after each inhalation to minimize dry mouth and throat irritation.
- Administer inhalant when arising in the morning and before meals.
- Do not increase dose in an attempt to obtain relief.

Adverse reactions
- Common: tremor.
- Serious: hypotension, bronchospasm.

Clinically important drug interactions:
- Drugs that increase effects/toxicity of β agonists: inatropium, MAO inhibitors, tricyclic antidepressants.
- Drugs that decrease activity of beta agonists: sympathomimetic drugs (nasal decongestants, weight loss drugs, eg, phenylpropanolamine), anticholinergic drugs, phenothiazines.

Parameters to monitor
- Monitor patient for possible development of tolerance with prolonged use. Discontinue drug temporarily and effectiveness will be restored.
- Signs of paradoxical bronchospasm.
- Pulmonary function on initiation and during bronchodilator therapy. Assess respiratory rate, sputum character (color, quantity), peak airway flow, O_2 saturation and blood gases.
- Efficacy of treatment: Improved breathing, prevention of bronchospasm, reduction of asthmatic attacks, prevention of exercise-induced asthma. If no relief is obtained from 3–5 aerosol inhalations within 6–12 hours, reevaluate effectiveness of treatment.
- FEV_1 rate to determine effectiveness of the drug to reverse bronchostriction. Efficacy is indicated by an increase in FEV_1 of 10–20%. In addition such patients, as well as those who have chronic disease, should be given a peak flow gauge and told to determine peak expiratory flow rate at least twice daily.

Editorial comments: For patients with acute asthma or acute exacerbation of COPD, reduce dose to minimum necessary to control condition after initial relief is achieved. For chronic conditions, the patient should be reassessed every 1–6 months following control of symptoms.

Alendronate

Brand name: Fosamax.
Class of drug: Bisphosphonate derivative/treatment for osteoporosis.
Mechanism of action: Inhibits osteoclast activity. Decreases bone resorption and increases bone mass.
Indications/dosage/route: Oral only.
• Treatment and prevention of osteoporosis
  – Adults: 10 mg/d.
  – Elderly: 10 mg/d.
  – Children: Safety and effectiveness not established in children <18 years.
• Paget's disease
  – Adults: 40 mg/d, 6 months.
Adjustment of dosage
• Kidney disease: Not given if creatinine clearance <35 mL/min. No adjustment of dosage needed for creatinine clearance >35 mL/min.
• Liver disease: None necessary.
• Elderly: None.
• Pediatric: See above.
Food: Drug must be taken at least 30 minutes before the first food, beverage, or medicine of the day with full glass of water. Must be in upright position for 30 minutes following ingestion.
Pregnancy: Category C.
Lactation: No data available. Best to avoid.
Contraindications: Hypersensitivity to biphosphonates, hypocalcemia, esophageal stricture or delayed esophageal emptying (achalasia), inability to sit or stand up for at least 30 minutes

following ingestion, marked renal impairment (serum creatinine >5 mg/dL, creatinine clearance <35 mL/min).

Warnings/precautions

- Safety of alendronate in combination with hormone replacement therapy has not been established.
- Hypocalcemia or vitamin D deficiency must be corrected prior to treatment.
- May cause severe esophagitis if adequate esophageal transient not present. Cases of GI bleeding due to esophageal irritation have been reported. Screen patients for symptoms of esophageal stricture or motility disorder (dysphagia, noncardiac chest pain) prior to use. Patients should be advised to report symptoms of chest pain, dysphagia, odynophagia, or GI bleeding if these occur while taking alendrondrate.
- Patient's with Paget's disease are at risk for GI side effects and muscle or bone pain.

Advice to patient

- Maintain adequate intake of calcium and vitamin D.
- Take calcium supplement at least 30 minutes after drug ingestion.
- Do not lie down until at least 30 minutes after taking this drug.
- Perform weight bearing exercises as a means of increasing bone mass.
- Stop smoking and decrease alcohol intake.

Adverse reactions

- Common: none.
- Serious: esophageal ulcer, GI bleeding.

Clinically important drug interactions

- Drugs that increase effects/toxicity of alendronate: ranitidine, aspirin.
- Drugs that decrease effects/toxicity of alendronate: concomitant calcium supplements, antacids.
- Because a variety of medications may decrease the absorption of alendronate, patients must wait at least 30 minutes after taking medications before taking alendronate.

Parameters to monitor

- Patient with Paget's disease: Check alkaline phosphatase levels periodically.

- Efficacy of treatment in patients with Paget's disease: Reduction in bone pain and headache, impaired visual or auditory acuity.
- Perform serial bone densitometry and or skeletal radiography.
- Monitor calcium phosphate on regular basis. Consider obtaining 24-hour urine calcium and vitamin D levels.

Editorial comments

- Before treating for osteoporosis, confirm diagnosis by measuring bone mass. History of bone fractures is also suggestive of osteoporosis.
- Diagnosis of Paget's disease depends on the following findings: alkaline phosphatase level at least twice that of the upper normal range, characteristic radiography.

Alfentanil

Brand name: Alfenta.
Class of drug: Narcotic analgesic, agonist.
Mechanism of action: Binds to opiate receptors and blocks ascending pain pathways. Reduces patient's perception of pain without altering cause of the pain.
Indications/dosage/route: IV only.
- Induction of anesthesia
  – Initial: 50–75 µg/kg, continuous infusion, ≥ 45 min. Maintenance (with nitrous oxide/oxygen): 0.5–3 µg/kg/min.
- Induction of anesthesia, ≥ 45 min.
  – Initial: 130–245 µg/kg. Maintenance: 0.5–1.5 µg/kg/min.
- Anesthetic adjunct, 30–60 minutes, incremental injection
  – Initial: 20–50 µg/kg. Maintenance: 5–15 µg/kg. Total dose: 75 µg/kg.
- Anesthetic adjunct, <30 min.
  – Initial: 8–20 µg/kg. Maintenance: 3–5 µg/kg. Total dose: 8–40 µg/kg.

Adjustment of dosage
- Kidney disease: None.
- Liver disease: None.
- Elderly: None.
- Pediatric: Not used in children <12.

Onset of Action	Peak Effect	Duration
Immediate	No data	No data

Food: Not applicable.

Pregnancy: Category C. Category D if prolonged use or if given in high doses at term.

Contraindications: Hypersensitivity to narcotics of the same chemical class.

Warnings/precautions
- Use with caution in patients with the following conditions: head injury with increased intracranial pressure, serious alcoholism, prostatic hypertrophy, chronic pulmonary disease, severe liver or kidney disease, postoperative patients with pulmonary disease, disorders of biliary tract.
- Administer drug before patient experiences severe pain for fullest efficacy of the drug.
- Nausea, vomiting, and orthostatic hypotension occur most prominently in ambulatory patients. If nausea and vomiting persist, it may be necessary to administer an antiemetic, eg, droperidol or prochlorperazine. This drug can cause severe hypotension in a patient who is volume depleted or if given along with a phenothiazine or general anesthesia.
- Careful diagnosis must be made of acute abdominal condition before this drug is administered.

Special considerations: This drug should be administered only by personnel who have experience in the use of IV and general anesthetics as well as in the management of possible respiratory depression by narcotic drugs. The following must be immediately available should the need arise: resuscitative and intubation equipment, oxygen, narcotic antagonist. Patient should be continuously monitored for oxygen saturation, vital signs, and signs of upper airway obstruction and hypotension.

Editorial comments
- This drug is listed without detail in *Physician's Desk Reference*, 54th edition, 2000.
- For additional information, see *morphine*, p. 633.

Allopurinol

Brand names: Zyloprim, Aloprim.

Class of drug: Treatment for gout, prophylaxsis for chemotherapy-induced hyperuricemia.

Mechanism of action: Inhibits xanthine oxidase, the enzyme that converts hypoxanthine to xanthine. Xanthine is a precursor for uric acid production; thus uric acid production is decreased.

Indications/dosage/route: Oral only.
- Mild gout
  - Adults: 200–300 mg/d.
- Moderate or severe gout
  - Adults: 400–600 mg/d.
- Prophylaxis against acute attack
  - 100 mg/d. Maximum: 800 mg/d.
- Prevention of hyperuricemia during cancer chemotherapy
  - Adults, children >10 years: 600–800 mg/d, 2–3 divided doses, 1–2 days before chemotherapy for 2–3 days. IV 200–400 mg/m^2/d.
  - Children <10 years: 200–300 mg/m^2/d, 2–4 divided doses. IV 200–300 mg/m^2/d.

Adjustment of dosage
- Kidney disease: Adjust dosage in relation to creatinine clearance. Reduce standard dose (300 mg/d) by 50 mg for each 20 mL/min. decrease in creatinine clearance below 100 mL/min. (Example: Creatinine clearance = 60; give 200 mg allopurinol/d). Creatinine clearance <20 mL/min: give q2d or q3d.

- Liver disease: None.
- Elderly: Maximum 200 mg/d.
- Pediatric: See above.

Onset of Action

48–72 h for decline of serum uric acid level,
1–3 wk to achieve proper level

Food: Take with meals or immediately after eating. Have patient drink large amounts of fluids.

Contraindications: Hypersensitivity to allopurinol; idiopathic hemochromatosis.

Warnings/precautions
- Discontinue at first sign of rash.
- Use drug in children only to treat hyperuricemia associated with chemotherapy.

Advice to patient
- Avoid driving and other activities requiring mental alertness or that are potentially dangerous until response to drug is known.
- Limit foods with high purine content (liver or other organ meats, salmon, sardines).
- Drink large quantities of water (10–12 glasses per day).
- Do not take large amounts of vitamin C.
- Avoid alcohol and other CNS depressants such as opiate analgesics and sedatives (eg, diazepam [Valium]) when taking this drug.
- Do not take iron salts while on allopurinol.
- Limit intake of caffeine and alcohol.
- Limit exposure to UV light as this may increase the risk of cataracts.

Pregnancy: Category C.

Lactation: Appears in breast milk. Considered compatible by American Academy of Pediatrics.

Adverse reactions
- Common: skin rash (generally maculopapular).

- Serious: agranulocytosis, aplastic anemia, thrombocytopenia, hepatic injury, Stevens–Johnson syndrome, vasculitis, toxic epidermal necrolysis, neuritis, cataracts, renal toxicity.

Clinically important drug interactions

- Drugs that increase effects/toxicity of allopurinol: thiazide diuretics, ACE inhibitors, vitamin C.
- Allopurinol increases effects/toxicity of the following: ampicillin, amoxicillin, oral anticoagulants, 6-mercaptopurine, cyclophosphamide, theophylline, chlorpropamide, alcohol.

Parameters to monitor

- Serum BUN and creatinine, CBC with differential and platelets, liver enzymes.
- Renal function and liver enzymes.
- Check urinary pH for excessive alkalinity.
- Monitor for acute attacks of gout during first 4–6 weeks of therapy. Consider colchicine as additional treatment.
- Serum uric acid levels for evidence of efficacy of treatment. These should be determined every 1–2 weeks after beginning therapy.
- Other evidence of efficacy of treatment: decrease in size of tophi, relief of joint pain, increased joint mobility, reduction in joint inflammation.
- Skin rashes: If they occur, drug may have to be discontinued permanently. If mild, reinstitute therapy at one-half initial dose, but if rash reappears, discontinue permanently.
- Change in vision: An ophthalmologic exam is indicated.

Editorial comments: Because the incidence of acute attacks of gout may increase during the first few months of treatment with allopurinol, colchicine, a uricosuric agent, or an NSAID should be added to the regimen as a prophylactic measure.

Alprazolam

Brand name: Xanax.

Class of drug: Antianxiety agent, hypnotic.

Mechanism of action: Potentiates effects of GABA in limbic system and reticular formation.

Indications/dosage/route: Oral only.
- Anxiety disorder
  - Adults: Initial: 0.25–0.5 mg t.i.d. Maximum: 4 mg/d.
  - Elderly or debilitated: Initial: 0.25 mg b.i.d. to t.i.d.
- Panic disorder
  - Adults: 0.5 mg t.i.d., increase to maximum of 10 mg/d.

Adjustment of dosage
- Kidney disease: Use caution.
- Liver disease: Initial: 0.25 mg, b.i.d. or t.i.d.
- Elderly: See above.
- Pediatric: Safety and efficacy have not been established in children under 18 years.

Food: No restrictions

Pregnancy: Category D.

Lactation: Appears in breast milk. Potentially toxic to infant. Avoid breastfeeding.

Contraindications: Hypersensitivity to benzodiazepines, pregnancy.

Warnings/precautions
- Use with caution in patients with the following conditions: history of drug abuse, severe renal and hepatic impairment, elderly, neonates, infants.
- Benzodiazepines may cause psychologic and physical dependence.
- These drugs may cause paradoxical rage.
- It is best not to prescribe this drug for more than 6 months. If there is a need for long-term therapy, evaluate patient frequently.
- Use only for patients who have significant anxiety without medication, do not respond to other treatment, and are not drug abusers.

Advice to patient
- Avoid driving and other activities requiring mental alertness or that are potentially dangerous until response to drug is known.
- Avoid alcohol and other CNS depressants such as narcotic

analgesics, alcohol, antidepressants, antihistamines, and barbiturates when taking this drug.

- Use OTC medications only with approval from the treating physician.
- Cigarette smoking will decrease drug effect. Do not smoke when taking this drug.
- Do not stop drug abruptly if taken for more than 1 month. If suddenly withdrawn, there may be recurrence of the original anxiety or insomnia. A full-blown withdrawal may occur consisting of vomiting, insomnia, tremor, sweating, muscle spasms. After chronic use, decrease drug dosage slowly, ie, over a period of several weeks at a rate of 25% per week.
- Avoid excessive use of xanthine-containing foods (regular coffee, tea, chocolate) as these may counteract the action of the drug.

Adverse reactions
- Common: drowsiness, lightheadedness, depression, headache.
- Serious: **depression**, respiratory depression, apnea, hallucinations, hepatitis, seizures, hostile behavior, Stevens–Johnson syndrome.

Clinically important drug interactions
- Drugs that increase effects/toxicity of benzodiazepines: CNS depressants (alcohol, antihistamines, narcotic analgesics, tricyclic antidepressants, SSRIs, MAO inhibitors), cimetidine, disulfiram.
- Drugs that decrease effects/toxicity of benzodiazepines: flumazenil (antidote for overdose), carbamazepine.

Parameters to monitor
- Signs of chronic toxicity: ataxia, vertigo, slurred speech.
- Monitor dosing to make sure amount taken is as prescribed particularly if patient has suicidal tendencies.
- Monitor patient for efficacy of treatment: reduced symptoms of anxiety and tension, improved sleep.
- Signs of physical/psychologic dependence, particularly if patient is addiction-prone and requests frequent renewal of prescription or is experiencing a diminished response to the drug.

- Patient's neurologic status including the following: memory (anterograde amnesia), disturbing thoughts, unusual behavior.
- Possibility of blood dyscrasias: fever, sore throat, upper respiratory infection. Perform total and differential WBC counts.

Editorial comments
- Alprazolam appears to have some antidepressant effects and is indicated for anxiety associated with depression.
- The side effect profile of alprazolam appears better than that of some other benzodiazepines.
- Seizures may occur if flumazenil is given after long term use of benzodiazepines.

Alprostadil

Brand names: Caverject, Prostin VR Pediatric, Muse (urethral suppository).
Class of drug: Prostaglandin; vasodilator for erectile dysfunction.
Mechanism of action: Causes vasodilation by activating prostaglandin receptors in blood vessels, increases nitric oxide in smooth muscle.
Indications/dosage/route: IV, intracavernosal, suppository.
- Maintenance of ductus arteriosus in neonate before cardiac surgery
  - Continuous IV into large vein or umbilical artery: 0.05–0.1 µg/kg/min. Reduce dose after achieving therapeutic goal. Maintain at 0.01–0.4 µg/kg/min.
- Erectile dysfunction: intracavernosal before intercourse.
  - 1–400 mg. Initial: 2.5 µg. Inject over 5–10 s. Incremental increases by 10–15 µg performed in physicians office.
  - Urethral suppository: 125, 250,500, or 1000 µg.

Adjustment of dosage
- Kidney disease: None.
- Liver disease: None.
- Elderly: Higher doses may be required. Use same initial doses.
- Pediatric: Contraindicated.

Onset of Action
15 min– 3 h

Pregnancy: Category X.

Lactation: No data available. Do not breastfeed.

Contraindications: Hyaline membrane disease in neonate, penile implant, adult respiratory distress syndrome, bleeding tendencies, pregnancy.

Warnings/precautions

- Use with caution in patients with the following conditions: neonates with bleeding tendencies, history of leukemia, sickle cell disease.
- Apnea may occur in greater than 10% of neonates with congenital heart defects, especially those <2 kg at birth. This usually presents during the first hour of infusion of alprostadil.
- Priapism may occur with intracavernous injections and must be treated quickly to avoid permanent penile damage.
- Do not use intercavernous injections more than 3 or 4 times a week.
- Use alternate sides of penis for injection.
- When drug is administered for maintenance of ductus arteriosus, equipment for artificial ventilation should be immediately available.

Advice to patient

- Use two forms of birth control including hormonal and barrier methods.
- Contact physician if priapism lasts more than 6 hours or if patient observes presence of nodules in penis or swelling or curvature of the erect penis.

Adverse reactions

- Common: IV: flushing, fever. Intracavernosal: penile pain, URI.
- Serious: IV: **apnea, depression**, cardiac arrest, DIC, seizures, hypotension, cerebral bleeding, arrythmia, hypokalemia, shock, hypoglycemia, peritonitis. Intracavernosal: prolonged erection, priapism.

Parameters to monitor
- For IV administration: Monitor arterial pressure (umbilical artery) and respiratory status, respiratory rate, lung sounds, arterial blood gases.
- Signs and symptoms of overdose in infant receiving the drug for ductus arteriosus treatment: bradycardia, apnea, flushing, hyperpyrexia, hypotension. Stop if apnea or bradycardia occurs. Otherwise, reduce rate of administration.
- Efficacy of treatment for ductus arteriosus: closure of ductus about 1–2 hours after administration as indicated by improved oxygenation, improved urine output, improved circulation to extremities.
- Rectal temperature for hyperpyrexia.
- Signs and symptoms of catheter displacement for IV administration.
- Efficacy in treatment of erectile dysfunction: Erection 5–20 minutes after administration, duration no more than 1 hour.
- Monitor for possible erectile dysfunction, cavernosal fibrosis, Peyronie's disease, penile angulation.

Editorial comments: The first injection to determine proper dose for erectile dysfunction should be done in the office under physician supervision.

Alteplase

Brand name: Activase.
Class of drug: Thrombolytic agent.
Mechanism of action: Converts fibrin-bound plasminogen to plasmin, which initiates local fibrinolysis (clot dissolution).
Indications/dosage/route: IV only.
- Acute myocardial infarction: accelerated infusion:
  – Adults weighing more than 65 kg: Infuse 15 mg over 1–2 minutes; infuse 50 mg over next 30 min. Begin heparin

5000–10,000 units IV bolus followed by continuous infusion of 1000 units/h. Infuse 35 mg alteplase over next hour.

 – Adults weighing less than 65 kg: Infuse 15 mg over 1–2 minutes; follow with 0.75 mg/kg over next 30 minutes. Begin heparin 5000–10,000 units by IV bolus followed by continuous infusion of 1000 units/h. Infuse 0.5 mg/kg alteplase over next hour.

• Acute myocardial infarction: 3-hour infusion
 – Adults weighing more than 65 kg: 60 mg over the first hour, of which 6–10 mg is administered as bolus over first 1–2 minutes, 20 mg over the second hour and 20 mg over the third hour.
 – Adults weighing less than 65 kg: 1.25 mg/kg over 3 hours as described for those weighing more than 65 kg.

• Acute ischemic stroke (acute ischemic stroke in highly selected populations is still under investigation though early reports are excellent)
 – Adults: 0.9 mg/kg infused over 60 minutes; 10% of the dose should be given as bolus over the first minute. Maximum dose 90 mg.

• Pulmonary embolism
 – Adults: 100 mg by IV infusion over 2 hours. Begin heparin, continuous infusion, 1300 units/h when PT or PTT falls to less than twice the control time.

Adjustment of dosage
• Kidney disease: Use with caution.
• Liver disease: Use with caution.
• Elderly: Use with caution.
• Pediatric: Safety and effectiveness have not been determined for children.

Onset of Action	Peak Effect	Duration
Immediate	40–50 min	No known

Food: Not applicable.

Pregnancy: Category B (listed as C by manufacturer).

Lactation: It is not known whether alteplase is excreted in breast milk. However, not likely to be relevant.

Contraindications

• Patients treated for acute MI, pulmonary embolism, active internal bleeding, history of cerebrovascular accident, recent intracranial or intraspinal surgery or trauma, intracranial neoplasm, arteriovenous malformation or aneurysm, known bleeding diathesis, severe uncontrolled bleeding, severe uncontrolled hypertension.

• Patients treated for acute ischemic stroke: intracranial hemorrhage, recent intracranial or intraspinal surgery, serious head trauma, previous stroke, uncontrolled hypertension (systolic >185, diastolic >110), seizure at onset of stroke, active internal bleeding, intracranial neoplasm, arteriovenous aneurysm, known bleeding diathesis, heparin administration within 48 hours preceding stroke, platelet count <100,000/mm^3.

Warnings/precautions

• Use with caution in patients with the following conditions: internal bleeding (intracranial, retroperitoneal, gastrointestinal, genitourinary, or respiratory tracts), superficial bleeding (venous cutdown sites, arterial punctures), recent major surgery (coronary artery bypass graft, obstetric delivery), cerebrovascular disease, mitral stenosis with atrial fibrillation, acute pericarditis, hemorrhagic ophthalmic conditions, concomitant administration of anticoagulants.

• Cardiac and blood pressure monitors are required when using this drug.

• Dose should be limited to 100 mg. Doses of 150 mg or greater have been shown to increase intracranial bleeding.

• Administer with great caution during the first 10 days postpartum.

• Discontinue administration immediately if local pressure does not control bleeding.

• Initiate therapy as soon as possible after stroke symptoms are apparent and no more than 3 hours after onset of stroke symptoms. After MI, therapy should be initiated within 7 hours.

- An electronic measuring devise should be used for IV infusions.
- Invasive procedures such as arterial puncture or venipuncture should be conducted with care when administering this drug.
- Obtain values for the following parameters before administering this drug: CBC, PT, PTT, creatinine phosphokinase, fibrinogen, cardiac isoenzymes.

Advice to patient: Not applicable.

Adverse reactions
- Common: None.
- Serious: GU, retroperitoneal, intracranial bleeding, anaphylactic reactions, urticaria, worsening cardiovascular, cerebrovascular or pulmonary conditions (may be due to underlying illness).

Clinically important drug interactions: The following drugs increase effects/toxicity of alteplase: warfarin, aspirin, ticlopidine, dipyridamole, heparin.

Parameters to monitor
- Coagulation parameters: CBC, PT, PTT, INR, fibrinogen. PT or PTT should be less than twice control values for those patients treated for pulmonary embolism.
- Monitor BP frequently and maintain at less than 180 mm systolic, 100 mm diasystolic.
- Monitor ECG for signs of reperfusion after coronary thrombolysis and for arrhythmias, eg, sinus bradycardia, ventricular arrhythmias.

Editorial comments
- Thrombolytic therapy has been thoroughly investigated. Large randomized trials have been completed and clearly indicate the efficacy of alteplase and streptokinase.
- Alteplase is easy to infuse and the sooner an effective steady state of the drug is achieved, the more rapidly an occluded artery opens. There is a higher risk of intracerebral hemorrhage with tPA (about 1%) when compared with streptokinase or its derivatives.
- Efficacy is enhanced with rapid administration of heparin following a bolus over 90 minutes or 3 hours depending on the clinical circumstances.

• Frequent and timely monitoring of coagulation parameters is essential to minimize risk of side effects of thrombolytic therapy.

Amantadine

Brand name: Symmetrel.
Class of drug: Treatment for Parkinson's disease, antiviral agent.
Mechanism of action: Anti-Parkinson action: promotes release of dopamine in substantia nigra. Antiviral action: prevents viral penetration of influenza A virus into target host cells.
Indications/dosage/route: Oral only.
• Parkinson's disease
  – Adults: 100 mg b.i.d., may be titrated up. Maximum: 400 mg/d.
• Influenza A:
  – Adults: 200 mg/d, single or divided dose.
  – Children 1–9 years: 4.4–8.8 mg/d. Maximum: 150 mg/d.
Adjustment of dosage:
• Kidney disease: reduce dose as follows. Creatinine clearance 30–50 mL/min: initial 200 mg, then 100 mg/d; creatinine clearance 15–29 mL/min: initial 200 mg, then 100 mg q.i.d.; creatinine clearance <15 mL/min: 200 mg q7d.
• Liver disease: None
• Elderly: Dosage should be divided as twice daily administration.
• Pediatric: See above

Onset of Action:

Parkinson's disease: <2 d.

Food: No information available.
Pregnancy: Category C.

Lactation: Appears in breast milk; best to avoid.

Contraindications: Hypersensitivity to amantadine, untreated angle-closure glaucoma.

Warnings/precautions

- Use with caution in patients with the following conditions: psychiatric disorders, liver or kidney disease, history of epilepsy, peripheral edema, orthostatic hypotension, severe psychosis, eczematoid dermatitis, exposure to rubella.
- There is a possibility of seizures if given with CNS stimulants or in patients with history of epilepsy.
- Do not stop abruptly when treating Parkinson's disease.
- Deaths from amantadine overdose have been reported. Suicide attempts in patients taking amantadine have been reported. The cause of these has not been determined.

Advice to patient

- Change position slowly, in particular from recumbent to upright to minimize orthostatic hypotension.
- Sit at the edge of the bed for several minutes before standing, and lie down if feeling faint or dizzy.
- Avoid hot showers or baths and standing for long periods. Male patients with orthostatic hypotension may be safer urinating while seated on the toilet rather than standing.
- Avoid alcohol and other CNS depressants (see Drug Interactions) when taking this drug.
- Avoid driving and other activities requiring mental alertness or that are potentially dangerous until response to drug is known.
- Immunocompromised, elderly patients should avoid crowds, particularly during the flu season; obtain immunizations against influenza and pneumonia on an annual basis.
- Take last dose well before bedtime to avoid insomnia.

Adverse reactions

- Common: dizziness, insomnia.
- Serious: CHF, seizures, hallucinations, depression, psychosis, bone marrow depression, livedo reticularis, renal toxicity.

Clinically important drug interactions

- Drugs that increase effects/toxicity of amantadine: anticholinergic drugs (benztropine, trihexphenidyl), CNS stimulants, thioridizine, possibly other phenothiazines, potassium-sparing diuretics, alcohol.

Parameters to monitor

- Serum BUN and creatinine, CBC with differential and platelets.
- Watch for increased incidence of seizures if history of epilepsy.
- Signs and symptoms of psychological problems: depression, confusion, or other new symptoms.
- Intake of fluids and urinary and other fluid output to minimize renal toxicity. Closely monitor electrolyte levels.
- Symptoms of CHF.
- Signs and symptoms of livedo reticularis: red or rose-colored mottling of skin usually in lower extremities but may also appear on arms. This condition is more prominent when patient is exposed to cold. This side effect generally appears within 1–12 months of treatment.
- Efficacy of treatment for Parkinson's disease: decrease in abnormal muscle movements, in particular akinesia, rigidity, tremors. Discontinue drug if no improvement within 1–2 weeks.

Editorial comments:

- Be advised that for amantadine to be effective in treating influenza, it must be administered not later than 48 hours after symptoms are noted.
- Amantadine is recommended for prophylactic use in patients at high risk who cannot be administered influenza vaccine. Such prophylactic therapy should be given for up to 90 days.
- This drug should be administered for Parkinsonian patients only under close medical supervision. Although there may be a satisfactory relief of Parkinsonian symtoms within a few days, effectiveness may diminish after 6–8 weeks of treatment. If this occurs, a decision will have to be made whether to increase the dose or discontinue drug administration and use another anti-Parkinson drug.

Amikacin

Brand name: Amikin.
Class of drug: Antibiotic, aminoglycoside.
Mechanism of action: Binds to ribosomal units in bacteria, inhibits protein synthesis.
Susceptible organisms *in vivo*: Staphylococci (penicillinase and nonpenicillinase), *Staphylococcus epidermidis, Acinetobacter* sp, *Citrobacter* sp, *Enterobacter* sp, *Escherichia coli, Klebsiella* sp, *Proteus* sp, *Providencia* sp, *Pseudomonas* sp, *Serratia* sp.
Indications/dosage/route: IM, IV.
- Bacterial septicemia (including neonatal sepsis); serious infections of the respiratory tract, bones, joints, skin, soft tissue, and CNS (eg, meningitis); burns; serious complicated infections of the urinary tract
  - Adults, children, older infants: 15 mg/kg in 2–3 divided doses, 7–10 days. Maximum: 15 mg/kg/d.
- Uncomplicated UTIs
  - Adults: 250 mg b.i.d.
  - Newborns: loading dose of 10 mg/kg, then 7.5 mg/kg q12h.
Adjustment of dosage: Kidney disease: initial: 7.5 mg/kg (loading dose); maintenance: divide normal recommended dose by patient's serum creatinine level, administer calculated dose q12h.
Food: No restrictions.
Pregnancy: Category D.
Lactation: Appears in breast milk in small amounts. Potentially toxic to infant. Best to avoid.
Contraindications: Hypersensitivity to aminoglycoside antibiotics.
Warnings/precautions
- Use with caution in patients with the following conditions: renal disease, neuromuscular disorders (eg, myasthenia gravis, parkinsonism), hearing disorders.
- Do not combine this drug with any other drug in the same IV bag.

Adverse reactions
- Common: None.
- Serious: renal toxicity, ototoxicity, neuromuscular paralysis, respiratory depression (infants), superinfection.

Clinically important drug interactions
- Drugs that decrease effects/toxicity of aminoglycosides: penicillins (high dose), cephalosporins.
- Drugs that increase effects/toxicity of aminoglycosides: loop diuretics, amphotericin B, enflurane, vancomycin, NSAIDs.

Parameters to monitor
- Determine peak and trough serum levels 48 hours after beginning therapy and every 3–4 days thereafter as well as after changing doses.
- Monitor patient for ototoxicity: tinnitus, vertigo, hearing loss. The drug should be stopped if tinnitus occurs. Limit administration to 7–10 days to decrease the risk of ototoxicity.
- Monitor patient's renal function periodically. If serum creatinine increases by more than 50% over baseline value, it may be advisable to discontinue drug treatment and use a less nephrotoxic agent, eg, a quinolone or cephalosporin.
- Efficacy of drug action: If there is no response in 3–7 days, reculture and consider another drug.
- Monitor neuromuscular function when administering the drug IV. Too rapid administration may cause paralysis and apnea. Have calcium gluconate or pyridostigmine available to reverse such an effect.
- Monitor patient's neurologic status if the drug is given for hepatic encephalopathy.
- Monitor patient for signs and symptoms of allergic reaction.

Editorial comments: Once daily dosing of amikacin has been advocated by some authors to increase efficacy and reduce toxicity.

Amiloride

Brand name: Midamor.
Class of drug: Potassium-sparing diuretic.

Mechanism of action: Acts on distal renal tubules to inhibit sodium–potassium exchange.

Indications/dosage/route: Oral only.

- Hypertension, alone or with other diuretics (loop or thiazide)
  – Adults: Initial: 5–10 mg/d. Maximum: 20 mg/d.

Adjustment of dosage

- Kidney disease: creatinine clearance 10–50 mL/min: reduce dose by 50%; creatinine clearance <10 mL/min: do not use.
- Liver disease: None.
- Elderly: None.
- Pediatric: Safety and efficacy in children have not been established.

Onset of Action	Peak Effect	Duration
<2 h	6–10 h	24 h

Food: Take with food or milk.

Pregnancy: Category B.

Lactation: No data available. Best to avoid.

Contraindications: Anuria, hyperkalemia, severe renal insufficiency, serum potassium level >5 mEq/L, patients receiving other potassium-sparing diuretics or potassium supplements, hypersensitivity to amiloride.

Editorial comments: For additional information, see *spironolactone*, p. 849.

Amiodarone

Brand name: Cordarone.

Class of drug: Antiarrhythmic, Class III.

Mechanism of action: Prolongs action potential duration as well as refractory period.

Indications/dosage/route: Oral, IV.
- Ventricular arrhythmias after MI
  - Adults: Loading dose: IV 5 mg/kg over 25–50 minutes. Maintenance: 10–15 mg/kg/d. Further data needed to clarify proper dosages.
- Intractable ventricular tachycardia or fibrillation
  - Adults: PO 800–1600 mg/day loading dose for 1–3 weeks, then for 4–14 days, 5 mg/kg/d for 2–4 weeks. Maintenance: 2.5 mg/kg.
  - Children: PO 10–15 mg/kg/d, loading dose, as single or divided dose, daily or 5 of 7 days weekly.

Onset of Action	Peak Effect
3 d to 3 wk	1 wk to 5 mo

Adjustment of dosage
- Kidney disease: None.
- Liver disease: None.
- Elderly: None.
- Pediatric: Safety and efficacy have not been established.

Food: To be taken with food.

Pregnancy: Category C.

Lactation: Appears in breast milk. Potentially toxic to infant. Avoid breastfeeding until several months after discontinuation of drug.

Contraindications: Sinus node dysfunction, bradycardia accompanied by syncope, AV block (second or third degree).

Warnings/precautions
- Use with caution in patients with the following conditions: CHF, hypersensitivity to iodine.
- A number of potentially fatal toxic effects are associated with use of amiodarone. Up to 17% of patients receiving this medication may develop pulmonary toxicity characterized by hypersensitivity pneumonitis or interstitial pneumonitis. Other potentially serious side effects with this medication include

hepatotoxicity, exacerbation of arrhythmia, and loss of vision due to optic neuritis or optic neuropathy. Neonatal hypo- or hyperthyroidism may occur if amiodarone is administered during pregnancy.

- This is not a first line antiarrhythmic drug; it is used when others fail.
- Because of extremely long half-life (100 days), extreme care must be used when other antiarrhythmic drugs are given after discontinuing amiodarone. Approximately 75% of patients receiving more than 400 mg/d experience adverse effects over time. Patients should be monitored in the hospital during administration of loading doses. Note that severe and life-threatening toxic effects are associated with the loading phase and chronic use of amiodorane.
- Evaluate patient for orthostasis with BP measurements in the sitting, lying, and standing positions repeatedly before and after initiating therapy.
- Hypokalemia or hypomagnesemia should be corrected before amiodarone is administered.

Advice to patient

- Use sunscreen or protective clothing in strong sunlight. These precautions should be maintained for up to 4 months following discontinuation of drug therapy.
- There may be a bluish discoloration, mainly in the face, arms, and neck. This will disappear after drug is discontinued.

Adverse reactions

- Oral
  - Common: headache, dizziness, fatigue, muscle weakness, solar dermatitis, photosensitivity, discoordination, hyperlipidemia, nausea, vomiting, constipation, anorexia, tremor, paresthesias,visual disturbances.
  - Serious: **pulmonary fibrosis and/or interstitial pneumonitis (17%), hepatotoxicity, hypotension (16%),** pulmonary infiltrates, dysrhythmias, hypothyroidism, cardiovascular collapse, CHF, thrombocytopenia, optic neuritis or neuropathy, corneal microdeposits, peripheral neuropathy.

• Intravenous: **Cardiovascular collapse, asystole, heart failure.**

Clinically important drug interactions

- Drugs that increase effects/toxicity of amiodarone: calcium channel blockers, cimetidine, ritonavir, volatile anesthetics.
- Amiodarone increases effects/toxicity of the following drugs: oral anticoagulants, β blockers, digoxin, phenytoin, quinidine, cyclosporine, procainamide, flecainide, cisapride, methotrexate theophylline.
- Drugs that decrease effects/toxicity of amiodarone: cholestyramine.

Parameters to monitor

- Baseline and follow-up serum electrolytes, BUN and creatinine, thyroid functions, liver enzymes.
- Ophthalmic examinations for signs of granular corneal deposits (brown colored). Advise patient to instill methycellulose ophthalmic solution frequently to minimize problem.
- Signs and symptoms of psychiatric symptoms or neurotoxicity: depression, insomnia, headache, hallucinations, muscle weakness, ataxia, paresthesia of fingers, toes. If these occur, consider changing medication.
- Pulmonary function test to monitor signs and symptoms of pulmonary toxicity.
- ECG for the following parameters: heart rate and rhythm, reduction of T-wave amplitude, Q-T prolongation.
- Signs and symptoms of thyroid dysfunction, including both hyper- and hypothyroidism, weight gain, pale skin, edema of extremities and periorbital region.

Editorial comment

- Oral: Bioavailability of amiodarone is 40–60% depending on absorption. Iodine dose is about 40 mg/pill and this likely contributes to the most common adverse reaction: thyroid dysfunction. Most adverse end-organ problems are cumulative dose-related and therefore lower maintenance doses have been better tolerated for longer periods. Loading should always be performed in the hospital if the patient has left ventricular dysfunction due to potential proarrhythmia in this group. If the heart structure is well preserved, then low-dose (200 mg t.i.d.) loading with gradual decrease can safely be done as an outpatient over 2 months as long as the ECG and clinical status are stable. Pulmonary toxicity can often be managed as an outpatient with or without home O_2.

- IV: The loading dose of IV amiodarone is not as large as in-hospital oral amiodarone loading. IV amiodarone should always be given in a monitored setting preferably in the intensive care unit or skilled telemetry ward. A central line is essential to decrease the phlebitis that accompanies infusion.
- ACLS protocol has now replaced bretylium with amiodarone IV in the treatment of malignant hemodynamically compromised ventricular tachyarrhythmia.
- It is recommended that patients undergoing general anesthesia while receiving amiodarone therapy should be monitored carefully in the perioperative period. These patients may be at higher risk for conduction abnormalities and myocardial dysfunction secondary to anesthetic agents. Additionally, episodes of ARDS and post-bypass hypotension have been noted in patients undergoing surgery when receiving amiodarone.

Amitriptyline

Brand name: Elavil.
Class of drug: Tricyclic antidepressant.
Mechanism of action: Inhibits reuptake of CNS neurotransmitters, primarily serotonin and norepinephrine.
Indications/dosage/route: Oral, IM.
- Depression
  – Adults (outpatients): Initial: PO 75 mg/d in divided doses; increase to 150 mg/d if needed.

- Hospitalized patients. PO—Initial: 100 mg/d, may be increased to 200–300 mg/d. IM—20–30 mg q.i.d.; change to oral drug as quickly as possible. Maintenance: 40–100 mg/d.
- Adolescents and elderly: PO 10 mg t.i.d. with 20 mg at bedtime. Maximum: 100 mg/d.
- Children 6–12 years: PO 10–30 mg/d, up to 4 divided doses.
- Chronic pain
  - Adults: PO 50–100 mg/d.
- Enuresis
  - Children >6 years: PO 10 mg/day at bedtime; increase to maximum of 25 mg/day if needed.
  - Children <6 years: PO 10 mg/day at bedtime.

Adjustment of dosage
- Kidney disease: None.
- Liver disease: None.
- Elderly: See above.
- Pediatric: Not recommended for children <12 years old except for treatment of enuresis.

Food: No restriction.

Pregnancy: Category C.

Lactation: Appears in breast milk. American Academy of Pediatrics expresses concern over use when breastfeeding.

Contraindications: Hypersensitivity to tricyclic antidepressants, acute recovery from MI, concurrent MAO inhibitor.

Warnings/precautions
- Use with caution in patients with the following conditions: epilepsy, angle-closure glaucoma, cardiovascular disease, history of urinary retention, suicidal tendencies, benign prostatic hypertrophy, concurrent anticholinergic drugs, hyperthyroid patients receiving thyroid drugs, alcoholism, schizophrenia.
- May cause psychosis in schizophrenic patients.
- May unmask mania or hypomania.

Advice to patient
- Avoid alcohol and other CNS depressants such as opiate analgesics and sedatives (eg, diazepam) when taking this drug.
- Avoid driving and other activities requiring mental alertness or that are potentially dangerous until response to drug is known.

- Change position slowly, in particular from recumbent to upright, to minimize orthostatic hypotension. Sit at the edge of the bed for several minutes before standing, and lie down if feeling faint or dizzy. Avoid hot showers or baths and standing for long periods. Male patients should sit on the toilet while urinating rather than standing.
- If mouth is dry rinse with warm water frequently, chew sugarless gum, suck on ice cube, or use artificial saliva. Carry out meticulous oral hygiene (floss teeth daily).
- To minimize possible photosensitivity reaction, apply adequate sunscreen and use proper covering when exposed to strong sunlight.
- If constipation develops, increase fiber and fluid intake. Notify physician if constipation is severe.

Adverse reactions
- Common: sedation, anticholinergic effects (dry mouth, constipation), nausea, dizziness, headache, taste disturbance, weight gain.
- Serious: orthostatic hypotension, arrhythmias, extrapyramidal symptoms, seizures, bone marrow depression, hepatitis, increased intraocular pressure, allergic reactions.

Clinically important drug interactions
- Drugs that increase effects/toxicity of tricyclic antidepressants: MAO inhibitors, cimetidine, SSRIs, β blockers, estrogens.
- Drugs that decrease effects/toxicity of tricyclic antidepressants: barbiturates, cholestyramine.
- Tricyclic antidepressants increase effects/toxicity of following drugs: CNS depressants (alcohol, sedatives, hypnotics), oral anticoagulants, carbamazepine, sympathomimetic amines (dobutamine, dopamine, epinephrine, ephedrine), opioids (morphine-type drugs), drugs with anticholinergic activity (atropine, anti-Parkinson drugs).
- Tricyclic antidepressants decrease effects/toxicity of following drugs: clonidine, guanethidine.

Parameters to monitor
- CBC with differential and platelets, liver enzymes.

- Suicidal ideation: Advise patient's family to remove firearms from the home.
- Signs and symptoms of hepatotoxicity.
- Monitor drug levels: therapeutic level: 160–250 mg/mL; toxic level: >500 mg/mL.
- Evaluate neurologic and mental status: mood changes, agitation. May require dose reduction. Hypomania, mania, or delusions: stop medication.
- Monitor patient for signs and symptoms of angle-closure glaucoma and visual or other ophthalmic disturbances, eg, halos, eye pain, dilated pupils.
- Signs and symptoms of bone marrow depression.
- Monitor patient with history of hyperthyroidism or cardiovascular disease for arrhythmias.
- Monitor patient for efficacy of treatment: increased appetite and energy level and sense of well-being, renewed interest in environment, improved sleep.

Editorial comments
- Patients with depression are at increased risk of suicide. To reduce this risk as well as the chance of overdose, prescribe limited amounts.
- Withdrawal symptoms have been reported after abrupt cessation of administration. These include nausea, headaches, irritability, and sleep disturbances.
- It may take several months for maximum response to be realized.

Amlodipine

Brand name: Norvasc.
Class of drug: Calcium channel blocker.
Mechanism of action: Inhibits calcium movement across cell membranes.

Indications/dosage/route: Oral only.
• Hypertension
  – Adults: Individualize: 2.5–5 mg/d. Maximum: 10 mg/d.
• Angina
  – Adults: 5–10 mg.
  – Elderly: 5 mg.
Adjustment of dosage
• Kidney disease: Use with caution.
• Liver disease: Initial dose 2.5 mg/d.
• Elderly: Initial dose 2.5 mg/d.
• Pediatric: Safety and efficacy have not been established in children.

Onset of Action	Peak Effect	Duration
1–2 h	6–12 h	24 h

Food: No restriction.
Pregnancy: Category C.
Lactation: Probably appears in breast milk. Potentially toxic to infant. Avoid breastfeeding.
Contraindications: Hypersensitivity to calcium blockers.
Warnings/precautions
• Use with caution in patients with the following conditions: CHF, severe left ventricular dysfunction, concomitant use with β blockers or digoxin.
• Do not withdraw drug abruptly, since this may result in increased frequency and intensity of angina.
• For the diabetic patient, amlodipine may interfere with insulin release and therefore produce hyperglycemia.
• Patient should be tapered off β blockers before beginning calcium channel blockers to avoid exacerbation of angina due to abrupt withdrawal of the β blocker.
Advice to patient
• Use two forms of birth control including hormonal and barrier methods.

- Change position slowly, in particular from recumbent to upright, to minimize orthostatic hypotension. Sit at the edge of the bed for several minutes before standing, and lie down if feeling faint or dizzy. Avoid hot showers or baths and standing for long periods. Male patients should sit on the toilet while urinating rather than standing.
- Avoid driving and other activities requiring mental alertness or that are potentially dangerous until response to drug is known.
- Avoid use of OTC medications without first informing the treating physician.
- Determine blood pressure and heart rate aproximately at the same time each day and at least twice a week, particularly at the beginning of therapy.
- Be aware of the fact that this drug may also block or reduce anginal pain, thereby giving a false sense of security on severe exertion.
- Include high-fiber foods to minimize constipation.
- Limit consumption of xanthine-containing drinks: regular coffee (fewer than 5 cups/day), tea, cocoa.

Adverse reactions
- Common: headache, edema.
- Serious: CHF, arrhythmias, hypotension, depression.

Clinically important drug interactions
- Drugs that increase effects/toxicity of calcium blockers: cimetidine, β blockers, cyclosporine.
- Drugs that decrease effects of calcium blockers: barbiturates.

Parameters to monitor
- Patient's BP during initial administration and frequently thereafter. Ideally, check BP close to the end of dosage interval or before next administration.
- Status of liver and kidney function. Impaired renal function prolongs duration of action and increases tendency for toxicity.
- Intake of fluids and urinary and other fluid output to minimize renal toxicity. Increase fluid intake if inadequate. Closely monitor electrolyte levels.

- Efficacy of treatment for angina: decrease in frequency of angina attacks, need for nitroglycerin, episodes of PST segment deviation, anginal pain.
- If anginal pain is not reduced at rest or during effort reassess patient as to medication.
- GI side effects: use alternative.
- Monitor ECG for development of heart block.
- Symptoms of CHF.

Amoxapine

Brand name: Asendia.
Class of drug: Tricyclic antidepressant.
Mechanism of action: Inhibits reuptake of CNS neurotransmitters, primarily serotonin and norepinephrine.
Indications/dosage/route: Oral only.
- Depression
  - Adults: Initial: 50 mg t.i.d.; increase to 100 mg t.i.d. during first week. Maintenance: 300 mg as single dose at bedtime.
  - Hospitalized patients: up to 150 mg q.i.d.
  - Elderly: Initial: 25 mg b.i.d. to t.i.d.; increase to 50 mg b.i.d. to t.i.d. after first week. Maintenance: ≤ 300 mg/d at bedtime.
Adjustment of dosage
- Kidney disease: None.
- Liver disease: None.
- Elderly: Lower doses recommended.
- Pediatric: Not recommended for children <12 years.
Food: No restriction.
Pregnancy: Category C
Lactation: Appears in breast milk. American Academy of Pediatrics expresses concern over use when breastfeeding.
Contraindications: Hypersensitivity to tricyclic antidepressants, acute recovery from MI, concurrent MAO inhibitor.

Editorial comments
- This drug is not listed in *Physicians' Desk Reference*, 54th edition, 2000.
- For additional information, see *amitriptyline*, p. 39.

Amoxicillin

Brand name: Amoxil.
Class of drug: Antibiotic, penicillin family, aminopenicillin.
Mechanism of action: Inhibits bacterial cell wall synthesis.
Susceptible organisms *in vivo*: [same as ampicillin] *Streptococcus pneumoniae*, beta-hemolytic streptococci, *Enterococcus faecalis*, viridans streptococci, *Escherichia coli*, *Hemophilus influenzae*, *Neisseria gonorrhoeae*, *Proteus mirabilis*, *Salmonella* (often resistant), *Shigella* (often resistant), *Listeria monocytogenes*, *Neisseria meningitidis*.
Indications/dosage/route: Oral only.
- Ear, nose, and throat infections, mild/moderate; GU tract infections, mild/moderate
  – Adults: 500 mg q12h.
  – Children >3 months: 25 mg/kg/d, divided doses q12h.
- Ear, nose and throat infections, severe; GU tract infections, severe
  – Adults: 875 mg q12h.
  – Children >3 months: 45 mg/kg, divided doses q12h.
- Lower respiratory tract infections
  – Adults: 875 mg q12h.
  – Children >3 months: 45 mg/kg, divided doses q12h.
- Skin, skin structure infections, mild/moderate
  – Adults: 500 mg q12h.
- Children >3 months: 25 mg/kg/d, divided doses q12h.
- Skin, skin structure infections, severe
  – Adults: 875 mg q12h.

 – Children >3 months: 45 mg/kg/d, divided doses q8h.
• Acute gonorrhea, uncomplicated anogenital and urethral infections
 – Adults: 3 mg as single dose.
 – Children >2 years: 50 mg/kg plus 25 mg probenecid as single dose.

Adjustment of dosage
• Kidney disease: creatinine clearance 10–30 mL/min: 250 or 500 mg q12h; creatinine clearance <10 mL/minute: 250 or 500 mg q24h.
• Liver disease: None.
• Elderly: None.
• Pediatric: Contraindicated for children <2 years.

Food: No restrictions.

Pregnancy: Category B.

Lactation: Appears in breast milk. Considered compatible by American Academy of Pediatrics.

Contraindications: Hypersensitivity to penicillin or cephalosporins.

Warnings/precautions
• Use with caution in patients with mononucleosis.
• Allergic reactions are more likely to occur in patients with the following conditions: asthma, hay fever, allergy to cephalosporins, history of allergy to penicillin. Consider skin testing, with major and minor antigenic components, of penicillin hypersensitivity in patients with β-lactamase allergy who require amoxicillin for life-threatening infections, to assess possibility of a hypersensitivity reaction. If patient is given drug parenterally, observe for at least 20 minutes for possible anaphylactic reaction. Negative history of penicillin hypersensitivity does not prelude a patient from reacting to the drug.
• Administer at least 1 h before a bacteriostatic agent is given (eg, tetracycline, erythromycin, chloramphenicol).
• For IV infusion: Make sure no other drugs are added or mixed into the infusing solution. Do not use solution containing precipitates or foreign matter.
• Do not use a penicillin to test *Enterobacter* or *Citrobacter* infections because of inducible β-lactamase.

Advice to patient
- If you are using an oral contraceptive, use an additional method of birth control as efficacy of oral contraceptive may be reduced.
- If you are allergic to a penicillin or cephalosporin, carry an identification card with this information.

Adverse reactions
- Common: None.
- Serious: Stevens–Johnson syndrome, anaphylaxis, angioedema, laryngospasm, pseudomembraneous colitis.

Clinically important drug interactions
- Drugs that increase effects/toxicity of penicillins: probenecid, disufiram (increase levels).
- Drugs that decrease effects/toxicity of penicillins: antacids, tetracyclines.
- Penicillins increase effects of following drugs: oral anticoagulants, heparin.
- Penicillins decrease effects of following drugs: oral contraceptives.

Parameters to monitor
- Signs and symptoms of anaphylactic shock.
- Signs and symptoms of allergic reaction.
- Signs and symptoms of pseudomembranous colitis.
- Patient's intake/output of fluid.
- Renal, hepatic, and hematologic status for patients on high-dose prolonged therapy.

Editorial comments
- Amoxicillin is preferred over ampicillin for oral use because incidence of diarrhea is less. Ampicillin is preferred for intravenous use.
- Amoxicillin and ampicillin are the first choice for *Enterococcus faecalis* and *Listeria monocytogenes* infections. Amoxicillin is also used orally for prophylaxis of endocarditis after dental procedures in high-risk patients. Dosage is 2 g PO 1 h prior to procedure.

• The American Association of Pediatrics recommends amoxicillin for the treatment of otitis media due to cost-effectiveness. However, resistant organisms are clearly an important problem.

Amoxicillin/Clavulanate

Brand name: Augmentin.

Class of drug: Antibiotic, penicillin family plus β-lactamase inhibitor (clavulanate).

Mechanism of action: Inhibits bacterial cell wall synthesis. Clavulanate inhibits the β-lactamase of methicillin-susceptible *Staphylococcus aureus*, *Hemophilis infuenzae*, *Branhamella catarrhalis*, anaerobic organisms, *Neisseria gonorrhoeae*.

Susceptible organisms *in vivo*: *Staphylococcus aureus* (not MRSA), *Hemophilis infuenzae*, *Branhamella catarrhalis*, *Streptococcus pneumoniae*, *Enterococcus faecalis*, betahemolytic streptococci, viridans streptococci. Resistance is increasing in *E. coli* even in the community.

Indications/dosage/route: Oral only.

• All infections
 – Adults, children >40 kg: 500-mg tablet q12h or 125- to 250-mg chewable tablet q8h.
• Severe infections
 – Adults, children >40 kg: 500-mg tablet q8h or 875 mg every 12 h.
• Otitis media, sinusitis, lower respiratory tract infections, severe infections
 – Children <40 kg: 45 mg/kg/d in divided doses q12h or 40 mg/kg/d q8h.
• Less severe infections
 – Children <40 kg: 25 mg/kg/d in divided doses q12h or 20 mg/kg/d q8h.

Adjustment of dosage
- Kidney disease: creatinine clearance 10–30 mL/min: 250 or 500 mg q12h; creatinine clearance <10 mL/min: 250 or 500 mg q24h.
- Liver disease: None.
- Elderly: None.
- Pediatric: Contraindicated for children <2 years.

Food: No restrictions.

Pregnancy: Category B.

Lactation: Appears in breast milk. Considered compatible by American Academy of Pediatrics.

Contraindications: Hypersensitivity to penicillin or cephalosporins.

Warnings/precautions
- Diarrhea is more common with amoxicillin–clavulanate than with amoxicillin alone.
- Allergic reactions are more likely to occur in patients with the following conditions: asthma, hay fever, allergy to cephalosporins, history of allergy to penicillin. Consider skin testing, with major and minor antigenic components, of penicillin hypersensitivity patients with β-lactamase allergy who require amoxicillin for life-threatening infections, to assess the possibility of a hypersensitivity reaction. If patient is give the drug parenterally, observe for at least 20 min for possible anaphylactic reaction. Negative history of penicillin hypersensitivity does not prelude a patient from reacting to the drug. Administer at least 1 hour before a bacteriostatic agent is given (eg, tetracycline, erythromycin, chloramphenicol).
- For IV infusion: Make sure no other drugs are added or mixed into the infusing solution. Do not use solution containing precipitates or foreign matter.

Advice to patient
- If you are receiving an oral contraceptive, use an alternative method of birth control.
- If you are allergic to a penicillin or cephalopsporin, carry an identification card with this information.

Adverse reactions
- Common: Diarrhea.

- Serious: Stevens–Johnson syndrome, anaphylaxis, angioedema, laryngospasm, pseudomembraneous colitis.

Clinically important drug interactions
- Drugs that increase effects/toxicity of penicillins: probenecid.
- Drugs that decrease effects/toxicity of penicillins: antacids, tetracyclines.
- Penicillins increase effects of following drugs: oral anticoagulants, heparin.
- Penicillins decrease effects of following drugs: oral contraceptives.

Parameters to monitor
- Signs and symptoms of anaphylactic shock.
- Signs and symptoms of allergic reaction.
- Signs and symptoms of pseudomembranous colitis.
- Patient's intake/output of fluid.
- Renal, hepatic, and hematologic status for patients on high-dose prolonged therapy.

Editorial comments
- Amoxicillin–clavulanate is used for complicated or chronic sinusitis and otitis media because its spectrum includes *S. pneumoniae*, *H. influenzae*, *B. catarrhalis*, and anaerobic organisms.
- It is also appropriate for GI infections (eg, diverticulitis), exacerbations of COPD, aspiration pneumonia, head and neck infections. It is the drug of choice for bite-related infections, as it provides coverage for oral anaerobes, streptococci, and Pasteurella multocida.

Amphotericin B

Brand names: Abelcet, Ambisome.
Class of drug: Systemic and topic antifungal agent.
Mechanism of action: Increases fungal cell membrane permeability causing cell death.

Indications/dosage/route: IV, intrathecal, topical.
• Systemic fungal infections
  – Adults: Initial: IV 0.25 mg/kg q2–6h. Maintenance: IV 0.25–1 mg/kg/d.
  – Infants, children: Initial: IV 0.25 mg/kg/d. Maintenance: IV 0.25–1 mg/kg/d.
• Fungal meningitis
  – Adults: Initial: intrathecal 50 µg. Maintenance: 25 µg q2–3wk.
• Topical fungal infections
  – Adults: Initial: 3% cream 2–4 times per day. Maintenance: 2–4 times per day.

Adjustment of dosage
• Kidney disease: Decrease by 50%.
• Liver disease: No information available.
• Elderly: May be at high risk for toxicity.
• Pediatric: See above.

Duration of therapy: 2 weeks to 3 months.

Pregnancy: Category B.

Lactation: No data available. Best to avoid.

Contraindications: Hypersensitivity to amphotericin B.

Warnings/precautions
• Avoid other nephrotoxic drugs. Avoid rapid IV infusion.
• Use caution in renal disease. Discontinue if BUN increases to >40 mg/dL or serum creatinine rises above 3 mg/dL.

Adverse reactions
• Common: increased liver enzymes, tachycardia, azotemia, hypokalemia, hypotension, chills, fever, nausea, hyperbilirubinemia.
• Serious: **hypokalemia, hypokalemia, nephrotoxicity (renal tubular acidosis, renal failure)**, convulsions, hypersensitivity reaction, anaphylaxis, arrythmia, multiple organ failure, bone marrow depression, cardiac arrest.

Clinically important drug interactions
• Drugs that increase effects/toxicity of amphotericin B: aminoglycosides, cisplatin and other antineoplastic drugs, cyclosporine, corticosteroids, nephrotoxic drugs.

- Amphotericin B increases effects/toxicity of following drugs: digoxin, skeletal muscle relaxants (nondepolarizing, succinyl-choline), thiazide diuretics, AZT.

Parameters to monitor

- Serum electrolytes, especially magnesium and potassium.
- Creatinine clearance (determine weekly), serum creatinine, BUN.
- Liver enzymes (weekly).
- Urine output.
- CBC with differential and platelets.

Editorial comments

- Currently two forms of amphotericin B are available on the market. While Ambisome is incorporated into a liposomal drug delivery system, Abelcet is combined with phospholipid. It appears that the liposomal product may have fewer adverse reactions. Fevers and chills have been reported to occur 1–2 hours after beginning intravenous infusion with Abelcet.
- Parenteral amphotericin B is to be used for severe lifethreatening infections.

Ampicillin

Brand names: Totacillin, Omnipen.

Class of drug: Antibiotic, penicillin family plus β-lactamase inhibitor.

Mechanism of action: Inhibits bacterial cell wall synthesis.

Susceptible organisms *in vivo*: *Streptococcus pneumoniae*, beta-hemolytic streptococci, *Enterococcus faecalis*, viridans streptococci, *Escherichia coli*, *Hemophilus influenzae*, *Neisseria gonorrhoeae*, *Proteus mirabilis*, *Salmonella* (often resistant), *Shigella* (often resistant), *Listeria monocytogenes*, *Neisseria meningitidis*.

Indications/dosage/route: Oral, IV, IM.

- Respiratory tract and soft tissue infections
  - Children >20 kg: PO 250 mg q6h.

- Children <20 kg: PO 50 mg/kg/d in divided doses q6–8h.
- Children >40 kg: IV, IM 250–500 mg q6h.
- Children <40 kg: IV, IM 25–50 mg/kg/d in divided doses q6–8h.
- Bacterial meningitis (to cover for *Listeria monocytogenes* in neonates, adults >50 years, and immunocompromised individuals)
  - Adults and children: IV 150–200 mg/kg/d in divided doses, then IM q3–4h.
- Prophylaxis bacterial endocarditis, dental, oral, or upper respiratory tract procedures (amoxicillin PO preferred unless NPO)
  - Patients at moderate risk: *Adults*: IM, IV, 2 gm 30 minutes prior to procedure *Children*: 50 mg/kg 30 minutes prior to procedure.
  - Patients at high risk: *Adults*: IM, IV, 2 gm ampicillin plus gentamicin, 1.5 mg/kg 30 minutes before procedure followed in 6 hours by ampicillin, 1 gm IM or IV, or ampicillin, 1 gm PO *Children*: IM, IV ampicillin 50 mg/kg plus gentamicin 1.5 mg/kg, 30 min prior to procedure, followed in 6 hours by ampicillin 25 mg/kg IM or IV or amoxicillin 25 mg/kg PO.
- Septicemia
  - Adults, children: IV 150–200 mg/kg/d first 3 days, then IM q3–4h.
- GI and GU infections other than *N. gonorrhoeae*
  - Adults, children >20 kg: PO 500 mg q6h.
  - Children <20 kg: 100 mg/kg/d q6h.
- *N. gonorrhoeae* infections (non-penicillinase-producing): PO single dose of 3.5 g together with probenecid 1 g
  - Adults, children >40 kg: IV or IM 500 mg q6h.
  - Children <40 kg: 50 mg/kg/d IV or IM in divided doses q6–8h.
- Urethritis in males caused by N. *gonorrhoeae*
  - Males >40 kg: IV or IM 1 g at an interval of 8–12 hours; repeat if necessary.

Adjustment of dosage

- Kidney disease: creatinine clearance <10 mL/min: increase dosing interval to 12 h.

• Liver disease: None.
• Elderly: None.
• Pediatric: Contraindicated for children <2 years.

Food: Take on empty stomach, 1 hour before or 2 hours after eating.

Pregnancy: Category B.

Lactation: Appears in breast milk. Use with caution.

Contraindications: Hypersensitivity to penicillin or cephalosporins.

Warnings/precautions

• Use with caution in patients with mononucleosis.
• Allergic reactions are more likely to occur in patients with the following conditions: asthma, hay fever, allergy to cephalosporins, history of allergy to penicillin. Consider skin testing, with major and minor antigenic components, of penicillin hypersensitivity in such patients to assess the possibility of a hypersensitivity reaction. If patient is given drug parenterally, observe for at least 20 minutes for possible anaphylactic reaction.
• Negative history of penicillin hypersensitivity does not prelude a patient from reacting to the drug.
• Administer at least 1 hour before a bacteriostatic agent is given (eg, tetracycline, erythromycin, chloramphenicol).
• For IV infusion: Make sure no other drugs are added or mixed into the infusing solution. Do not use solution containing precipitates or foreign matter.

Advice to patient

• If you are receiving an oral contraceptive, use an alternative method of birth control.
• If you are allergic to a penicillin or cephalosporin, carry an identification card with this information.

Adverse reactions

• Common: None.
• Serious: Stevens–Johnson syndrome, anaphylaxis, angioedema, laryngospasm, pseudomembraneous colitis, seizures (high dose).

Clinically important drug interactions

• Drug that increases effects/toxicity of penicillins: probenecid.
• Drugs that decrease effects/toxicity of penicillins: antacids, tetracyclines.

- Penicillins increase effects of following drugs: oral anticoagulants, heparin.
- Penicillins decrease effects of following drugs: oral contraceptives.

Parameters to monitor

- Signs and symptoms of anaphylactic shock.
- Signs and symptoms of allergic reaction.
- Signs and symptoms of pseudomembranous colitis.
- Patient's intake/output of fluid.
- Signs of bleeding, particularly in patients on high-dose therapy.
- Monitor bleeding time in these patients.
- Renal, hepatic, and hematologic status for patients on high-dose prolonged therapy.

Editorial comments

- Ampicillin is added empirically for acute meningitis to cover for *Listeria* when the organism is a possible pathogen (neonate, adults >50 years, and immunocompromised patients).
- Ampicillin is also used with an aminoglycoside to treat subacute bacterial endocarditis before the blood culture results are known. This regimen covers the viridans streptococci, *Enterococcus faecalis*, and the HACEK organisms.
- Ampicillin is no longer adequate monotherapy for the treatment of UTI since *E. coli* frequently is resistant.
- Surgeons frequently use ampicillin, gentamicin, and metronidazole for surgical intraabdominal infections. Ampicillin in this regimen covers *Enterococcus faecalis*, a frequent pathogen.

Ampicillin/Sulbactam

Brand name: Unasyn.
Class of drug: Antibiotic, penicillin family plus β-lactamase inhibitor.
Mechanism of action: Inhibits bacterial cell wall synthesis.
Susceptible organisms *in vivo*: See *ampicillin*. The addition of sulbactam inhibits the penicillinase of anaeorbes (oral anaeorbes, *Bacteroides fragilis*), MSSA, *Hemophilus influenzae*, Branhamella catarrhalis, *Escherichia coli*.

Indications/dosage/route: IM, IV.
- Adults, children >12 years: 1.5 g (1 g ampicillin, 0.5 g sulbactam) q6–8h.
- Children (3 months to 12 years): 100–200 mg ampicillin/kg/d, plus 50–100 mg sulbactam/kg/day, divided every 8 h. Maximum: 8 g ampicillin/d.

Adjustment of dosage
- Kidney disease: creatinine clearance: 15–30 mL/min, dose every 12 hours; creatinine clearance: 5–14 mL/min, dose every 24 hours.
- Liver disease: None.
- Elderly: None.
- Pediatric: See above.

Food: Not applicable.
Pregnancy: Category B.
Lactation: Appears in breast milk. Considered compatible by American Academy of Pediatrics.
Contraindications: Hypersensitivity to penicillin or cephalosporins, IV injections.

Editorial comments
- This antibiotic is used in mixed infections when *Pseudomonas aeruginosa* is not a pathogen.
- As a single agent, it is effective in animal and human bites, complicated otitis media, sinusitis, oral and neck infections, and community-acquired pneumonia when aspiration is suspected. All these infections are caused mainly by oral flora.
- With the addition of an aminoglycoside, it is very appropriate for the treatment of pelvic inflammatory disease and other gynecologic infections.
- For additional information, see *ampicillin*, p. 53.

Amrinone

Brand name: Inocor.
Class of drug: Phosphodiesterase inhibitor, inotropic agent.
Mechanism of action: Increases myocardial cyclic AMP in cardiac tissue by phosphodiesterase inhibition.

Indications/dosage/route: IV only.
- CHF low cardiac output (sepsis), poor responders to digitalis
  – Adults: Initial: 0.75 mg/kg bolus over 2–3 min. Maintenance:
    5–10 µg/kg/min. Maximum: 10 mg/kg/d.

Adjustment of dosage
- Kidney disease: Reduce dose by 50–75% in renal failure.
- Liver disease: None
- Elderly: Reduce dose relative to renal function.
- Pediatric: Safety and efficacy have not been established.

Onset of Action	Peak Effect	Duration
2–5 min	10 min	30 min–2h, depending on dose

Pregnancy: Category C.
Lactation: No data available. Best to avoid.
Contraindications: Hypersensitivity, severe pulmonary or aortic valvular disease, acute MI.

Warnings/precautions
- Use with caution in patients with the following conditions: atrial fibrillation or flutter, hypertrophic obstructive cardiomyopathy.
- Reduce dose as cardiac function improves.
- Decreased efficacy (tachphylaxis) may occur during first few days of treatment.
- Monitor for allergic reaction to preservative (sodium metabisulfite).
- Correct hypokalemia before instituting therapy with this drug.
- For patients receiving amrinone plus diuretic, make sure patient is sufficiently hydrated so there will be sufficient cardiac filling pressure.

Adverse reactions
- Common: fever, nausea.
- Serious: thrombocytopenia, hypersensitivity reactions, hypercalcemia, hepatotoxicity.

Clinically important drug interactions
- Do not mix with furosemide; precipitate forms.
- Amrinone increases effects/toxicity of disopyramide.

Parameters to monitor

- Cardiac output, stroke volume, pulmonary capillary wedge pressure, potassium, other electrolytes.
- Signs and symptoms of thrombocytopenia. Discontinue this medication if platelet count falls below 100,000/mm^3.
- Signs and symptoms of hepatotoxicity.
- Cardiac function: cardiac output static volume, pulmonary capillary pressure.
- Heart rate and BP continuously during infusion. Reduce rate if there is a significant fall in BP or if arrhythmias occur.
- Serum potassium levels. Correct if hypokalemia is observed.
- Possible tachyphylaxis to antiarrhythmic action. This generally occurs within 72 hours of beginning drug therapy.

Editorial comments

- Amrinone is generally prescribed for patients with CHF who have not responded satisfactorily to diuretics, vasodilators, or cardiac glycosides.
- Amrinone and the phosphodiesterase inhibitors in general have been double-edged swords. While they enhance contractility and lower vascular resistance, they also have been associated with sudden death likely due to increasing metabolic demand. These effects can occur even after infusion has ceased.
- This drug is not listed in the *Physician's Desk Reference*, 54th edition, 2000.

Amyl Nitrite

Class of drug: Antianginal, nitrate vasodilator, antidote to cyanide poisoning.

Mechanism of action: As antianginal agent, reduces peripheral resistance (arterial and venous) by vasodilation; decreases left ventricular pressure. As antidote for cyanide poisoning, produces methemoglobin which binds and inactivates cyanide.

Indications/dosage/route: Inhalation only.
• Angina pectoris
  – Adults: 2–6 inhalations. Repeat in 3–5 minutes if necessary.
• Antidote for cyanide poisoning
  – Adults: Inhalation for 15–30 seconds q 1 minute until IV sodium nitrite (10 ml of 3% solution) is administered over 2.5–5 minutes. This is followed immediately by 50 ml of 25% sodium thiosulfate. If signs of poisoning reappear, administer 50% of initial dose of sodium nitrite and sodium thiosufate.

Adjustment of dosage
• Kidney disease: None.
• Liver disease: None.
• Elderly: Lower doses may be required.
• Pediatric: Safety and efficacy have not been established in children.

Onset of Action	Peak Effect	Duration
0.5 min	—	3–5 min

Food: Not applicable.
Pregnancy: Category C.
Lactation: No data available. Best to avoid.
Contraindications: Hypersensitivity to nitrates or nitrites, very low blood pressure, shock, acute MI with low ventricular filling pressure.
Advice to patient: Advise patient that if pain is not relieved after 3 doses, call paramedics or to emergency room immediately.
Editorial comments
• This drug is highly flammable. Keep away from flame and extinguish cigarettes before using.
• This drug is not listed in the *Physician's Desk Reference*, 54th edition, 2000.
• For additional information, see *isosorbide dinitrate*, p. 473.

Atenolol

Brand name: Tenormin.
Class of drug: β-Adrenergic receptor blocker.
Mechanism of action: Competitive blocker of β-adrenergic receptors in heart and blood vessels.
Indications/dosage/route: Oral, IV.
• Hypertension
  – Initial: PO 50 mg/d. Maximum: 100 mg/d.
• Angina
  – Initial: PO 50 mg/d. Maintenance: 100–200 mg/d.
• Ventricular arrhythmias
  – PO 50–100 mg/d.
• Acute MI
  – Initial: IV 5 mg over 5 min, followed by second 5-mg dose 10 min later; then 50-mg tablet 10 min after last IV dose, then another 50-mg dose 12 hours later, then 100 mg/d or 50 mg b.i.d. for 6–9 days.
Adjustment of dosage
• Kidney disease: creatinine clearance 15–35 mL/min: 50 mg/d; creatinine clearance <15 mL/min : 25 mg/d.
• Liver disease: None.
• Elderly: None.
• Pediatric: Safety and efficacy have not been established in children.
Food: No restriction.
Pregnancy: Category B.
Lactation: Appears in breast milk. Considered compatible by the American Academy of Pediatrics. Observe infant for hypotension, bradycardia, cyanosis.
Contraindications: Cardiogenic shock, asthma, CHF unless it is secondary to tachyarrhythmia treated with a β blocker, sinus bradycardia and AV block greater than first degree, severe COPD.

Warnings/precautions
- Use with caution in patients with the following conditions: diabetes, kidney disease, liver disease, COPD, peripheral vascular disease.
- Do not stop drug abruptly as this may precipitate arrhythmias, angina, MI or cause rebound hypertension. If necessary to discontinue, taper as follows: Reduce dose by 25–50% and reassess after 1–2 weeks. If status is unchanged, reduce by another 50% and reassess after 1–2 weeks.
- Drug may mask the symptoms of hyperthyroidism, mainly tachycardia.
- Drug may exacerbate symptoms of arterial insufficiency in patients with peripheral or mesenteric vascular disease.

Advice to patient
- Avoid driving and other activities requiring mental alertness or that are potentially dangerous until response to drug is known.
- Change position slowly, in particular from recumbent to upright, to minimize orthostatic hypotension. Sit at the edge of the bed for several minutes before standing, and lie down if feeling faint or dizzy. Avoid hot showers or baths and standing for long periods. Male patients should sit on the toilet while urinating rather than standing.
- Dress warmly in winter and avoid prolonged exposure to cold as drug may cause increased sensitivity to cold.
- Avoid drinks that contain xanthines (caffeine, theophylline, theobromine) including colas, tea, and cocoa because they may counteract effect of drug.
- Restrict dietary sodium to avoid volume expansion.
- Drug may blunt response to usual rise in BP and chest pain under stressful conditions such as vigorous exercise and fever.

Adverse reactions
- Common: fatigue, headache, impotence.
- Serious: symptomatic bradycardia, CHF, pulmonary edema.

Clinically important drug interactions
- Drugs that increase effects/toxicity of β blockers: reserpine, bretylium, calcium channel blockers.

- Drugs that decrease effects/toxicity of β blockers: aluminum salts, calcium salts, cholestyramine, barbiturates, NSAIDs, rifampin.

Parameters to monitor

- Liver enzymes, serum BUN and creatinine, CBC with differential and platelets.

- Pulse rate near end of dosing interval or before the next dose is taken. A reasonable target is 60–80 bpm for resting apical ventricular rate. If severe bradycardia develops, consider treatment with glucagon, isoproterenol, IV atropine (1–3 mg in divided doses). If hypotension occurs despite correction of bradycardia, administer vasopressor (norephinephrine, dopamine, or dobutamine).

- Symptoms of CHF. Digitalize patient and administer a diuretic or glucagon.

- Efficacy of treatment: decreased BP, decreased number and severity of anginal attacks, improvement in exercise tolerance. Confirm control of arrhythmias by ECG, apical pulse, BP, circulation in extremities, and respiration. Monitor closely when changing dose.

- CNS effects. If patient experiences mental depression reduce dosage by 50%. The elderly are particularly sensitive to adverse CNS effects.

- Signs of bronchospasm. Stop therapy and administer large doses of β-adrenergic bronchodilator, eg, albuterol, terbutaline, or aminophylline.

- Signs of cold extremities. If severe, stop drug. Consider β blocker with sympathomimetic property.

Editorial comments

- Stopping a β blocker before surgery is controversial. Some advocate discontinuing the drug 48 hours before surgery; others recommend withdrawal for a considerably longer time. Notify anesthesiologist that patient has been on β blocker.

- β blockers are drugs of first choice for hypertension, particularly in patients with the following conditions: previous MI, ischemic heart disease, aneurysm, atrioventricular arrhythmias, migraine. These drugs are also first choice for chronic stable angina, used in conjunction with nitroglycerin.

- Following a MI, patients should be administered a β blocker.

• β blockers are considered to be first-line drugs for prophylaxis of migraine headache in patients who have two or more attacks per month.

Atorvastatin

Brand name: Lipitor.
Class of drug: Antilipidemic agent.
Mechanism of action: Inhibits HMG-CoA reductase. Reduces total LDL, cholesterol, serum triglyceride levels. There is little if any effect on serum HDL levels.
Indications/dosage/route: Oral only.
• Hyperlipidemia
 – Adults: Initial: 10 mg/d. Maintenance: 10–80 mg/d.
• Homozygous familial hypercholesterolemia
 – Adults: 10–80 mg/d.
Adjustment of dosage
• Kidney disease: None.
• Liver disease: None.
• Elderly: None.
• Pediatric: Limited data available.
Food: No restriction.
Pregnancy: Category X—contraindicated.
Lactation: Appears in breast milk. Contraindicated.
Contraindications: Hypersensitivity to statins, active liver disease or unexplained persistent elevations of serum transaminase, pregnancy, lactation.
Warnings/precautions
• Use with caution in patients with the following conditions: renal insufficiency, history of liver disease, alcohol abusers.
• Discontinue if drug-induced myopathy develops. This is characterized by myalgia, creatinine kinase levels >10x normal.

May cause acute renal failure from rhabdomyolysis. May occur more frequently when drug is combined with gemfibrozil or niacin.

- Discontinue drug if patient experiences severe trauma, surgery, or serious illness.

Advice to patient

- Avoid alcohol.
- Use of OTC medications only with approval from treating physician.
- Exercise regularly, reduce fat and alcohol intake, and stop smoking.

Adverse reactions

- Common: None.
- Serious: myopathy, rhabdomyolysis, neuropathy, cranial nerve abnormalities, hypersensitivity reactions, pancreatitis, hepatic injury including hepatic necrosis and cirrhosis, lens opacities.

Clinically important drug interactions

- Drugs that increase effects/toxicity of HMG-CoA reductase inhibitors: gemfibrozil, clofibrate, erythromycin, cyclosporin, niacin, clarithromycin, itraconazole, protease inhibitors.
- HMG-CoA reductase inhibitors increase effects/toxicity of oral anticoagulants.

Parameters to monitor

- Total cholesterol, LDL and HDL cholesterol, triglycerides. Values should be obtained prior to and periodically after treatment begins to ascertain drug efficacy.
- Serum BUN and creatinine.
- Monitor liver enzymes before beginning therapy, at 3, 6, and 12 months thereafter, and semiannually afterward.
- Signs and symptoms of myopathy: unexplained skeletal muscle pain, muscle tenderness or weakness particularly when accompanied by fever or fatigue. Check creatinine kinase levels. If these are markedly elevated or patient is symptomatic, discontinue drug.

- Discontinue drug if transaminase levels exceed three times normal values. It may be advisable to take a liver biopsy if transaminase elevation persists after drug is discontinued.
- Patient's ophthalmic state should be evaluated once a year following treatment. If lens opacity occurs, consider discontinuing drug.

Editorial comments: Current literature suggests that the most effective reduction of total and LDL cholesterol occurs with a combination of exercise, weight reduction, low-fat diet, and lipid-lowering agents.

Atracurium

Brand name: Tacrium Injection.
Class of drug: Nondepolarizing neuromuscular blocker.
Mechanism of action: Blocks nicotinic acetylcholine receptors at neuromuscular junction resulting in skeletal muscle relaxation and paralysis.
Indications/dosage/route: IV only.
- Intubation and maintenance of neuromuscular blockade
  – Adults, children >2 years: Initial: IV bolus 0.4–0.5 mg/kg. Maintenance: 0.08–0.1 mg/kg q12–25min.
- Muscle relaxation during anesthesia
  – Adults IV bolus: 0.25–0.35 mg/kg.
  – Adults IV infusion: 9–10 µg/kg.

Adjustment of dosage: None.
Food: Not applicable.
Pregnancy: Category C.
Lactation: Best to avoid.
Contraindications: Hypersensitivity to acracurium and chemically related drugs.
Editorial comments
- This drug is not listed in *Physician's Desk Reference*, 54th edition, 2000.
- For additional information, see *rocuronium*, p. 824.

Atropine

Brand names: Atropisol, Isopto, Atropine.
Class of drug: Cholinergic blocking agent.
Mechanism of action: Blocks acetylcholine effects at muscarinic receptors throughout the body.
Indications/dosage/route: IV, IM, SC, oral, topical (ophthalmic).

- Anticholinergic or antispasmodic
  - Adults: PO, 0.3–1.2 mg q 4–6 hr.
  - Children >41 kg: same as adult.
  - Children 29.5–41 kg: PO 0.4 mg q4–6h.
  - Children 8.2–29.5 kg: PO 0.3 mg q4–6h.
  - Children 7.4–8.1 kg: PO 0.15 mg q4–6h.
  - Children 3.2–7.3 kg: PO 0.1 mg q4–6h.
- Prophylaxis of respiratory tract secretions and excess salivation during anesthesia
  - Adults: IM, IV SC 0.4–0.6 mg 30–60 min before surgery. Repeat doses as needed q4–6h.
  - Children <5 kg: IM, IV, SC 0.02 mg/kg 30–60 minutes before surgery. Repeat doses as needed q4–6h.
  - Children >5 kg: IM, IV, SC 0.01–0.02 mg/kg, 30–60 minutes before surgery. Repeat doses as needed q4–6h.
- Parkinsonism
  - Adults: PO 0.1–025 mg q.i.d.
- Reversal of curariform blockade
  - Adults: IV 0.5–1.2 mg plus 0.5–2 mg neostigmine methylsulfate.
- Toxicity from cholinesterase inhibitor
  - Adults: IV 2–4 mg, then 2 mg repeated q5–10min until muscarinic symptoms disappear.
  - Children: IM, IV 1 mg, then 0.5–2 mg q5–10min until muscarinic symptoms disappear.
- Treatment of mushroom poisoning due to muscarine
  - Adults: IM, IV 1–2 mg every hour until respiratory effects decrease.
- Treatment of organophosphate poisoning

– Adults: IM, IV 1–2 mg, then repeat in 10–20 minutes.
• Arrhythmias
  – Children: IV 0.01–0.03 mg/kg.
• Uveitis
  – Adults: 1–2 drops in each eye.
  – Children: 1–2 drops in each eye up to t.i.d.
• Refraction
  – Adults: 1–2 drops of the 1% solution in each eye 1 hour before refraction.
  – Children: 1–2 drops of the 0.5% solution in each eye 1–3 hours before refraction.

Adjustment of dosage
• Kidney disease: None.
• Liver disease: None.
• Elderly: Use with caution; higher incidence of side effects.
• Pediatric: See above.

	Onset of Action	Peak Effect	Duration
Mydriasis	Rapid	30–40 min	12 d
PO use	—	—	4–6 h

Pregnancy: Category C.
Lactation: Limited data available. Potentially toxic to infant. Considered compatible by the American Academy of Pediatrics.
Contraindications: Myasthenia gravis, narrow-angle glaucoma, GI obstruction, megacolon, active ulcerative colitis, obstructive uropathy, hypersensitivity to atropine-type compounds (belladonna alkaloids).
Warnings/precautions
• Use with caution in patients with the following conditions: GI infections, chronic biliary disease, CHF, arrhythmias, pulmonary disease, benign prostatic hypertrophy, hyperthyroidism, coronary artery disease, hypertension, seizures, psychosis, spastic paralysis.
• Anticholinergic psychosis can occur in sensitive individuals.

- Elderly may react with agitation and excitement even to small doses of anticholinergic drugs.
- Ophthalmic atropine produces weaker effects in dark-eyed individuals whereas the following types of patients are highly sensitive to the drug: infants and children with Down syndrome, spastic paralysis, brain damage, blond blue-eyed individuals.
- More than half of deaths from ophthalmic atropine in infants have been the result of systemic absorption of the drug.

Advice to patient

- Take medication exactly as directed. If dose is missed, do not double subsequent dose when it is remembered.
- Avoid driving and other activities requiring mental alertness or that are potentially dangerous until response to drug is known.
- Use caution when exercising in hot weather as this might cause heat prostration.
- Avoid alcohol and other CNS depressants such as opiate analgesics and sedatives (eg, diazepam) when taking this drug.
- If mouth is dry, rinse with warm water frequently, chew sugarless gum, suck on an ice cube, or use artificial saliva. Carry out meticulous oral hygiene (floss teeth daily).
- Visual acuity will be impaired for several days after pharmacologic treatment. Protect eyes from strong light by wearing dark glasses.

Adverse reactions

- Common: Dry mouth, blurred vision (decreased accommodation), drowsiness, tachycardia, urinary hesitancy, dry skin, constipation.
- Serious: Disorientation, hallucinations, acute narrow-angle glaucoma, orthostatic hypotension, arrhythmia.

Clinically important drug interactions

- Drugs that increase effects/toxicity of systemic anticholinergics: phenothiazines, amantadine, other antipsychotic agentics, thiazide diuretics, tricyclic antidepressants, MAO inhibitors, quinidine, procainamide.
- Drugs that increase effects/toxicity of ophthalmic anticholinergics: corticosteroids, haloperidol.

- Drugs that decrease effect /toxicity of systemic anticholinergics: antacids, cholinergic ents.

Parameters to monitor
- Signs and symptoms of severe toxicity: tachycardia, supraventricular arrythmias, delirium, seizures, agitation, hyperthermia. Use physostigmine (Eserine) as antidote only for life-threatening toxicity. Discontinue physostigmine if patient experiences dizziness, palpitations, rapid pulse.
- Intake of fluids and urinary and other fluid output. Increase fluid intake if inadequate. Signs of urinary retention: pelvic pain and distention, decreased urine output. This is particularly important in elderly with benign prostatic hypertrophy. Determine whether there is a need for catherization.
- Opthalmic status: Intraocular pressure before and during treatment, accommodation, pupillary response to light, visual acuity (blurred vision). Discontinue administration if the following occur: eye pain, conjunctivitis.

Editorial comments
- This drug is not listed in the *Physician's Desk Reference*, 54th edition, 2000.

Auranofin

Brand name: Ridaira.
Class of drug: Antirheumatic agent, gold compound.
Mechanism of action: Inhibits phagocytosis, stabilizes lysosomal membranes, decreases rheumatoid factor levels.
Indications/dosage/route: Oral only.
- Rheumatoid arthritis or psoriatric a ritis that does not respond to other agents
  - Adults: Initial: 6 mg/d as single or divided doses; increase to 9 mg/d if needed (maximum dose).
  - Children >6 years: Initial: 0.1 mg/kg/d; increase to 0.10 mg/kg/d if needed (maximum dose).

Adjustment of dosage
- Kidney disease: creatinine clearance 50–80 mL/min: reduce dose by 50%; creatinine clearance less than 50 mL/min: do not use.
- Liver disease: No adjustment necessary.
- Pediatric: Not recommended for children <6 years.

Onset of Action
≤3 mo

Food: Take shortly after eating. Take with milk or full glass of water.

Pregnancy: Category C.

Lactation: Gold salts appear in breast milk. Potentially toxic to infant. Related compounds considered compatible with breast-feeding by the American Academy of Pediatrics.

Contraindications: History of gold-associated disorders such as necrotizing enterocolitis, exfoliative dermatitis, pulmonary fibrosis, bone marrow insufficiency, drugs known to cause blood dyscrasias (antimalarials, pyrazolones, immunosuppressants).

Warnings/precautions
- Use with caution in patients with the following conditions: hepatic, renal, inflammatory bowel disease.
- Advise patient which drugs to avoid that cause blood dyscrasias.
- In general, administer along with salicylates or NSAIDs for first few weeks or months of therapy.
- Diabetic patients or those with CHF must be well controlled before beginning therapy with this drug.

Advice to patient: Use sunscreen and protective clothing to avoid photosensitivity reactions.
- A blue-gray coloration (chrysiasis) may occur on exposed surfaces and mucous membranes. Treat with Lugol's solution (strong iodine solution).

Adverse reactions
- Common: diarrhea (47%), abdominal cramping (14%), nausea, vomiting, rash (24%), pruritus (17%), stomatitis.

- Serious: seizures, hemorrhagic colitis, acute renal failure, nephrotic syndrome, glomerulonephritis, pulmonary fibrosis, eosinophilic pneumonia, thrombocytopenia, bone marrow depression, exfoliative dermatitis, hepatotoxicity, peripheral neuropathy.

Clinically important drug interactions
- Drugs that increase effects/toxicity of auranofin: penicillamine, immunosuppressants, cytotoxic drugs.

Parameters to monitor
- Signs and symptoms of nititoid reactions following IV injection: dizziness, sweating, fainting, flushing, nausea, vomiting. Maintain patient in recumbent position for about 15 minutes after the injection. This reaction is transient and administration should not be discontinued.
- Signs and symptoms of bone marrow depression.
- Urinalysis for presence of proteinuria.
- Signs and symptoms of neuropathy.

Editorial comments: This drug is not listed in the *Physician's Desk Reference*, 54th edition, 2000.

Azatadine

Brand names: Rynatan, Trinalin.
Class of drug: H_1 receptor blocker.
Mechanism of action: Antagonizes histamine effects on GI tract, respiratory tract, blood vessels.
Indications/dosage/route: Oral only.
- Allergic rhinitis, relief of nasal congestion.
  – Adults, children >12 years: 1 mg b.i.d.

Adjustment of dosage
- Kidney disease: None.
- Liver disease: None.
- Elderly: Use caution. At higher risk for side effects.
- Pediatric: See above.

Food: No restriction.
Pregnancy: Category C.
Lactation: No data available. Potentially toxic to infant. Avoid breastfeeding.
Contraindications: Hypersensitivity to antihistamines, acute asthma, narrow-angle glaucoma, concurrent use of MAO inhibitor.
Editorial comments
• Usually available in combination with other agents, including pseudoephedrine, phenylephrine, and phenylpropanolamine. Warnings and precautions, side effects, etc, of other ingredients should be kept in mind when prescribing.
• For additional information, see *brompheniramine*, p. 107.

Azathioprine

Brand name: Imuran.
Class of drug: Immunosuppressant, antirheumatic agent.
Mechanism of action: Blocks purine metabolism, inhibits DNA synthesis, inhibits mitosis.
Indications/dosage/route: Oral, IV.
• Immunosuppressant, to prevent renal transplant rejection
  – Initial: IV, PO 3–5 mg/kg/d. Maintenance: IV, PO 1–3 mg/kg/d.
• Severe rheumatoid arthritis not responsive to other drugs
  – Initial: PO 1 mg/kg/d. Maintenance: PO 2–5 mg/kg/d.
Adjustment of dosage
• Kidney disease: creatinine clearance 10–50 mL/min: reduce dose by 25%; creatinine clearance <10 mL/min: reduce dose by 50%.
• Liver disease: None.
• Elderly: None.
• Pediatric: Safety and efficacy have not been established in children.

Onset of Action
≤12 wk

There may be a prolonged delay prior to onset of antiinflammatory action. Do not discontinue unless no effect occurs after 3 months of use for rheumatoid arthritis.

Food: No restriction.

Pregnancy: Category D. Avoid pregnancy for 4 months after stopping drug.

Lactation: No data available. Potentially toxic to fetus. Avoid breastfeeding.

Contraindications: Hypersensitivity to azathioprine, pregnancy.

Warnings/precautions

• Use with caution in patients with the following conditions: liver and renal disease.

• With chronic use there is an increased risk of neoplasms, opportunistic infections.

• May cause severe bone marrow depression.

• Patients who have previously received alkylating agents such as cyclophosphamide, chlorambucil, and melphalan may be at increased risk for carcinogenesis from azathioprine.

Advice to patient

• Use two forms of birth control including hormonal and barrier methods.

• Male patients should use condoms if engaging in sexual intercourse while using this medication.

• Avoid crowds as well as persons who may have a contagious disease.

• Receive vaccinations (particularly live attenuated viruses) only with permission from treating physician.

• Avoid the use of OTC medications without first informing the treating physician.

Adverse reactions

• Common: nausea, vomiting.

- Serious: **bone marrow depression (thrombocytopenia, leukopenia, anemia)**, pancreatitis hepatotoxicity, systemic infections, hypotension, retinopathy, hypersensitivity reactions.

Clinically important drug interactions

- Drugs that increase effects/toxicity of azathioprine: allopurinol, methotrexate, ACE inhibitors, other immunosuppressants, alkylating agents.
- Azathioprine decreases effects/toxicity of following drugs: anticoagulants, corticosteroids, nondepolarizing neuromuscular blockers.

Parameters to monitor

- Frequent monitoring of CBC with differential and platelet count, liver enzymes.
- Signs and symptoms of hepatotoxicity.
- Efficacy in rheumatoid arthritis: increased range of motion, decreased swelling and joint pain.
- Nausea and vomiting. If necessary, administer antiemetic drug.
- Liver enzymes.

Editorial comments

- Because of risk of severe bone marrow depression, frequent monitoring of complete blood counts and platelet counts are recommended. It is suggested that these should be performed weekly for the first month, twice monthly for the second and third months, and then monthly thereafter. Additionally they should be monitored if dosage changes are made. Discontinuation of the drug is recommended if there is rapid development of leukopenia, thrombocytopenia, or other signs of bone marrow depression.
- Azathioprine is used as a steroid-sparing agent in a variety of autoimmune disorders including inflammatory bowel disease. The active metabolite of azathioprine is 6-mercaptopurine. Randomized, double blind placebo controlled trials have demonstrated efficacy of 6-mercaptopurine and azathioprine in active or quiescent Crohn's disease. Patients in these trials were often able to taper prednisone doses to 5 mg/d or less. Doses for

6-mercpatopurine were generally 1.5 mg/kg/d and for azathioprine 2.5 mg/kg/d.

• Cytotoxic drug. Use latex gloves and safety glasses when handling parenteral form of this medication. Avoid contact with skin and inhalation. If possible prepare in biologic hood.

Azithromycin

Brand name: Zithromax.
Class of drug: Antibiotic, macrolide.
Mechanism of action: Inhibits RNA-dependent protein synthesis at the level of the 50S ribosome.
Susceptible organisms *in vivo*: Like erythromycin but less active against gram-positive bacteria and more active against gram-negative bacteria. Better against *Hemophilus influenzae* and *Moraxella catarrhalis.* Also useful against *Mycobacterium avium-intracellulare* and *Helicobacter pylori.*
Indications/dosage/route: Oral, IV.

• Community-acquired pneumonia
  – Adults: IV 500 mg as single daily dose, at least 2 days. Follow by oral dosing 500 mg/d, 7–10 days.
• Acute pelvic inflammatory disease
  – IV 500 mg as single daily dose, 1 or 2 days. Follow by oral dosing 250 mg/d 7 days.
• Mild to moderate acute exacerbation of COPD, community-acquired pneumonia (mild to moderate), pharyngitis/tonsillitis (second-line therapy), uncomplicated skin and skin structure infections
  – Adults: PO 500 mg as single dose on first day, then 250 mg/d, days 2–5.
• Genital ulcer disease (chanchroid), nongonoccocal urethritis and cervicitis
  – Adults: PO 1 g as single dose.
• Urethritis and cervicitis (Neisseria gonorrhoeae)
  – Adults: PO 2 g as single dose. (Note: resistance is a problem.)

- Acute otitis media, community-acquired pneumonia
  - Children: Oral suspension 10 mg/kg as single dose on first day, then 5 mg/kg days 2–5. Maximum: 250 mg/d.
- Pharyngitis/tonsillitis
  - Children >2 years: Oral suspension 12 mg/kg once daily, days 1–5.

Adjustment of dosage
- Kidney disease: None.
- Liver disease: None.
- Elderly: None.
- Pediatric: Safety and efficacy have not been established for children <6 months for treatment of acute otitis media and <2 years for treatment of pharyngitis/tonsillitis.

Food: Should be taken on empty stomach, 1–2 hours after meals.

Pregnancy: Category B.

Lactation: No data available. May appear in breast milk. Best to avoid.

Contraindications: Hypersensitivity to macrolide antibiotics.

Warnings/precautions: Use with caution in patients with hepatic dysfunction.

Adverse reactions
- Common: None.
- Severe: pseudomembranous colitis, ventricular arrhythmias, nephritis, cholestatic jaundice, angioedema.

Clinically important drug interactions
- Drugs that decrease effects/toxicity of macrolides: rifampin, antacids (aluminum, magnesium).
- Macrolides increase effects/toxicity of following drugs: oral anticoagulants, astemizole, benzodiazepines, bromocriptine, buspirone, carbamazepine, cisapride, cyclosporine, digoxin, ergot alkaloids, felodipine, grepafloxacin, statins, pimozide, sparfloxacin, tacrolimus.

Parameters to monitor
- Signs and symptoms of superinfection, in particular pseudomembranous colitis.
- Signs and symptoms of renal toxicity.

- Signs and symptoms of hearing impairment. Patients with kidney or liver disease are at highest risk.

Editorial comments

- Azithromycin has the advantage of improved compliance compared with erythromycin because of better tolerability, daily dosage, and shorter course of therapy.
- Often used as outpatient medication and inpatient for community-acquired pneumonia.
- It may be combined with ceftriaxone or cefuroxime for community-acquired pneumonia.
- Increasing resistance in *Streptococcus* pneumoniae is a problem.
- It is also useful for otitis media, sinusitis, and as single 1-g dose for nongonoccocal urethritis.

Bacampicillin

Brand name: Spectrobid.
Class of drug: Antibiotic, penicillin family.
Mechanism of action: Inhibits bacterial cell wall synthesis.
Susceptible organisms *in vivo*: staphylococci, *Streptococcus pneumoniae*, beta-hemolytic streptococci, *Streptococcus faecalis, Streptococcus viridans, Escherichia coli, Hemophilus influenzae, Neisseria gonorrhoeae, Proteus mirabilis, Salmonella* sp, *Shigella* sp.
Indications/dosage/route: Oral only.
• Severe upper respiratory tract, urinary tract, skin and skin structure infections:
Adults: 800 mg q12h.
Children >25 kg: 50 mg/kg/d, two equal doses.
• Lower respiratory tract infections
Adults: 800 mg q12h.
Children >25 kg: 50 mg/kg/d, two equal doses
• Gonorrhea, acute uncomplicated urogenital infections
Adults: 1.6 g plus 1 g probenecid as single dose.
Adjustment of dosage: None.
Food: No restrictions.
Pregnancy: Category B.
Lactation: Appears in breast milk. Use with caution.
Contraindications: Hypersensitivity to penicillin or cephalosporins.
Editorial comments
• Bacampicillin has no advantage over ampicillin and has a similar spectrum of activity. 1 g of bacampicillin $\cong$ 700 mg of ampicillin.
• For additional information, see *ampicillin*, p. 53.

Baclofen

Brand name: Lioresal.

Class of drug: Skeletal muscle relaxant.

Mechanism of action: Inhibits mono- and polysynaptic reflexes within the spinal cord resulting in decreased spasticity.

Indications/dosage/route: Oral only.

• Spasticity of multiple sclerosis and spinal cord lesion
  – Adults: Initial: 15 mg/d, may increase dose every 3 days by 5–15 mg/d. Maximum: 80 mg/d, q8h.
  – Children 2–7 years: Initial: 10–15 mg/kg/d, may increase dose every 3 days by 5–15 mg/d. Maximum: 40 mg/d.
  – Children >8 years: Initial: 10–15 mg/d, titrate dose as above. Maximum: 80 mg/d.

Adjustment of dosage

• Kidney disease: reduce dose.
• Liver disease: no reduction required.
• Elderly: reduce dose.
• Pediatric: see above.

Onset of Action	Peak Effect
3–4 d	5–10 d

Food: Take with food or milk.

Pregnancy: Category C.

Lactation: Appears in breast milk. Considered compatible by American Academy of Pediatrics.

Contraindications: Hypersensitivity to baclofen.

Warnings/precautions

• Use with caution in patients with the following conditions: seizures, decreased renal function.
• Seizure threshold may be lowered in epileptics.
• Patients requiring spasticity to maintain posture and balance may worsen with treatment.
• Avoid abrupt withdrawal.

Advice to patient

• Avoid alcohol and other CNS depressants such as opiate analgesics and sedatives (eg, diazepam) when taking this drug.

- Change position slowly, in particular from recumbent to upright, minimizing orthostatic hypotension. Sit at the edge of the bed for several minutes before standing, lie down if feeling faint or dizzy. Avoid hot showers or baths and standing for long periods. Male patients with orthostatic hypotension may be safer urinating while seated on the toilet rather than standing.
- Avoid driving and other activities requiring mental alertness or that are potentially dangerous until response to drug is known.
- Do not stop drug abruptly as this may precipitate withdrawal reaction (anxiety, hallucinations, tachycardia, seizures).

Adverse reactions
- Common: slurred speech, dizziness, drowsiness.
- Serious: **psychiatric abnormalities**, confusion, syncope, dyspnea, hallucinations, depression.

Clinically important drug interactions
- Drugs that increase effects/toxicity of balclofen: antihistamines, sedatives, opioids, CNS depressants, alcohol, MAO inhibitors.

Parameters to monitor
- Evaluate patient for orthostasis.
- Monitor for sedation and CNS side effects.
- Signs of hypersensitivity reactions.

Editorial comments: Balclofen appears to also be an effective treatment for refractory hiccups (singultus).
- This drug is listed without details in *Physician's Desk Reference*, 54th edition, 2000.

Beclomethasone

Brand names: Beclovent, Vanceril, Beconase, Vancenase.
Class of drug: Inhalation corticosteroid.
Mechanism of action: Inhibits elaboration of many of the mediators of allergic inflammation, eg, leukotrienes and other products of the arachidonic acid cascade.
Indications/dosage/route: Metered dose inhaler.
- Asthma
  - Adults, children ≥ 12 years: 2–4 inhalations t.i.d. to q.i.d.

– Children 6–12 years: 1–2 inhalations. Maximum: 10 inhalations.
- Severe asthma
  – Adults: Initial: 12–16 inhalations/d, decrease according to response. Maximum: 20 inhalations/d.
- Seasonal or perennial rhinitis
  – Adults, children ≥ 12 years 1 inhalation, each nostril b.i.d. to q.i.d.
  – Children 6–12 years: 1 inhalation, each nostril, t.i.d.

Adjustment of dosage
- Kidney disease: None.
- Liver disease: None.
- Elderly: None.
- Pediatric: Safety and efficacy have not been established in children <6 years.

Pregnancy: Category C.

Lactation: Present in breast milk. Safe to use.

Contraindications: Untreated fungal, bacterial, or viral infections, untreated infections of nasal mucosa, hypersensitiv' to corticosteroids.

Warnings/precautions
- Use with caution in patients with the following c tuberculosis of the respiratory tract (active or quiescent), exposure to measles or chicken pox.
- If a patient is transferred from systemic corticosteroid to inhalation drug, symptoms of steroid withdrawal may result. These include muscle and joint pain, depression. Alternatively, adrenal insufficiency may occur: weakness, fatigue, nausea, anorexia.
- Provide patient with instructions for use of the inhaler or nasal spray and make sure patient completely understands these instructions.
- Provide patient with a list of side effects and note those that require immediate reporting to the physician.
- Patients on long-term inhaled or intranasal corticosteroic may require steroid pulsing during stress, eg, surgery or infection.

Advice to patient

- Rinse mouth and gargle with warm water after each inhalation. This may minimize the development of dry mouth, hoarseness, and oral fungal infection.
- This drug should be inhaled 5 minutes after a previously inhaled bronchodilator, eg, albuterol.
- Do not exceed recommended dosage of the drug. Excessive doses have been associated with adrenal insufficiency.
- Notify physician if worsening symptoms occur.
- Carry a card indicating your condition, drugs you are taking, and need for supplemental steroid in the event of a severe asthmatic attack. Attempt to decrease dose once the desired clinical effect is achieved. Decrease dose gradually every 2–4 weeks. Return to initial starting dose if symptoms recur.
- Stop smoking.
- Do not overuse the inhaler.

Adverse reactions

- Common: nasal irritation, cough, pharyngitis, sneezing attacks.
- Serious: adrenal insufficiency, hypercorticism, urticaria, angioedema, bronchospasm, increased intraocular pressure, cataracts, pharyngeal or esophageal candidiasis.

Clinically important drug interactions: None.

Parameters to monitor

- Signs and symptoms of acute adrenal insufficiency, particularly in response to stress.
- Child growth: Drug may suppress growth.
- Changes in nasal mucosa in patients on long-term drug therapy.
- Signs of localized infection in mouth and pharynx, eg, red membranes with vesicular eruptions. Treat with appropriate antifungal drug, eg, nystatin, or discontinue treatment.
- When switching from systemic inhalation therapy, monitor patient for symptoms of adrenal insufficiency: hypotension, weight loss, muscular and joint pain. If these occur, the dose of systemic steroid should be increased followed by slower withdrawal. It may require up to 12 months for HPA function to fully recover.

Editorial comments

- Inhaled corticosteroids are the drug of choice for patients with refractory symptoms on prn adrenergic agonist bronchodilators.
- Inhalation steroids are useful in reducing the dose or discontinuing use of oral corticosteroids. However, there is considerable controversy with respect to the beneficial use of higher than recommended inhalation doses of these drugs.
- Doses for beclomethasone are 42 μg per bronchial and nasal inhalation. Double-strength forms are available for both (84 μg/dose).

Benazepril

Brand name: Lotensin.

Class of drug: ACE inhibitor.

Mechanism of action: Inhibits ACE, thereby preventing conversion of angiotensin I to angiotensin II, resulting in decreased peripheral arterial resistance.

Indications/dosage/route: Oral only.

- Hypertension: Patients receiving a diuretic
  - Initial: 10 mg/d. Maintenance: 20–40 mg/d.
- Hypertension: Patients receiving a diuretic
  - Initial: 5 mg/d.

Adjustment of dosage

- Kidney disease: Creatinine clearance <30 mL/min: initial dose 5 mg/d.
- Liver disease: None.
- Elderly: None.
- Pediatric: Safety and efficacy in children have not been established.

Onset of Action	Duration
1 h	24 h

Food: No restrictions.

Pregnancy: Category C first trimester, Category D second and third trimesters.

Lactation: Appears in breast milk. Considered compatible by American Academy of Pediatrics.

Contraindications: Hypersensitivity to ACE inhibitors, hereditary or idiopathic angioedema, second and third trimesters of pregnancy.

Warnings/precautions

- Use with caution in patients with the following conditions: kidney disease, especially renal artery stenosis, drugs that cause bone marrow depression, hypovolemia, hyponatremia, cardiac or cerebral insufficiency, collagen vascular disease, lupus erythematosus, scleroderma, patients undergoing dialysis.
- ACE inhibitors have been associated with anaphylaxis and angioedema.
- Use extreme caution in combination with potassium-sparing diuretics (high risk of hyperkalemia).
- Sodium- or volume-depleted patients may experience severe hypotension. Lower initial doses are advised.
- During surgery/anesthesia, the drug may increase hypotension. Volume expansion may be required.
- There may be a profound drop in BP after the first dose is taken. Close medical supervision is necessary once therapy is begun.

Advice to patient

- Do not use salt substitutes containing potassium.
- Use two forms of birth control including hormonal and barrier methods.
- Avoid NSAIDs; may be present in OTC preparations.
- Take BP periodically and report to treating physician if significant changes occur.

- Stop drug if prolonged vomiting or diarrhea occurs. These symptoms may indicate plasma volume reduction.
- Discontinue drug immediately if signs of angioedema (swelling of face, lips, extremities; breathing or swallowing difficulty) become prominent, and notify physician immediately if this occurs. If chronic cough develops, notify treating physician.

Adverse reactions
- Common: none.
- Serious: bone marrow depression (neutropenia, agranulocytosis), hypotension, angioedema, tachycardia, hyperkalemia, oliguria, autoimmune symptom complex (see Editorial Comments), elevated liver enzymes, asthma.

Clinically important drug interactions
- Drugs that increase effects/toxicity of benazepril: potassium-sparing drugs, other diuretics, guanethidine.
- Drugs that decrease effectiveness of benazepril: NSAIDs, antacids, cyclosporine.
- Benazepril increases effects/toxicity of following drugs: lithium, azothioprine, allopurinol, digoxin.

Parameters to monitor
- Patient's electrolytes, CBC with differential and platelet count, BUN, and creatinine.
- Signs and symptoms of angioedema: swelling of face, lips, tongue, extremities, glottis, larynx. Observe in particular for obs-truction of airway, difficulty in breathing. If symptoms are not relieved by an antihistamine, discontinue drug.
- Patient's BP closely, particularly at beginning of therapy. Observe for evidence of severe hypotension. Patients who are hypovolemic due to GI fluid loss or diuretics may exhibit severe hypotension. Also monitor for orthostatic changes.
- Signs of persistent, nonproductive cough; this may be drug-induced.
- Changes in weight in patients with CHF. Gain of more than 2 kg/wk may indicate development of edema.
- Signs and symptoms of infection.
- Possible antinuclear antibody development.

- WBC monthly (first 3–6 months) and at frequent intervals thereafter for patients with collagen vascular disease or renal insufficiency. Discontinue therapy if neutrophil count drops below 1000.
- Signs and symptoms of bone marrow depression.
- Intake of fluids and urinary and other fluid output to minimize renal toxicity. Increase fluid intake if inadequate. Closely monitor electrolyte levels.
- Signs and symptoms of renal toxicity.

Editorial comments

- Unlabeled uses of ACE inhibitors include hypertensive crisis, diagnosis of renal artery stenosis, hyperaldosteronism, Raynaud's phenomenon, angina, diabetic nephropathy.
- ACE inhibitors have been associated with an autoimmune-type symptom complex including fever, positive antinuclear antibody, titers, myositis, vasculitis, and arthritis.
- Once daily dosing to twice daily dosing improves compliance.
- The ACE inhibitors have been a highly efficacious and well-tolerated class of drugs. Nearly every large randomized clinical trial examining their use has been favorable. First, a consensus trial proved that enalapril decreases mortality and increases quality of life in class II and III CHF patients. Then the SOLVE trial and others proved their benefits in remodeling myocardium post MI. The DCCT trial of diabetic patients demonstrated the ability of ACE inhibitors to decrease the small vessel damage to retinas and glomeruli. Clinical trials looking into primary prevention of cardiac effects are ongoing. Treatment with this class of drugs is the gold standard in patients with left ventricular systolic dysfunction. The two most common adverse effects of ACE inhibitors are cough and angioedema. Transient and persistent rises in antinuclear antibody have been noted. As drugs in this class are vasodilators, orthostasis is another potential problem.

Bendroflumethiazide

Brand name: Naturectin.
Class of drug: Thiazide diuretic.
Mechanism of action: Inhibits sodium resorption in distal tubule, resulting in increased urinary excretion of sodium, potasssium, and water.
Indications/dosage/route: Oral only.
• Diuretic
  – Adults: Initial: 2.5–20 mg once or twice daily, once every other day, or once a day for 3–5 weeks. Maintenance: 2.5–5 mg/d.
  – Children: Initial: 0.4 mg/kg, as single dose or two divided doses.
• Hypertension
  – Adults: Initial: 2.5–20 mg/d. Adjust to response.
  – Children: Initial: 0.005–0.4 mg/kg. Adjust to response.
  – Elderly: Use lower doses. Risk of postural hypotension.
Adjustment of dosage
• Kidney disease: Use with caution. Ineffective in severe renal failure.
• Liver disease: Use with caution. May cause electrolyte imbalance.
• Elderly: Use with caution. Risk of postural hypotension.
• Pediatric: See above.

Onset of Action	Peak Effect	Duration
1–2 h	4 h	6–24 h

Food: Should be taken with food.
Pregnancy: Category C. Use only if potential benefit to mother outweighs risk to fetus.
Lactation: No data available. Hydrochlorothiazide (another thiazide diuretic) is considered compatible with breastfeeding by the American Academy of Pediatrics. Thiazide diuretics may suppress lactation.

Contraindications: Anuria, hypersensitivity to thiazides or sulfonamide-derived drugs.

Editorial comments
- Do not coadminister with allopurinol as the combination may lead to severe hypersensitivity vasculitis.
- For additional information, see *hydrochlorothiazide*, p. 426.

Benztropine

Brand name: Cogentin.
Class of drug: Cholinergic blocking agent.
Mechanism of action: Blocks acetylcholine effects at muscarinic receptors throughout the body.
Indications/dosage/route: Oral, IM.
- Idiopathic parkinsonism
  - Adults: PO 0.5–6 mg/d.
- Postencephalitic parkinsonism
  - Adults: IM, PO 2 mg/d in one or more doses.
- Drug-induced extrapyramidal effects
  - Adults: IM, PO 1–4 mg, 1–2 times/d.

Adjustment of dosage
- Kidney disease: None.
- Liver disease: None.
- Elderly: Use with caution; higher incidence of side effects.
- Pediatric: Contraindicated in children under 3. Use with extreme caution in older children.

Onset of Action	Peak Effect	Duration
1–2 h	—	2–3 days

Pregnancy: Category C.
Lactation: No data available. Potentially toxic to infant. Avoid breastfeeding.

Contraindications: Myasthenia gravis, narrow-angle glaucoma, GI obstruction, megacolon, colitis, ulcerative colitis, obstructive uropathy, hypersensitivity to atropine-type compounds (belladonna alkaloids), children <3 years.

Warnings/precautions

- Use with caution in patients with the following conditions: GI infections, chronic biliary disease, CHF, arrhythmias, pulmonary disease, benign prostatic hypertrophy, hyperthyroidism, coronary artery disease, hypertension, seizures, psychosis, spastic paralysis.
- Anticholinergic psychosis can occur in sensitive individuals.
- Elderly may react with agitation and excitement even to small doses of anticholinergic drugs.

Advice to patient

- Take medication exactly as directed. If dose is missed, do not double subsequent dose when it is remembered.
- Avoid driving and other activities requiring mental alertness or that are potentially dangerous until response to drug is known.
- Use caution when exercising in hot weather as this might cause heat prostration.
- Avoid alcohol and other CNS depressants such as opiate analgesics and sedatives (eg, diazepam) when taking this drug.
- If mouth is dry, rinse with warm water frequently, chew sugarless gum, suck on an ice cube, or use artificial saliva. Carry out meticulous oral hygiene (floss teeth daily).
- Patients with Parkinson's disease should not stop this drug abruptly.

Adverse reactions

- Common: dry mouth, blurred vision (decreased accommodation), drowsiness, tachycardia, urinary hesitancy, dry skin, constipation.
- Serious: disorientation, hallucinations, acute narrow-angle glaucoma, orthostatic hypotension, arrhythmia.

Clinically important drug interactions

- Drugs that increase effects/toxicity of systemic anticholinergics: phenothiazines, amantadine, other antipsychotic agentics,

thiazide diuretics, tricyclic antidepressants, MAO inhibitors, quinidine, procainamide.
• Drugs that decrease effects/toxicity of systemic anticholinergics: antacids, cholinergic agents.

Parameters to monitor
• Signs and symptoms of severe toxicity: tachycardia, supraventricular arrythmias, delirium, seizures, agitation, hyperthermia. Discontinue if patient experiences dizziness, palpitations, rapid pulse. Use physostigmine (Eserine) as antidote only for life-threatening toxicity.
• Intake of fluids and urinary and other fluid output. Increase fluid intake if inadequate.
• Signs of urinary retention: pelvic pain and distention, decreased urine output. This is particularly important in elderly with benign prostatic hypertrophy. Determine whether there is a need for catherization.
• Ophthalmic status: intraocular pressure before and during treatment, accommodation, pupillary response to light, visual acuity (blurred vision). Discontinue administration if the following occur: eye pain, conjunctivitis.

Editorial comments: IV administration of benztropine offers no advantage over IM. It is therefore recommended not to use IV benztropine.

Bepridil Hydrochloride

Brand name: Vascor.
Class of drug: Calcium channel blocker.
Mechanism of action: Inhibits calcium movement across cell membranes.
Indications/dosage/route: Oral only.
• Angina
  – Adults: Initial: 200 mg once daily. Maintenance: 200–300 mg/d. Maximum: 400 mg/d.

Adjustment of dosage
- Kidney disease: Use with caution. Guidelines have not been established.
- Liver disease: Use with caution. Guidelines have not been established.
- Elderly: Use normal dose with caution.
- Pediatric: Safety and efficacy have not been established in children.

Onset of Action	Peak Effect	Duration
0.5–1 h	2–3 h	4–8 h

Food: No restriction.
Pregnancy: Category C.
Lactation: Probably appears in breast milk. Potentially toxic to infant. Avoid breastfeeding.
Contraindications: Hypersensitivity to calcium blockers.
Editorial comments: For additional information, see *felodipine*, p. 346.

Betamethasone

Brand names: Celestone, Diprosone, Uticort, Valisone, Diprolene.
Class of drug: Topical and systemic antiinflammatory glucocorticoid.
Mechanism of action: Inhibits migration of polymorphonuclear leukocytes; stabilizes lysomal membranes; inhibits production of products of arachidonic acid cascade.
Indications/dosage/route: IM, topical, intraarticular, intrabursal, intradermal. Dosages of corticosteroids are variable. These should be individualized according to the disease being treated and the response of the patient.
- Adrenal insufficiency

   – Initial: IM 0.5 mg/d.
- Bursitis, peritendinitis, tenosynovitis
  – Intrabursal: 3 mg (1 mL).
- Rheumatoid arthritis and osteoarthritis
  – Intraarticular: 0.75–6 mg (0.25–2 mL).
- Acute gouty arthritis
  – Intraarticular 1.5–3 mg (0.5–1 mL).
- Dermatologic conditions
  – Intradermal: 0.2 mL/cm^2, not to exceed 1 mL/wk.
- Corticosteroid-responsive dermatoses
  – Apply thin layer to affected area once or twice a day.

Adjustment of dosage
- Kidney disease: None.
- Liver disease: None.
- Elderly: None.
- Pediatric: Systemic use: Children on long-term therapy must be monitored carefully for growth and development. Topical use: Safety and efficacy have not been established in children <12.

Food: Not applicable.

Pregnancy: Category C.

Lactation: No data available. Best to avoid.

Contraindications: Systemic use: fungal, viral, or bacterial infections, Cushing's syndrome. Topical use: hypersensitivity to corticosteroids, markedly impaired circulation, occlusive dressing if primary skin infection is present, monotherapy in primary bacterial infections, eg, impetigo, cellulitis, rosacea, ophthalmic use, plaque psoriasis (widespread).

Warnings/precautions
- Use with caution in patients with the following conditions: diabetes mellitus, cardiovascular disease, hypertension, thrombophlebitis, renal or hepatic insufficiency. Topical agent: Use with caution in patients with primary skin infections and those receiving other immunosuppressant drugs.
- Skin test patient for tuberculosis before beginning treatment if patient is at high risk.
- For long-term treatment consider alternative-day dosing; however, if the disease flares, may need to return to initial daily dose.

- Observe neonates for signs of adrenal insufficiency if mother has taken steroids during pregnancy.
- Tapering is always required when administration of a steroid is stopped. A variety of procedures for tapering after long-term therapy have been suggested. For example, taper dose by 5 mg/wk until 10 mg/d is reached. Then 2.5 mg/wk until therapy is discontinued or lowest dosage giving relief is reached. Longer tapering periods may be required for some patients. Adrenal insufficiency may persist for up to 1 year.
- Attempt dose reduction periodically to determine if disease can be controlled at a lower dose. When every-other-day therapy is initiated, twice the daily dose should be administered on alternate days in the morning.
- Check whether patient is allergic to tartrazine which is present in some of these drugs.

Adverse reactions
- Common: dyspepsia, appetite stimulation, insomnia, anxiety, fluid retension, cushinoid facies.
- Serious: Cushing-like syndrome, adrenocortical insufficiency, muscle wasting, osteoporosis, immunosuppression with increased susceptibility to infection, potassium loss, glaucoma, cataracts (nuclear, posterior, subcapsular), hyperglycemia, hypercorticism, peptic ulcer, psychosis, insomnia, skin atrophy, thrombosis, seizures, angioneuritic edema. *Children*: Growth suppression, pseudotumor cerebri (reversible papilledema, visual loss, nerve paralysis [abducens or oculomotor]), vascular bone necrosis, pancreatitis.
- Topical: Common: itching, burning, skin dryness, erythema, folliculitis, hypertrichosis, allergic contact dermatitis, skin maceration, secondary infection, striae, millaria, skin atrophy. Serious: HPA axis suppression, Cushing's syndrome.

Clinically important drug interactions
- Systemic
  – Drugs that increase effects/toxicity of corticosteroids: broad-spectrum antibiotics, anticholinergics, oral contraceptives, cyclosporine, loop diuretics, thiazide diuretics, NSAIDs, tricyclic antidepressants.

 – Drugs that decrease effects/toxicity of corticosteroids: barbiturates, cholestyramine, ketoconazole, phenytoin, rifampin.
 – Corticosteroids increase effects/toxicity of following drugs: digitalis glycosides, neuromuscular blocking drugs.
 – Corticosteroids decrease effects of vaccines, toxoids.
• Topical: None.

Editorial comments: Corticoid treatment remains challenging for clinicians due to commonly occurring short-term and long-term side effects. With chronic use, adrenal suppression may persist for up to 1 year. The agents produce accelerated bone resorption as well as decreased bone formation, resulting in overall bone loss with chronic use. Ongoing monitoring is suggested and treatment with bisphosphonates or calcitonin is suggested when decreased bone mineral density occurs.

Betaxolol

Brand names: Kerlone, Betoptic.
Class of drug: β-Adrenergic receptor blocker.
Mechanism of action: Competitive blocker of β-adrenergic receptors in heart, blood vessels, and eyes.
Indications/dosage/route: Oral, topical (ophthalmic).
• Hypertension
 – Adults: Initial: PO 10–20 mg/d. Maximum: 20 mg/d.
 – Elderly: Initial: PO 5 mg/d. Maximum: 10 mg/d.
• Glaucoma
 – Ophthalmic preparations: 1–2 drops b.i.d. in affected eye.
Adjustment of dosage
• Kidney disease (severe): PO initial dose 5 mg q.d.
• Liver disease: None.
• Elderly: See above.

- Pediatric: Safety and efficacy have not been established in children.

Food: No restriction.

Pregnancy: Category C.

Lactation: Appears in breast milk. Potentially toxic to infant. Best to avoid.

Contraindications: Cardiogenic shock, CHF unless it is secondary to tachyarrhythmia treated with a β blocker, sinus bradycardia and AV block greater than first degree, severe COPD.

Warnings/precautions

- Use with caution in patients with the following conditions: diabetes, kidney disease, liver disease, COPD, peripheral vascular disease.
- Do not stop drug abruptly as this may precipitate arrhythmias, angina, MI or cause rebound hypertension. If necessary to discontinue, taper as follows: Reduce dose and reassess after 1–2 weeks. If status is unchanged, reduce by another 50% and reassess after 1–2 weeks.
- Drug may mask symptoms of hyperthyroidism, mainly tachycardia.
- Drug may exacerbate symptoms of arterial insufficiency in patients with peripheral or mesenteric vascular disease.

Advice to patient

- Avoid driving and other activities requiring mental alertness or that are potentially dangerous until response to drug is known.
- Dress warmly in winter and avoid prolonged exposure to cold as drug may cause increased sensitivity to cold.
- Avoid drinks that contain xanthines (caffeine, theophylline, theobromine) including colas, tea, and cocoa because they may counteract the effect of drug.
- Restrict dietary sodium to avoid volume expansion.
- Drug may blunt response to usual rise in BP and chest pain under stressful conditions such as vigorous exercise and fever.

Adverse reactions
- Common: headache, dizziness.
- Serious: symptomatic bradycardia, CHF, worsened AV block, hypotension, depression, bone marrow, depression, SLE-like syndrome, bronchospasm, Peyronie's disease, hepatitis.

Clinically important drug interactions
- Drugs that increase effects/toxicity of β blockers: reserpine, bretylium, calcium channel blockers.
- Drugs that decrease effects/toxicity of β blockers: aluminum salts, calcium salts, cholestyramine, barbiturates, NSAIDs, rifampin.

Parameters to monitor
- Liver enzymes, serum BUN and creatinine, CBC with differential and platelets.
- Patient's pulse rate near end of dosing interval or before next dose is taken. A reasonable target is 60–80 bpm for resting apical ventricular rate. If severe bradycardia develops, consider treatment with glucagon, isoproterenol, IV atropine (1–3 mg in divided doses). If hypotension occurs despite correction of bradycardia, administer vasopressor (norephinephrine, dopamine, or dobutamine).
- Symptoms of CHF. Digitalize patient and administer a diuretic or glucagon.
- Efficacy of treatment: decreased BP, decreased number and severity of anginal attacks, improvement in exercise tolerance. Confirm control of arrhythmias by ECG, apical pulse, BP, circulation in extremities, and respiration. Monitor closely when changing dose.
- CNS effects. If patient experiences mental depression reduce dosage by 50%. The elderly are particularly sensitive to adverse CNS effects.
- Signs of bronchospasm. Stop therapy and administer large doses of β-adrenergic bronchodilator, eg, albuterol, terbutaline, or aminophylline.
- Signs of cold extremities. If severe, stop drug. Consider β blocker with sympathomimetic property.

- Intraocular pressure (ophthalmic use): If inadequately controlled, administer another narcotic concomitantly (pilocarpine, epinephrine or acetazolamide).

Editorial comments
- Stopping a β blocker before surgery is controversial. Some advocate discontinuing the drug 48 hours before surgery; others recommend withdrawal for a considerably longer time. Notify anesthesiologist that patient has been on β blocker.
- β blockers are first-line treatments for hypertension particularly in patients with the following conditions: previous MI, ischemic heart disease, aneurysm, atrioventricular arrhythmias, migraine. These are drugs of first choice for chronic stable angina, used in conjunction with nitroglycerin.
- Many studies indicate benefit from administration of a β blocker following an MI.
- β blockers are considered to be first-line drugs for prophylaxis of migraine headache in patients who have two or more attacks per month.

Bethanechol

Brand name: Urecholine.
Class of drug: Cholinergic agonist, parasympathomimetic.
Mechanism of action: Stimulant of postsynaptic cholinergic receptors in urinary bladder and GI tract. This causes increased contractility and peristalsis.
Indications/dosage/route: Oral, SC.
- Urinary retention due to neurogenic bladder and other nonobstructive causes, GI prokinetic
  - Adults: PO 10–50 mg, b.i.d. to q.i.d. SC 7.5–20 mg/d, divided as t.i.d. or q.i.d. doses. Maximum SC dose: 10 mg 0.4 h for neurogenic bladder.
  - Children: PO 0.6 mg/kg/d, divided as t.i.d. or q.i.d. doses. SC 0.15–0.2 mg/kg/d.

Adjustment of dosage
• Kidney disease: None.
• Liver disease: None.
• Elderly: May be at higher risk for side effects.
• Pediatric: Safety and efficacy have not been established in children <5 years.

	Onset of Action	Duration
Oral	30–90 min	6 h
SC	5–15 min	2 h

Food: Should be taken 1 hour before or 2 hours after meals when given orally. For SC administration, take 2 hours before meals.
Pregnancy: Category C.
Lactation: No data available. Potentially toxic to infants. Avoid breastfeeding.
Contraindications: IV, IM use, hypersensitivity to bethanecol, mechanical obstruction of GI tract, active peptic ulcer disease, COPD, epilepsy, bradycardia, Parkinson's disease, AV block, hypotension, hypertension.

Warnings/precautions
• Use with caution in patients with the following conditions: epilepsy, hyperthyroidism.
• Observe patient closely for 30–60 minutes for possible side effects after drug administration.
• Atropine should be available for treating side effects.

Advice to patient: Change position slowly, in particular from recumbent to upright, to minimize orthostatic hypotension. Sit at the edge of the bed for several minutes before standing and lie down if feeling faint or dizzy. Avoid hot showers, or baths and standing for long periods. Male patients with orthostatic hypotension may be safer urinating while seated on the toilet rather than standing.

Adverse reactions
• Common: None.
• Serious: hypotension, cardiac arrest, bronchial constriction.

Clinically important drug interactions
- Drugs that increase effects/toxicity of bethanechol: cholinesterase inhibitors (contraindicated).
- Drugs that decrease effects/toxicity of bethanechol: procainamide, quinidine.

Parameters to monitor
- Intake of fluids and urinary and other fluid output to minimize renal toxicity. Closely monitor electrolyte levels.
- Signs of abdominal distention. Effectiveness of treatment is indicated by reduction in abdominal distention and decreased bowel activity.

Editorial comments: Because of the potential for life-threatening complications from this drug, the editors recommend administration only by experienced practitioners.

Bitolterol

Brand name: Tornalate.
Class of drug: β-Adrenergic agonist, bronchodilator.
Mechanism of action: Relaxes smooth muscles of the bronchioles by stimulating β_2-adrenergic receptors.
Indications/dosage/route: Inhalation only.
- Bronchodilation
  – Adults, children >12 years: Initial: 2 inhalations at interval of 1–3 minutes q8h; third inhalation may be taken. Maximum: 3 inhalations q6h or 2 inhalations q4h.
- Prophylaxis of bronchospasm
  – Adults, children >12 years: 2 inhalations q8h.

Adjustment of dosage
- Kidney disease: None.
- Liver disease: None.
- Elderly: Lower doses may be required.
- Pediatric: See above. Safety and efficacy have not been established in children <12 years.

Onset of Action	Peak Effect	Duration
3–4 min	—	5–8 h

Food: Not applicable.
Pregnancy: Category C.
Lactation: No data available. Best to avoid.
Contraindications: Hypersensitivity to adrenergic compounds, tachycardia (idiopathic or from digitalis).
Editorial comments
• This agent appears to cause tremor and palpitations more frequently than isoproterenol. Headache appears less common.
• For additional information, see *metaproterenol*, p. 575.

Bleomycin

Brand name: Blenoxane.
Class of drug: Antineoplastic, antitumor antibiotic, sclerosing agent.
Mechanism of action: Inhibits synthesis of DNA.
Indications/dosage/route: IV, IM, SC, intracavitary.
• Chemotherapy regimens for Hodgkin's and non-Hodgkin's lymphoma, testicular cancer, squamous cell carcinoma, melanoma, sarcoma
  – Adults: IV, IM, SC 0.25–0.5 units/kg, 1–2 times per week. Maintenance: IM or IV 1 unit/d or 5 units/wk.
  – Adults: Continuous IV infusion of 15 units/m^2/d for 4 days. Maximum lifetime dose: 400 units.
• Malignant pleural effusion.
  – Adults: intracavitary 60 units.
Adjustment of dosage
• Kidney disease: creatinine clearance 10–50 mL/min: reduce dose by 25%; creatinine clearance <10 mL/min: reduce dose by 50%.

Onset of action: Parenteral; 2–3 wks.
Pregnancy: Category D.
Lactation: No data available. Potentially toxic to infant. Do not breastfeed.
Contraindications: Hypersensitivity to bleomycin, severe pulmonary disease.

Warnings/precautions

• Use caution in patients with kidney impairment, compromised pulmonary function.
• High-percentage oxygen inhalation in patients who have received bleomycin has been associated with pulmonary failure.

Advice to patient

• Use two forms of birth control including hormonal and barrier methods.
• Do not receive any vaccinations (particularly live attenuated viruses) without permission from treating physician.
• Do not smoke.

Adverse reactions

• Common: Raynaud's phenomenon, febrile allergic reactions, nausea, vomiting, anorexia, stomatitis, thickening bronchial secretions, alopecia, dermatologic changes (erythema, peeling, hyperkeratosis, induration in 50% of patients).
• Serious: **pulmonary toxicity, interstitial pneumonitis, pulmonary fibrosis,** hypoxia, myelosuppression, MI, anaphylaxis reaction. Severe idiosyncratic reaction: mental confusion, fever, hypotension, particularly in lymphoma patients.

Clinically important drug interactions

• Drugs that increase effects/toxicity of bleomycin: cisplatin.
• Bleomycin decreases effects/toxicity of following: digitalis, phenytoin.

Parameters to monitor

• CBC, serum BUN and creatinine, liver enzymes.
• Signs and symptoms of anaphylactic reaction, pulmonary toxicity, hepatotoxicity, bone marrow depression.

- Signs and symptoms of stomatitis. Treat with peroxide, tea, topical anesthetics such as benzocaine, lidocaine, or antifungal drug.

Editorial comment

- Use latex gloves and safety glasses when handling this medication; avoid contact with skin as well as inhalation. If possible prepare in biologic hood.
- Although cumulative doses of 400 units/m^2 increase the risk of pulmonary fibrosis, this toxic effect can occasionally occur at much lower cumulative doses. Corticosteroids are sometimes helpful in treating this problem, but it may also be fatal.

Bretylium

Brand name: Bretylol.

Class of drug: Antiarrhythmic agent, Class III.

Mechanism of action: Depletes adrenergic nerve terminals of norepinephrine; this decreases adrenergic stimulation of the myocardium.

Indications/dosage/route: IV and IM only.

- Ventricular arrhythmias (resistant to lidocaine).
  - Adults: IV bolus 5 mg/kg over 1 minute. Repeat if necessary at 15- to 30-minute intervals. Total dose: 30–35 mg/kg. Maintenance: 5–10 mg/kg q6–8h.
  - Pediatric dose: IM 2–5 mg/kg; IV 5 mg/kg. Repeat every 10–20 minutes if necessary. Maximum: 30 mg/kg. Maintenance: 5 mg/kg q6–8h.

Adjustment of dosage

- Kidney disease: creatinine clearance 10–60 mL/min; reduce dose by 50–75%; creatinine clearance <10 mL/min: reduce dose by 75%.
- Liver disease: None.
- Elderly: May be at higher risk for toxicity.
- Pediatric: See above.

	Onset of Action	Peak Effect	Duration
IV	6–20 min	6–9 h	6–24 h

Pregnancy: Category B.
Lactation: No data available. Potentially toxic to infant. Avoid breastfeeding.
Contraindications: Arrhythmias induced by digitalis. Severe pulmonary hypertension. For treatment of ventricular fibrillation or life-threatening refractory ventricular arrhythmias, there is no contraindication to using bretylium.

Warnings/precautions
• Use with caution in patients with the following conditions: hypotension, pulmonary hypertension, aortic stenosis.
• Reduce dose gradually (over 3–5 days) with ECG monitoring.

Advice to patient: If ambulation is permitted, change position slowly, in particular from recumbent to upright, to minimize orthostatic hypotension.

Adverse reactions
• Common: hypotension.
• Serious: **hypotension (50–75%)**, bradycardia, syncope, confusion, kidney damage, respiratory depression.

Clinically important drug interactions
• Other antiarrhythmic agents increase effects/toxicity of bretylium.
• Bretylium increases effects/toxicity of sympathomimetics, digoxin.

Parameters to monitor
• Monitor patient's BP very carefully. If supine systolic pressure is lower than 75 mm Hg, carefully administer an IV infusion of dopamine or norepinephrine and titrate to increase BP.
• ECG, heart rate, BP. Patient should be on continuous cardiac monitoring. Additional hemodynamic monitoring also recommended.

Editorial comments
• Adequate facilities, equipment, and personnel must be available for constant ECG and BP monitoring when bretylium is used.

- Tolerance to the hypotensive action of bretylium may occur after several days. Patient should remain in supine position under close supervision for postural hypotension until tolerance develops to this effect. If severe hypotension occurs, the patient should be administered IV infusion of dopamine or norepinephrine as well as volume replacement with blood or plasma if necessary.
- Bretylium is only for short-term use and should be discontinued after 3–5 days with gradual dose reduction and replaced by an orally effective antiarrhythmic drug if necessary.
- Bretylium is currently not used clinically as a cardiac drug since IV amiodarone became available. It will likely be removed from the ACLS training protocol and transitional from crash carts.
- This drug is not listed in the *Physician's Desk Reference*, 54th edition, 2000.

Bromocriptine

Brand name: Parlodel.
Class of drug: Anti-Parkinson agent, prolactin inhibitor.
Mechanism of action: Prolactin inhibition: inhibits prolactin secretion from anterior pituitary. Anti-Parkinson effects: stimulates dopamine receptors in the brain, thus improving symptoms of Parkinson's disease.
Indications/dosage/route: Oral only.
- Parkinson's disease (usually used in combination with levodopa–carbidopa)
  – Adults: 1.25 mg b.i.d. or t.i.d. increase dosage by 2.5 mg/d every 2–4 weeks. Maintenance: 10–40 mg/d.
- Hyperprolactinemia
  – Adults: 0.5–2.5 mg b.i.d. or t.i.d. Maintenance: 2.5–15 mg/d. Maximum: 6 months.
- Acromegaly

– Adults: Initial: 1.25–2.5 mg/d; increase dose by 2.5 mg/d q3–7d as needed. Maintenance: 20–30 mg/d.

Adjustment of dosage
• Kidney disease: Use with caution.
• Liver disease: May require lower doses.
• Elderly: May require lower doses.
• Pediatric: No data available.

	Onset of Action	Duration
Hyperprolactinemia	2 h	24 h
Parkinson's disease	30–90 min	No data
Acromegaly	1–2 h	4–8 h

Food: Take with food or milk.

Pregnancy: Category C.

Lactation: Suppresses lactation. Contraindicated by the American Academy of Pediatrics.

Contraindications: Severe ischemic heart disease, peripheral vascular disease, sensitivity to ergot alkaloids.

Warnings/precautions: Use with caution in patients with kidney disease, liver disease.

Advice to patients
• Avoid driving and other activities requiring mental alertness or that are potentially dangerous until response to drug is known.
• Avoid alcohol.
• Use two forms of birth control including hormonal and barrier methods.

Adverse reactions
• Common: decreased BP (28%), headache (10%), dizziness, nausea.
• Serious: Seizures, CVA, prolonged hypotension, depression, hallucinations, syncope, MI, liver toxicity.

Clinically important drug interactions
• Drugs that increase effects/toxicity of bromocriptine: sympathomimetics, diuretics.

- Drugs that decrease the antiprolactin action of bromocriptine: phenothiazines, butyrophenones, reserpine, amitriptyline, imipramine, methyldopa.
- Bromocriptine increases effects/toxicity of following: antihypertensive drugs, alcohol, ergot alkaloids.

Parameters to monitor
- CBC with differential and platelets, liver enzymes.
- Evaluate patient for orthostasis with BP measurements in the sitting, lying, and standing positions repeatedly before and after initiating therapy.
- Monitor tumor enlargement for patient with pituitary tumor: sudden headache, severe nausea and vomiting, visual disturbances.

Editorial comments: A large percentage of patients will experience mild to moderate side effects from bromocriptine, particularly with higher doses (>20 mg/d). In postpartum studies, only 3% of patients needed to discontinue therapy because of side effects.
- This drug is listed without details in the *Physician's Desk Reference,* 54th edition, 2000.

Brompheniramine

Brand names: Dimetane, Bromfed.
Class of drug: H_1 receptor blocker.
Mechanism of action: Antagonizes histamine effects on GI tract, respiratory tract, blood vessels.
Indications/dosage/route: Oral only (capsules, syrup).
- Allergic rhinitis
  - Adults, children >12 years: 24 mg/d in divided doses q4–12h. Maximum: 48 mg/d.
  - Children 6–12 years: 12 mg/d in divided doses q4–12h.
  - Children 2–4 years: 1 mg (syrup) q4h.
  - Children <2 years: Doses not established.

Adjustment of dosage
- Kidney disease: None.
- Liver disease: None.

- Elderly: Use caution. At higher risk for side effects.
- Pediatric: See above.

Onset of Action	Peak Effect	Duration
—	3–9 h	4–25 h

Food: No restriction.

Pregnancy: Category C.

Lactation: Appears in breast milk. Potentially toxic to infant. Although brompheniramine is considered compatible with breastfeeding by the American Academy of Pediatrics, it is stated to be contraindicated by one manufacturer.

Contraindications: Hypersensitivity to antihistamines, acute asthma, narrow-angle glaucoma, concurrent use of MAO inhibitor.

Warnings/precautions

- Use with extreme caution in patients with active peptic ulcer, severe coronary artery disease, symptomatic prostatic hypertrophy.
- Use with caution in patients with the following conditions: hypertension, hyperthyroidism, asthma, heart disease, diabetes, increased intraocular pressure.
- Do not use in neonates or premature infants.
- Infants and young children are at risk for overdosage.

Advice to patient

- Avoid driving and other activities requiring mental alertness or that are potentially dangerous until response to drug is known.
- Use caution if used along with alcohol and other CNS depressants such as narcotic analgesics and sedatives (eg, diazepam).
- Drink large quantities of water to minimize drying of secretions.
- If mouth is dry, rinse with warm water frequently, chew sugarless gum, suck on an ice cube, or use artificial saliva. Carry out meticulous oral hygiene (floss teeth daily).
- Discontinue drug at least 4 days before skin testing (for allergies) to avoid the possibility of false-negative results.

Adverse reactions
• Common: drowsiness, dry mouth and throat, nervousness.
• Serious: Palpitations.
Clinically important drug interactions
• Drugs that increase effects/toxicity of antihistamines: CNS depressants (barbiturates, benzodiazepines, narcotic analgesics), MAO inhibitors (combination contraindicated).
• Antihistamines decrease effects of sulfonylureas.
Parameters to monitor
• Signs of dry mouth, eg, thickened secretions. Increase fluid intake to decrease viscosity of secretion.
• Signs and symptoms of severe CNS depression, dilated pupils, or flushing as symptoms of overdose. Administer syrup of ipecac if necessary.
Editorial comments: This drug is available in combination with other agents, including pseudoephedrine, phenylephrine, phenylpropanolamine, aspirin, acetaminophen. Warnings and precautions, side effects, etc, of other ingredients should be kept in mind when prescribing.

Budesonide

Brand names: Rhinocort, Pulmicort.
Class of drug: Inhalation corticosteroid.
Mechanism of action: Inhibits elaboration of many of the mediators of allergic inflammation, eg, leukotrienes and other products of the arachidonic acid cascade.
Indications/dosage/route: Inhalation aerosol.
• Asthma
  – Adults: 200–800 µg b.i.d. (1–4 inhalations morning and evening).
  – Children >6 years: 200–400 µg b.i.d. (1–2 inhalations, morning and evening).
• Seasonal or perennial rhinitis

– Adults, children ≥6 years: Initial: 256 µg/d, 2 sprays in each nostril in morning and evening. Maintenance: reduce initial dose to smallest amount necessary to control symptoms.

Adjustment of dosage
• Kidney disease: None.
• Liver disease: None.
• Elderly: None.
• Pediatric: Safety and efficacy have not been established in children <6 years.

Pregnancy: Category C.

Lactation: Present in breast milk. Safe to use.

Contraindications: Hypersensitivity to corticosteroids.

Warnings/precautions
• If patient is transferred from systemic corticosteroid to inhalation drug, symptoms of steroid withdrawal may result. These include muscle and joint pain, depression. Alternatively, adreneal insufficiency may occur: weakness, fatigue, nausea, anorexia.
• Provide patient with instructions for use of the inhaler or nasal spray and make sure patient completely understands these instructions.
• Provide patient with a list of side effects and note those that require immediate reporting to the physician.
• Patients on long-term inhaled or intranasal corticosteroids may require steroid pulsing during stress, eg, surgery or infection.

Advice to patient
• Rinse mouth and gargle with warm water after each inhalation. This may minimize the development of dry mouth, hoarseness, and oral fungal infection.
• This drug should be inhaled 5 minutes after a previously inhaled bronchodilator, eg, albuterol.
• Do not exceed recommended dosage of the drug. Excessive doses have been associated with adrenal insufficiency.
• Notify physician if symptoms worsen.

• Carry a card indicating your condition, drugs you are taking, and need for supplemental steroid in the event of a severe asthmatic attack. Attempt to decrease dose once the desired clinical effect is achieved. Decrease dose gradually every 2–4 weeks. Return to initial starting dose if symptoms recur.
• Stop smoking.
• Do not overuse the inhaler.

Adverse reactions
• Common: pharyngitis, headache.
• Serious: potential for hypercorticism, adrenal insufficiency.

Clinically important drug interactions: None.

Parameters to monitor
• Signs and symptoms of acute adrenal insufficiency, particularly in response to stress.
• Child growth: Drug may suppress growth.
• Changes in nasal mucosa in patients on long-term drug therapy.
• Signs of localized infection in mouth and pharynx, eg, red membranes with vesicular eruptions. Treat with appropriate antifungal drug, eg, nystatin, or discontinue treatment.
• When switching from systemic inhalation therapy, monitor patient for symptoms of adrenal insufficiency: hypotension, weight loss, muscular and joint pain. If these occur, the dose of systemic steroid should be increased followed by slower withdrawal. It may require up to 12 months for HPA function to fully recover.

Editorial comments
• Inhaled corticosteroids are the drugs of choice for patients with refractory symptoms on prn adrenergic agonist bronchodilators.
• Inhalation steroids are useful in reducing the dose or discontinuing use of oral corticosteroids. However, there is considerable controversy with respect to the beneficial use of higher than recommended inhalation doses of these drugs.

Bumetanide

Brand name: Bumex.

Class of drug: Loop diuretic.

Mechanism of action: Inhibits sodium and chloride resorption in proximal part of ascending loop of Henle.

Indications/dosage/route: Oral, IV, IM.

• Edema (CHF, nephrotic syndrome, hepatic disease)
  – Adults: PO 0.5–2 mg/d; if response is inadequate, give additional dose q4–5h. Maximum: 10 mg/d.
  – Adults: IV, IM 0.5–1 mg; if response is inadequate, give additional dose q2–3h. Maximum: 10 mg/d.

Adjustment of dosage

• Kidney disease: None.
• Liver disease: Use with caution. At higher risk for toxicity.
• Elderly: Use with caution. At higher risk for toxicity.
• Pediatric: Safety and efficacy have not been established in children <18 years.

	Onset of Action	Peak Effect	Duration
Oral	30–60 min	60–120 min	4–6 h
IV	Within minutes	15–30 min	0.5–1 h

Food: Take with food or milk.

Pregnancy: Category D.

Lactation: No data available. Suppresses lactation. Avoid breast-feeding.

Contraindications: Hypersensitivity to sulfonamides, anuria, hepatic coma, severe electrolyte depletion.

Editorial comments

• This drug is listed without detail in the *Physician's Desk Reference*, 54th edition, 2000.
• For additional information, see *furosemide*, p. 394.

Bupivacaine

Brand names: Marcaine, Sensorcaine.

Class of drug: Local and regional anesthetic

Mechanism of action: Reversibly inhibits initiation and conduction of nerve impulses near site of injection.

Indications/dosage/route: Local injection only.

• Caudal, epidural anesthesia, peripheral nerve block
  – Adults: Usual dose 225 mg plus epinephrine 1:200,000 or 175 mg without epinephrine. Repeat after 3 hours as needed. Maximum: 400 mg/24 h.

Adjustment of dosage

• Kidney disease: None.
• Liver disease: Use with extreme caution in severe liver disease.
• Elderly: None.
• Pediatric: Not recommended for use in children <12 years.

Food: Not applicable.

Pregnancy: Category C.

Lactation: No data available. Use with caution.

Contraindications: Hypersensitivity for amide-type local anesthetic (eg, lidocaine), sensitivity to sodium metabisulfate (in preparations containing epinephrine), obstetrical paracervical block.

Warnings/precautions

• Use local anethetics plus vasoconstrictor (eg, epinephrine, norepinephrine) with caution in patients with the following conditions: peripheral vascular disease, hypertension, administration of general anesthetics.

• Use local anesthetics with or without vasoconstrictor with caution in patients with severe liver disease. Use with extreme caution for lumbar and caudal epidural anesthesia in patients with the following conditions: spinal deformities, existing neurologic disease, severe uncontrolled hypotention, septicemia.

• For epidural anesthesia: A test dose of the local anesthetic should first be given before the full dose is administered to ensure that the catheter is not within a blood vessel. The test dose should include 10–15 µg epinephrine. Any increase in heart rate and systolic pressure within 45 seconds (the epinephrine response) would indicate that the injection is intravascular.

- Local anesthetics can trigger familial malignant hyperthermia. Symptoms of this condition include tachycardia, labile BP, tachypnea, muscle rigidity. The necessary means must be available to manage this condition (dantrolene, oxygen, supportive measures).
- A local anesthetic containing a vasoconstrictor should be injected with great caution into areas of the body supplied by end-organ arteries (nose, ears, penis, digits).

Advice to patient: Be aware that there will be a loss of sensation for several hours after the injection.

Adverse reactions
- Common: None.
- Serious: CNS toxicity, tremors, seizures, arrhythmias (local anesthetics plus vasoconstrictors), cardiovascular toxicity (bradycardia, hypotension, cardiovascular collapse), allergic reactions, apnea.

Clinically important drug interactions
- MAO inhibitors, tricyclic antidepressants, ergot-type oxytocic drugs increase toxicity/effects of local anesthetics containing a vasoconstrictor.

Parameters to monitor
- Respiratory and cardiovascular function. At the first sign of a change that suggests onset of toxicity, administer oxygen and stop drug. Do not administer a respiratory stimulant. Control symptoms by supportive means. Establish and maintain a patent airway, begin assisted ventilation, and administer 100% oxygen.
- Signs of convulsions. If these occur, inject by IV bolus one or more of the following: 5–10 mg diazepam, 50–100 mg thiopental, 50–100 mg succinylcholine.

Editorial comments
- A local anesthetic should be administered with caution. Toxicity arises primarily because of excessively high doses, inadvertent intravascular injection, too rapid rate of injection, injection into

tissue that is highly vascular, and idiosyncratic reactions of the patient.
- Injection should be made slowly with frequent aspiration to ensure that the needle or catheter is not in a blood vessel. Resuscitation equipment and drugs, as well as oxygen, should be available for immediate use.

Buprenorphine

Brand name: Buprenex.
Class of drug: Narcotic analgesic, agonist.
Mechanism of action: Binds to opiate receptors and blocks ascending pain pathways. Reduces patient's perception of pain without altering cause of the pain.
Indications/dosage/route: IV, IM.
- Moderate to severe pain
  - Adults, children >13 years: IV, IM 0.3 mg q6h. Repeat once 30–60 minutes after initial dose if needed. Maximum: 0.6 mg, single dose.
  - Children 2–12 years: IV, IM 2–6 µg/kg q4–6h.

Adjustment of dosage
- Kidney disease: creatinine clearance <30 mL/min: 50–100 mg q12h Maximum: 200 mg.
- Liver disease: Use with caution.
- Elderly: Use with caution. Reduce dose by 50%.
- Pediatric: Not recommend for children <2 years.

Onset of Action	Peak Effect	Duration
15 min	60 min	6 h

Food: Not applicable.
Pregnancy: Category C. Category D if prolonged use or if given in high doses at term.

Lactation: Appears in breast milk. Potentially toxic to infant. Avoid breastfeeding.

Contraindications: Hypersensitivity to buprenorphine.

Warnings/precautions

- Use with caution in patients with the following conditions: head injury with increased intracranial pressure, serious alcoholism, prostatic hypertrophy, chronic pulmonary disease, severe liver or kidney disease, postoperative patients with pulmonary disease, disorders of biliary tract.
- Administer drug before patient experiences severe pain for fullest efficacy of the drug.
- Have the following available when treating patient with this drug: means of administering oxygen and support of respiration.
- Nausea, vomiting, and orthostatic hypotension occur most prominently in ambulatory patients. If nausea and vomiting persist, it may be necessary to administer an antiemetic, eg, droperidol or prochlorperazine. This drug can cause severe hypotension in a patient who is volume depleted or if given along with a phenothiazine or general anesthesia.
- Careful diagnosis must be made of acute abdominal condition before this drug is administered.

Editorial comments

- Naloxone may not be effective in reversing respiratory depression from buprenorphine. Overdose is best managed by using mechanically assisted ventilation.
- Avoid using buprenorphine and diazepam or lorazepam as the combination may cause respiratory and cardiovascular collapse.
- Administration of buprenorphine in narcotic-dependent individuals may result in withdrawal reaction.
- For additional information, see *morphine*, p. 633.

Bupropion

Brand names: Welbutrin, Zyban.
Class of drug: Antidepressant, smoking cessation adjunct.

Mechanism of action: Not completely known. Blocks serotonin and norepinepherine receptors in the brain. Mild dopamine reuptake inhibitor.

Indications/dosage/route: Oral only.

• Depression
  – Adults: Initial, 100 mg b.i.d. Increase gradually to maximum 150 mg t.i.d. Maximum: 150 mg t.i.d.
• Smoking cessation
  – 150 mg/d for 3 days, then 150 mg b.i.d. for 7–12 weeks. Minimum of 8 hours between doses.

Adjustment of dosage

• Kidney disease: Reduced dose initially, monitor closely.
• Liver disease: Reduced dose initially, monitor closely.
• Elderly: Reduced dose initially, monitor closely.
• Pediatric: Safety and efficacy have not been determined in children under 18 years.

Food: No restrictions.

Pregnancy: Category B.

Lactation: Appears in breast milk. Best to avoid. American Academy of Pediatrics expresses concern regarding antidepressants and breastfeeding.

Contraindications: Bulimia, anorexia nervosa, head trauma, seizure disorders, concurrent use of an MAO inhibitor, hypersensitivity to Bupropion.

Warnings/precautions: Use with caution in patients with history of unstable heart disease, recent MI, renal or hepatic impairment, history of seizures.

Advice to patient

• Avoid driving and other activities requiring mental alertness or that are potentially dangerous until response to drug is known.
• Do not discontinue without consulting treating physician.
• Avoid alcohol.
• For symptomatic relief of xerostomia (dry mouth): Rinse mouth with warm water frequently, chew sugarless gum, suck on ice cube, use artificial saliva if necessary, carry out meticulous oral hygiene (floss teeth daily).

- Be aware that it may take considerable time (up to 3 weeks) for the drug to be effective in deterring smoking.

Adverse reactions
- Common: dizziness, headache, insomnia, dry mouth, nausea/vomiting, diaphoresis, constipation, tremor, agitation, weight change, sedation.
- Serious: **tachycardia**, other arrhythmias, seizures, psychosis, syncope, confusion, hostility.

Clinically important drug interactions
- Drugs that increase effects/toxicity of buproprion: MAO inhibitors, cimetidine, phenothiazines, SSRI antidepressants, levodopa, ritonavir.
- Drugs that decrease effects/toxicity of buproprion: carbamazepine, phenytoin, phenobarbital.

Parameters to monitor
- Suicidal tendencies until there is improvement of depression.
- Manic episodes if patient has a bipolar disorder.
- Body weight: May be loss or gain of weight because of change in taste perception.
- Possible mood changes such as insomnia, increased anxiety.

Editorial comments
- High doses of bupropion (up to 450 mg/d) increase seizure potential 4 times greater than other antidepressants.
- Patients using bupropion for smoking cessation require additional physician counseling and/or an established smoke-ending program for best results.
- Clinicians should note that Welbutrin, a treatment for depression, and Zyban, a smoke ending therapy, are both trade names for bupropion. Therefore, these two treatments should not be combined in the same patient.

Buspirone

Brand name: BuSpar.

Class of drug: Antianxiety agent, nonsedating.

Mechanism of action: Not entirely known. Appears to inhibit 5-HT_A serotonin receptors and possibly D_2 dopamine receptors in the brain.

Indications/dosage/route: Oral only.

• Anxiety disorders
  – Adults: Initial: 5 mg t.i.d., increase daily dose by 5 mg/d every 2–3 days to achieve desired effect. Maximum: 60 mg/d. Maintenance: 20–30 mg/d, divided doses.

Adjustment of dosage

• Kidney disease: Decrease dose. Do not use in severe renal impairment.
• Liver disease: Decrease dose. Do not use in severe hepatic insufficiency.
• Elderly: None.
• Pediatric: Safety and effectiveness have not been established in children <18 years.

Food: No restriction.

Pregnancy: Category B.

Lactation: Appears in breast milk in animal studies. American Academy of Pediatrics expresses concern regarding antianxiety drugs and breastfeeding.

Contraindications: Concomitant MAO inhibitor, hypersensitivity to buspirone.

Warnings/precautions

• Use with caution in patients with the following conditions: kidney disease (see above), liver disease (see above).
• Restrict amount of drug prescribed at any given time for patients who have a history of drug abuse.

Advice to patient

• Avoid driving and other activities requiring mental alertness or that are potentially dangerous until response to drug is known.
• Avoid alcohol and other CNS depressants such as opiate analgesics and sedatives (eg, diazepam) when taking this drug.

Adverse reactions

• Common: drowsiness, dizziness.
• Serious: none.

Clinically important drug interactions
- Drugs that increase effects/toxicity of busipirone: MAO inhibitors, phenothiaznes, other CNS depressants.
- Buspirone increases effects/toxicity of following: digoxin, haloperidol, warfarin.

Parameters to monitor: Relief of symptoms of anxiety.

Editorial comments: This drug has not been proven to be effective for long-term use.

Busulfan

Brand name: Myleran.

Class of drug: Alkylating antineoplastic agent.

Mechanism of action: Intercalates and crosslinks strands of DNA. Blocks replication of DNA and transcription of RNA.

Indications/dosage/route: Oral only.
- Chronic myelogenous leukemia
  - Adults: 4–8 mg/d. Maximum: 12 mg/d. Maintenance: 1–3 mg/d or as little as 2 mg/wk. Used to keep WBC <50,000 mm^3. Dosage stopped when WBC <10,000 mm^3.
  - Children: 0.06-0.12 mg/kg/d. Dosage adjusted to keep WBC <40,000 mm^3. Drug stopped if WBC <20,000 mm^3.
- Myelofibrosis, polycythemia vera, thrombocytosis
  - Adults: 2–8 mg, 2–3 weeks.
- Pre-bone marrow transplantation
  - Adults: 1 mg/kg q6h. Total: 16 doses.

Onset of Action
1–2 w.

Pregnancy: Category D.

Lactation: No data available. Contraindicated.

Contraindications: Failure to respond to previously adminis-tered drug, hypersensitivity to busulfan.

Warnings/precautions

• Use with caution in patients with the following conditions: previous radiation treatment, recently administered immuno-suppressive drugs and other agents that are toxic to bone marrow.

• A most frequent and serious side effect of busulfan therapy is the induction of bone marrow failure and subsequent severe pancytopenia.

• Busulfan therapy is also rarely associated with bronchopul-monary dysplasia and pulmonary fibrosis. This may occur shortly after therapy or up to 10 years after therapy.

• Busulfan therapy may result in the development of secondary malignancy. This treatment has also been associated with menopausal symptoms, hepatic veno-occlusive disease, and possibly cardiac tamponade.

Advice to patient

• Male patients should use condoms if engaging in sexual inter-course while using this medication.

• Female patients should use two forms of birth control includ-ing hormonal and barrier methods.

• Discontinue at first sign of pulmonary fibrosis (shortness of breath, fever).

• Do not receive any vaccinations (particularly live attenuated viruses) without permission from treating physician.

Adverse reactions

• Common: alopecia, hyperpigmentation of the skin, amenorrhea, azoospermia.

• Serious: **bone marrow depression** (severe pancytopenia), **testic-ular atrophy, sterility**, "busulfan lung" (fever, cough, dyspnea, pulmonary fibrosis), endocardial fibrosis, GU tumors, seizures (high dose), adrenal suppression, testicular atrophy, cataracts, secondary malignancies, cardiac tamponade, cataracts, hepatic veno-occlusive disease.

Clinically important drug interactions: None reported.

Parameters to monitor
- CBC with differential and platelets, liver enzymes.
- Signs and symptoms of thrombocytopenia. Discontinue this medication if platelet count falls below 100,000/mm^3.
- Signs of hyperuricemia: gouty arthritis, uric acid kidney stones. Administer allopurinol.
- Signs and symptoms of anemia.
- Signs and symptoms of pulmonary toxicity.
- Signs and symptoms of bone marrow depression.

Editorial comments
- Busulfan is used only rarely now. Interferon-α and hydroxyurea are much more commonly used.
- Use latex gloves and safety glasses when handling cytotoxic drugs. Avoid contact with skin as well as inhalation.

Butabarbital

Brand names: Phrenilin, Esgic, Zebutal.
Class of drug: Sedative, hypnotic.
Mechanism of action: Facilitates action of GABA at its receptor. Depresses sensory cortex, cerebellum; decreases motor activity.
Indications/dosage/route: Oral only.
- Daytime sedation
  – Adults: 15–30 mg b.i.d. or q.i.d.
- Hypnotic:
  – Adults: 50–100 mg h.s.
- Preoperative sedation
  – Adults: 50–100 mg 60–90 min before surgery.
  – Children: 2–6 mg/kg. Maximum: 100 mg.

Adjustment of dosage
- Kidney disease: Reduce dose.
- Liver disease: Reduce dose.
- Elderly: Reduce dose.
- Pediatric: See above.

Onset of Action	Duration
10–15 min	3–4 h

Food: No information available.

Pregnancy: Category D. Causes fetal abnormalities. Infants with chronic *in utero* barbiturate exposure are at risk for withdrawal. Administration during labor may cause infant respiratory depression.

Lactation: Appears in breast milk. Classified by American Academy of Pediatrics as potentially causing major adverse effects on infant when breastfeeding. Avoid breastfeeding.

Contraindications: Hypersensitivity to barbiturates, porphyria, preexisting CNS depression, hepatic encephalopathy, severe respiratory disease, compromised respiration, previous addiction to a barbiturate or other sedative hypnotics (eg, benzodiazepines), pregnancy.

Editorial comments

- This drug is not listed in the *Physician's Desk Reference,* 54th edition, 2000.
- For additional information, see *phenobarbital,* p. 728.

Butorphanol

Brand name: Stadol.

Class of drug: Narcotic analgesic, agonist/antagonist.

Mechanism of action: Binds to opiate receptors and blocks ascending pain pathways. Reduces patient's perception of pain without altering cause of the pain.

Indications/dosage/route: Nasal spray, IM, IV.

- Pain
  - Adults: Initial: 1 mg (1 spray in one nostril). Repeat in 60–90 minutes if needed. This sequence may be repeated in 3–4 hours.
- Severe pain

– Adults: Initial: 2 mg (1 spray in each nostril). Repeat in 3–4
hours if needed. IM 1–4 mg q3–4h as needed. IV 0.5–2 mg
q3–4h as needed.

Adjustment of dosage
• Kidney disease: None.
• Liver disease: None.
• Elderly: IM, IV 0.5–1 mg every 4–6 hours as needed. Increase
dose gradually as tolerated.
• Pediatric: Safety and efficacy have not been established in chil-
dren <18.

Onset of Action	Peak Effect	Duration
10–15 min	30–60 min	3–4 h

Food: May be taken with food to lessen GI upset.
Pregnancy: Category B. Category D if prolonged use or if given
in high doses at term.
Lactation: Appears in breast milk. Potentially toxic to infant.
Considered compatible with breastfeeding by the American
Academy of Pediatrics.
Contraindications: Hypersensitivity to butorphanol or benzeme-
thonium (preservative).

Warnings/precautions
• Use with caution in patients with the following conditions:
head injury with increased intracranial pressure, serious alcoholism, prostatic hypertrophy, chronic preliminary disease,
severe liver or kidney disease, postoperative patients with pulmonary disease, disorders of biliary tract.
• It is not recommended in patients who received chronic narcotics as it may precipitate a withdrawal reaction.
• Administer drug before patient experiences severe pain for
fullest efficacy of the drug.
• Have the following available when treating patient with this
drug: naloxone (Narcan) or other antagonist, means of administering oxygen, and support of respiration.

- Nausea, vomiting, and orthostatic hypotension occur most prominently in ambulatory patients. If nausea and vomiting persist, it may be necessary to administer an antiemetic, eg, droperidol or prochlorperazine.
- This drug can cause severe hypotension in a patient who is volume depleted or if given along with a phenothiazine or general anesthesia.
- Careful diagnosis must be made of acute abdominal condition before this drug is administered.

Advice to patient

- Avoid alcohol and other CNS depressants such as sedatives (eg, diazepam) when taking this drug.
- Avoid driving and other activities requiring mental alertness or that are potentially dangerous until response to drug is known.
- Change position slowly, in particular from recumbent to upright, to minimize orthostatic hypotension. Sit at the edge of the bed for several minutes before standing, and lie down if feeling faint or dizzy. Avoid hot showers or baths and standing for long periods. Male patients should sit on the toilet while urinating rather than standing.
- Do not increase dose if you are not experiencing sufficient pain relief without approval from treating physician.
- Do not stop medication abruptly when you have been taking it for 2 or more weeks. If so, a withdrawal reaction may occur within 24–48 hours. The following are typical symptoms: irritability, perspiration, rhinorrhea, lacrimation, dilated pupils, piloerection ("goose flesh"), bone and muscle aches, restless sleep ("yen"), increased systolic pressure, hyperpyrexia, diarrhea, hyperglycemia, spontaneous orgasm.
- Take OTC drugs only with approval by treating physician. Some of these may potentiate the CNS depressant effects of the drug.
- If dizziness persists for more than 3 days, decrease dose gradually (over 1–2 days).
- Attempt to void every 4 hours.

Adverse reactions
• Common: drowsiness.
• Serious: **hypotension, bradycardia**, tachycardia, confusion, respiratory depression, physical and psychologic dependence, addiction.

Clinically important drug interactions: Drugs that increase effects/toxicity of narcotic analgesics: Alcohol, benzodiazepines, antihistamines, phenothiazines, butyrophenones, triyclic antidepressants, MAO inhibitors.

Parameters to monitor
• Signs and symptoms of pain: restlessness, anorexia, elevated pulse, increased respiratory rate. Differentiate restlessness associated with pain and that caused by CNS stimulation caused by the drug. This paradoxical reaction is seen mainly in women and elderly patients.
• Monitor respiratory status prior to and following drug administration. Note rate, depth, and rhythm of respirations. If rate falls below 12/min, withhold drug unless patient is receiving ventilatory support. Consider administering an antagonist, eg, naloxone 0.1–0.5 mg IV every 2–3 min. Be aware that respiratory depression may occur even at small doses. Restlessness may also be a symptom of hypoxia. Monitor character of cough reflex. Encourage postoperative patient to change position frequently (at least every 2 hours), breathe deeply, and cough at regular intervals, unless coughing is contraindicated. These steps will help prevent atelectasis.
• Signs and symptoms of urinary retention, particularly in patients with prostatic hypertrophy or urethral stricture. Monitor output/intake and check for oliguria or urinary retention.
• Signs of tolerance or dependence. Determine whether patient is attempting to obtain more drug than prescribed as this may indicate onset of tolerance and possibility of dependence. If tolerance develops to one opiate, there is generally cross-tolerance to all drugs in this class. Physical dependence is generally not a problem if the drug is given for less than 2 weeks.

- Monitor patient's BP. If systolic pressure falls below 90 mm Hg, do not administer the drug unless there is ventilatory support. Be aware that the elderly and those receiving drugs with hypotensive properties are most susceptible to sharp fall in BP.
- Patient's heart rate. Withhold drug if adult pulse rate is below 60 bpm. Alternatively, administer atropine.
- Respiratory status of newborn baby and possible withdrawal reaction. If the mother has received an opiate just prior to delivery, the neonate may experience severe respiratory depression. Resuscitation, as well as a narcotic antgonist, eg, Narcan, may be necessary. Alternatively, the neonate may experience severe withdrawal symptoms 1–4 days after birth. In such circumstances, administer opium tincture or paregoric.
- Signs and symptoms of constipation. If patient is on drug for more than 2–3 days, administer a laxative. For patients on long-term therapy, administer a bulk or fiber laxative, eg, psyllium, 1 teaspoon in 240 mL liquid/d. Encourage patient to drink large amounts of fluid, 2.5 to 3 L/d.

Editorial comments: This drug is indicated for treatment of moderate to severe pain. Intranasal formulation allows for rapid onset of pain relief.

Calcitonin

Brand names: Calcimar (salmon), Cibacalcin (human), Miacalcin (salmon).

Class of drug: Calcium-lowering agent, treatment for Paget's disease, antiosteoporosis agent.

Mechanism of action: Promotes renal excretion of calcium and phosphate, inhibits osteoclastic bone resorption

Indications/dosage/route: IM, SC, intranasal. *Note*: Prior to treatment, a skin test must be performed (see Warnings/ Precautions).

• Paget's disease
  – Adults, salmon calcitonin: Initial: SC or IM 100 units/d. Maintenance: 50 units/d.
  – Adults, human calcitonin: Initial: SC 0.5 mg/d. Maintenance: 0.5 mg 2 or 3 times/wk.

• Hypercalcemia
  – Adults, salmon calcitonin: IM, SC 4 units/kg q12h. Maximum: 8 units/kg q6h.

• Postmenopausal osteoporosis
  – Adults, salmon calcitonin: IM, SC 100 units/d.
  – Intranasal: 1 spray (200 units)/day. Combine with oral calcium carbonate, vitamin D.

• Osteogenesis imperfecta
  – Adults: IM, SC 2 units/kg 3 times/wk. Combine with oral calcium.
  – Children: Safety and efficacy have not been established.

	Onset of Action	Duration
Hypercalcemia	2 h	6–8 h

Pregnancy: Category C.

Lactation: No data available. Best to avoid.

Contraindications: Hypersensitivity reaction to salmon calcitonin or its gelatin diluent.

Warnings/precautions
- When using salmon calcitonin determine whether patient is allergic by performing skin test before administration. One unit is injected into the skin. Observe for 15 minutes for development of erythema or wheal. Have emergency equipment available during administration.
- Potential for hypocalcemic tetany.

Advice to patient
- Learn the correct way to use the nasal spray.
- Calcium and vitamin D supplements are part of the treatment for osteoporosis.
- Employ sterile techniques for injection.
- Alternate injection sites.

Adverse reactions
- Common: None.
- Serious: Allergic reactions, hypocalcemia, tetany (overdose).

Clinically important drug interactions: None reported.

Parameters to monitor
- Serum electrolytes, calcium, alkaline phosphatase.
- Signs of hypersensitivity reactions.
- BP, pulse, ECG.
- Signs and symptoms of hypercalcemia: bone pain, thirst, nausea, vomiting, anorexia, constipation.
- Signs and symptoms of hypocalcemic tetany: convulsions, tetanic spasms, muscle twitching. Administer calcium parenterally.

Editorial comments
- The most frequent use for calcitonin is postmenopausal osteoporosis. It is also useful to prevent and treat corticosteroid-induced osteoporosis. Consider an alternative drug such as alendronate (Fosamax) for these indications.

Calcitriol

Brand names: Calcijex, Rocaltrol.

Class of drug: Vitamin D analog, calcium-raising agent.

Mechanism of action: Promotes intestinal absorption of calcium. Promotes renal calcium resorption.

Indications/dosage/route: Oral, IV.

• Hypocalcemic patients undergoing chronic dialysis
  – Adults, PO: Initial: 0.25 µg/d. Maintenance: 0.25 µg/d 2 days, increase dose up to 1 µg/d by 0.25 µg/d. Check serum calcium levels q2wk during titration.
  – Children, PO: 0.25–2 µg/d; 0.014–0.041 µg/kg/d (not on dialysis).
  – Adults, IV dosing for hypocalcemia Initial: 0.5 µg 3 times/wk. Maintenance: 0.5–3 µg 3 times/wk.
  – Children, IV: 0.01–0.05 µg/kg 3 times/wk.
• Hypoparathyroidism
  – Adults, children >5 years: Initial: PO 0.25 µg/d. Maintenance: 0.5–2.0 µg/d.
  – Children <1 year, PO 0.04–0.08 µg/kg/d.
  – Children 1–5 years: PO 0.25–0.75 µg/d.
• Vitamin D-dependent rickets
  – PO 1 µg/d.

Adjustment of dosage

• Kidney disease: Reduce dose in severe disease.
• Liver disease: None.
• Elderly: None.
• Pediatric: Safety and efficacy have not been established.

	Onset of Action	Peak Effect	Duration
Treatment of Hypocalcemia	Approx 2–6 h	10 h	3–5 d

Food: Patient should have diet rich in calcium.

Pregnancy: Category C. Could be toxic to fetus if dose exceeds recommended dose.

Lactation: Appears in breast milk. Contraindicated.

Contraindications: Hypercalcemia, vitamin D toxicity, hypersensitivity to calcitriol.

Warnings/precautions
- This drug must be given with calcium supplements.
- Serum phosphate must be controlled before initiating therapy. Instruct patient how to avoid excessive phosphorus intake.
- May produce vitamin D overdose: Do not allow serum [Ca] × [phosphate] to exceed 70 (see Parameters to monitor).

Advice to patient
- Limit intake of vitamin D, ie, avoid megavitamins and limit intake of vitamin D-rich foods: fortified milk, fish liver oils, cereals.
- Avoid magnesium-containing antacids.
- Maintain a high fluid intake.
- Avoid excessive phosphorus intake.

Adverse reactions
- Common: None.
- Serious (seen with hypervitaminosis only): hypertension, arrhythmias, hypotension, hyperthermia, psychosis, pancreatitis, hematitis, ectopic calcification, nephrocalciumesis.

Clinically important drug interactions
- Drugs that increase effects/toxicity of calcitriol: thiazide diuretics.
- Drugs that decrease effects/toxicity of calcitriol: cholestyramine, cholestipol, barbiturates, phenytoin, corticosteroids.

Parameters to monitor
- Serum calcium, phosphorus, albumin, BUN and creatinine.
- Urinary output, fluid intake.
- Calcium concentration should be maintained between 9 and 10 mg/dL. If the product of calcium (mg/dL) and phosphate (mg/dL) is greater than 70, discontinue therapy.
- Urinary calcium and creatinine. If the calcium:creatinine ratio is less than 0.18, discontinue therapy.
- Serum alkaline phosphatase levels. If enzyme level falls significantly, this may be a sign of impending hypercalcemia.
- Signs of hypocalcemia: laryngospasm, paresthesia, arrhythmia, Chvostek's or Trousseau's sign.
- Signs of hypercalcemia: Early: headache, anorexia, weakness, dry mouth, metallic taste, abdominal cramps, ataxia. Later:

nephrocalcinosis, polyuria, polydipsia, proteinuria, osteoporosis (adults), decreased growth (children).

Candesartan

Brand name: Atacand.
Class of drug: Angiotension II receptor antagonist.
Mechanism of action: Inhibits binding of angiotension II to AT_1 receptor thereby blocking the actions of angiotensin II.
Indications/dosage/route: Oral only.
 – Adults: Initial: 16 mg once daily. Maintenance dosage range: 8–32 mg once daily.
Adjustment of dosage
• Kidney disease: None for mild disease.
• Liver disease: None for mild disease. Consider lower doses if intravascular volume is depleted (eg, by diuretic).
• Elderly: None.
• Pediatric: Safety and efficacy have not been established.
Food: No restriction.
Pregnancy: Category C, first trimester; Category D, second and third trimesters.
Lactation: No data available. Best to avoid.
Contraindications: Hypersensitivity to candesartan.
Editorial comments
• This drug has been used as an alternative in patients who are unable to tolerate ACE inhibitors.
• Discontinue this drug immediately if pregnancy is detected.
• For additional information, see *losartan*, p. 541.

Capreomycin

Brand name: Capastat.

Class of drug: Antitubercular.

Mechanism of action: Unknown. Has bacteriostatic action.

Indications/dosage/route: IM, IV.

• Treatment of tuberculosis
  – Adults: 10–20 mg/kg/d; maximum 1 g/d, continue 60–120 days; followed by 1 g 2–3 times/week. Treatment for 12–24 months.

Adjustment of dosage

• Kidney disease: Dosage reduced based on creatinine clearance. In general, individual doses reduced with increased interval. For example, creatinine clearance 50 mL/min: 14 mg/kg q48h; creatinine clearance 30 mL/min: 10 mg/kg q48h; creatinine clearance 10–20 mL/min: 7–10 mg/kg q48h; creatinine clearance <10 mL/min: 4 mg/kg. q48h.

• Liver disease: None.

• Pediatric: Safety and efficacy have not been established.

Pregnancy: Category C.

Lactation: No data available. Best to avoid.

Contraindications: Hypersensitivity to capreomycin.

Warnings/precautions: Use with caution in patients with the following conditions: renal insufficiency, auditory impairment, concurrent use of nephrotoxic drugs (eg, gentamicin) or ototoxic drugs (eg, streptomycin, viomycin).

Adverse reactions

• Common: skin rash, pain or bleeding at injection site, vertigo, tinnitus.

• Serious: **nephrotoxicity (36%), ototoxicity (11%)**, bone marrow depression, hypersensitivity reactions, eosinophilia.

Clinically important drug interactions: Capreomycin increases effects/toxicity of aminoglycosides, other ototoxic and nephrotoxic agents, neuromuscular blocking drugs.

Parameters to monitor

• CBC with differential and platelets, serum BUN, and creatinine.

• Pretreatment audiometry and periodic hearing tests thereafter.

• Signs and symptoms of ototoxicity: tinnitus, vertigo, hearing loss, initially in range of 4000–8000 Hz.

• Signs and symptoms of renal toxicity.
• Signs and symptoms of bone marrow depression.
Editorial comments: Used in combination regimens for resistant *Mycobacterium tuberculosis* infections.

Captopril

Brand name: Capoten.
Class of drug: ACE inhibitor.
Mechanism of action: Inhibits ACE, thereby preventing conversion of angiotensin I to angiotensin II, resulting in decreased peripheral arterial resistance.
Indications/dosage/route: Oral only.
• Hypertension
  – Initial: 25 mg b.i.d. to t.i.d. Increase to 50 mg b.i.d. to t.i.d.
• Accelerated or malignant hypertension
  – Initial: 25 mg b.i.d. to t.i.d.
• Heart failure
  – Initial: 25 mg t.i.d. Maintenance: 50–100 mg t.i.d.
• Left ventricular dysfunction after MI
  – Initial: 6.25 mg/d, then begin 12.5 mg t.i.d. and increase to 25 mg t.i.d. Maintenance: 50 mg t.i.d.
• Diabetic nephropathy
  – 25 mg t.i.d.
• Hypertensive crisis
  – Initial: 25 mg/d, then 100 mg 90–120 min later. Maintenance: 200–300 mg/d.
• Severe childhood hypertension
  – Initial: 0.3 mg/kg titrated to 6 mg or less in b.i.d. to t.i.d. doses.
Adjustment of dosage
• Kidney disease: Reduce initial daily dose, use smaller increments for titration. Titrate slowly (1- to 2-week intervals).
• Liver disease: None.

- Elderly: May need smaller initial and titrating doses.
- Pediatric: Safety and efficacy have not been fully established. Newborns and infants are at higher risk of toxicity.

Onset of Action	Peak Effect	Duration
15–60 min	60–90 min	6–12 h

Food: Administer 1 hour before meals.

Pregnancy: Category C first trimester, Category D second and third trimesters.

Lactation: Not excreted in breast milk. Considered compatible by the American Academy of Pediatricians.

Contraindications: Previous history of ACE inhibitor-induced angioedema, second and third trimesters of pregnancy.

Warnings/precautions

- Use with caution in patients with the following conditions: kidney disease, especially renal artery stenosis, drugs that cause bone marrow depression, hypovolemia, hyponatremia, cardiac or cerebral insufficiency, collagen vascular disease, patients undergoing dialysis.
- ACE inhibitors have been associated with anaphylactic reactions and angioedema.
- Use extreme caution in combination with potassium-sparing diuretics (high risk of hyperkalemia).
- Sodium- or volume-depleted patients may experience severe hypotension. Lower initial doses are advised.
- Neutropenia most often seen in patients with renal disease.
- During surgery/anesthesia, the drug may increase hypotension. Volume expansion may be required.
- There may be a profound drop in BP after the first dose is taken. Close medical supervision is necessary once therapy is begun.
- Proteinurea with nephrotic syndrome has occurred.

Advice to Patient

- Do not use salt substitutes containing potassium.

- Use two forms of birth control including hormonal and barrier methods.
- Avoid NSAIDs; may be present in OTC preparations.
- Take BP periodically and report to treating physician if significant changes occur.
- Stop drug if the following occurs: prolonged vomiting or diarrhea. These symptoms may indicate plasma volume reduction.
- Discontinue drug immediately if signs of angioedema (swelling of face, lips, extremities, breathing or swallowing difficulty) become prominent, and notify physician immediately if this occurs.
- If chronic cough develops, notify treating physician.

Adverse reactions
- Common: None.
- Serious: bone marrow depression (neutropenia, agranulocytosis), hypotension, angioedema, hyperkalemia, oliguria, chest pain, angina, tachycardia, palpitations, proteinuria, autoimmune symptom complex (see Editorial Comments).

Clinically important drug interactions
- Captopril increases toxicity of following drugs: lithium, azothioprine, allopurinol, potassium-sparing diuretics, digoxin.
- Drugs that increase toxicity of captopril: potassium-sparing drugs, phenothiazines (eg, chlorpromazine).
- Drugs that decrease effectiveness of captopril: NSAIDs, antacids, cyclosporine.

Parameters to monitor
- Patient's electrolytes, CBC with differential and platelets, BUN, and creatinine.
- Signs and symptoms of angioedema: swelling of face, lips, tongue, extremities, glottis, larynx. Observed in particular for obstruction of airway, difficulty in breathing. If symptoms are not relieved by an antihistamine, discontinue drug.
- BP closely, particularly at beginning of therapy. Observe for evidence of severe hypotension. Patients who are hypovolemic as a result of GI fluid loss or diuretics may exhibit severe hypotension. Also monitor for orthostatic changes.
- Signs of persistent, nonproductive cough; this may be drug-induced.

- Changes in weight in patients with CHF. Gain of more than 2 kg/wk may indicate edema development.
- Signs and symptoms of infection.
- Possible antinuclear antibody development.
- Monitor WBC monthly (first 3–6 months) and at frequent intervals thereafter for patients with collagen vascular disease or renal insufficiency. Discontinue therapy if neutrophil count drops below 1000.
- Signs and symptoms of bone marrow depression.
- Intake of fluids and urinary and other fluid output to minimize renal toxicity. Increase fluid intake if inadequate. Closely monitor electrolyte levels.
- Signs and symptoms of renal toxicity.

Editorial comments

- Unlabeled uses of ACE inhibitors include hypertensive crisis, diagnosis of renal artery stenosis, hyperaldosteronism, Raynaud's phenomenon, angina, diabetic nephropathy.
- ACE inhibitors have been associated with an autoimmune type symptom complex including fever, positive antinuclear antibody, myositis, vasculitis, arthritis.
- Captopril is widely used especially when starting treatment in patients with high BP in the hospital.
- Shorter half-life has allowed more rapid titration.
- The ACE inhibitors have been a highly efficacious and well-tolerated class of drugs. Nearly every large randomized clinical trial examining their use has been favorable. First, a consensus trial proved that enalapril decreased mortality and increased quality of life in class II and III CHF patients. Then the SOLVE trial and others proved their benefits in remodeling myocardium post MI. The DCCT trial of diabetic patients demonstrated the ability of ACE inhibitors to decrease the small vessel damage to retinas and glomeruli. Clinical trials looking into primary prevention of cardiac effects are ongoing. Treatment with this class of drugs is the gold standard in patients with left venricular systolic dysfunction. The two most common adverse effects of ACE inhibitors are cough and angioedema. Transient and persistent rises in antinuclear

antibody have been noted. As drugs in this class are vasodilators, orthostasis is another potential problem.

Carbachol

Brand names: Carboptic, Miostat.
Class of drug: Cholinergic agonist, miotic agent.
Mechanism of action: Reduces intraocular fluid, contracts sphincter muscle of iris producing myosis, stimulates muscarinic receptors in eye.
Indications/dosage/route: Topical (ophthalmic).
• Open-angle or narrow-angle glaucoma: ophthalmic solution
  – Adults: 1–2 drops of 0.75–3% solution, q4–8h.
• Ocular surgery
  – Adults: 0.5 mL of 0.01% intraocular form into anterior chamber; instill before or after suturing.
Adjustment of dosage
• Kidney disease: None.
• Liver disease: None.
• Elderly: None.
• Pediatric: Safety and efficacy have not been established.

Onset of Action	Peak Effect
10–20 min	<4 h

Pregnancy: Category C.
Lactation: No data available. Best to avoid.
Contraindications: Acute iritis, secondary glaucoma, acute inflammatory disease of the anterior chamber, acute or anterior uveitis, hypersensitivity to carbachol.

Warnings/precautions
- Use with caution in patients with the following conditions: acute heart failure, peptic ulcer, bronchial asthma, hyperthyroidism, Parkinson's disease, urinary tract obstruction.
- Use with caution if there is corneal abrasion and in patients undergoing general anesthesia.

Advice to patient
- May cause decreased night vision and alter distance vision. Use caution while night driving or carrying on hazardous tasks in dim light.
- Avoid potential exposure to bright light and wear sunglasses.
- Avoid organophosphate insecticides while taking this drug.

Adverse reactions
- Common: transient stinging and burning of the eye.
- Serious: corneal clouding, keratitis, retinal detachment, ciliary spasm.

Clinically important drug interactions: Cholinergic blocking agents, ophthalmic atropine-like compounds decrease effects/ toxicity of carbachol.

Parameters to monitor
- Evaluate patient for orthostasis with BP measurements in the sitting, lying, and standing positions before and after initiating therapy.
- Signs and symptoms of pulmonary toxicity: basilar rales, tachypnea, cough, fever, exertional dyspnea.
- Symptoms of systemic absorption: diarrhea, abdominal pain, nausea, vomiting, increased sweating.

Carbamazepine

Brand name: Tegretol.
Class of drug: Anticonvulsant, analgesic.
Mechanism of action: Anticonvulsant action: blocks polysynptatic transmission by inhibiting influx of sodium ions across the

cell membrane. Analgesic action: blocks polysynpatic transmission within the CNS. Also has anticholinergic, antidiuretic, antiarrythmic, muscle relaxant properties.

Indications/dosage/route: Oral only.

• Epilepsy: tonic–clonic, partial seizures with complex symptoms (psychomotor or temporal lobe seizures)

 – Adults, children >12 years: Initial: 200 mg b.i.d.; increase dose weekly by 200 mg/d maximum. Maintenance: 800–1200 mg/d. Maximum: 1600 mg/d.

 – Children 6–12 years: Initial: 100 mg b.i.d.; increase dose weekly by 100 mg/d. Maintenance: 400–800 mg/d. Maximum: 1000 mg/d.

• Trigeminal neuralgia (unlabeled use)

 – Adults: Initial: 100 mg b.i.d. Maintenance: 200 mg–1.2 g/d. Maximum: 1.2 g/d.

Adjustment of dosage

• Kidney disease: creatinine clearance <10 mL/min: 75% of standard dose.

• Liver disease: None.

• Elderly: Reduce dose and monitor carefully.

• Pediatric: Safety and efficacy have not been established in children <6 years.

Food: Should be taken with food to prevent GI upset.

Pregnancy: Category C. Should be continued during pregnancy if favorable benefits versus risk.

Lactation: Present in breast milk. Considered compatible by American Academy of Pediatrics. Should be continued during lactation if favorable benefits versus risk.

Contraindications: Bone marrow depression, use of MAO inhibitor within 14 days, cross-sensitivity with tricyclic antidepressants, hypersensitivity to carbamazepine.

Warnings/precautions

• Use with caution in patient with the following conditions: mixed type seizures, liver and cardiac disease.

• Carbamazepine should be discontinued if WBC is <3000 and neutrophils ≦1500.

- Abrupt withdrawal may precipitate seizures.
- Aplastic anemia and agranulocytosis are significant risks in using carbamazepine.

Advice to patient

- To minimize possible photosensitivity reaction, apply adequate sunscreen and use proper covering when exposed to strong sunlight.
- If you are receiving an oral contraceptive, use an alternative method of birth control.
- Avoid alcohol and other CNS depressants such as opiate analgesics and sedatives (eg, diazepam) when taking this drug.
- Avoid driving and other activities requiring mental alertness or that are potentially dangerous until response to drug is known.
- Notify dentist or treating physician prior to surgery if taking this medication.
- Do not stop taking this drug without consulting treating physician.

Adverse reactions

- Common: drowsiness, dizziness, ataxia, confusion, nausea, vomiting, rash, blurred vision, nystagmus.
- Serious: worsening of seizures, bone marrow depression (including aplastic anemia), hepatitis, Stevens–Johnson syndrome, toxic epidermal necrolysis, CHF, heart block, arrhythmia.

Clinically important drug interactions

- Drugs that increase effects/toxicity of carbamazepine: isoniazid, cimetidine, diltiazem, verapamil, erythromycin, propoxyphene, danazol.
- Drugs that decrease effects/toxicity of carbamazepine: phenobarbital, phenytoin, primidone, theophylline.
- Carbamazepine increases effects/toxicity of following: primidone, clomipramine, lithium, phenytoin.
- Carbamazepine decreases effects/toxicity of following: phenytoin, warfarin, doxycycline, theophylline, alprazolam, rifampin, cisplatin, oral contraceptives, cyclosporine, clonazepam, valproic acid.

Parameters to monitor
- CBC with differential and platelets, liver enzymes.
- Serum drug levels (trough): Therapeutic: 4–12 µg/mL. Toxic: >15 µg/mL.
- Discontinue if signs of active liver disease or dysfunction appear.
- ECG.
- Kidney function tests before and after initiating drug treatment.
- Response to therapy.
- Signs and symptoms of bone marrow depression.
- EEG evaluation before and periodically after initiating drug treatment.
- Signs and symptoms of activation of psychosis.

Editorial comments
- Carbamazepine has not been shown to be efficacious for the treatment of myoclonic, akinetic, or absence seizures. Exacerbation of mixed type seizures with this agent has been seen in pediatric patients.
- Unlabeled uses for this medication include: relief of pain from trigeminal neuralgia or diabetic neuropathy, psychotic behavior associated with dementia, alcohol withdrawal, resistance schizophrenia, and bipolar disorders.

Carbenicillin

Brand name: Geocillin.
Class of drug: Antibiotic, penicillin family, carboxypenicillin.
Mechanism of action: Inhibits bacterial cell wall synthesis.
Susceptible organisms *in vivo*: Staphylococci, *Streptococcus pneumoniae,* beta-hemolytic streptococci, *Escherichia coli, Proteus mirabilis, Morganella morganii, Proteus vulgaris, Providencia rettgeri, Enterobacter* sp, *Pseudomonas aeruginosa.* Is destroyed by β-lactamases.

• Less effective than ampicillin against *Streptococcus pyogenes* (Group A), *Streptococcus pneumoniae, Enterococcus faecalis.* Most *Staphylococcus aureus* are resistant. Inactive against *Klebsiella.*

Indications/dosage/route: Oral only (to treat UTI and prostatitis due to aerobic gram-negative bacteria).

• UTIs due to *Escherichia coli, Proteus*
  – 382-764 mg q.i.d.
• UTIs caused by *Pseudomonas,* enterococci
  – 764 mg q.i.d.
• Prostatitis caused by *E. coli, Proteus mirabilis, Enterobacter,* enterococci
  – 764 mg q.i.d.

Adjustment of dosage

• Kidney disease: creatinine clearance 10–20 mL/min: dosage adjustment may be necessary, exact guidelines are not available; creatinine clearance <10 mL/min: therapeutic urine levels will not be achieved.
• Liver disease: Increase dosage.
• Elderly: None.
• Pediatric: Safety and efficacy have not been established.

Food: Take on empty stomach, 1 hour before or 2 hours after eating.

Pregnancy: Category B.

Lactation: No data available. Best to avoid.

Contraindications: Hypersensitivity to penicillin or cephalosporins.

Editorial comments: This was the first penicillin with activity against *Pseudomonas aeruginosa.* It is not used frequently because other more effective drugs are available. Oral carbenicillin is currently used to treat UTIs and prostatitis. The parenteral form is no longer available in the United States. In general, carbenicillin is not used in patients with kidney disease because of the requirement for large doses, increased toxicity, and the availability of better alternatives.

For additional alternatives see *penicillin* G, p. 708.

Carboplatin

Brand name: Paraplatin.
Class of drug: Alkylating antineoplastic agent.
Mechanism of action: Crosslinks DNA strands resulting in inhibition of strands to divide.
Indications/dosage/route: IV only.
- Initial and secondary treatment of ovarian carcinoma
  - Adults: Initial: 360 mg/m^2 q3wk, as single agent. In combination with cyclophosphamide: 300 mg/m^2 q4wk + 600 mg/m^2 cyclophosphamide. Intermittent courses generally repeated after neutrophil count ≥2000 mm^3, platelet count ≥100,000 mm^3.

(See Editorial Comments.)
Adjustment of dosage
- Bone marrow depression based on nadir blood counts: platelets <50,000 mm^3, neutrophils <500/mm^3: reduce dose by 25% of standard.
- Kidney disease: creatinine clearance between 41 and 59 mL/min: initial 250 mg/m^2; creatinine clearance between 16 and 40 mL/min: initial 200 mg/m^2; creatinine clearance 5 mL/min: avoid.
- Liver disease: None.
- Elderly: Possible higher risk for neurotoxicity. Consider dose reduction.
- Pediatric: Safety and efficacy have not been established.

Pregnancy: Category D.
Lactation: No data available. Do not breastfeed.
Contraindications: History of hypersensitivity to mannitol, carboplatin, or related compounds, severe bone marrow depression, acute bleeding.
Warnings/precautions
- Use with caution in patients with the following conditions: kidney disease, prior chemotherapy.

- Dose-limiting toxic effect of carboplatin is bone marrow depression.
- Blood transfusions may be required in patients on prolonged therapy.
- Avoid combining with potentially ototoxic or nephrotoxic agents such as aminoglycosides.
- Severe emesis may occur with administration of carboplatin.
- Do not use needles made of aluminum for injecting purpose.

Advice to patient

- Use two forms of birth control including hormonal and barrier methods.
- Carry out good personal oral hygiene.
- Drug may cause you to bruise easily.
- Maintain adequate fluid intake.
- Do not receive any vaccinations (particularly live attenuated viruses) without permission from treating physician.

Adverse reactions

- Common: nausea (10–18%), vomiting (65–80%), electrolyte abnormalities (see below), bone marrow depression (see below).
- Serious: **bone marrow depression (thrombocytopenia 60–70%), neutropenia (95%), anemia (88%), hypocalcemia, hypomagnesemia (30–60%), hyponatremia (10–50%), hypokalemia (10–50%),** neurotoxicity (only after prior cisplatin), nephrotoxicity, ototoxicity, cardiac failure, hepatitis, bleeding.

Clinically important drug interactions: Nephrotoxic agents, eg, aminoglycosides, aluminum increase effects/toxicity of carboplatin.

Parameters to monitor

- Serum electrolytes including calcium, magnesium, sodium, and potassium.
- CBC with differential and platelets, liver enzymes.
- Signs of hypersensitivity reaction.
- Signs and symptoms of bone marrow depression.
- Signs and symptoms of anemia.

- Signs and symptoms of neuropathy.
- Signs and symptoms of stomatitis. Treat with peroxide, tea, topical anesthetics such as benzocaine, lidocaine, or antifungal drug.

Editorial comments

- It is recommended that this drug be administered only by physicians who are well versed in the use of alkylating agents of this type.
- Use latex gloves and safety glasses when handling cytotoxic drugs. Avoid contact with skin as well as inhalation. If possible, prepare in biologic hood.
- This drug is also used widely in the treatment of lung cancer.
- The Calvert formula is commonly used to dose carboplatin: total dose (mg) – (target AUC) × (GFR + 25). This dosage calculation (in mg) is based on a target AUC of 4–6 mg/mL/min.

Carboprost

Brand name: Hemabate.

Class of drug: Oxytocic, postpartum hemostatic agent, abortant.

Mechanism of action: Oxytocic: stimulates uterine contraction by altering calcium transport. Uterine hemostatic: causes uterine contraction, which stops bleeding.

Indications/dosage/route: IM only.

- Abortion between 13th and 20th weeks
  - Adults: Initial: deep IM 250 μg. If ineffective, 250 μg at intervals of 1.5–3.5 hours. May be followed by 500 μg-doses. Total: 12 mg. Use no longer than 2 days.
- Postpartum hemorrhage
  - Adults: Deep IM 250 μg. Repeat dose at 15- to 90-minute intervals. Maximum: 2 mg.

Pregnancy: Category X.

Adjustment of dosage. None.

Contraindications: Hypersensitivity to carboprost, acute pelvic inflammatory disease.

Warnings/precautions

• Use with caution in patients with the following conditions: asthma, hypotension, renal or hepatic disease, diabetes, epilepsy, cardiac or adrenal disease. Also in patients with anemia, jaundice, uterine compromise. If abortion is incomplete use other measures to ensure expulsion of the fetus.

Advice to patient: Use two forms of birth control including hormonal and barrier methods.

• Avoid taking NSAIDs together with this drug.

Adverse reactions

• Common: vomiting, diarrhea, nausea.

• Serious: hypotension, hypertension, hematemesis, dystonia, asthma, respiratory distress, septic shock.

Clinically important drug interactions: Carboprost increases effects/toxicity of oxytocin and other oxytocic drugs.

Parameters to monitor

• Evaluate patient for orthostasis with BP measurements in the sitting, lying, and standing positions repeatedly before and after initiating therapy.

• For abdominal cramps, administer meperidine (Demerol).

Carisoprodol

Brand name: Soma.

Class of drug: Skeletal muscle relaxant.

Mechanism of action: Blocks interneuronal activity in spinal cord, and reticular formation, causing muscle relaxation (animal data).

Indications/dosage/route: Oral only.

• Acute painful musculoskeletal conditions
   – Adults, children >12 years: 350 mg t.i.d. and h.s.

Adjustment of dosage
- Kidney disease: Use with caution.
- Liver disease: Use with caution.
- Elderly: Use with caution.
- Pediatric: See above.

Onset of Action	Duration
30 min	4–6 h

Food: Administer with food if gastric upset occurs.
Pregnancy: Category C.
Lactation: Appears in breast milk. Best to avoid.
Contraindications: Hypersensitivity to carisoprodol, aspirin, or related compounds, eg, meprobamate; acute intermittant porphyria, bleeding disorders.

Warnings/precautions
- Use with caution in patients with the following conditions: kidney or liver disease, history of drug abuse.
- Psychologic dependence, although rare, may occur when used long term. Withdrawal symptoms have not been reported to occur if drug is stopped abruptly.
- An acute idiosyncratic effect of the first dose has been reported to occur rarely. This is characterized by weakness, quadriplegia, visual disturbance, confusion, dysarthria. These symptoms resolve after several hours. Close observation and supportive care are required if episode occurs.

Advice to patient
- This drug may cause dizziness and faintness especially at the beginning of use.
- Avoid alcohol and other CNS depressants such as opiate analgesics and sedatives (eg, diazepam) when taking this drug.
- Avoid driving and other activities requiring mental alertness or that are potentially dangerous until response to drug is known.

Adverse reactions
• Common: drowsiness, dizziness.
• Serious: allergic reactions characterized by skin eruption, erythema multiforme, asthma, angioneurotic edema, anaphylaxis; idiosyncratic reactions (see Warnings/Precautions), postural hypotension, bone marrow suppression.

Clinically important drug interactions: Drugs that increase effects/toxicity of carisprodol: CNS depressants (narcotic analgesies, antipsychotics, tricyclics, antianxiety drugs), and MAO inhibitors.

Parameters to monitor
• Signs of idiosyncratic and allergic reactions.
• CNS side effects: ataxia, tremor, vertigo, headache, syncope.

Carmustine

Brand name: BiCNU.
Class of drug: Alkylating antineoplastic agent.
Mechanism of action: Crosslinks DNA; metabolites interfere with DNA formation.
Indications/dosage/route: IV only.
• Brain tumors, Hodgkin's disease, multiple myeloma, non-Hodgkin's lymphoma
  – Adults: 150–200 mg/m^2, slow IV infusion; repeat in 6 weeks if platelet count >100,000/mm^3 and WBC >4000 mm^3.

Adjustment of dosage
• Leukocyte nadir 2000–3000 m^3, platelets 25,000–75,000 mm^3: reduce dose to 70% of standard; leukocytes <2000: reduce dose to 50% of standard.
• Kidney disease: None.
• Liver disease: None.
• Elderly: None.
• Pediatric: Safety and efficacy have not been established.

Pregnancy: Category D.

Lactation: No data available. Potentially toxic to infant. Avoid breastfeeding.

Contraindications: Hypersensitivity to carmustine, bone marrow depression from various causes including previous chemotherapy, previous resistance to the drug.

Warnings/precautions

- Use with caution in patients with the following conditions: history of seizures, head trauma, potential epileptogenic drugs, renal or hepatic disease, bone marrow depression.
- Drug should not be administered more often than every 6 weeks.
- Baseline pulmonary function testing is advisable.
- Children appear to be at extremely high risk for delayed-onset pulmonary fibrosis.

Advice to patient

- Use two forms of birth control including hormonal and barrier methods.
- Avoid alcohol.
- Receive any vaccinations (particularly live attenuated viruses) only with permission from treating physician.

Adverse reactions

- Common: nausea, vomiting, pain at infusion site, dizziness, ataxia, alopecia, flushing.
- Serious: **bone marrow depression especially cumulative thrombocytopenia**, renal failure, pulmonary fibrosis, hepatotoxicity, neuroretinitis, hypotension.

Clinically important drug interactions: Cimetidine, etoposide increase effects/toxicity of carmustine.

Parameters to monitor

- CBC with differential and platelets, serum BUN and creatinine, liver enzymes.
- Signs and symptoms of bone marrow depression.
- Signs and symptoms of pulmonary toxicity.
- Signs and symptoms of anemia.
- Intake of fluids and urinary and other fluid output to minimize renal toxicity. Closely monitor electrolyte levels.
- Signs of hyperuricemia: gouty arthritis, uric acid kidney stones.

- Signs and symptoms of hepatotoxicity.
- Signs and symptoms of renal toxicity.

Editorial comments

- It is essential to perform a complete hematologic evaluation every 2 weeks for patients on this drug. Clinicians should consult published protocols for current dosages of this and other chemotherapeutic agents as well as the method and sequence of drug administration.
- Use latex gloves and safety glasses when handling cytotoxic drugs. Avoid contact with skin as well as inhalation. If possible, prepare in biologic hood.

Carteolol

Brand name: Cartrol.

Class of drug: β-Adrenergic receptor blocker.

Mechanism of action: Competitive blocker of β-adrenergic receptors in heart and blood vessels.

Indications/dosage/route: Oral only.

- Hypertension
  - Adults: Initial: 2.5 mg/d. Maintenance: 2.5–5 mg/day. Maximum: 10 mg/d.
- Reduce frequency of anginal attacks
  - 10 mg/d.

Adjustment of dosage

- Kidney disease: creatinine clearance >60 mL/min: dose q24h; creatinine clearance >20–60 mL/min: dose q48h; creatinine clearance <20 mL/min: dose q72h.
- Liver disease: None.
- Elderly: None.
- Pediatric: Safety and efficacy have not been established.

Food: No restriction.

Pregnancy: Category C.

Lactation: Appears in breast milk. Potentially toxic to infant. Best to avoid.

Contraindications: Cardiogenic shock, asthma, CHF unless it is secondary to tachyarrhythmia treated with a β blocker, sinus bradycardia and AV block greater than first degree, severe COPD.

Editorial comments: For additional information, see *propranolol*, p. 790.

Cefaclor

Brand name: Ceclor.

Class of drug: Cephalosporin, second generation.

Mechanism of action: Binds to penicillin-binding proteins and disrupts or inhibits bacterial cell wall synthesis.

Susceptible organisms *in vivo*: Comparable to cefuroxime axetil, but less active against *Hemophilus influenzae* and *Moraxella catarrhalis*.

Indications/dosage/route: Oral only.

Capsules, oral suspension: all uses
  – Adults: 250 mg q8h.
  – Children: 20 mg/kg in divided doses q8h.
• More severe infections
  – Adults: 500 mg q8h.
  – Children: 40 mg/kg in divided doses q8h.
• Otitis media, pharyngitis
  – Children: give total daily dose q12h.

Extended-release tablets: all uses
• Acute exacerbations (bacterial), chronic bronchitis, secondary bacterial infections of acute bronchitis
  – Adults: 500 mg q12h, 10 days.
• Pharyngitis, tonsillitis
  – Adults: 375 mg q12h, 10 days.
• Uncomplicated skin and skin structure infections
  – Adults: 375 mg q12h, 7–10 days.

Adjustment of dosage
- Kidney disease: creatinine clearance <50 mL/min: 250–500 mg q8h; creatinine clearance 10–50 mL/min: 125–500 mg q8h.
- Liver disease: None.
- Elderly: None.
- Pediatric: See above.

Food: Take with yogurt or buttermilk (4 oz/d) to maintain bacterial flora and reduce the possibility of severe GI effects.

Pregnancy: Category B.

Lactation: Appears in breast milk. American Academy of Pediatrics considers cephalosporins to be compatible with breastfeeding.

Contraindications: Hypersensitivity to other cephalosporins or related antibiotics, eg, penicillin.

Warnings/precautions
- Use with caution in patients with the following condition: kidney disease.
- It is recommended to continue therapy for at least 2–3 days after symptoms are no longer present. For group A beta-hemolytic streptococcal infections, therapy should be continued for 10 days.
- Before use, determine if patient had previous hypersensitivity reaction to cephalosporins or penicillins. Incidence of cross-sensitivity to penicillins is 1–16%. A negative response to penicillin does not preclude allergic reaction to a cephalosporin.

Advice to patient: Allow at least 1 hour between taking this medication and a bacteriostatic antibiotic, eg, tetracycline or amphenicol.

Adverse reactions
- Common: none.
- Serious: hypersensitivity, serum sickness, hepatitis, confusion, bone marrow suppression, renal dysfunction, seizures.

Clinically important drug interactions: Cefaclor increases effects/toxicity of oral anticoagulants.

Parameters to monitor
- CBC with differential and platelets, serum BUN and creatinine, PT, PTT, and INR (if patient on anticoagulants).

- Serum glucose levels initially and periodically during therapy.
- Temperature for sign of drug-induced persistent fever.
- Signs and symptoms of antibiotic-induced bacterial or fungal superinfection.
- Signs and symptoms of renal toxicity.

Editorial comments: Cefuroxime is more effective than cefaclor for otitis media and pharyngitis due to improved coverage for *Hemophilus influenzae* and *Moraxella catarrhalis*.

Cefadroxil

Brand name: Duricef.
Class of drug: Cephalosporin, first generation.
Mechanism of action: Binds to penicillin-binding proteins and disrupts or inhibits bacterial cell wall synthesis.
Susceptible organisms *in vivo*: Similar to cephalexin.
Indications/dosage/route: Oral only.
- Pharyngitis, tonsillitis
  – Adults: 1 g/d in single or two divided doses for 10 days.
  – Children: 30 mg/kg/d in single or two divided doses.
- Skin and skin structure infections
  – Adults: 1 g/d in single or two divided doses.
  – Children: 30 mg/kg/d in divided doses.
- UTIs
  – Adults: 1–2 g/d in single or two divided doses for uncomplicated lower UTI (eg, cystitis). For all other UTIs, the usual dose is 2 g/d in two divided doses.
  – Children: 30 mg/kg/d in divided doses.

Adjustment of dosage
- Kidney disease: creatinine clearance <50 mL/min: no adjustment; creatinine clearance 25–50 mL/min: 12-hour intervals; creatinine clearance 10–25 mL/min: 24-hour intervals; creatinine clearance 0–10 mL/min: 36-hour intervals.
- Liver disease: None.
- Elderly: None.

• Pediatric: See above.

Food: Take with yogurt or buttermilk (4 oz/d) to maintain bacterial flora and reduce the possibility of severe GI effects.

Pregnancy: Category B.

Lactation: Appears in breast milk. American Academy of Pediatrics considers cephalosporins to be compatible with breast-feeding.

Contraindications: Hypersensitivity to other cephalosporins or related antibiotics, eg, penicillin.

Editorial comments

• Oral first-generation cephalosporins are used for *Staphylococcus aureus* and streptococcal infection when penicillins are to be avoided, generally due to rash. Common uses are cellulitis, other infections of the skin, osteomyelitis, streptococcal pharyngitis. They should not be used for sinusitis, otitis media, or lower respiratory infections because of poor coverage of *Streptococcus pneumoniae* and especially *Moraxella catarrhalis* and *Hemophilus influenzae*. They are not suitable coverage for bite wounds as they do not cover *Pasteurella multocida*.

• For additional information, see *cefuroxime*, p. 182.

Cefamandole

Brand name: Mandol.

Class of drug: Cephalosporin, second generation.

Mechanism of action: Binds to penicillin-binding proteins and disrupts or inhibits bacterial cell wall synthesis.

Susceptible organisms *in vivo*: Comparable to cefuroxime axetil, but less active against *Hemophilus influenzae* and *Moraxella catarrhalis*.

Indications/dosage/route: IV, IM (same dose both routes).

• Uncomplicated pneumonia, skin structure infections
  – Adults: 500 mg to 1 gm q4–8h.

• Uncomplicated UTIs

– Adults: 500 mg q8h.
• Severe infections
  – Adults: 1 g q4–6h.
• Life-threatening infections
  – Adults: 2 g q4h.
• Most infections
  – Children, infants: 50–100 mg/d, in equally divided doses q4–8h. Maximum: 150 mg/kg.

Adjustment of dosage
• Kidney disease: creatinine clearance 50–80 mL/min: less severe infections 0.75–1.5 g q6h, life-threatening infections 1.5 g q4h; creatinine clearance 25–50 mL/min: less severe infections 0.75–1.5 g q8h, life-threatening infections 1.5 g q6h, creatinine clearance 10–25 mL/min: less severe infections 0.5–1 g q8h, life-threatening infections 1 g q6h; creatinine clearance 2–10 mL/min: less severe infections 0.5–0.75 g q12h, life-threatening infections 0.67 g q8h; creatinine clearance <2 mL/min: less severe infections 0.25–0.5 g q12h, life-threatening infections 0.5 g q8h.
• Liver disease: None.
• Elderly: None.
• Pediatric: See above.

Food: Take with yogurt or buttermilk (4 oz/d) to maintain bacterial flora and reduce the possibility of severe GI effects.

Pregnancy: Category B.

Lactation: Appears in breast milk. American Academy of Pediatrics considers cephalosporins to be compatible with breastfeeding.

Contraindications: Hypersensitivity to other cephalosporins or related antibiotics, eg, penicillin.

Editorial comments
• Oral first-generation cephalosporins are used for *Staphylococcus aureus* and streptococcal infection when penicillins are to be avoided, generally due to rash. Common uses are cellulitis, other infections of the skin, osteomyelitis, streptococcal pharyngitis. They should not be used for sinusitis, otitis media, or lower respiratory infections because of poor coverage of *Strepto-coccus*

pneumoniae and especially *Moraxella catarrhalis* and *Hemophilus influenzae.* They are not suitable coverage for bite wounds as they do not cover *Pasteurella multocida.*

• For additional information, see *cefuroxime,* p. 182.

Cefazolin

Brand name: Ancef.
Class of drug: Cephalosporin, first generation, parenteral.
Mechanism of action: Binds to penicillin-binding proteins and disrupts or inhibits bacterial cell wall synthesis.
Susceptible organisms *in vivo*: Very effective against staphylococci and streptococci, potentially active against *Streptococcus pneumoniae*, active against *enterococci.* Not effective against MRSA. Gram-negative spectrum is limited to community-acquired *Escherichia coli, Moraxella catarrhalis,* indole-negative *Proteus mirabilis*, and some *Klebsiella pneumoniae.* Not useful against nosocomial gram-negative oral anaerobes.
Indications/dosage/route: IM, IV (same dose both routes).

• Mild infections
  – Adults: 250–500 mg q8h.
  – Children >1 month: 25–50 mg/kg/d in three to four doses.
• Moderate to severe infections
  – Adults: 0.5–1 g q6–8h.
• Acute, uncomplicated UTIs
  – Adults: 1 g q12h, severe infections, up to 100 mg/kg/d.
• Endocarditis, septicemia (especially staphylococci or streptococci when allergic to penicillin)
  – Adults: 1–1.5 g q6h (rarely, up to 12 g/d).
• Preoperative prophylaxis (not for procedures involving the colon, rectum, or appendix)
  – Adults: 1 g 30–60 min prior to surgery.
• Postoperative prophylaxis
  – Adults: 0.5–1 g q6–8h for 24 hours.

Adjustment of dosage
Kidney disease: creatinine clearance <10 mL/min: 250–500 mg q18–24h; creatinine clearance 11–34 mL/min: 250–500 mg q12h; creatinine clearance 35–54 mL/min: 500–1000 mg q8h.
• Liver disease: None.
• Elderly: None.
• Pediatric: See above.

Food: Not applicable.

Pregnancy: Category B.

Lactation: Appears in breast milk. American Academy of Pediatrics considers cephalosporins to be compatible with breastfeeding.

Contraindications: Hypersensitivity to other cephalosporins or related antibiotics, eg, penicillin.

Warnings/precautions
• Use with caution in patients with the following condition: kidney disease.
• It is recommended therapy be continued for at least 2–3 days after symptoms are no longer present. For group A beta-hemolytic streptococcal infections, therapy should be continued for 10 days.
• Before use, determine if patient had previous hypersensitivity reaction to cephalosporins or penicillins. Incidence of cross-sensitivity to penicillins is 1–16%. A negative response to penicillin does not preclude allergic reaction to a cephalosporin.

Advice to patient:
Allow at least 1 hour between taking this medication and a bacteriostatic antibiotic, eg, tetracycline or amphenicol.

Adverse reactions
• Common: None.
• Serious: Hypersensitivity reactions, seizures, confusion, bone marrow suppression, liver toxicity.

Clinically important drug interactions
• Drug that increases effects/toxicity of cefazolin: probenecid.
• Cefazolin increases effects/toxicity of following: furosemide.

Parameters to monitor
• CBC with differential and platelets, serum BUN and creatinine, liver enzymes.

- Temperature for sign of drug-induced persistent fever.
- Signs and symptoms of antibiotic-induced bacterial or fungal superinfection.
- Signs and symptoms of renal toxicity.
- Signs and symptoms of fluid retention, particularly in patients receiving sodium salts of cephalosporins.

Editorial comments

- Cefazolin is the prophylactic antibiotic of choice for surgery, foreign body implantation, and clean or clean/contaminated procedures (cardiac surgery, orthopedic device implantation, head and neck surgery with opening of the oropharyngeal mucosa, gastric surgery, biliary surgery, hysterectomy, cesarean section). It is not used for colon surgery because it does not cover *Bacteroides fragilis* or when MRSA is a likely pathogen in postsurgical infections.
- Parenteral cephalosporins do not give adequate CSF levels and, therefore, are not used in CNS infections.
- Effective against uncomplicated UTIs but other antibiotics are preferable.
- Not effective in nosocomial infections caused by gram-negative organisms (eg, UTI).

Cefdinir

Brand name: Omnicef.
Class of drug: Cephalosporin, third generation.
Mechanism of action: Binds to penicillin-binding proteins and disrupts or inhibits bacterial cell wall synthesis.
Susceptible organisms *in vivo*: Comparable to cefixime, but less active against gram-negative organisms.
Indications/dosage/route: Oral only.

- Community-acquired pneumonia, skin and skin structure infections
  - Adults, children >13 years: 300 mg q12h for 10 days.

- Acute exacerbations of chronic bronchitis, acute maxillary sinusitis, pharyngitis/tonsillitis
  - Adults, children >13 years: 300 mg q12h or 600 mg q24h for 10 days.
- Acute bacterial otitis media, acute maxillary sinusitis, pharyngitis/tonsillitis
  - Children 6–12 years: 7 mg/kg q12h or 14 mg/kg q24h for 10 days.
- Skin and skin structure infections
  - Children 6–12 years: 7 mg/kg q12h for 10 days.

Adjustment of dosage
- Kidney disease: creatinine clearance <30 mL/min: 300 mg, once/daily.
- Liver disease: None.
- Elderly: None.
- Pediatric: See above.

Food: Take with yogurt or buttermilk (4 oz/d) to maintain bacterial flora and reduce the possibility of severe GI effects.

Pregnancy: Category B.

Lactation: Apparently not present in breast milk. American Academy of Pediatrics considers cephalosporins to be compatible with breastfeeding.

Contraindications: Hypersensitivity to other cephalosporins or related antibiotics, eg, penicillin.

Editorial comments: For additional information, see *cefixime*, p. 163.

Cefepime

Brand name: Maxipime.

Class of drug: Cephalosporin, fourth generation (with antipseudomonal activity and improved gram-positive activity).

Mechanism of action: Binds to penicillin-binding proteins and disrupts or inhibits bacterial cell wall synthesis.

Susceptible organisms *in vivo*: Compared with ceftazidime, cefepime has much improved gram-positive coverage including *Staphylococcus aureus* (not MRSA), streptococci, *Streptococcus pneumoniae*; comparable *Pseudomonas aeruginosa* activity; superior activity against ESBL-producing Enterobacteriaceae.

Indications/dosage/route: IV (should be used in severe infections only), IM.

- Mild to moderate uncomplicated or complicated UTIs caused by *Escherichia coli, Klebsiella pneumoniae*, or *Proteus mirabilis* (should be used in severe infections only)
  – Adults, children >12 years: IV or IM 0.5–1 g q12h for 7–10 days.
- Severe UTIs caused by *E. coli* or *K. pneumoniae*
  – Adults, children >12 years: IV 2 g q12h for 10 days.
- Moderate to severe pneunomia caused by *S. pneumoniae, P. aeruginosa, K. pneumoniae*, or *Enterobacter* species
  – Adults, children >12 years: IV 1–2 g q12h for 10 days.
- Skin and skin structure infections caused by *S. aureus* or *Streptococcus pyogenes*
  – Adults, children >12 years: IV 2 g q12h for 10 days.
- Febrile neutropenia (severe infections caused by *Pseudomonas aeruginosa*)
  – IV 2 g q8h for 7 days.

Adjustment of dosage

- Kidney disease: creatinine clearance <60 mL/min: 500 mg q12h; creatinine clearance 30–60 mL/min: 500 mg q24h; creatinine clearance 11–29 mL/min: 500 mg q24h; creatinine clearance >10 mL/min: 250 mg q24h. At higher risk for CNS toxicity.
- Liver disease: None.
- Elderly: None.
- Pediatric: See above.

Food: Not applicable.

Pregnancy: Category B.

Lactation: Appears in breast milk. American Academy of Pediatrics considers cephalosporins to be compatible with breastfeeding.

Contraindications: Hypersensitivity to other cephalosporins or related antibiotics, eg, penicillin.

Warnings/precautions

- It is recommended to continue therapy for at least 2–3 days after symptoms are no longer present. For group A beta-hemolytic streptococcal infections, therapy should be continued for 10 days.
- Before use, determine if patient had previous hypersensitivity reaction to cephalosporins or penicillins. Incidence of cross-sensitivity to penicillins is 1–5%. A negative response to penicillin does not preclude allergic reaction to a cephalosporin.

Advice to patient: None.

Adverse reactions

- Common: Positive Coombs' test.
- Serious: encephalopathy, myoclonus, seizures, bone marrow suppression, hypersensitivity reactions, hepatitis, hemolytic anemia.

Clinically important drug interactions: Cefepime increases effects/toxicity of aminoglycosides, loop diuretics.

Parameters to monitor

- CBC with differential and platelets, serum BUN and creatinine, liver enzymes.
- Patient's temperature for signs of drug-induced persistent fever.
- Signs and symptoms of antibiotic-induced bacterial or fungal superinfection.
- Signs and symptoms of renal toxicity.
- Signs and symptoms of fluid retention, particularly in patients receiving sodium salts of cephalosporins.

Editorial comments

- Use of cefepime should be reserved to noscomial infections especially when constant gram-negative infections are suspected or proven (preferably).
- Also useful in neutropenic fever as monotherapy and in mixed infection, such as nosocomial pneumonia and line infections.

• Like all cephalosporins, cefepime does not cover enterococci and MRSA.

Cefixime

Brand name: Suprax.
Class of drug: Cephalosporin, third generation.
Mechanism of action: Binds to penicillin-binding proteins and disrupts or inhibits bacterial cell wall synthesis.
Susceptible organisms *in vivo*: Highly effective against beta-hemolytic streptococci, penicillin-susceptible *Streptococcus pneumoniae, Hemophilus influenzae, Moraxella catarrhalis, Neisseria gonorrhoeae*, and many Enterobacteriaceae. Poor activity against *Staphylococcus aureus*.
Indications/dosage/route: Oral only.
• Uncomplicated UTIs, otitis media, pharyngitis, tonsillitis, acute bronchitis, acute exacerbations of or chronic bronchitis
  – Adults: 400 mg once daily or 200 mg q12h.
  – Children: 8 mg/kg/d or 4 mg/kg q12h.
• Uncomplicated gonorrhea
  – 400 mg/d.
Adjustment of dosage
• Kidney disease: creatinine clearance <60 mL/min: standard dosage; creatinine clearance 21–60 mL/min: 75% of standard dosage; creatinine clearance >20 mL/min: 50% of standard dosage.
• Liver disease: None.
• Elderly: None.
• Pediatric: See above.
Food: Take with yogurt or buttermilk (4 oz/d) to maintain bacterial flora and reduce the possibility of severe GI effects.
Pregnancy: Category B.
Lactation: No data available. American Academy of Pediatrics considers cephalosporins compatible with breastfeeding.

Contraindications: Hypersensitivity to other cephalosporins or related antibiotics, eg, penicillin.

Warnings/precautions
- Use with caution in patients with the following condition: kidney disease.
- It is recommended to continue therapy for at least 2–3 days after symptoms are no longer present. For group A beta-hemolytic streptococcal infections, therapy should be continued for 10 days.
- Before use, determine if patient had previous hypersensitivity reaction to cephalosporins or penicillins. Incidence of cross–sensitivity to penicillins is 1–16%. A negative response to penicillin does not preclude allergic reaction to a cephalosporin.

Advice to patient: Allow at least 1 hour between taking this medication and a bacteriostatic antibiotic, eg, tetracycline or amphenicol.

Adverse reactions
- Common: diarrhea, other GI symptoms.
- Serious: pseudomembranous colitis, hypersensitivity reactions, hepatitis, nephrotoxicity, bone marrow suppression, increased PT, seizures.

Clinically important drug interactions: Cefixime increases effects/toxicity of carbamazepine.

Parameters to monitor
- CBC with differential and platelets, PT, serum BUN and creatinine, liver enzymes.
- Temperature for signs of drug-induced persistent fever.
- Signs and symptoms of antibiotic-induced bacterial or fungal superinfection.
- Signs and symptoms of renal toxicity.
- Signs and symptoms of fluid retention, particularly in patients receiving sodium salts of cephalosporins.

Editorial comments: Uses of cefixime include single-dose therapy of gonorrhea, upper and lower respiratory infections, UTIs, respiratory infections, COPD exacerbators.

Cefoperazone

Brand name: Cefobid.

Class of drug: Cephalosporin, third generation.

Mechanism of action: Binds to penicillin-binding proteins and disrupts or inhibits bacterial cell wall synthesis.

Susceptible organisms *in vivo*: Has activity against >50% of *Pseudomonas aeruginosa* strains but is less effective than cefotaxime and ceftriaxone against gram-positive and gram-negative bacteria other than *P. aeruginosa*.

Indications/dosage/route: IV, IM.

• Respiratory tract infections, peritonitis and other intraabdominal infections, bacterial septicemia, skin and skin structure infections, pelvic inflammatory disease, UTIs.

   – Adults: 2–4 g/d in equally divided doses. Maximum: 12–16 g/d.

Adjustment of dosage

• Kidney disease: None.

• Liver disease: Advanced cirrhosis: 50% of usual dose. Maximum: 4 g/d.

• Elderly: None.

• Pediatric: Safety and efficacy have not been established.

Food: Not applicable.

Pregnancy: Category B.

Lactation: Appears in breast milk. American Academy of Pediatrics considers cephalosporins to be compatible with breastfeeding.

Contraindications: Hypersensitivity to other cephalosporins or related antibiotics, eg, penicillin.

Editorial comments

• Monitor PT for coagulation abnormalities.

• This drug significantly inhibits vitamin K activation.

• A disulfiram-like effect occurs when cefoperazone is combined with alcohol.

• For additional information, see *ceftriaxone axetil*, p. 180.

Cefotaxime

Brand name: Claforan.
Class of drug: Cephalosporin, third generation.
Mechanism of action: Binds to penicillin-binding proteins and disrupts or inhibits bacterial cell wall synthesis.

Susceptible organisms *in vivo*

- Gram-positive: excellent against streptococci and *Streptococcus pneumoniae*. Does not cover staphylococci and *Enterococcus*.
- Gram-negative: excellent against *Neisseria meningitidis, Neisseria gonorrhoeae, Escherichia coli, Proteus mirabilis, Klebsiella pneumoniae, Morganella* sp.

Indications/dosage/route: IV, IM.

- Gonococcal urethritis
  - Adults, males and females: IM 0.5 g, single dose.
- Rectal gonorrhea
  - Adults, female: IM 0.5 g, single dose.
  - Adults, male: IM 1 g, single dose.
- Disseminated gonococcal infection
  - IV 500 mg, 4 times/d (CDC recommendation).
- Uncomplicated infections
  - Adults: IM or IV 1 g q12h.
- Moderate to severe infections
  - Adults: IM or IV 1–2 g q8h.
- Septicemia
  - Adults: IV, 2 g q6–8h.
- Life-threatening infections
  - Adults: IV 2 g q4h.
- Pediatric patients, uncomplicated infections
  - Infants 0–1 wk: IV 50 mg/kg q12h.
  - Infants 1–4 wks: IV 50 mg/kg q8h.
  - Children 1 month to 12 years: IV or IV 50–100 mg/kg/d in 4–6 divided doses.

Adjustment of dosage
- Kidney disease: creatinine clearance <20 mL/min: reduce dose by 50%.
- Liver disease: None.
- Elderly: None.
- Pediatric: See above.

Food: Not applicable.

Pregnancy: Category B.

Lactation: Appears in breast milk. American Academy of Pediatrics considers cephalosporins to be compatible with breastfeeding.

Contraindications: Hypersensitivity to other cephalosporins or related antibiotics, eg, penicillin.

Warnings/precautions
- It is recommended to continue therapy for at least 2–3 days after symptoms are no longer present. For group A beta-hemolytic streptococcal infections, therapy should be continued for 10 days.
- Before use, determine if patient had previous hypersensitivity reaction to cephalosporins or penicillins. Incidence of cross-sensitivity to penicillins is 1–16%. A negative response to penicillin does not preclude allergic reaction to a cephalosporin.

Advice to patient: None.

Adverse reactions
- Common: None.
- Serious: bone marrow suppression, hepatitis, nephrotoxicity.

Clinically important drug interactions
- Drug that increases effects/toxicity of cefotaxime: probenecid.
- Cefotetan increases effects/toxicity of following: aminoglycosides, loop diuretics.

Parameters to monitor
- CBC with differential and platelets, serum BUN and creatinine, liver enzymes.
- Temperature for signs of drug-induced persistent fever.
- Signs and symptoms of antibiotic-induced bacterial or fungal superinfection.
- Use with caution in patient with penicillin allergy, kidney disease.

- Signs and symptoms of renal toxicity.
- Signs and symptoms of fluid retention, particularly in patients receiving sodium salts of cephalosporins.

Editorial comments

- Cefotaxime is used similarly to ceftriaxone except less useful for home antibiotic therapy because of the higher frequency of dosing.
- Useful in liver transplant patients because hepatobiliary toxicity is rare.

Cefotetan

Brand name: Cefotan.

Class of drug: Cephalosporin, second generation (a cephamycin, like cefoxitin, and not a true cephalosporin).

Mechanism of action: Binds to penicillin-binding proteins and disrupts or inhibits bacterial cell wall synthesis.

Susceptible organisms *in vivo*

- As compared with first-generation cefazolin and second-generation true cephalosporins, less active against gram-positive organisms, more active against gram-negative organisms. More active against anaerobes, especially *Bacteroides fragilis.*
- As compared with cefoxitin, not as active against *Bacteroides* of the "DOT" group: *B. distasoris, B. ovatus, B. thetacotaomicron.* More active against gram-negative organisms. Less effective against *Hemophilus influenzae* than cefuroxime.

Indications/dosage/route: IV, IM.

- UTIs
  - Adults: IV or IM 500 mg q12h or 1–2 g q24h.
- Skin and structure infections, mild to moderate
  - Adults: IV 2 g q24h or IV, IM 1 g q12h.
  - Severe infections: Adults: IV 2 g q12h.
- Infections at other sites, mild to moderate
  - Adults: IV or IM 1 or 2 g q12h.

  – Severe infections: IV 2 g q12h.
  – Life-threatening infections: IV 3 g q12h.

Adjustment of dosage

• Kidney disease: creatinine clearance <30 mL/min: usual recommended dose q12h; creatinine clearance 10–30 mL/min: usual recommended dose q24h; creatinine clearance >10 mL/min: usual recommended dose q48h.
• Liver disease: None.
• Elderly: None.
• Pediatric: Safety and efficacy have not been established.

Food: Not applicable.

Pregnancy: Category B.

Lactation: Appears in breast milk. American Academy of Pediatrics considers cephalosporins to be compatible with breastfeeding.

Contraindications: Hypersensitivity to other cephalosporins or related antibiotics, eg, penicillin.

Warnings/precautions

• Use with caution in patients with the following condition: kidney disease.
• It is recommended to continue therapy for at least 2–3 days after symptoms are no longer present. For group A beta-hemolytic streptococcal infections, therapy should be continued for 10 days.
• Before use, determine if patient had previous hypersensitivity reaction to cephalosporins or penicillins. Incidence of cross-sensitivity to penicillins is 1–16%. A negative response to penicillin does not preclude allergic reaction to a cephalosporin.

Advice to patient: None.

Adverse reactions

• Common: None.
• Serious: hypersensitivity reactions, anaphylaxis, nephrotoxicity, bone marrow suppression, thrombocytosis, hemolytic anemia, pseudomembranous colitis, seizures.

Clinically important drug interactions: Cefotetan increases effects/toxicity of aminoglycosides.

Parameters to monitor
- Serum BUN and creatinine, CBC with differential and platelets, PT, liver enzymes.
- Bleeding due to MTT chain.
- Patient's temperature for signs of drug-induced persistent fever.
- Signs and symptoms of antibiotic-induced bacterial or fungal superinfection.
- Signs and symptoms of renal toxicity.
- Signs and symptoms of fluid retention, particularly in patients receiving sodium salts of cephalosporins.

Editorial comment
- Cefotetan is used in antibiotic prophylaxis of colorectal surgery and appendectomy because of its superiority to cefazolin in these settings (better anaerobic and gram-negative coverage).
- Cefotetan has a MTT chain that inhibits the activator of vitamin K, causing occasional bleeding with prolonged use.
- Cefotetan is effective in treating diabetic foot infection, pelvic inflammatory disease (with doxycycline), gonorrhea, intrabdominal infections, pelvic infections, infected decubitus ulcer. Avoid in nosocomial infections.

Cefoxitin

Brand name: Mefoxin.
Class of drug: Cephalosporin, second generation (a cephamycin, like cefotetan, and not a true cephalosporin).
Mechanism of action: Binds to penicillin-binding proteins and disrupts or inhibits bacterial cell wall synthesis.
Susceptible organisms *in vivo*: Comparable to cefotetan, except cefoxitin covers *Bacteroides* species. Not as effective as cefotetan against gram-negative organisms.
Indications/dosage/route: IV, IM.
- Uncomplicated infections (pneumonia, UTI, cutaneous)
  - Adults: IV, 1 g q6–8h.

- Infants >3 months, children, mild to moderate infections: IV, IM 80–100 mg/kg, divided doses q4–6h.
- Moderately severe or severe infections
  - Adults: IV 1 g q2h or 2 g q6–8h.
- Severe infections
  - Adults: IV 2 g q4h or 3 g q6h.
  - Infants >3 months, children: IV, IM 100–160 mg/kg, divided doses q4–6h. Maximum: 12 g/d.
- Gonorrhea
  - Adults: IM 2 g with 1 g probenecid PO.
- Prophylaxis in surgery
  - Adults: IV 2 g 30–60 min before surgery, then 2 g q6h for 24 hours only.
- Cesarean section, prophylaxis
  - IV, 2 g when cord is clamped, then 2 doses IV 4 and 8 hours later.

Adjustment of dosage
- Kidney disease: Creatinine clearance 30–50 mL/min: 1–2 g q8–12h; creatinine clearance 10–29 mL/min: 1–2 g q12–24h; creatinine clearance 5–9 mL/min: 0.5–1 g q12–24h; creatinine clearance >5 mL/min: 0.5–1 g q24–48h.
- Liver disease: None.
- Elderly: None.
- Pediatric: See above.

Food: Not applicable.

Pregnancy: Category B.

Lactation: Appears in breast milk. American Academy of Pediatrics considers cephalosporins to be compatible with breastfeeding.

Contraindications: Hypersensitivity to other cephalosporins or related antibiotics, eg, penicillin.

Warnings/precautions
- Use with caution in patients with the following condition: kidney disease.
- It is recommended to continue therapy for at least 2–3 days after symptoms are no longer present. For group A beta-hemolytic streptococcal infections, therapy should be continued for 10 days.

- Before use, determine if patient had previous hypersensitivity reaction to cephalosporins or penicillins. Incidence of cross-sensitivity to penicillins is 1–16%. A negative response to penicillin does not preclude allergic reaction to a cephalosporin.

Advice to patient: Allow at least 1 hour between taking this medication and a bacteriostatic antibiotic, eg, tetracycline or amphenicol.

Adverse reactions
- Common: None.
- Serious: hypersensitivity reactions, pseudomembranous colitis, hepatotoxicity, renal toxicity, bone marrow suppression, seizures.

Clinically important drug interactions: Cefoxitin increases the effects/toxicity of aminoglycosides, loop diuretics.

Parameters to monitor
- CBC with differential and platelets, serum BUN and creatinine, liver enzymes.
- Temperature for sign of drug-induced persistent fever.
- Signs and symptoms of antibiotic-induced bacterial or fungal superinfection.
- Signs and symptoms of renal toxicity.
- Signs and symptoms of fluid retention, particularly in patients receiving sodium salts of cephalosporins.

Editorial comments: Uses for cefoxitin are similar to those for cefotetan.

Cefpodoxime

Brand name: Vantin.
Class of drug: Cephalosporin, third generation.
Mechanism of action: Binds to penicillin-binding proteins and disrupts or inhibits bacterial cell wall synthesis.

Susceptible organisms *in vivo*: Comparable to cefixime with, however, moderate antistaphlococcal activity.

Indications/dosage/route: Oral only.

• Acute community-acquired pneumonia
  – Adults, children >13 years: 200 mg q12h for 14 days.
• Exacerbations of chronic bronchitis
  – Adults, children >13 years: 200 mg q12h for 10 days.
• Gonorrhea and rectal gonococcal infections (women)
  – Adults, children >13 years: single dose of 200 mg/d.
• Skin and skin structure infections
  – Adults, children >13 years: 400 mg q12h for 7–14 days.
• Pharyngitis, tonsillitus
  – Adults, children >13 years: 100 mg q12h for 5–10 days.
  – Children 5 months–12 years: 5 mg/kg q12h. Maximum: 200 mg/d for 5–10 days.
• Uncomplicated UTIs
  – Adults, children >13 years: 100 mg q12h for 7 days.
• Acute otitis media
  – Children 5 months–12 years: 5 mg/kg q12h or 10 mg/kg q24h for 10 days.

Adjustment of dosage

• Kidney disease: Creatinine clearance <30 mL/min: dosing interval 24 hours.
• Liver disease: None.
• Elderly: None.
• Pediatric: See above.

Food: Take with yogurt or buttermilk (4 oz/d) to maintain bacterial flora and reduce the possibility of severe GI effects.

Pregnancy: Category B.

Lactation: Appears in breast milk. American Academy of Pediatrics considers cephalosporins to be compatible with breast-feeding.

Contraindications: Hypersensitivity to other cephalosporins or related antibiotics, eg, penicillin.

Editorial comments: For additional information, see *cefixime*, p. 163.

Cefprozil

Brand name: Cefzil.
Class of drug: Cephalosporin, second generation.
Mechanism of action: Binds to penicillin-binding proteins and disrupts or inhibits bacterial cell wall synthesis.
Susceptible organisms *in vivo*: Comparable to cefuroxime axetil, but less effective against *Hemophilus influenzae* and *Moraxella catarrhalis*.
Indications/dosage/route: Oral only.

• Pharyngitis, tonsillitis
  – Adults, children >13 years: 500 mg q24h for at least 10 days.
  – Children 2–12 years: 7.5 mg/kg q12h for at least 10 days.
• Acute sinusitis (cefuroxime axetil preferred)
  – Adults, children >13 years: 250 mg q12h or 500 mg q12h for 10 days.
  – Children 6 months–12 years: 7.5 mg/kg q12h or 15 mg/kg q12h for 10 days.
• Acute bronchitis and acute bacterial exacerbation of chronic bronchitis
  – Adults, children >13 years: 500 mg q12h for 10 days.
• Skin and skin structure infections
  – Adults, children >13 years: 250–500 mg q12h.
  – Children 2–12 years: 20 mg/kg q24h for 10 days.
• Otitis media (cefuroxime axetil preferred)
  – Infants, children 6 months–12 years: 15 mg/kg q12h for 10 days.

Adjustment of dosage

• Kidney disease: Creatinine clearance 30–120 mL/min: standard dosage; creatinine clearance 0–30 mL/min: 50% of standard dosage.
• Liver disease: None.
• Elderly: None.
• Pediatric: See above.

Food: Take with yogurt or buttermilk (4 oz/d) to maintain bacterial flora and reduce the possibility of severe GI effects.

Pregnancy: Category B.
Lactation: Appears in breast milk. American Academy of Pediatrics considers cephalosporins to be compatible with breast-feeding.
Contraindications: Hypersensitivity to other cephalosporins or related antibiotics, eg, penicillin.
Editorial comments: For additional information, see *cefuroxime*, p. 182.

Ceftazidime

Brand names: Fortaz, Tazicef, Tazidime.
Class of drug: Cephalosporin, third generation with antipseudomonal activitiy.
Mechanism of action: Binds to penicillin-binding proteins and disrupts or inhibits bacterial cell wall synthesis.
Susceptible organisms *in vivo*
• Excellent activity against gram-negative bacteria including *Pseudomonas aeruginosa*.
• Poor antistaphylococcal activity.
• Poor activity against *Bacteroides fragilis*.
• Not as effective as cefotaxime and ceftriaxone against *Streptococcus pneumoniae* and other streptococci.
Indications/dosage/route: IV, IM.
• Most infections
 – Neonates (0–4 weeks): IV 30 mg/kg q12h.
 – Infants and children 1 month–12 years: IV 30–60 mg/kg q8h. Maximum: 6 g.
• Uncomplicated UTIs
 – Adults: IV or IM 250 mg q12h.
• Complicated UTIs
 – Adults: IV or IM 500 mg q8–12h.
• Bone and joint infections
 – Adults: IV 2 g q12h.

- Uncomplicated pneumonia, mild skin and skin structure infections
  – Adults: IV or IM 500 mg–1 g q8h.
- Serious gynecologic and intraabdominal infections, meningitis, severe life-threatening infections
  – Adults: IV 2 g q8h.

Adjustment of dosage

- Kidney disease: Creatinine clearance 31–50 mL/min: 1 g q12h; creatinine clearance 16–30 mL/min: 1 g q24h; creatinine clearance 6–15 mL/min: 500 mg q24h; creatinine clearance >5 mL/min: 500 mg q48h.
- Liver disease: None.
- Elderly: None.
- Pediatric: See above.

Food: Not applicable.

Pregnancy: Category B.

Lactation: Appears in breast milk. American Academy of Pediatrics considers cephalosporins to be compatible with breastfeeding.

Contraindications: Hypersensitivity to other cephalosporins or related antibiotics, eg, penicillin.

Warnings/precautions

- Use with caution in patients with the following condition: kidney disease.
- It is recommended to continue therapy for at least 2–3 days after symptoms are no longer present. For group A beta-hemolytic streptococcal infections, therapy should be continued for 10 days.
- Before use, determine if patient had previous hypersensitivity reaction to cephalosporins or penicillins. Incidence of cross-sensitivity to penicillins is 1–16%. A negative response to penicillin does not preclude allergic reaction to a cephalosporin.

Advice to patient:

Allow at least 1 hour between taking this medication and a bacteriostatic antibiotic, eg, tetracycline or amphenicol.

Adverse reactions

- Common: None.

- Serious: hypersensitivity reactions, bone marrow suppression, hemolytic anemia, pseudomembranous colitis, nephrotoxicity.

Clinically important drug interactions
- Drugs that decrease the effects/toxicity of ceftazidime: chloramphenical.
- Ceftazidime increases effects/toxicity of following drugs: aminoglycosides, loop diuretics.

Parameters to monitor
- CBC with differential and platelets, serum BUN and creatinine, liver enzymes.
- Temperature for sign of drug-induced persistent fever.
- Signs and symptoms of antibiotic-induced bacterial or fungal superinfection.
- Signs and symptoms of renal toxicity.
- Signs and symptoms of fluid retention, particularly in patients receiving sodium salts of cephalosporins.

Editorial comments
- Ceftazidime has excellent antipseudomonal activity (better than all other cephalosporins except for cefepime). It is used mainly for the coverage of *P. aeruginosa*, either empirically (as in neutropenic fever nosocomial pneumonia) or based on culture and susceptibility.
- It is combined with an aminoglycoside in severe *Pseudomonas* infections.

Ceftibuten

Brand name: Cedax.
Class of drug: Cephalosporin, third generation.
Mechanism of action: Binds to penicillin-binding proteins and disrupts or inhibits bacterial cell wall synthesis.
Susceptible organisms *in vivo*
- Not active against *Staphylococcus aureus*.

- Poor activity against *Streptococcus pneumoniae* and *Moraxella catarrhalis*.
- Very active against Enterobacteriaceae.

Indications/dosage/route: Oral only.

- Acute bacterial infections as indicated above
  - Adults, children >12 years: 400 mg/d for 10 days. Maximum daily dose: 400 mg.

Adjustment of dosage

- Kidney disease: Creatinine clearance <50 mL/min: 9 mg/kg or 500 mg q24h (normal dosing schedule); creatinine clearance 30–49 mL/min: 4.5 mg/kg or 200 mg q24h; creatinine clearance 5–29 mL/min: 2.25 mg/kg or 100 mg q24h.
- Liver disease: None.
- Elderly: None.
- Pediatric: See above.

Food: Take with yogurt or buttermilk (4 oz/d) to maintain bacterial flora and reduce the possibility of severe GI effects.

Pregnancy: Category B.

Lactation: No data available. American Academy of Pediatrics considers cephalosporins to be compatible with breastfeeding.

Contraindications: Hypersensitivity to other cephalosporins or related antibiotics, eg, penicillin.

Editorial comments

- Use of ceftibuten is limited to Enterobacteriaceae infection, eg, UTI, bacterial colitis, epiglottis.
- For additional information see *cefuroxime*, p. 182.

Ceftizoxime

Brand name: Cefizox.
Class of drug: Cephalosporin, third generation.
Mechanism of action: Binds to penicillin-binding proteins and disrupts or inhibits bacterial cell wall synthesis.

Susceptible organisms *in vivo*: Spectrum similar to those of cefotaxime and ceftriaxone except that it is less potent against *Streptococcus pneumoniae* (therefore not indicated for meningitis) and it has more anaerobic activity including a majority of strains of *Bacteroides fragilis.*

Indications/dosage/route: IM, IV.

- Uncomplicated UTIs
  - Adults: IM, IV 0.5 g q12h.
- Severe or resistant infections
  - Adults: IM, IV 1 g q8h or 2 g q8–12h.
- Life-threatening infections
  - Adults: IV 3–4 q8h.
- Pelvic inflammatory disease
  - Adults: IV 2 g q8h.
- Infections or other sites
  - Adults: IM, IV 1 g q8–12h.
- Gonorrhea
  - Adults: IM 1 g as a single dose.
- Children: all uses

Adjustment of dosage

- Kidney disease: Creatinine clearance 50–79 mL/min: less severe infections 500 mg q8h; life-threatening infections 750 mg–1.5 g q8h; creatinine clearance 5–49 mL/min: less severe infections 250–500 mg q12h; life-threatening infections 500 mg–1 g q12h; creatinine clearance 0–4 mL/min: less severe infections 500 mg q48h or 250 mg q24h, life-threatening infections 500 mg–1 g q48h or 500 mg q24h.
- Liver disease: None.
- Elderly: None.
- Pediatric: Children >6 months: 50 mg/kg q6–8h. Maximum: 200 mg/kg/d. Dose not to exceed maximum adult dose.

Food: Not applicable.

Pregnancy: Category B.

Lactation: Appears in breast milk. American Academy of Pediatrics considers cephalosporins to be compatible with breastfeeding.

Contraindications: Hypersensitivity to other cephalosporins or related antibiotics, eg, penicillin.

Editorial comments

• Ceftizoxime has significant anaerobic activity. However, up to one third of *Bacteroides fragilis* colonies are resistant.

• It does not cover *Pseudomonas*.

• It is also not indicated in bacterial meningitis because of its weaker activity against *Streptococcus pneumoniae,* but is otherwise adequate for *Neisseria meningitidis* and *Streptococcus pneumoniae*.

• For additional information, see c*eftriaxone*, p. 180.

Ceftriaxone

Brand name: Rocephin.

Class of drug: Cephalosporin, third generation.

Mechanism of action: Binds to penicillin-binding proteins and disrupts or inhibits bacterial cell wall synthesis.

Susceptible organisms *in vivo*

• Gram positive: excellent against streptococci and *Streptococcus pneumoniae*. Does not cover staphylococci and *Enterococcus*.

• Gram negative: excellent against *Neisseria meningitidis, Neisseria gonorrhoeae, Escherichia coli, Proteus mirabilis, Klebsiella pneumoniae, Morganella*.

Indications/dosage/route: IV or IM.

• General infections

– Adults: IV, IM 1–2 g/d q24h. Maximum: 4 g/d.

– Children, other than meningitis: IV, IM 50–75 mg/d in divided doses. Maximum: 2 g/d.

• Meningitis

– Adults: IV, IM 2 g/d q12h (or 1 g/d q12h).

– Children: IV, IM 100 mg/kg/d, once daily or 2 doses/d. Maximum: 4 g/d. Usual duration of therapy: 7–14 days.

• Serious miscellaneous infections other than meningitis including skin and skin structure infections

– Children: IV, IM 50–75 mg/kg/d, divided doses q12h. Maximum: 2 g/d.
- Acute otitis media (bacterial)
  – Children: IM 50 mg/kg as single dose. Maximum: 1 g.
  – Uncomplicated gonorrhea
  – Adults: IM 250 mg as single dose.

Adjustment of dosage: None.

Food: Not applicable.

Pregnancy: Category B.

Lactation: Appears in breast milk. American Academy of Pediatrics considers cephalosporins to be compatible with breastfeeding.

Contraindications: Hypersensitivity to other cephalosporins or related antibiotics, eg, penicillin.

Warnings/precautions
- Use with caution in patients with the following conditions: kidney disease, penicillin allergy, elderly.
- Avoid in orthotopic liver transplant because of the risk of biliary sludge formation.
- It is recommended to continue therapy for at least 2–3 days after symptoms are no longer present. For group A beta-hemolytic streptococcal infections, therapy should be continued for 10 days.
- Before use, determine if patient had previous hypersensitivity reaction to cephalosporins or penicillins. Incidence of cross-sensitivity to penicillins is 1–16%. A negative response to penicillin does not preclude allergic reaction to a cephalosporin.
- Watch bilirubin levels if the use is prolonged.

Advice to patient: None.

Adverse reactions
- Common: None.
- Serious: hepatitis, hypersensitivity reactions, pseudomembranous colitis, nephrotoxicity, bone marrow suppression, hemolytic anemia.

Clinically important drug interactions
- Drug that increases effects/toxicity of ceftriaxone: probenecid.

- Ceftriaxone increases effects/toxicity of following drugs: aminoglycosides, loop diuretics.

Parameters to monitor

- CBC with differential and platelets, serum BUN and creatinine, liver enzymes.
- Temperature for sign of drug-induced persistent fever.
- Signs and symptoms of antibiotic-induced bacterial or fungal superinfection.
- Signs and symptoms of renal toxicity.
- Signs and symptoms of fluid retention, particularly in patients receiving sodium salts of cephalosporins.

Editorial comments

- Uses for ceftriaxone are as follows: Acute bacterial meningitis: effective against *Neisseria meningitidis*, *Hemophilus influenzae*, and, most importantly, *Streptococcus pneumoniae* even when not susceptible to penicillin. It does not cover *Listeria*. Community-acquired pneumonia: effective against all important pathogens other than atypical organisms for which a macrolide or a quinolone is added (*Legionella, Mycloplasma, Chlamydia*). Nosocomial infection, eg, pneumonia; not recommended as monotherapy because of resistance from *Pseudomonas aeruginosa* and ESBL-producing Enterobacteriaceae.
- A great advantage of ceftriaxone is once-a-day use (other than in meningitis). It is therefore often used for home IV infusion.

Cefuroxime

Brand names: Ceftin, Kefurox, Zinacef.
Class of drug: Cephalosporin, second generation.
Mechanism of action: Binds to penicillin-binding proteins and disrupts or inhibits bacterial cell wall synthesis.
Susceptible organisms *in vivo*: *Staphylococcus aureus, Streptococcus pneumoniae*, beta-hemolytic streptococci, gram-negative

organisms (especially *Hemophilus influenzae, Moraxella catarrhalis, Escherichia coli, Proteus mirabilis, Klebsiella, Citrobacter, Morganella, Neisseria gonorrhoeae, Neisseria meningitidis.*

Indications/dosage/route: Oral, IV, IM.

Cefuroxime axetil tablets

- Pharyngitis, tonsillitis
  - Adults, children >13 years: 250 mg q12h for 10 days.
  - Children, under 3 years: 125 mg q12h for 10 days.
- Exacerbations of chronic bronchitis, secondary bacterial infections of acute bronchitis, uncomplicated skin and skin structure infections
  - Adults, children >13 years: 250 or 500 mg q12h for 10 days.
- Uncomplicated UTIs (other agents more cost effective)
  - Adults, children >13 years: 125 or 250 mg q12h for 7–10 days.
  - Children <12 years: 125 mg b.i.d.
- Acute otitis media
  - Children: 250 mg b.i.d. for 10 days.
- Uncomplicated gonorrhea
  - Adults, children >13 years: 1000 mg as a single dose.
- Early Lyme disease (alternative treatment, doxycycline is first line)
  - 500 mg/d for 20 days.

Cefuroxime suspension

- Pharyngitis, tonsillitis
  - Children 3 months–12 years: 20 mg/kg/d in 2 divided doses. Maximum: 500-mg total dose/d, for 10 days.
- Acute otitis media, impetigo
  - Children 3 months–12 years: 30 mg/kg/d in 2 divided doses. Maximum: 1000-mg total dose/d, for 10 days.

Cefuroxime sodium

- UTI, uncomplicated pneumonia, disseminated gonococcal, skin and skin structure infections
  - Adults: IV, IM 750 mg q8h.
  - Children >3 months: IV, IM 50–100 mg/kg/d in divided doses q6–8h (not to exceed adult dose of severe infections).

- Severe complicated infections, bone and joint infections
  – Adults: IV, IM 1.5 g q8h.
  – Children >3 months: IV 150 mg/kg/d in divided doses q8h (not to exceed adult dose).
- Life-threatening infections
  – Adults: IV, IM 1.5 g q6h.
- Bacterial meningitis
  – Adults: IV, IM 1–3 g q8h.
  – Children >3 months: Initial: IV 200–240 mg/kg in divided doses q6–8h, then 100 mg/kg/d.
- Gonorrhea (uncomplicated)
  – Adults: IM 1.5 g, single dose, two different sites along with 1 g probenecid PO.
- Prophylaxis in surgery
  – Adults: IV 1.5 g 30–60 min before surgery.
- Open heart surgery, prophylaxis
  – Adults: IV 1.5 g at initiation of anesthesia, then 1.5 g q12h. Total: 6 g.

Adjustment of dosage
- Kidney disease: Creatinine clearance <20 mL/min: 750 mg–1.5 g q8h; creatinine clearance l0–20 mL/min: 750 mg q12h; creatinine clearance >l0 mL/min: 750 mg q24h.
- Liver disease: None.
- Elderly: None.
- Pediatric: See above.

Food: Take with yogurt or buttermilk (4 oz/d) to maintain bacterial flora and reduce the possibility of severe GI effects.

Pregnancy: Category B.

Lactation: Appears in breast milk. American Academy of Pediatrics considers cephalosporins to be compatible with breastfeeding.

Contraindications: Hypersensitivity to other cephalosporins or related antibiotics, eg, penicillin.

Warnings/precautions
- Use with caution in patients with the following condition: kidney disease.

- It is recommended to continue therapy for at least 2–3 days after symptoms are no longer present. For group A beta-hemolytic streptococcal infections, therapy should be continued for 10 days.
- Before use, determine if patient had previous hypersensitivity reaction to cephalosporins or penicillins. Incidence of cross-sensitivity to penicillins is 1–16%. A negative response to penicillin does not preclude allergic reaction to a cephalosporin.

Advice to patient: Allow at least 1 hour between taking this medication and a bacteriostatic antibiotic, eg, tetracycline or amphenicol.

Adverse reactions
- Common: None.
- Serious: hepatotoxicity, nephrotoxicity, pseudomembranous colitis, hypersensitivity reactions, bone marrow suppression.

Clinically important drug interactions
- Drug that increases effects/toxicity of cefuroxime: probenecid.
- Cefuroxime increase effects/toxicity of following drugs: aminoglycosides, loop diuretics.

Parameters to monitor
- CBC with differential and platelets, serum BUN and creatinine, liver enzymes.
- Temperature for sign of drug-induced persistent fever.
- Signs and symptoms of antibiotic-induced bacterial or fungal superinfection.
- Signs and symptoms of renal toxicity.
- Signs and symptoms of fluid retention, particularly in patients receiving sodium salts of cephalosporins.

Editorial comments
- Cefuroxime axetil is the best oral second-generation cephalosporin for treatment of otitis media, sinusitis, COPD exacerbation, and streptococcal pharyngitis.
- The oral second-generation cephalosporins are also effective in skin, soft tissue, and urinary tract infections, but other antibiotics are more cost effective.

• IV cefuroxime is effective in meningitis caused by *Hemophilus influenzae* and *Neisseria meningitidis*. In children, however, ceftriaxone is superior to cefuroxime in the treatment of *H. influenzae* meningitis.

Celecoxib

Brand name: Celebrex.
Class of drug: Antiinflammatory, analgesic, COX-2 inhibitor.
Mechanism of action: Selective inhibitor of COX-2, the enzyme required for synthesis of prostaglandins and other products of the arachidonic acid cascade.
Indications/dosage/route: Oral only.
• Osteoarthritis
 – Adults: 100 mg b.i.d. or 200 mg as single dose.
• Rheumatoid arthritis
 – Adults: 100–200 mg b.i.d.
Adjustment of dosage
• Kidney disease: None. Potentially toxic to kidney.
• Liver disease: Reduce dosage. Monitor carefully.
• Elderly: Use lowest recommended dose.
• Pediatric: Safety and efficacy have not been determined in children <18 years.
Food: May be taken with or without food.
Pregnancy: Category C. Category D in third trimester and near delivery.
Lactation: No data available. Best to avoid.
Contraindications: Severe liver disease, history of allergic reaction to aspirin or other NSAIDs.
Warnings/precautions
• Use with caution in patients with the following conditions: active gastric ulcer, history of ulcer disease or GI bleeding, active asthma, hypertension, fluid retention, chronic kidney or liver disease.

- Celecoxib can cause significant GI bleeding despite being a specific COX-2 inhibitor.
- Potentially toxic to kidneys, particularly when prostaglandins maintain renal blood flow (renal and heptatic insufficiency), CHF.
- Avoid in patients with kidney or severe hepatic dysfunction.

Advice to patient: Report to treating physician if you experience any of the following symptoms: dyspepsia, changes in stool, abdominal pain, swelling of ankles.

Adverse reactions
- Common: Headache.
- Severe: GI bleeding, hypertension, angina, hypersensitivity reactions, hepatitis, nephrotoxicity, anemia, neuropathy.

Clinically important drug interactions
- Drugs that increase effects/toxicity of celecoxib: rifampin, aspirin, fluconazole, inhibitors of cytochrome P450 2C9.
- Drugs that decrease effects/toxicity of celecoxib: antacids.
- Celecoxib increases effects/toxicity of following drugs: methotrexate, warfarin, lithium.
- Celecoxib decreases effects/toxicity of following drugs: fureosemide, thiazide diuretics, ACE inhibitors.

Parameters to monitor
- Improvement in pain and inflammation.
- Signs and symptoms of salt and water retention.
- Signs and symptoms of GI toxicity.
- Signs and symptoms of renal toxicity.

Editorial comments
- Celecoxib is as effective as other NSAIDs in osteoarthritis and is associated with a lower incidence of GI toxicity than the older drugs. However, the incidence of long-term GI effects has not been determined as compared with older NSAIDs or other COX-2 inhibitors.
- Celecoxib was recently approved as chemoprophylaxsis for adenoma development in patients with familial adenomatous polyposis. Dosage for this indication is 400 mg b.i.d.

Cephalexin

Brand names: Keftab, Keflet.

Class of drug: Cephalosporin, first generation.

Mechanism of action: Binds to penicillin-binding proteins and disrupts or inhibits bacterial cell wall synthesis.

Susceptible organisms *in vivo*
- Very active against *Staphylococcus aureus* and streptococci.
- Moderately active against *Streptococcus pneumoniae.*
- Moderately active against community-acquired *Escherichia coli, Hemophilus influenzae, Moraxella catarrhalis*, and indole-negative *Proteus mirabilis.*
- Inactive against *Bacteroides fragilis.* As with other cephalosporins, inactive against enterococci.

Indications/dosage/route: Oral only.
- General infections
  - Adults: Usual dose: 250 mg q6h. Maximum: 4 g/d.
  - Children: 25–50 mg/kg/d in 4 divided doses.
- Infections of skin and skin structures, streptococcal pharyngitis, uncomplicated cystitis in patients >15 years
  - Adults: 500 mg q12h.
- Streptococcal pharyngitis, skin and skin structure infections
  - Children >1 year: Divide total daily dose and give q12h.

Adjustment of dosage
- Kidney disease: Creatinine clearance 50–80 mL/min: 2 g q6h; creatinine clearance 25–50 mL/min: 1.5 g q6h; creatinine clearance 10–25 mL/min: 1 g q6h; creatinine clearance 2–10 mL/min: 0.5 g q6h; creatinine clearance >2 mL/min: 0.5 g q8h.
- Liver disease: None.
- Elderly: None.
- Pediatric: See above.

Food: Take on empty stomach unless drug causes gastric distress. Consume yogurt or buttermilk (4 oz/d) to maintain bacterial flora and reduce the possibility of severe GI effects.

Pregnancy: Category B.

Lactation: Appears in breast milk. American Academy of Pediatrics considers cephalosporins to be compatible with breastfeeding.

Contraindications: Hypersensitivity to other cephalosporins or related antibiotics, eg, penicillin.

Warnings/precautions

• Use with caution in patients with the following condition: kidney disease.

• It is recommended to continue therapy for at least 2–3 days after symptoms are no longer present. For group A beta-hemolytic streptococcal infections, therapy should be continued for 10 days.

• Before use, determine if patient had previous hypersensitivity reaction to cephalosporins or penicillins. Incidence of cross-sensitivity to penicillins is 1–16%. A negative response to penicillin does not preclude allergic reaction to a cephalosporin.

Advice to patient: Allow at least 1 hour between taking this medication and a bacteriostatic antibiotic, eg, tetracycline or amphenicol.

Adverse reactions

• Common: None.

• Serious: pseudomembranous colitis, hypersensitivity reactions, bone marrow suppression, hepatitis.

Clinically important drug interactions: Probenecid increases effects/toxicity of cephalexin.

Parameters to monitor

• CBC with differential and platelets, liver enzymes.

• Temperature for sign of drug-induced persistent fever.

• Signs and symptoms of antibiotic-induced bacterial or fungal superinfection.

• Signs and symptoms of renal toxicity.

• Signs and symptoms of fluid retention, particularly in patients receiving sodium salts of cephalosporins.

Editorial comments

• Oral cephalosporins are used for *Staphylococcus aureus* and streptococcal infection, when penicillins are to be avoided. Common uses are cellulitis, other infections of the skin,

osteomyelitis, streptococcal pharyngitis. They should not be used for sinusitis, otitis media, or lower respiratory infections because of poor coverage of *Streptococcus pneumoniae, Moraxella catarrhalis,* and *Hemophilus influenzae*. They are not suitable coverage for bite wounds as they do not cover *Pasteurella multocida*.
- Cephalexin uses are similar to those of cefadroxil.

Cephalothin

Brand name: Keflin.
Class of drug: Cephalosporin, first generation, parenteral.
Mechanism of action: Binds to penicillin-binding proteins and disrupts or inhibits bacterial cell wall synthesis.
Susceptible organisms *in vivo*
- Very effective against staphylococci and streptococci, potentially active against *Streptococcus pneumoniae*, active against enterococci. Not effective against MRSA.
- Gram-negative spectrum is limited to community-acquired *Escherichia coli, Moraxella catarrhalis*, indole-negative *Proteus mirabilis,* and some *Klebsiella pneumoniae*. Not useful for nosocomial gram-negative oral anaerobes.
Indications/dosage/route: IV, IM.
- Serious respiratory, GU, GI, skin and soft tissue, bone, and joint infections, septicemia, endocarditis
  - Adults: IV, IM 500 mg–1 g q4–6h. Life-threatening infections: ≤2 g q4h.
Adjustment of dosage
- Kidney disease: Creatinine clearance less than 80 mL/min: usual adult dose; creatinine clearance 50–80 mL/min: ≤2 g q6h; creatinine clearance 25–50 mL/min: up to 1.5 g q6h; creatinine clearance 10–25 mL/min: up to 1 g q6h; creatinine clearance 2–10 mL/min: ≤ 500 mg q6h; creatinine clearance <2 mL/min: ≤500 mg q8h.

- Liver disease: None.
- Elderly: None.
- Pediatric: See above.

Food: No applicable.

Pregnancy: Category B.

Lactation: Appears in breast milk. American Academy of Pediatrics considers cephalosporins to be compatible with breast-feeding.

Contraindications: Hypersensitivity to other cephalosporins or related antibiotics, eg, penicillin.

Editorial comments

- Cephalothin has poor CNS penetration and should therefore not be used for CNS infections.
- This drug is not listed in the *Physician's Desk Reference*, 54th edition, 2000.
- For additional information, see *cefazolin*, p. 157.

Cerivastatin

Brand name: Baycol.

Class of drug: Antilipidemic agent.

Mechanism of action: Inhibits HMG-CoA reductase. Reduces total LDL, cholesterol, serum triglyceride levels. There is little if any effect on serum HDL levels.

Indications/dosage/route: Oral only.

– Adults, elderly: 0.4 mg h.s. Maximum: 0.8 mg/d.

Adjustment of dosage

- Kidney disease, severe: Initial: 0.2 mg. Safety and effectiveness of higher doses are under investigation.
- Liver disease: Reduce dose in chronic liver disease.
- Elderly: See above.
- Pediatric: Safety and efficacy have not been established in children.

Food: No restriction.

Pregnancy: Category X. Contraindicated.

Lactation: Appears in breast milk. Contraindicated.
Contraindications: Hypersensitivity to statins, active liver disease or unexplained persistent elevations of serum transaminase, pregnancy, lactation.

Editorial comments

• It remains to be established whether cerivastatin has a significant effect on morbidity and mortality from coronary heart disease. Older HMG-CoA reductase inhibitors have been shown to cause regression of coronary lesions and some have been shown to reduce coronary and total mortality. It is presumed that cerivastatin would probably have similar effects.

• Cerivastatin at approved dosage appears to be less effective than maximum FDA-approved doses of other HMG-CoA reductase inhibitors. Until the safety and effectiveness of higher doses of cerivastatin have been determined, older drugs are preferred.

• For additional information, see *lovastatin*, p. 543.

Cetirizine

Brand name: Zyrtec.
Class of drug: H_1 receptor blocker, nonsedating.
Mechanism of action: Antagonizes histamine effects on GI tract, respiratory tract, blood vessels.
Indications/dosage/route: Oral only.

• Rhinitis (seasonal), chronic urticaria
  – Adults, children >6 years: 5–10 mg/d.
  – Children 2–5 years: 2.5 mg/d. Maximum: 5 mg/d.

Adjustment of dosage

• Kidney disease: Creatinine clearance <31 mL/min: reduce dose to 5 mg/d. Do not use if <6 years old.
• Liver disease: Reduce dose to 5 mg/d. Do not use if <6 years old.
• Elderly: None.

- Pediatric: Safety and efficacy have not been established in children <2 years.

Food: No restriction.

Pregnancy: Category B.

Lactation: Appears in breast milk. Avoid breastfeeding.

Contraindications: Hypersensitivity to cetirizine.

Warnings/precautions: Use caution in kidney, liver disease.

Advice to patient

- Avoid driving or other activities requiring mental alertness or that are potentially dangerous until response to drug is known.
- Avoid alcohol and other drugs causing sleepiness.

Adverse reactions

- Common: Drowsiness.
- Serious: heart failure, discoordination, confusion, hepatitis, renal toxicity.

Clinically important drug interactions: None.

Parameters to monitor: Efficacy of treatment: improvement of symptoms of rhinitis including sneezing, rhinorrhea, itchy/water eyes.

Editorial comments

- Cetirizine does not cause the prolongation of the QT interval seen with some nonsedating antihistamines.
- Interactions with erythromycin, cimetidine, and ketoconazole do not appear to be clinically significant.

Chlorambucil

Brand name: Leukeran.

Class of drug: Alkylating antineoplastic agent (nitrogen mustard type).

Mechanism of action: Crosslinks DNA strands, thereby interfering with DNA replication and RNA transcription.

Indications/dosage/route: Oral only.

- Hodgkin's and non-Hodgkin's lymphoma, chronic lympho-cytic leukemia, breast and ovarian cancer (generally used to palliate symptoms)
  - Adults: Initial: 0.1–0.2 mg/kg/d. Maintenance: 4–6 mg/d. Alternate: monthly doses of 0.4 mg/kg.

Adjustment of dosage
- Kidney disease: None.
- Liver disease: None
- Elderly: None
- Pediatric: Safety and efficacy have not been established in children.

Food: Administer on empty stomach; food will decrease absorption.

Pregnancy: Category D.

Lactation: No data available. Avoidance of breastfeeding suggested.

Contraindications: Hypersensitivity to chlorambucil or other alkylating agents, patient who did not respond to previous course of therapy.

Warnings/precautions
- Use with caution in patients with the following conditions: bone marrow depression, history of seizures or head trauma, administration of potential epileptogenic drugs.
- This agent has carcinogenic potential and secondary malignancies have occurred in patients receiving chlorambucil.
- Chlorambucil has been associated with chromosomal damage in humans and may produce sterility in males or females.
- Dose-related neutropenia develops commonly after 3 weeks of treatment and persists for up to 2 weeks after discontinuation.
- Dosage should be reduced if patient has been receiving radio-therapy. Avoid full dosage within 4 weeks of radiation therapy because of high risk of bone marrow depression.
- Irreversible bone marrow depression can occur, particularly if total dose is 6.5 mg/kg.

Advice to patient
- Use two forms of birth control including hormonal and barrier methods.
- Drink at least 2 L of fluid per day.

Adverse Reactions
- Common: See serious.
- Serious: **bone marrow depression**, pulmonary fibrosis, interstitial pneumonia, seizures, allergic reactions including drug-induced hepatitis, skin rash, Stevens–Johnson syndrome, paralysis, infertility, hepatic necrosis, secondary malignancies, confusion, hallucinations, peripheral neuropathy.

Clinically important drug interactions: None.

Parameters to monitor
- CBC with differential and platelets, liver enzymes.
- Signs and symptoms of thrombocytopenia.
- Signs and symptoms of anemia.
- Signs and symptoms of infection.
- Signs and symptoms of Stevens–Johnson syndrome: urticaria, edema of mucous membranes including lips and genital organs, headache, high fever, conjunctivitis, rhinitis, stomatitis.
- Signs of hypersensitivity reactions.
- Signs and symptoms of pulmonary toxicity.

Editorial comments
- Use latex gloves and safety glasses when handling cytotoxic drugs. Avoid contact with skin as well as inhalation.
- Careful monitoring of CBC is essential during administration of this medication. It has been suggested that for the first 3–6 weeks of therapy, WBC counts should be checked every 3–4 days as should complete weekly blood counts. All patients should have CBC at least every 2 weeks and frequent clinical examinations while undergoing therapy with chlorambucil.

Chloramphenicol

Brand name: Chloromycetin.
Class of drug: Systemic, ophthalmic, otic antibiotic.
Mechanism of action: Inhibits bacterial protein synthesis.

Susceptible organisms (*in vitro*)

• *Bacillus anthracis, Bordteella peretussis, Ehrlichia* species, *Hemophilus* influenzae, *Neisseria meningitidis, Rickettsia rickettsii, Salmonella* species, *Streptococcus pneumoniae.*

Indications/dosage/route: IV, topical (eye, ear).

• Most infections
  – Adults, children with normal renal and hepatic function: IV 50 mg/kg in equal doses q6h.
  – Neonates, children with undeveloped liver/kidney function: IV 25 mg/kg/d in equal doses q6h.
• Severe and exceptional infections (meningitis, brain abscess)
  – Adults: Initial: IV 75 mg/kg/d. Increase to 100 mg/kg/d if needed.
• Gonococcal meningitis caused by susceptible *Neisseria gonorrhoeae* when drug of first choice cannot be used
  – Adults: IV 4–6 g/d.
  – Children <45 kg: IV 100 mg/d in divided doses q6h for at least 10 days.
• External ear canal infection
  – Adults, children: 2 drops of otic solution, t.i.d. or q.i.d.
• Bacterial infection of eye (cornea or conjunctiva)
  – Adults, children: 2 drops of ophthalmic solution in infected eye q3–6h or more frequently if necessary. Continue for at least 48 hours after the eye appears to be normal.

Adjustment of dosage

• Kidney disease: Adjust dose according to blood levels (see Parameters to Monitor).
• Liver disease: Initial: 1 g followed by 500 mg q.i.d.
• Elderly: None.
• Pediatric: See above. Neonates are at risk for gray baby syndrome. Plasma drug levels must be monitored carefully in such patients (see Parameters to Monitor).

Food: Take on empty stomach or with food if there is GI upset.

Pregnancy: Category C.

Lactation: Appears in breast milk. Potentially toxic to fetus. Considered an agent of concern by American Academy of Pediatrics. Avoid breastfeeding.

Contraindications: Hypersensitivity to chloramphenicol, proplylaxis of bacterial infection, treatment of trivial infections (cold, influenza).

Warnings/precautions

- Use with caution in patients with the following conditions: liver or kidney disease, bone marrow depression, other drugs that suppress bone marrow function, glucose-6-phosphate dehydrogenase deficiency, acute intermittent porphyria.
- Ophthalmic preparation has been shown to cause aplastic anemia.
- Ophthalmic preparation may retard corneal wound healing.
- It is essential to determine bacterial sensitivity to chloramphenicol before administering this drug.

Adverse reactions

- Common: none.
- Serious: bone marrow suppression, gray baby syndrome (vasomotor collapse, cyanosis, abdominal distention, respiratory distress, acidosis, cardiac decompression, coma, death), aplastic anemia, peripheral neuropathy, optic neuritis.

Clinically important drug interactions

- Drugs that increase effects/toxicity of chloramphenicol: aminoglycosides, polymyxin, nondepolarizing muscle relaxants, succinylcholine, cephalothin.
- Chloramphenicol increases effects/toxicity of following drugs: phenytoin, oral anticoagulants, chlorpropamide, tolbutamide.
- Chloramphenicol decreases effects/toxicity of following drugs: phenobarbital, rifampin.

Parameters to monitor

- CBC with differential and platelets, liver enzymes.
- Therapeutic blood levels of chloramphenicol: peak 15–25 µg/mL, trough 5–15 µg/mL, toxic >40 µg/mL. It is essential to monitor blood levels in the newborn to avoid gray baby syndrome.
- Signs and symptoms of bone marrow depression.
- Signs and symptoms of antibiotic-induced bacterial or fungal superinfection. Use of yogurt (4 oz/d) may be helpful in prevention of superinfection.

- Signs and symptoms of neuropathy.
- Optic neuritis: bilateral reduced visual accuity.
- Gray baby syndrome in neonates and prematures.
- Signs and symptoms of hepatotoxicity.
- Symptoms of aplastic anemia. CBC monitoring is recommended for 1 year following treatment.

Editorial comments
- This drug is to be used only for severe infections that do not respond to other antibiotics or would be expected to respond best to chloramphenicol infections. Detailed knowledge of proper dosing and acute awareness of toxic effects of chloramphenicol are strongly advised prior to clinical use.
- Important use for the VRE and often resistant infections. Use of last resort because of narrow therapeutic index.
- Reserved for treatment of serious infections with organisms that are resistant to agents with less toxicity or when agent is superior in penetrating affected tissue.
- The oral form of this drug is no longer available.
- This drug is not listed in the *Physician's Desk Reference*, 54th edition, 2000.

Chlordiazepoxide

Brand name: Librium.
Class of drug: Antianxiety agent, hypnotic.
Mechanism of action: Potentiates effects of GABA in limbic system and reticular formation.
Indications/dosage/route: Oral, IV, IM.
- Anxiety and tension, mild to moderate
  – Adults: PO 5–25 mg t.i.d. to q.i.d.; reduce dose to 5 mg b.i.d. to q.i.d.
  – Children >6 years: PO 5 mg b.i.d or q.i.d.
  – Geriatric or debilitated patients: PO 5 mg b.i.d or q.i.d.
- Alcohol withdrawal/sedative hypnotic

– Adults: PO 50–300 mg; reduce to maintenance levels.
- Acute/severe agitation, anxiety
  – Adults: Initial: IV, IM 50–100 mg. Maintenance: 25–50 mg t.i.d. to q.i.d.
- Preoperative sedation
  – Adults: IM 50–100 mg 1 hour before surgery.
- Alcohol withdrawal
  – Adults: IM, IV 50–100 mg. Repeat in 2–4 hours if necessary. Maximum: 300 mg/d.

Adjustment of dosage
- Kidney disease: None.
- Liver disease: Use caution.
- Elderly: Use lower doses (see above).
- Pediatric: See above. Safety and efficacy have not been established in children <6 years old.

Food: Effects may be counteracted by grapefruit juice, xanthines.

Pregnancy: Category D.

Lactation: Appears in breast milk. Potentially toxic to infant. American Academy of Pediatrics expresses concern about breastfeeding while taking benzodiazepines. Avoid breastfeeding.

Contraindications: Hypersensitivity to benzodiazepines, pregnancy.

Warnings/precautions
- Use with caution in patients with the following conditions: history of drug abuse, severe renal and hepatic impairment, elderly, neonates and infants.
- Benzodiazepines may cause psychologic and physical dependence.
- Benzodiazepines may cause paradoxical rage.
- It is best not to prescribe this drug for more than 6 months. If there is a need for long-term therapy, evaluate patient frequently.
- Use only for patients who have significant anxiety without medication, do not respond to other treatment, and are not drug abusers.

Advice to patient
- Avoid driving and other activities requiring mental alertness or that are potentially dangerous until response to drug is known.

- Avoid alcohol and other CNS depressants such as narcotic analgesics, alcohol, antidepressants, antihistamines, barbiturates, when taking this drug.
- Avoid use of OTC medications without first informing the treating physician.
- Cigarette smoking decreases drug effect. Do not smoke when taking this drug.
- Do not stop drug abruptly if taken for more than 1 month. If suddenly withdrawn, there may be recurrence of the original anxiety or insomnia. A full-blown withdrawal symptom may occur consisting of vomiting, insomnia, tremor, sweating, muscle spasms. After chronic use, decrease drug dosage slowly, ie, over a period of several weeks at the rate of 25% per week.
- Avoid excessive use of xanthine-containing food (regular coffee, tea, chocolate) as these may counteract the action of the drug.

Adverse reactions
- Common: None.
- Serious: respiratory depression, apnea, bone marrow depression, hypotension, drug dependence, rigidity, hostile behavior, hypotension, syncope.

Clinically important drug interactions
- Drugs that increase effects/toxicity of benzodiazepines: CNS depressants (alcohol, antihistamines, narcotic analgesics, tricyclic antidepressants, SSRIs, MAO inhibitors), cimetidine, disulfiram.
- Drugs that decrease effects/toxicity of benzodiazepines: flumazenil (antidote for overdose), carbamazepine.

Parameters to monitor
- Signs of chronic toxicity: ataxia, vertigo, slurred speech.
- Monitor dosing to make sure amount taken is as prescribed particularly if patient has suicidal tendencies.
- Monitor for efficacy of treatment: reduced symptoms of anxiety and tension, improved sleep.
- Signs of physical/psychologic dependence, particularly if patient is addiction-prone and requests frequent renewal of

prescription or is experiencing a diminished response to the drug.

- Neurologic status including memory (anterograde amnesia), disturbing thoughts, unusual behavior.
- Possibility of blood dyscrasias: fever, sore throat, upper respiratory infection. Perform total and differential WBC counts.

Editorial comments

- Because of the long half-life of chlordiazepoxide and desmethyldiazepam (its active metabolite), prolonged sedation may occur. The elderly are particularly at risk. Shorter-acting benzodiazepines are suggested for the elderly.
- Overdose from a benzodiazepine is characterized by the following: hyptension, respiratory depression, cardiac arrhythmias, coma.
- Treatment is supportive, generally without mechanical ventilation.
- Flumazenil, a benzodiazepine antagonist, has been used successfully to reverse the CNS depression but its effectiveness in reversing respiratory depression is in doubt. The physician should be thoroughly familiar with the risks involved in using flumazenil, including the possibility of drug-induced seizures.
- See entry for *flumazenil*, p. 369, or package insert before using this drug.
- The *Physician's Desk Reference*, 54th edition, 2000, lists no drug interactions for chlordiazepoxide or other benzodiazepines.

Chloroquine

Brand name: Aralen.
Class of drug: Antimalarial, amebicide, antiinflammatory.
Mechanism of action: For malaria and amebiasis, inhibits protein synthesis by inhibiting DNA and RNA polymerase.

Indications/dosage/route: Oral, IV, IM, SC.
- Acute attack of malaria
  - Adults: Initial: IM 200–250 mg; repeat in 6 hours if needed.
  - Infants, children: IM, SC 6.25 mg/kg; repeat in 6 hours if needed.
  - Adults: PO 1 g (day 1), 500 mg/day (days 2 & 3).
  - Adults: IV, 16.6 mg/kg over 8 hours, then 8.3 mg/kg q6–8h (continuous infusion).
- Extraintestinal amebiasis
  - Adults: PO 200–250 mg/d, 10–12 days.
  - Children: PO 7.5 mg/kg/d, 10–12 days.
- Prophylaxis of malaria
  - Adults: PO 500 mg/week.
  - Children: PO 50 mg/kg/week.

Adjustment of dosage
- Kidney disease: For severe kidney failure, 50% of usual adult dose should be used. Creatinine clearance <10 mL/min: 50% of dose.
- Liver disease: Use caution, no specific recommendations available.
- Elderly: None.
- Pediatric: See above.

	Onset of Action	Peak Effect	Duration
PO	Rapid	1–2 h	Days–weeks
IM	Rapid	Unknown	Days–weeks

Food: Take with food or milk to reduce stomach distress. Foods that increase urinary acidity may decrease effectiveness of chloroquine. Such foods include cheeses, cranberries, eggs, grains.
Pregnancy: Category C.
Lactation: Appears in breast milk; best to avoid.
Contraindications: Porphyria, retinal or visual field impairment, hypersensitivity to other 4-aminoquinolones (eg, hydroxychloroquine).
Warnings/precautions
- Use with caution in patients with the following conditions: neurologic, GI, blood disorders, kidney, liver disease, alcoholism,

G6PD deficiency, psoriasis, colchicine, use of other hepatotoxic agents.
- Avoid IV and IM administration if possible.

Advice to patient
- Substances (drugs or foods) that increase urinary acidity may increase renal excretion and thereby decrease effectiveness.
- For prophylaxis of malaria, start therapy 2 weeks before exposure and continue for 6 weeks after leaving infested area.
- Use dark glasses to avoid ocular damage caused by bright sunlight.
- Keep this drug out of reach of children.
- Inform treating physician if severe GI distress occurs.

Adverse reactions
- Common: none.
- Serious: retinal damage, visual disturbances, scotomatous vision, visual blurring, deafness, hypotension, muscle weakness, decreased ankle reflexes, seizures, bone marrow depression.

Clinically important drug interactions
- Drugs that decrease effects/toxicity of chloroquine: kaolin, magnesium trisilicate.
- Drug that increases effects/toxicity of chloroquine: cimetidine.

Parameters to monitor
- CBC with differential and platelets.
- Periodic ophthalmologic examinations for signs and symptoms of ocular toxicity: reduced visual acuity, floaters, eye pain. Monitor for symptoms of retinopathy periodically as this may be irreversible if it occurs.
- Periodic audiologic examinations.
- Signs and symptoms of bone marrow depression.
- Determine if patient has muscle weakness. If so, discontinue therapy.
- Monitor joint pain and range of motion when treating rheumatoid arthritis.

Editorial comments
- Used in malaria when chloroquine refractoriness is not a concern.

- Used in sarcoidosis (cutaneous) for its antiinflammatory effects.
- Patients undergoing therapy with this agent should have initial and periodic ophthalmologic examinations including tests of visual acuity, slit lamp, fundoscopic examination, and digital field testing.
- Fatalities from accidental pediatric ingestion of this agent have been reported.

Chlorothiazide

Brand name: Diuril.
Class of drug: Thiazide diurectic.
Mechanism of action: Inhibits sodium resorption in distal tubule resulting in increased urinary excretion of sodium, potasssium, and water.
Indications/dosage/route: Oral, IV.

- Diuretic, hypertension
  - Adults: PO 125 mg/d as single or divided doses: IV 500 mg – 1 g daily in one or two divided doses.
  - Children: IV administration not recommended.
  - Children ≤6 months: 10–20 mg/kg daily in 2 divided doses.
  - Children >6 months: 10–30 mg/kg daily in 2 divided doses.

Adjustment of dosage

- Kidney disease: Use with caution. Ineffective in severe renal failure.
- Liver disease: Use with caution. May cause electrolyte imbalance.
- Elderly: Use with caution. Risk of postural hypotension.
- Pediatric: See above.

	Onset of Action	Peak Effect	Duration
Oral	2 h	4 h	16–12 h

Food: Should be taken with food.

Pregnancy: Category D.

Lactation: Excreted in breast milk. Considered compatible by American Academy of Pediatrics. Thiazide diuretics may suppress lactation.

Contraindications: Anuria, hypersensitivity to thiazides or sulfonamide-derived drugs.

Editorial comments: For additional information, see *hydrochlorothiazide*, p. 426.

Chlorpheniramine

Brand names: Chlor-Trimeton, Teldrin.

Class of drug: H_1 receptor blocker.

Mechanism of action: Antagonizes histamine effects on GI tract, respiratory tract, blood vessels.

Indications/dosage/route: Oral only.

• Allergic rhinitis
  – Adults, children >12 years: 4 mg q6h. Maximum: 24 mg/d.
  – Children 6–12 years: 2 mg q6h. Maximum: 12 mg/d.
  – Children 2–6 years: 1 mg q6h.

• Extended-release tablets
  – Adults, children >12 years: 8 mg q12h. Maximum: 24 mg/d.
  – Children 6–12 years: 4 mg q12h.
  – Children <6 years: Dosage not established.

Adjustment of dosage

• Kidney disease: None.

• Liver disease: None.

• Elderly: Use with caution, at higher risk for toxicity.

• Pediatric: See above. Avoid in neonates, premature infants. Infants and young children are at increased risk of overdose.

Food: No restriction.

Pregnancy: Category B.

Lactation: No data available. Potentially toxic to infant. Avoid breastfeeding.

Contraindications: Hypersensitivity to antihistamines, acute asthma, narrow-angle glaucoma, concurrent use of MAO inhibitors.

Editorial comments

- Chlorpheniramine has antiserotonergic as well as antihistaminic properties. It has also been used as an appetite stimulant and sedative (nonapproved).
- For additional information, see *brompheniramine*, p. 107.

Chlorpromazine

Brand name: Thorazine.

Class of drug: Phenothiazine antipsychotic (neuroleptic).

Mechanism of action: Antagonizes dopamine at dopaminergic receptors in CNS neurons.

Indications/dosage/route: Oral, IV, IM.

- Psychotic disorders, less acutely disturbed
  - Adults, adolescents: PO 25 mg t.i.d.; increase by 20–50 mg/d q3–4d as needed. Maximum: 400 mg/d.
- Nausea and vomiting
  - Adults, adolescents: PO 10–25 mg q4h.
  - Children: PO 0.5 mg/kg q4–6h.
- Preoperative sedation
  - Adults, adolescents: PO 25–50 mg 2–3h before surgery.
  - Children: PO 0.5 mg/kg 2–3h before surgery.
- Hiccoughs or porphyria
  - Adults, adolescents: PO 25–50 mg t.i.d. to q.i.d.
- Psychotic disorders, acutely manic or disturbed
  - Adults: Initial: IM 25 mg; if needed, additional 25–50 mg in 1h; increase up to 400 mg q4–6h.
  - Children >6 months: IM 0.5 mg/kg q6–8h. Maximum: 75 mg/d for children 5–12 years, 40 mg/d for children ≤5 years.
- Preoperative sedative

- Adults: IM 12.5–25 mg 1–2 hours before surgery.
- Children: IM 0.5 mg/kg 1–2 hours before surgery.
- Hiccoughs
  - Adults: IM 25–50 mg t.i.d. to q.i.d.
- Acute intermittent porphyria
  - Adults: IM 25 mg q6–8h; change to oral dosing as soon as possible.
- Tetanus
  - Adults: PO 25–50 mg t.i.d. to q.i.d. IV, IM 25–50 mg injected at 1 mg/min.
  - Pediatric: IV, IM 0.5 mg/kg injected at 1 mg/2 min.

Adjustment of dosage
- Kidney disease: Use with caution. Guidelines not available.
- Liver disease: Use with caution. Guidelines not available.
- Elderly: Use lower doses. Increase dosage more gradually.
- Pediatric: See above.

Food: No restrictions. Oral concentrate should be diluted in 2–4 oz of liquid or pudding.

Pregnancy: Category C.

Lactation: No data available. Considered to be an agent of concern by American Academy of Pediatrics. Avoid breast-feeding.

Contraindications: Hypersensitivity to phenothiazines, concurrent use of high-dose CNS depressants (alcohol, barbituates, benzodiazepines, narcotics), CNS depression, comatose state.

Warnings/precautions
- Use with caution in patients with the following conditions: cardiovascular, liver, kidney disease, glaucoma, chronic respiratory disorders, exposure to extreme heat, organophosphate insecticides or atropine-type drugs.
- Tardive dyskinesia, a syndrome associated with involuntary movements, occurs frequently after long-term administration of neuroleptic agents. Because this syndrome is potentially irreversible, close monitoring for drug-induced movement disorders is mandatory for all patients. Elderly women appear to be at highest risk. Medication must be discontinued if tardive dyskinesia develops.

- NMS is a potentially fatal symptom complex seen with administration of antipsychotic drugs. Symptoms include fever, muscular rigidity, and autonomic instability, including arrhythmias and BP disturbances. Patients with suggestive symptoms must be evaluated immediately. Management includes drug discontinuation, close monitoring, and symptom-directed therapy including administration of dantrolene.
- Pharmacotherapies for NMS is not standardized at present.
- Make sure patient swallows drug and does not hoard tablets. Suicide attempts by drug overdose may occur even when patient's symptoms appear to be improving.
- Be aware of danger of aspiration of vomitus.
- Some preparations contain tartrazine (FD&C Yellow No. 5). This dye can cause a severe allergic reaction, even an asthmatic attack, in susceptible patients, particularly those who are allergic to aspirin. Prescribe drug preparation that does not contain this dye for these individuals.
- Use lower doses initially in patients with prior insulin reactions and those receiving electroconvulsive therapy.
- Be aware that this drug, because of its antiemetic action, may obscure diagnosis and treatment of overdose of other drugs as well as diagnosis and treatment of such conditions as Reye's syndrome and intestinal obstruction.
- IM injections should be made slowly in upper quadrant of buttocks. Avoid SC injection.

Advice to patient

- Avoid driving and other activities requiring mental alertness or that are potentially dangerous until response to drug is known.
- Patient and family members should avoid contact of the drug with skin or eyes as it can cause contact dermatitis or conjunctivitis.
- Discard if drug solution is any color other than yellow.
- Keep up compliance with dosing regimen and do not increase dose without approval of treating physician.
- Do not take any other medication including OTC products without approval from treating physician.

- Swallow enteric-coated tablets whole; do not crush or chew.
- This drug may make you feel cold. If this occurs, use extra blankets only, not a hot water bottle, heating pad, or electric blanket.
- Do not expose yourself to very high temperatures, ie, above 105°F (hot baths, sun lamps, sauna, whirlpool) as the drug may cause heat stroke. Symptoms of this condition include red, dry skin, dyspnea, strong pulse, body temperature >105°F (40.6°C). Contact physician immediately. In the event of heat stroke, treatment includes body ice packs and antihypertensive drugs to rapidly lower body temperature.
- If mouth is dry, rinse with warm water frequently, chew sugarless gum, suck on ice cube, or use artificial saliva. Carry out meticulous oral hygiene (floss teeth daily).
- Do not stop taking drug abruptly as this may precipitate a withdrawal reaction, particularly extrpyramidal symptoms. Other symptoms of withdrawal include abdominal discomfort, dizziness, headache, tachycardia, insomnia. Reduce dosage gradually over several weeks, eg, 10–25% every 2 weeks.
- Be aware that your skin may turn yellow-brown to grayish-purple. This is a temporary condition.

Adverse reactions
- Common: drowsiness.
- Serious: **hypotension, postural hypotension (IV injection), arrhythmias**, hepatitis, bone marrow depression, extrapyramidal reactions, dystonias, amenorrhea, galactorrhea, gynecomastia, tardive dyskinesia, NMS, hypersensitivity reaction, seizures, agranulocytosis, corneal and lens abnormalities, pigmentary retinopathy.

Clinically important drug interactions
- Drugs that increase effects/toxicity of phenothiazines: CNS depressants (barbiturates, opioids, general anesthetics, benzodiazepines, alcohol), quinidine, procainamide, anticholinergic agents, MAO inhibitors, antihistamines, nitrates, β blockers, tricyclic antidepressants, lithium, pimozide.

- Drugs that decrease effects/toxicity of phenothiazines: methyldopa, carbamazepine, barbiturates, aluminum- and magnesium- containing antacids, heavy smoking, amphetamines.
- Phenothiazines increase effects/toxicity of following drugs: hydantoins.
- Phenothiazines decrease effects/toxicity of following drugs: centrally acting antihypertensive drugs (guanethidine, clonidine, methyldopa), bromocriptine, levodopa.

Parameters to monitor

- CBC with differential and platelets, liver enzymes, serum BUN and creatinine.
- Observe patient receiving parenteral injection closely for hypotensive reaction. Patient should remain in recumbent position for at least 30 minutes following injection. If hypotensive reaction occurs, administer norepinephrine or phenylephrine; epinephrine is contraindicated under these conditions as it might cause a sudden drop in BP (vasomotor reversal). Recovery usually occurs spontaneously within 0.5 to 2 hours.
- Signs and symptoms of GI complications including fecal impaction and constipation. Urge patient to increase intake of fluids and bulk-containing food.
- Signs and symptoms of fluid extravasation from IV injection.
- Signs and symptoms of bronchial pneumonia as a result of suppression of cough reflex. This may be a particular problem in the elderly and severely depressed patient.
- Signs and symptoms of tardive dyskinesia: uncontrolled rhythmic movements of face, mouth, tongue, jaw, protrusion of tongue, uncontrolled rapid or wormlike movements of tongue, chewing movements. At first indication of tardive dyskinesia—vermicular movements of tongue—withdraw drug immediately. Tardive dyskinesia generally develops several months after treatment with a phenothiazine. Patient should be monitored every 6 months for possible development of tardive dyskinesia.
- Blood and urine glucose in diabetic or prediabetic patients on high-dose drug for loss of diabetes control. If control is lost, it

may be necessary to discontinue the drug and substitute another.
- Signs of agranulocytosis.
- Signs and symptoms of cholestatic jaundice: fever, flulike symptoms, pruritus, jaundice. These effects may occur between the second and fourth weeks of treatment.
- Signs and symptoms of overdose: somnolence, coma. Treat by gastric lavage and maintain patient airway. Do not induce vomiting.
- Ophthalmologic status, particularly in patients with glaucoma. Adverse ocular reactions include: increased intraocular pressure; particle deposition in the cornea and lens which may lead to venticular opacities; blurred vision; photophobia; ptosis.
- Signs of hypersensitivity reactions.
- Efficacy of treatment: improvement in mental status, including orientation, mood, general behavior, improved sleep, reduction in auditory and visual hallucinations, disorganized thinking, blunted affect, agitation.
- Signs and symptoms of NMS.

Editorial comments: Phenothiazines have been a mainstay of treatment for psychosis. They have wide-ranging CNS effects and have complex effects on a variety of neurotransmitters. These properties cause frequent and often severe side effects. Because of prominent anticholinergic effects, extrapyramidal symptoms are less frequent than for high-potency dopaminergic blocking agents such as haloperidol.

Chlorpropamide

Brand name: Diabinese.
Class of drug: Oral hypoglycemic agent.
Mechanism of action: Stimulates release of insulin from pancreatic beta cells; decreases glucose production in liver; increases

sensitivity of receptors for insulin, thereby promoting effectiveness of insulin.

Indications/dosage/route: Oral only.

• Diabetes, type II (non-insulin-dependent diabetes mellitus):
  – Adults, mild to moderate diabetes: Initial: 250 mg/d as a single or divided dose. Maintenance: 100–250 mg/d as single or divided doses. Maximum: 750 mg/d.
  – Elderly: Initial: 100–125 mg/d.

Adjustment of dosage

• Kidney disease: None.
• Liver disease: None.
• Elderly: See above.
• Pediatric: Not recommended.

Onset of Action	Duration
1 h	≤60 h

Food: No restriction. Patient should be told to eat regularly and not to skip meals. Sugar supply should be kept handy at all times. If stomach is upset, Tums should be taken with meal. Dose is best administered before breakfast or, if taken twice a day, before the evening meal.

Pregnancy: Category C.

Lactation: Appears in breast milk. Potentially toxic to infant. Avoid breastfeeding.

Contraindications: Hypersensitivity to chlorpropamide diabetes complicated by ketoacidosis.

Editorial comments

• A disulfirsam-like reaction may occur when chlorpropamide is combined with alcohol. Because of the long half-life, prolonged hypoglycemia is an important potential adverse effect of chlorpropamide.

• For additional information, see *glyburide*, p. 409.

Chlorthalidone

Brand names: Hygroton, Thalitone.
Class of drug: Thiazide diurectic.
Mechanism of action: Inhibits sodium resorption in distal tubule, resulting in increased urinary excretion of sodium, potasssium, and water.
Indications/dosage/route: Oral only.
- Diuretic
  - Adults: 25–50 mg/d, 50–100 mg once every other day, or once a day for 3 d/wk.
- Hypertension
  - Adults: 12.5–25 mg/d.
- Diuretic, hypertension
  - Children: 1–2 mg/kg, once per day for 3 d/wk.

Adjustment of dosage
- Kidney disease: Use with caution. Ineffective in severe renal failure.
- Liver disease: Use with caution. May cause electrolyte imbalance.
- Elderly: Use with caution because of age-related impairment of kidney function.
- Pediatric: See above.

	Onset of Action	Peak Effect	Duration
Diuretic:	2 h	2–6 h	24–48 h

Food: Should be taken with food.
Pregnancy: Category D.
Lactation: Excreted in breast milk. Considered compatible by American Academy of Pediatrics. Thiazide diuretics may suppress lactation.
Contraindications: Anuria, hypersensitivity to thiazides or sulfonamide-derived drugs.

Editorial comments: For additional information, see *hydrochloroth-iazide*, p. 426.

Cholestyramine

Brand names: Questran, LoCholest, Prevalite.
Class of drug: Lipid-lowering agent.
Mechanism of action: Binds bile acids, forming a non-absorbable complex in the intestinal lumen, resulting in increased fecal bile acid excretion and increased cholesterol metabolism, and dec-reased LDL, VLDL cholesterol and total cholesterol levels in the serum.
Indications/dosage/route: Oral only.
• Primary hypercholestermia with or without associated hyper-triglyceridemia that is not responsive to dietary measures alone, relief of pruritis associated with partial biliary obstruction.
  – Adult: 1 pouch or scoopful contains 1 g powder and 4 g cho-lesteramine resin. Maintenance: 2–4 packets or scoopfuls per day.
  – Children 6–12: 80 mg/kg divided in 2 doses.
• Treatment of digitalis overdose
  – Adults: Initial: 4 g 1–2 times/d. Maintenance: 8–16 g/d, two divided doses.
Adjustment of dosage: None.
Food: Take with meals.
Pregnancy: Category C. May cause decreased absorption of fat-soluble vitamins with potential adverse fetal effects.
Lactation: Use with caution. Effect of vitamin malabsorption in nursing infants unknown.
Contraindications: Hypersensitivity to cholestyramine and other bile acid-sequestering resins, complete biliary obstruction, type III, IV, or V hyperlipoproteinemia.
Warnings/precautions
• Use with caution in patients with the following conditions: con-stipation, phenylketonuria (Prevalite contains phenylalanine).

- Chronic use of cholestyramine may result in increased tendency to bleed because of vitamin K deficiency as well as deficiency of other fat-soluble vitamins.
- High doses may potentially cause hyperchloremic acidosis in patients with renal insufficiency or volume depletion in patients taking spironolactone.
- Provide patient a list of drugs whose absorption is reduced by cholestyramine.

Advice to patient
- Always mix drug with 60–180 mL water or noncarbonated drink. Place contents of packet on fluid surface and stir slowly after 2–4 min.
- Take other drugs 1 hour before or 4–6 hours after cholestyramine.
- Supplement your diet with vitamins A,D,E,K.
- If experiencing constipation increase intake of fluids.

Adverse reactions
- Common: constipation.
- Serious: fecal impaction, intestinal obstruction, fat-soluble vitamin deficiencies, steatorrhea, hypoprothrombinemia, hyperchloremic acidosis.

Clinically important drug interactions
Cholestyramine decreases effects/toxicity of following drugs: acetaminophen, amiodarone, cardiac glycosides, furosemide, corticosteroids, thyroid preparations, propranolol, estrogens, methotrexate, oral anticoagulants, penicillin G, phenobarbital, thiazide diuretics.

Parameters to monitor
- Levels of digitalis and other drugs to ensure appropriate drug levels. Use caution when discontinuing cholestyramine in patients using digitalis. Levels may be increased.
- Determine serum cholesterol levels.
- Signs of vitamin A, D, or K deficiency.

Editorial comments
- Cholestyramine has procarcinogenic effects in laboratory animals, but this effect has not been demonstrated in humans.

- Treatment of hyperlipidemias is generally performed in a stepwise approach with dietary modification, weight reduction, and exercise as important initial components of treatment.
- Alternative drugs for treatment for hyperlipidemias include the various HMG-CoA reductase inhibitors.

Cimetidine

Brand name: Tagamet.
Class of drug: H_2 receptor blocker.
Mechanism of action: Competitively blocks H_2 receptors on parietal cells, thereby blocking gastric acid secretion.
Indications/dosage/route: Oral, IV, IM.
- Active duodenal ulcer.
  - Adults: PO 400–1600 mg h.s. Alternative: 300 mg q.i.d. with meals and h.s. Maintenance: 400 mg h.s.
- Active benign gastric ulcer:
  - Adults: PO 800 mg h.s.
- Pathologic hypersecretory conditions or intractable ulcers
  - Adults: IM or IV 300 mg q6–8h. If necessary, administer 300 mg more frequently than q6–8h. PO 300 mg q.i.d. Maximum: 2400 mg/d.
- Prophylaxis of upper GI bleeding
  - Adults: IV 50 mg/h by continuous infusion.
- Before anesthesia to prevent aspiration of gastric acid
  - Adults: IV 300 mg 60–90 min before induction with anesthetic.
Adjustment of dosage
- Kidney: Creatinine clearance <30 mL/min: use half recommended dose.
- Liver disease: None.
- Elderly: None.
- Pediatric: Not recommended for children <6 years.

	Onset of Action	Peak Effect	Duration
Oral	30 min	45–90 min	4–5 h

Food: Take with food.

Pregnancy: Category B.

Lactation: Appears in breast milk. Considered compatible by American Academy of Pediatrics.

Contraindications: Hypersensitivity to H_2 blockers.

Warnings/precautions

- Use with caution in the elderly, patients with hepatic or liver disease, immunocompromised patients.
- Symptomatic relief does not mean absence of gastric malignancy.
- Adverse reactions are most likely to occur in elderly and in patients who have impaired renal function.
- Discontinue drug for 24–72 h before performing skin test for allergens.
- Decreased gastric acidity may increase the possibility of intestinal parasites and bacterial overgrowth, particularly in immunocompromised patients.

Advice to patient

- Avoid driving and other activities requiring mental alertness or that are potentially dangerous until response to drug is known.
- Avoid alcohol and smoking.
- Avoid foods that might cause gastroesophageal reflux.
- Continue taking drug even after reduction in ulcer pain.
- Report ongoing use of OTC H_2 blockers to your physician.

Adverse reactions

- Common: none.
- Serious: arrythmia, jaundice, bone marrow suppression, aplastic anemia (rare), hypersensitivity reactions, gynecomastia.

Clinically important drug interactions: Cimetidine increases effects/toxicity of the following drugs: benzodiazepines, theophylline, tricyclic antidepressants, warfarin, β blockers, carbamazepine, carmustine, chlordiazepoxide, chloroquine, diazepam, lidocaine, calcium channel blockers, phenytoin, procainamide, quinidine.

Parameters to monitor

- Presence of *Helicobacter pylori*: This is a standard approach in patients with peptic ulcer disease.
- Efficacy of treatment: improved symptoms of GERD or peptic ulcer disease. Use endoscopy to prove healing of gastric ulcers. A nonhealing gastric ulcer may actually be caused by gastric cancer.
- Symptoms of serious underlying disease requiring further testing (weight loss, worsening abdominal pain, early satiety, etc).

Editorial comments

- Current management of peptic ulcer disease includes diagnosis and treatment of *H. pylori* infection. Check if patients are receiving NSAIDs and discontinue when possible. Hypersecretory states are uncommon causes of peptic ulcer disease.
- H_2 blockers are the drugs of choice for the following conditions: dyspepsia not evaluated by endoscopy (empirical), mild to moderate GERD, peptic ulcer disease not caused by *H. pylori* infection.
- Proton pump inhibitors are essentially replacing H_2 blockers for management of GERD.

Ciprofloxacin

Brand name: Cipro.
Class of drug: Broad-spectrum quinolone antibiotic.
Mechanism of action: Inhibits DNA gyrase, thereby blocking bacterial DNA replication.
Susceptible organisms *in vivo*: *Campylobacter* sp, *Citrobacter* sp, *Enterobacter, Escherichia coli, Hemophilus influenzae, Hemophilus parainfluenzae, Klebsiella pneumoniae, Morganella morganii, Proteus mirabilis, Proteus vulgaris, Providencia rettgeri, Providencia stuartii, Pseudomonas aeruginosa, Serratia,*

Marcescens, Shigella sp, *Staphylococcus aureus, Staphylococcus epidermidis, Legionella, Mycoplasma pneumoniae, Mycobacterium tuberculosis, Mycobacterium chelonae, Mycobacterium kansasii, Mycobacterium fortuitum.*

Indications/dosage/route: Oral, IV.

Oral
- Acute sinusitis
  - Adults: 500 mg q12h.
- Lower respiratory tract infections, COPD exacerbations
  - Adults: 500 mg q12h. Severe or more complicated infections (nosocomial): 750 mg q12h.
- Severe, complicated UTIs, 7–14 days
  - Adults: 500 mg q12h.
- Mild to moderate UTIs, 7–14 days
  - Adults: 250 mg q12h.
- Acute, uncomplicated cystitis
  - Adults, female: 100 mg q12h, 3 days.
- Chronic bacterial prostatis:
  - Adults: 500 mg q12h.
- Complicated intraabdominal infections (combination therapy)
  - Adults: 500 mg q12h plus metronidazole (given according to product labeling).
- Bone and joint infections, infectious diarrhea, typhoid fever
  - Adults: 500 mg q12h.
- Uncomplicated urethral and cervical gonococcal infections
  - Adults: single 250-mg dose.

IV
- Mild to moderate UTIs.
  - Adults: 200 mg q12h.
- Severe or complicated UTIs, lower respiratory tract infections, skin and skin structure infections, bone and joint infections (mild to moderate)
  - Adults: 400 mg 8–12h.
- Severe or complicated lower respiratory tract, infections, skin and skin structure infections, bone and joint infections, nosocomial pneumonia (mild, moderate, or severe)
  - 400 mg q8h.

- Complicated intraabdominal infections
  - Adults: 400 mg q8h plus IV metronidazole.
- Empirical therapy of febrile neutropenia
  - Adults: 400 mg q8h plus piperacillin 50 mg/kg IV q4h. Maximum: 24 g/d, 7–14 days.

Adjustment of dosage
- Kidney disease: Creatinine clearance >30 mL/min: usual dosages; creatinine clearance 5–29 mL/min: 200–400 q18–24h.
- Liver disease: None.
- Elderly: None.
- Pediatric: Safety and efficacy have not been established in children <18 years.

Food: Take 1 hour before or 2 hours after meals with a glass of water.

Pregnancy: Category C.

Lactation: Appears in breast milk. Potentially toxic to infant. Avoid breastfeeding.

Contraindications: Hypersensitivity to fluoroquinolone antibiotics or quinolone antibiotics, eg, cinoxacin, nalidixic acid.

Warnings/precautions
- Use with caution in patients with the following conditions: CNS disorders (epilepsy).
- Therapy should be continued for 2–4 days after symptoms have disappeared.
- Rupture of Achilles and other tendons has occurred in patients taking fluoroquinolones.
- Serious and even fatal hypersensitivity reactions have occurred with these drugs, even after the first dose.
- This drug is recommended as an alternative to aminoglycosides when clinically relevant.
- Reserve use of this drug for infections that are difficult to treat by other means.

Advice to patient
- Limit intake of caffeinated products including coffee, tea and colas.

- Drink a great deal of fluids during therapy with this drug.
- Do not undertake strenuous exercise while taking this drug.
- To minimize possible photosensitivity reaction, apply adequate sunscreen and use proper covering when exposed to strong sunlight.

Adverse reactions
- Common: None.
- Serious: hypersensitivity reaction (anaphylaxis), seizures, pseudomembraneous colitis, cholestatic jaundice, renal failure, pulmonary edema, pulmonary embolism, cardiovascular collapse, pharyngeal edema.

Clinically important drug interactions
- Drugs that increase effects/toxicity of fluoroquinolones: cyclosporine, probenecid.
- Drugs that decrease effects/toxicity of fluoroquinolones: antacids, antineoplastic agents, didanosine, sucralfate, iron salts, zinc salts, caffeine.
- Fluoroquinolones increase effects/toxicity of following drugs: oral anticoagulants, theophylline, caffeine.

Parameters to monitor
- Renal, hepatic, and hemopoietic systems should be monitored periodically during prolonged therapy.
- Intake of fluids and urinary and other fluid output to minimize renal toxicity. Increase fluid intake if inadequate. Closely monitor electrolyte levels.
- Signs of hypersensitivity reactions.
- Signs and symptoms of antibiotic-induced bacterial or fungal superinfection: Use of yogurt (4 oz/d) may be helpful in prevention of superinfection.
- Signs and symptoms of tendon pain. These may be an indication of tendon rupture.
- Evidence of development of microbial resistance: loss of effectiveness.

Editorial comments: Ciprofloxacin has excellent potency for gram-negative aerobes, including *Pseudomonas* and is the best quinolone for gram-negative coverage. As with quino-lones, ciprofloxacin is not appropriate monotherapy for community-acquired pneumonia because of poor activity against *Strepto-coccus pneumoniae*. These drugs are also not recommended for sinusitis or otitis media. Quinolones are very effective agents against atypical pneumonias and are used as treatments for GU infections.

Cisapride

Brand name: Propulsid.
Class of drug: Prokinetic drug.
Mechanism of action: Releases acetycholine within myenteric plexus; agonist at serotonin receptors.
Indications/dosage/route: Oral only.
- Heartburn, nocturnal; alkaline reflux gastritis; erosive and nonerosive esophagitis; gastroporesis; postoperative ileus
  - Adults: Initial: 10 mg q.i.d.; increase to 20–30 mg/q.i.d. Also may be administered as 10–40 mg b.i.d.
  - Children: 0.1–.3 mg/kg/d.
  - Elderly: 10 mg q.i.d. Maintenance: 20–30 mg/d.

Adjustment of dosage
- Kidney disease: None.
- Liver disease: 5 mg q.i.d.
- Elderly: See above.
- Pediatric: See above.

Onset of Action	Duration
30–60 min	No data

Food: Generally taken 15 minutes to 1 hour before meals and at bedtime. Grapefruit juice increases cisapride levels and should be avoided.
Pregnancy: Category C.
Lactation: Appears in breast milk. Best to avoid.

Contraindications: Mechanical obstruction of GI tract, hemorrhage or perforation of the GI tract, known family history of congenital prolonged QT intervals, clinically significant bradycardia, concomitant use with agents that increase cisapride levels (see Clinically Important Drug Interactions).

Warnings/precautions: Pretreatment ECG is required. Do not administer if QT interval is prolonged.

Advice to patient

• Avoid driving and other activities requiring mental alertness or that are potentially dangerous until response to drug is known.
• Avoid the use of OTC medications without first informing the treating physician.
• Avoid alcohol and benzodiazepines.

Adverse reactions

• Common: abdominal discomfort, diarrhea, headache.
• Serious: cardiac arrythmias, seizures, bone marrow depression, extrapyramidal reaction,.

Clinically important drug interactions

• Drugs that increase effects/toxicity of cisapride and are contraindicated in combination: ketoconazole, fluconazole, itraconazole, erythromycin, clarithromycin, troleandomycin, protease inhibitors, nefazodone.
• Drugs that decrease effects/toxicity of cisapride: anticholinergics.
• Cisapride increases effects/toxicity of oral anticoagulant agents that prolong the QT interval (class A and class III antiarrhythmics).

Parameters to monitor

• Relief of heartburn, relief of gastroporesis, ie, reduction of nausea and vomiting.
• ECG prior to initiating therapy.

Editorial comments

• Use of cisapride has been markedly restricted due to cardiac toxicity and is now only available in very special circumstances.
• Torsade de pointes (a potentially fatal ventricular arrhythmia) has occurred with the concomitant use of cisapride and drugs

that inhibit its metabolism (inhibitors of cytochrome P450 2A). Elevated cisapride levels are thought to result in arrhythmia. See Clinically Important Drug Interactions for drugs that should not be administered with cisapride.

Cisplatin

Brand name: Platinol.
Class of drug: Platinum-containing antineoplastic agent.
Mechanism of action: Forms irreversible covalent bond to DNA, preventing separation of the helical strands.
Indications/dosage/route: IV only. Dose is dependent on creatinine clearance, body surface area; laboratory parameters required prior to subsequent treatment (see Parameters to Monitor).
- Metastatic testicular cancer
  - Adults: 20 mg/m^2/d for 5 days, repeated q3–4wk.
- Metastatic ovarian cancer
  - Adults: 75–100 mg/m^2/d q3wk.
- Advanced bladder cancer
  - Adults: 50–70 mg/m^2/d q3–4wk.
- Head and neck cancer
  - Adults: 100–120 mg/m^2/d q3–4wk.
- Brain tumor recurrence
  - Adults: 60 mg/m^2/d for 2 days, then q3–4wk.

Adjustment of dosage
- Kidney disease: Creatinine clearance 10–50 mL/min: 50% of dose; creatinine clearance <10 mL/min: do not use.
- Liver disease: None.
- Elderly: Use with caution.
- Pediatric: Safety and efficacy have not been established in children.

Pregnancy: Category D.
Lactation: Appears in breast milk. Potentially toxic to infant. Avoid breastfeeding.

Contraindications: Hypersensitivity to cisplatin or other drugs containing platinum, severe renal insufficiency, creatinine clearance <10 mL/min, bone marrow depression, hearing impairment.

Warnings/precautions

• Patient must be well hydrated prior to and for 24 hours after treatment. It may be necessary to administer a diuretic to ensure good urine output (>100 mL/h), eg, mannitol or furosemide.

• An antiemetic should be administered with this drug.

• Cisplatin therapy commonly results in ototoxicity. This is usually noted only by high-frequency hearing loss on audiometry. However, severe hearing loss occasionally occurs.

• Cumulative nephrotoxicity is potentiated when combined with aminoglycoside antibiotics.

Advice to patient: Use two forms of birth control including hormonal and barrier methods.

Adverse reactions

• Common: hyperuricemia, tinnitus (9%), nausea and vomiting (76–100%) (antiemetics should always be administered with cisplatin).

• Serious: **bone marrow suppression, high-frequency hearing loss (24%), nephrotoxicity, acute renal failure, chronic renal insufficiency**, anaphylactic reaction, peripheral neuropathy, hypocalcemia, hypomagnesemia, hypokalemia, papilledema, optic neuritis, hepatotoxicity.

Clinically important drug interactions:

• Drugs that increase effects/toxicity of cisplatin: aminoglycosides, loop diuretics.

• Drug that decreases effects/toxicity of cisplatin: phenytoin.

Parameters to monitor:

• Serum BUN and creatinine, CBC with differential and platelets, liver enzymes, electrolytes (calcium, magnesium, potassium).

• Twenty-four-hour creatinine clearance at baseline and periodically with treatment (often done by calculated Cl_{CR}).

• Formal audiologic evaluation.

• Signs and symptoms of neuropathy.

• Intake of fluids and urinary and other fluid output to minimize renal toxicity.

- Signs and symptoms of ototoxicity: tinnitus, vertigo, hearing loss, initially in range 4000–8000 Hz.
- Signs and symptoms of fluid extravasation from IV injection.
- Signs and symptoms of infection.
- Signs and symptoms of anemia.
- Signs and symptoms of hypersensitivity reaction.
- Signs and symptoms of renal toxicity.

Editorial comments

- Cisplatin is one of the most emetogenic chemotherapy agents. Patient should receive an antiemetic prior to treatment, eg, a 5-HT$_3$ receptor antagonist, such as ondansetron, granisetron, or dolasetron is commonly combined with dexamethasone.
- This drug is also used for the treatment of small cell lung cancer, non-small cell lung cancer, sarcomas, esophageal cancer, and lymphoma.

Citalopram

Brand name: Celexa.
Class of drug: SSRI antidepressant.
Mechanism of action: Inhibits reuptake of serotonin into CNS neurons.
Indications/dosage/route: Oral only.

- Depression: DSM-III or DSM-R
  - Adults: Initial: 20 mg/d in am or pm. Maintenance: ≤40 mg/d. Maximum: 40 mg/d.

Adjustment of dosage

- Kidney disease: None.
- Liver disease: Decrease dose and/or interval in cirrhosis.
- Elderly: Consider lower dose.
- Pediatric: Safety and efficacy have not been established.

Food: May be taken with meals.
Pregnancy: Category B.

Lactation: Appears in breast milk. Best to avoid. American Academy of Pediatrics expresses concern with use during breast-feeding.

Contraindications: MAO inhibitor taken within 14 days, hypersensitivity to citalopram.

Warnings/precautions

- Use with caution in patients with the following conditions: diabetes mellitus, seizures, liver, kidney disease.
- Advise patient that effectiveness of the drug may not be apparent until 4 weeks of treatment.
- A withdrawal syndrome has been described after abrupt withdrawal of this drug. Symptoms include blurred vision, diaphoresis, agitation, and hypomania.
- Mania or hypomania may be unmasked by SSRIs.

Advice to patient

- Avoid driving and other activities requiring mental alertness or that are potentially dangerous until response to drug is known.
- Avoid alcohol and other CNS depressants such as opiate analgesics and sedatives (eg, diazepam) when taking this drug.
- Report excessive weight loss to treating physician.
- Take this drug in the morning as it may cause insomnia.

Adverse reactions

- Common: insomnia, drowsiness, nausea, dry mouth, excessive sweating.
- Serious: anaphylaxis, suicidal tendency, extrapyramidal reactions, orthostatic hypotension.

Clinically important drug interactions

- Drugs that increase effects/toxicity of SSRIs: MAO inhibitors (combination contraindicated), clarithromycin, tryptophan.
- SSRIs increase effects/toxicity of following drugs: tricyclic antidepressants, diazepam, dextromethorphan, encainide, haloperidol, perphenazine, propafenone, thioridizine, trazadone, warfarin, carbamazepine, lithium.
- Drug that decreases effects/toxicity of SSRIs: buspirone.

Parameters to monitor
- Progressive weight loss. Recommend dietary management to maintain weight. This may be particularly important in underweight patients.
- Signs of hypersensitivity reactions.

Editorial comment
- SSRIs are recommended for patients who are at risk for medication overdose because it is safer than tricyclic antidepressants and there have been no reported deaths from overdose with this drug.
- SSRIs may be a better choice than tricyclic antidepressants for the following patients: those who cannot tolerate the anticholinergic effects or excessive daytime sedation of tricyclic antidepressants, those who experience psychomotor retardation or weight gain. These drugs are generally well tolerated.
- If coadministered with tricyclic antidepressant, dosage of the latter may need to be reduced and blood monitored. Do not administer for at least 14 days after discontinuing a MAO inhibitor. Do not initiate MAO inhibitor until at least 5 weeks after discontinuing this agent.
- SSRIs have generally replaced other antidepressants (tricyclics, MAO inhibitors) as drugs of choice for this condition.
- Citalopram appears to have less of a tendency to produce altered bowel habits than other SSRIs.

Cladribine

Brand name: Leustatin.
Class of drug: Antineoplastic agent, antimetabolite.
Mechanism of action: Is converted to phosphorylated metabolite which causes a break in native DNA, thereby inhibiting synthesis of new DNA and DNA repair.

Indications/dosage/route: IV only.

- Hairy cell leukemia, chronic lymphocytic leukemia
  - Adults: 0.09–0.1 mg/kg/d, continuous infusion for 7 days or daily brief infusion for 7 days.

Adjustment of dosage

- Kidney disease: Use with caution.
- Liver disease: None.
- Elderly: None.
- Pediatric: Safety and efficacy have not been established in children.

Pregnancy: Category D.

Lactation: No information available. Potentially toxic to infant. Avoid breastfeeding.

Contraindications: Hypersensitivity to cladribine, pregnancy.

Warnings/precautions

- Use with caution in patients with the following conditions: kidney disease, active infection.
- This agent causes severe bone marrow depression.

Advice to patient: Use two forms of birth control including hormonal and barrier methods.

Adverse reactions

- Common: fever (66%), rash, nausea, pain at injection site, fatigue, headache.
- Serious: **bone marrow suppression (may persist for 1 year)**, tachycardia.

Clinically important drug interactions: None.

Parameters to monitor

- CBC with differential and platelets, serum uric acid.
- Signs and symptoms of thrombocytopenia. Discontinue this medication if platelet count falls below $100,000/mm^3$.
- Signs and symptoms of bone marrow depression.

Editorial comments

- Fever with temperature greater than 100°F occurs in about two thirds of patients in the first month of therapy.
- Because cladribine is a potent bone marrow suppressant, careful monitoring of blood counts is required. CBC with differential

and platelet counts should be checked for the first 4–8 weeks after therapy. Prolonged monitoring is necessary in some patients.

Clarithromycin

Brand name: Biaxin.
Class of drug: Antibiotic, macrolide.
Mechanism of action: Inhibits RNA-dependent protein synthesis at the level of the 50S ribosome.
Susceptible organisms *in vivo*: Similar to erythromycin but more effective against gram-negative organisms and more active against *Hemophilus influenzae*. Also used for *Mycobacterium avium-intracellulare* and *Helicobacter pylori*.
Indications/dosage/route: Oral only.
• Pharyngitis/tonsillitis
  – Adults: 250 mg q12h, 10 days.
• Acute maxillary sinusitis
  – Adults: 500 mg q12h, 14 days.
• Acute exacerbation of chronic bronchitis (*Streptococcus pneumoniae, Moraxella catarrhalis*), pneumonia (*S. pneumoniae, Mycoplasma pneumoniae*)
  – Adults: 250 mg q12h, 7–14 days.
• Acute exacerbation of chronic bronchitis (*H. influenzae*)
  – Adults: 500 mg q12h, 7–14 days.
• Uncomplicated skin and skin structure infections
  – Adults: 250 mg q12h.
• All infections
  – Children: 7.5 mg/kg q12h.
Adjustment of dosage
• Kidney disease: None.
• Liver disease: None.
• Elderly: None.

- Pediatric: Safety and efficacy have not been established for children <6 months.

Food: Taken without regard to food.

Pregnancy: Should not be used except if no alternative is available.

Lactation: No data available. May appear in breast milk. Best to avoid.

Contraindications: Hypersensitivity to macrolide antibiotics, concomitant administration of pimozide.

Warnings/precautions: Use with caution in patients with liver or kidney dysfunction.

Adverse reactions
- Common: diarrhea, nausea, abdominal pain.
- Severe: pseudomembranous colitis, ventricular arrhythmias, nephritis, cholestatic jaundice, angioedema.

Clinically important drug interactions
- Drugs that decrease effects/toxicity of macrolides: rifampin, aluminum, magnesium containing antacids.
- Macrolides increase effects/toxicity of following drugs: oral anticoagulants, astemizole, benzodiazepines, bromocriptine, buspirone, carbamazepine, cisapride, cyclosporine, digoxin, ergot alkaloids, felodipine, grepafloxacin, statins, pimozide, sparfloxacin, tacrolimus.

Parameters to monitor
- Signs and symptoms of superinfection, in particular pseudomembranous colitis.
- Signs and symptoms of renal toxicity.
- Signs and symptoms of hearing impairment. Patients with kidney or liver disease are at highest risk.

Editorial comments
- In general, clarithromycin has no major clinical advantages over azithromycin except in the treatment of pneumonia because of better *S. pneumoniae* activity.
- Like azithromycin, clarithromycin is used in *M. avium-intracellulare* infections in AIDS patients. It is also a component of many treatment regimens for *H. pylori*.

Clemastine

Brand name: Tavist.
Class of drug: H_1 receptor blocker.
Mechanism of action: Antagonizes histamine effects on GI tract, respiratory tract, blood vessels.
Indications/dosage/route: Oral only.
- Allergic rhinitis
  - Adults, children >12: Initial: syrup or tablets, 1.34 mg b.i.d. Maximum: 8.04 mg/d.
  - Children 6–12 years: Initial: syrup 0.67 mg b.i.d. Maximum: 4.02 mg/d.
- Urticaria, angioedema
  - Adults, children >12: syrup or tablets 2.68 mg, 1–3 times/d. Maximum: 8.04 mg/d.
  - Children 6–12 years: syrup 1.34 mg b.i.d. Maximum: 4.02 mg/d.

Adjustment of dosage
- Kidney disease: None.
- Liver disease: None.
- Elderly: None.
- Pediatric: Safety and efficacy have not been established in children <6 years.

Onset of Action	Peak Effect	Duration
—	5–7 h	10–12 h

Food: No restriction.
Pregnancy: Category B.
Lactation: Appears in breast milk. American Academy of Pediatrics suggests caution with use during breastfeeding.
Contraindications: Hypersensitivity to antihistamines, acute asthma, narrow-angle glaucoma, use in newborns, concurrent use of MAO inhibitor.

Editorial comments

• This drug is not listed in the *Physician's Desk Reference*, 54th edition, 2000.

• For additional information, see *brompheniramine*, p. 107.

Clofibrate

Brand name: Atromid-S.

Class of drug: Lipid-lowering agent.

Mechanism of action: Inhibits hepatic lipoprotein release, possibly potentiates lipoprotein lipase.

Indications/dosage/route: Oral only.

• Primary dysbetalipoproteinemia (type III) that does not respond to diet; some patients with refractory hyperlipedemia with elevated cholesterol and triglyceride levels (Type IV, V)
 – Adults: Usual: 2 g daily in divided doses.

Adjustment of dosage

• Kidney disease: Creatinine clearance >50 mL/min: dose q6–12h; creatinine clearance 10–50 mL/min: dose q12–18h; creatinine clearance <10 mL/min: avoid.

• Liver disease: Contraindicated if severe.

• Elderly: None

• Pediatric: Safety and efficacy have not been established in children.

Food: Take with food.

Pregnancy: Category C. Avoid in near-term pregnancy.

Lactation: Present in breast milk. Best to avoid.

Contraindications: Severe renal or hepatic dysfunction, primary biliary cirrhosis, hypersensitivity to clofibrate, pregnancy.

Warnings/precautions

• Use with caution in patients with the following conditions: gout, peptic ulcer.

• This drug is associated with increased rate of cholelithiasis.

Advice to patient
- Report muscle pain or weakness to treating physician.
- Use two forms of birth control including hormonal and barrier methods.

Adverse reactions
- Common: nausea, GI distress.
- Serious: cholethiasis, angina, arrhythmia, urticaria, bone marrow depression, renal toxicity, myopathy, rhabdomyolysis.

Clinically important drugs interactions
- Drug that increases effects/toxicity of clofibrate: probenicid.
- Clofibrate increases effects/toxicity of following drugs: oral anticoagulants, sulfonylureas, insulin, furosemide, phenytoin, lovastatin.

Parameters to monitor
- Serum lipid profile, CBC with differential and platelets, liver enzymes, serum BUN and creatinine, urine protein, cardiac function (for arrhythmias, angina).
- Signs and symptoms of renal toxicity.
- Signs and symptoms of hepatotoxicity.

Editorial comment: Use an alternative agent whenever possible as this drug is potentially carcinogenic and has not been shown to lessen cardiovascular mortality in hyperlipemic patients.

Clomiphene

Brand names: Clomid, Milophene, Serophene.
Class of drug: Ovulatory stimulant.
Mechanism of action: Stimulates release of pituitary gonadotropins (FSH, LH).
Indications/dosage/route: Oral only.
- Ovulation induction

– 50 mg/d, 5 days; if ovulation does not occur, 100 mg/d; 5-day course in another ovulatory cycle until conception occurs. Three courses should be adequate. If conception does not occur, reevaluate diagnosis. Begin drug on or about day 5 of menstrual cycle.

Pregnancy: Category X, contraindicated.

Lactation: Avoid, no information available.

Contraindications: hypersensitivity, pregnancy, abnormal uterine bleeding, liver disease, ovarian cysts, uncontrolled thyroid or adrenal dysfunction, organic intracranial lesion such as pituitary tumor.

Warnings/precautions

• Ovarian hyperstimulation syndrome (ovarian enlargement, GI symptoms, electrolyte disturbances) may occur with clomiphene. Start with lowest dose in patients with polycystic ovary syndrome.

• Inform patient of possibility of multiple births.

Advice to patient

• If visual disturbances occur (eg, blurred vision, spots), report to physician immediately for ophthalmologic evaluation.

• Avoid driving and other activities requiring mental alertness or that are potentially dangerous until response to drug is known.

Adverse reactions

• Common: ovarian enlargement, hot flashes.

• Serious: visual disturbances, ectopic pregnancy, pituitary hemorrhage, ovarian hyperstimulation syndrome, acute abdomen, severe allergic reactions, liver toxicity, secondary malignancies.

Clinically important drug interactions: None reported.

Parameters to monitor

• Visual disturbances.

• Weight gain.

• Abdominal pain or distention: possibility of tubal pregnancy. Perform frequent pregnancy tests to preclude pregnancy.

Editorial comments

• This drug has potential teratogenic effects. Inform patient of this hazard to pregnancy.

• If patients develops symptoms while receiving this agent, drug administration should be immediately discontinued and a complete ophthalmologic examination should be performed.

Clomipramine

Brand name: Anafranil.
Class of drug: Tricyclic antidepressant.
Mechanism of action: Inhibits reuptake of CNS neurotransmitters, primarily serotonin and norepinephrine.
Indications/dosage/route: Oral only.
  – Adults: Initial: 25 mg/d; increase to maximum of 250 mg/d.
  – Adolescents, children: Initial: 25 mg/d; increase to maximum of 200 mg.
  – Maintenance, adults and children: Lowest effective dose. Reassess to determine if continued therapy is needed.
Adjustment of dosage
• Kidney disease: None.
• Liver disease: None.
• Elderly: Lower doses recommended.
• Pediatric: Not recommended for children <12 years old.
Food: No restriction.
Pregnancy: Category C.
Lactation: Appears in breast milk. American Academy of Pediatrics expresses concern over use when breastfeeding.
Contraindications: Hypersensitivity to tricyclic antidepressants, acute recovery from MI, concurrent use of MAO inhibitor.
Editorial comments
• This drug is listed without details in the *Physician's Desk Reference*, 54th edition, 2000.
• For additional information, see *amitriptyline*, p. 39.

Clonidine

Brand name: Catapres.

Class of drug: Centrally acting antihypertensive, antiadrenergic.

Mechanism of action: Activates α_2 receptors in brain, resulting in an inhibitory effect on catecholamine release, thereby decreasing activity of CNS vasomotor center.

Indications/dosage/route: Oral, transdermal.

• Hypertension
  – PO: Initial: 0.1 mg b.i.d. a.m. and h.s.; increase dose to 0.1 mg/d as needed/tolerated. Maintenance: 0.2–0.6 mg/d. Maximum: 2.4 mg/d (rarely used at this dose).
  – Transdermal patch: Apply once q7d, start with 0.1 mg/d dose, increase dose as required q1–2wk. Allow 2–3 days for initial effect. Apply on upper arm or chest. Use a different site for each weekly application. Change q7d.

Adjustment of dosage

• Kidney disease: creatinine clearance <10 mL/min: 50–75% of normal initial dose.
• Liver disease: None.
• Elderly: May require lower doses. Initial: 0.1 mg q h.s.
• Pediatric: Safety and efficacy have not been established in children <12 years.

	Onset of Action	Peak Effect	Duration
Oral	30–60 min	2–4 h	12–24 h
Transdermal	2–3 d	No data	7 d

Food: No restriction.
Pregnancy: Category C.

Lactation: Appears in breast milk. Best to avoid.
Contraindications: Hypersensitivity to clonidine.

Warnings/precautions
- Use with caution in patients with the following conditions: severe coronary disease, recent MI, hepatic or renal disease, cerebral vascular disease.
- Localized contact dermatitis may occur with use of the clonidine patch.
- If hypertension is severe, another antihypertensive drug may be required.

Advice to patient
- Do not stop taking drug abruptly as this may precipitate a withdrawal reaction (eg, hypertensive crisis).
- Change position slowly, in particular from recumbent to upright, to minimize orthostatic hypotension. Sit at the edge of the bed for several minutes before standing, and lie down if feeling faint or dizzy. Avoid hot showers or baths and standing for long periods. Male patients with orthostatic hypotension may be safer urinating while seated on the toilet rather than standing.
- Apply patch at bedtime to clean, hairless area of upper arm or chest.
- Take last oral dose at bedtime to provide for continuing BP control during night hours.
- Avoid extremes of temperature, hot or cold.
- Do not discontinue drug suddenly. There may be a severe withdrawal reaction within 12–48 hours of the last dose. Drug dose should be gradually decreased over 3–4 days.
- Avoid driving and other activities requiring mental alertness or that are potentially dangerous until response to drug is known.
- For symptomatic relief of dry mouth, rinse mouth with warm water frequently, chew sugarless gum, suck on ice cube, use artificial saliva if necessary, carry out meticulous oral hygiene (floss teeth daily).
- Avoid alcohol and other CNS depressants such as opiate analgesics and sedatives (eg, diazepam) when taking this drug.

Adverse reactions
- Common: dizziness, sedation, drowsiness, dry mouth, constipation, weakness.
- Serious: orthostatic hypotension, rebound hypertension, tachycardia, sinus bradycardia, CHF, depression, AV block, urticaria, thrombocytopenia.

Clinically important drug interactions
- Drugs that decrease effects/toxicity of clonidine: tricyclic antidepressants.
- Clonidine increases toxicity/effects of the following: alcohol, barbiturates, and other sedative hyponotics, amitriptyline (corneal lesions), β blockers, narcotic analgesics, alcohol, barbiturates, CNS depressants including alcohol, other antihypertensive agents.

Parameters to monitor
- Signs and symptoms of depression, particularly in patient who has a history of this condition.
- BP.
- Signs and symptoms of CNS toxicity.

Editorial comments
- Clonidine has a number of non-FDA-approved uses including treatment for opiate withdrawal, smoking cessation, migraine headache, diabetic diarrhea.
- Generally not used as first-line therapy for hypertension.
- Taper oral dose gradually over one or more weeks to avoid rebound hypertension and withdrawal reaction.

Clorazepate

Brand name: Tranxene.
Class of drug: Antianxiety agent, hypnotic.
Mechanism of action: Potentiates effects of GABA in limbic system and reticular formation.

Indications/dosage/route: Oral only.
• Anxiety
  – Adults: Initial: 7.5–15 mg b.i.d. to q.i.d. Maintenance: 15–60 mg/d in divided dose.
  – Elderly, debilitated: Initial: 7.5–15 mg/d.
• Acute alcohol withdrawal
  – Day 1, initial: 30 mg; then 15 mg b.i.d. to q.i.d. Day 2: 45–90 mg in divided doses. Day 3: 22.5–45 mg in divided doses. Day 4: 15–30 mg in divided doses. Maximum: 90 mg/d.
• Adjunct to antiepileptic drugs
  – Adults, children >12: Initial: 7.5 mg t.i.d. Maximum: 90 mg/d.
  – Children 9–12 years: Initial: 7.5 mg b.i.d. Maximum: 60 mg/d.

Adjustment of dosage
• Kidney disease: Use with caution.
• Liver disease: Use with caution.
• Elderly: See above.
• Pediatric: Not recommended for children <9 years.

Food: No restrictions.

Pregnancy: Category D.

Lactation: Appears in breast milk. Potentially toxic to infant. American Academy of Pediatrics expresses concern about breast-feeding while taking benzodiazepines. Avoid breastfeeding.

Contraindications: Hypersensitivity to benzodiazepines, pregnancy.

Warnings/precautions
• Use with caution in patients with the following conditions: history of drug abuse, severe renal and hepatic impairment, elderly, neonates, infants.
• Benzodiazepines may cause psychologic and physical dependence.
• Benzodiazepines may cause paradoxical rage.
• It is best not to prescribe this drug for more than 6 months. If there is a need for long-term therapy, evaluate patient frequently.
• Use only for patients who have significant anxiety without medication, do not respond to other treatment, and are not drug abusers.

Advice to patient

• Avoid driving and other activities requiring mental alertness or that are potentially dangerous until response to drug is known.

• Avoid alcohol and other CNS depressants such as narcotic analgesics, alcohol, antidepressants, antihistamines, barbiturates, when taking this drug.

• Avoid use of OTC medications without first informing the treating physician.

• Cigarette smoking will decrease drug effect. Do not smoke when taking this drug.

• Do not stop drug abruptly if taken for more than 1 month. If suddenly withdrawn, there may be recurrence of the original anxiety or insomnia. A full-blown withdrawal symptom may occur consisting of vomiting, insomnia, tremor, sweating, muscle spasms. After chronic use, decrease drug dosage slowly, ie, over a period of several weeks at 25%/wk.

• Avoid excessive use of xanthine-containing foods (regular coffee, tea, chocolate) as these may counteract the action of the drug.

Adverse reactions

• Common: drowsiness, dizziness.

• Serious: respiratory depression, depression, apnea, hepatitis, worsened kidney function, anemia, hypotension.

Clinically important drug interactions

• Drugs that increase effects/toxicity of benzodiazepines: CNS depressants (alcohol, antihistamines, narcotic analgesics, tricyclic antidepressants, SSRIs, MAO inhibitors), cimetidine, disufiram.

• Drugs that decrease effects/toxicity of benzodiazepines: flumazenil (antidote or overdose), carbamazepine.

Parameters to monitor

• Liver enzymes, CBC with differential and platelets, serum BUN and creatinine.

• Signs of chronic toxicity: ataxia, vertigo, slurred speech.

• Dosing to make sure amount taken is as prescribed, particularly if patient has suicidal tendencies.

• Efficacy of treatment: reduced symptoms of anxiety and tension, improved sleep.

- Signs of physical/psychologic dependence, particularly if patient is addiction-prone and requests frequent renewal of prescription or is experiencing a diminished response to the drug.
- Patient's neurologic status including memory (anterograde amnesia), disturbing thoughts, unusual behavior.
- Possibility of blood dyscrasias: fever, sore throat, upper respiratory infection. Perform total and differential WBC counts.

Editorial comments: The side effect profile of clorazepate appears better than those of some other benzodiazepines. Seizures may occur if flumazenil is given after long-term use of benzodiazepines.

Cloxacillin

Brand names: Cloxapen, Togepen.
Class of drug: Antibiotic, penicillin family plus β-lactamase inhibitor.
Mechanism of action: Inhibits bacterial cell wall synthesis.
Susceptible organisms *in vivo*: MSSA, streptococci.
Indications/dosage/route: Oral only.
- Skin and soft tissue infections, mild to moderate upper respiratory tract infections
  – Adults, children >20 kg: 250 mg q6h.
  – Children <20 kg: 50 mg/kg/d in divided doses q6h.
- Lower respiratory tract infections or disseminated infections
  – Adults, children >20 kg: 500 mg q6h.
  – Children <20 kg: 100 mg/kg/d in divided doses q6h.

Adjustment of dosage: None.
Food: Take on empty stomach, 1 hour before or 2 hours after eating.
Pregnancy: Category B.
Lactation: No data available. Best to avoid.
Contraindications: Hypersensitivity to penicillin or cephalosporins.

Editorial comments
- This drug is not listed in the *Physician's Desk Reference*, 54th edition, 2000.
- For additional information, see *penicillin G*, p. 708.

Codeine

Class of drug: Narcotic analgesic, agonist.

Mechanism of action: Binds to opiate receptors and blocks ascending pain pathways; reduces patient's perception of pain without altering cause of the pain.

Indications/dosage/route: Oral, IM, IV, SC.
- Analgesia
  - Adults: All routes 15–60 mg q4–6h. Maximum: 360 mg/d.
  - Children >1 year: All routes 0.5 mg/kg q4–6h.
- Antitussive
  - Adults: All routes 10–20 mg q4–6h. Maximum: 120 mg/d.
  - Children 2–6 years: PO 2.5–5 mg q4–6h. Maximum: 30 mg/d.
  - Children 6–12 years: PO 5–10 mg q4–6h. Maximum: 60 mg/d.

Adjustment of dosage
- Kidney disease: None.
- Liver disease: None.
- Elderly: None.
- Pediatric: See above.

	Onset of Action	Peak Effect	Duration
oral	10–30 min	0.5–1 h	4–6 h

Food: May be taken with food to lessen GI upset.

Pregnancy: Category C. Category D if prolonged use or if given in high doses at term.

Lactation: Appears in breast milk. Potentially toxic to infant. Considered compatible with breastfeeding by American Academy of Pediatrics.

Contraindications: Hypersensitivity to narcotics of the same chemical class.

Warnings/precautions

• Use with caution in patients with the following conditions: head injury with increased intracranial pressure, serious alcoholism, prostatic hypertrophy, COPD, severe liver or kidney disease, postoperative patients with pulmonary disease, disorders of biliary tract.

• Administer drug before patient experiences severe pain for fullest efficacy of the drug.

• Have the following available when treating patient with this drug: naloxone (Narcan) or other antagonist, means of administering oxygen, and support of respiration.

• Nausea, vomiting, and orthostatic hypotension occur most prominently in ambulatory patients. If nausea and vomiting persist, it may be necessary to administer an antiemetic, eg, droperidol or prochlorperazine.

• This drug can cause severe hypotension in a patient who is volume depleted or if given along with a phenothiazine or general anesthesia.

• Careful diagnosis must be made of acute abdominal condition before this drug is administered.

• For additional information, see *morphine*, p. 633.

Colchicine

Class of drug: Antigout.

Mechanism of action: Inhibits leukocyte migration and lactic acid production. Exact mechanism in gout not established.

Indications/dosage/route: Oral, IV.

• Acute attack of gout or gouty arthritis

– Adult: Initial: PO 0.5–1.2 mg followed by additional dosages 0.5–0.6 mg every 1–2 hours until relief or GI side effects.
• Prevention of acute attacks of gout
– Adult: IV 0.5–0.6 mg once a day or every other day or 1–3 mg initial IV followed by 0.5 mg IV q6h until response. Maximum: 4 mg per 24 hours. May require 1–2 mg daily for several days.
• Prevention of attacks of gout in patients undergoing surgery
– Adults: PO 0.5–0.6 mg t.i.d. 3 days before and 3 days after surgery.
• Gouty arthritis or prophylaxis of recurrent attacks
– PO 0.5–6 mg/d or every other day.

Adjustment of dosage
• Kidney disease: Creatinine clearance <50 mL/min: Creatinine clearance <10 mL/min: decrease dose by 50% for acute attack.
• Liver disease: None.
• Elderly: Reduce dosages if symptoms of toxicity appear, eg, weakness, GI problems.
• Pediatric: Safety and efficacy have not been established. Has been used in children for familial Mediterranean fever.

Pregnancy: Category C by oral route. Category D by parenteral route.

Lactation: Appears in breast milk. Considered compatible by American Academy of Pediatrics.

Contraindications: Hypersensitivity to colchicine; pregnancy.

Warnings/precautions
• Use with caution in patients with the following conditions: renal, hepatic, GI disorders, debilitated and elderly patients.
• May produce severe local inflammation when given by SC or IM route.

Advice to patient
• Drink large amounts of fluids, 3–3.5 L/d.
• Use two forms of birth control including hormonal and barrier methods.

Adverse reactions
• Common: nausea, vomiting, diarrhea.

- Serious: aplastic anemia, agranulocytosis, thrombocytopenia (long-term administration), hepatotoxicity, myopathy, peripheral neuropathy.

Clinically important drug interactions
- Drugs that increase effects/toxicity of colchicine: alkalinizing agents.
- Drugs that decrease effects/toxicity of colchicine: acidifying agents.
- Colchicine increases effects/toxicity of sympathomimetic drugs.

Parameters to monitor
- CBC with differential and platelets, liver enzymes.
- Signs of toxicity: nausea, vomiting, diarrhea. Administer paragoric if diarrhea is severe.
- Signs of liver toxicity.
- Signs of myopathy, peripheral neuropathy.

Editorial comments: Animal studies suggest that colchicine is a mutagenic agent. The clinical significance of this not known.

Colestipol

Brand name: Colestid.
Class of drug: Lipid-lowering agent.
Mechanism of action: Binds bile acids, forming a non-absorbable complex in the intestinal lumen, resulting in inreased fecal bile acid excretion and increased cholesterol metabolism, decreased LDL, VLDL cholesterol, and total cholesterol levels in the serum.
Indications/dosage/route: Oral only.
- Primary hypercholestermia
  – Adults, tablets: Initial: 2 g once or twice daily. Maintenance: 2–16 g/d. Adults, granules: Initial, 5 g once or twice daily. Increase by 5 mg/d at 1- to 2-months intervals as needed. Total: 5–30 g once a day or 2–3 divided doses.

Adjustment of dosage: None.
Food: Take with meals.
Pregnancy: Category D. It is recommended to discontinue therapy during gestation.
Lactation: Use with caution. Effect of vitamin malabsorption in nursing infants unknown; however, not systemically absorbed.
Contraindications: Hypersensitivity to cholestyramine and other bile acid-sequestering resins; complete biliary obstruction; type III, IV, or V hyperlipoproteinemia.
Editorial comments: For additional information, see *cholestyramine*, p. 214.

Cortisone

Brand name: Cortone.
Class of drug: Topical, systemic antiinflammatory glucocorticoid.
Mechanism of action: Inhibits migration of polymorphonuclear leukocytes; stabilizes lysosomal membranes; inhibits production of products of arachidonic acid cascade.
Indications/dosage/route: Oral. Dosages of corticosteroids are variable. These should be individualized according to the disease being treated and the response of the patient.
• Replacement therapy
  – Initial or during crisis: 25–300 mg/d.
• Antiinflammatory
  – 25–150 mg/d.
• Acute rheumatic fever
  – Initial: 200 mg b.i.d. Maintenance: 200 mg/d.
Adjustment of dosage
• Kidney disease: None.
• Liver disease: None.
• Elderly: None.

- Pediatric: For systemic use: children on long-term therapy must be monitored carefully for growth and development.

Food: Administer with food to minimize GI upset.

Pregnancy: Category D.

Lactation: No data available. Best to avoid.

Contraindications: Systemic fungal, viral, or bacterial infections, Cushing's syndrome, hypersensitivity to corticosteroids.

Editorial comments

- Higher pregnancy category and increased reports of congenital defects with cortisone use may reflect higher frequency of use rather than increased risk compared with other corticosteroids.
- For additional information, see *prednisone*, p. 760.

Cromolyn

Brand names: Gastrocrom, Intal, Nasalcrom, Opticrom.

Class of drug: Inhalation and ophthalmic, antiallergic and antiasthmatic.

Mechanism of action

- Antiasthmatic: mast cell stabilizer, prevents release of histamine and other allergens from mast cells.
- Ocular antiallergic action: inhibits degranulation of sensitized mast cells.

Indications/dosage/route: Inhalation, topical (ophthalmic).

- Severe perennial bronchial asthma
  - Adults, children >6 years: Two inhalations q.i.d.
- Prevention and treatment of allergic rhinitis
  - Adults, children ≥6 years: One spray in each nostril t.i.d. or q.i.d. Maximum: 6 per day.
- Prevention of exercise-induced bronchospasm
  - Adults, children >5 years: Two sprays from inhaler, less than 1 hour before exercise.
- Allergic ocular disorders

– Adults, children >4 years: One or two drops in each eye, 4–6 times/d.

Adjustment of dosage
• Kidney disease: Reduce dosage.
• Liver disease: Reduce dosage.
• Pediatric: Use of ophthalmic preparations has not been established in children <4 years. Use of nasal preparation has not been established in children <6 years. Use of inhaled preparation has not been established in children <2 years.

Pregnancy: Category B.

Lactation: No data available. Use with caution.

Contraindications: Hypersensitivity to cromolyn.

Warnings/precautions
• Cromolyn is to be used prophylactically; it has no benefit for acute asthma or status asthmaticus.
• Bronchospasm may occur occasionally following inhalation. Inhaled β_2 agonist should be administered to counteract.
• Continue corticosteroid administration after beginning cromolyn and taper steroid slowly. Steroid may have to be given again at times of stress.

Advice to patient
• Do not discontinue inhalation product without consulting treating physician. Inhalation product should be reduced progressively over a 1-week period, eg, decrease daily dose by one puff every 2 days.
• Take inhalation product 15 minutes before exercise for best results.
• Ophthalmic solution should be kept in a dark place and discarded 4 weeks after container is opened.
• Do not use soft contact lenses when using ophthalmic preparation without consulting treating physician.

Adverse reactions
• Common: cough (transient).
• Serious: bronchospasm, angioedema.

Clinically important drug interactions: None.

Parameters to monitor: Pulmonary status before and shortly after initiating therapy. Monitor for coughing or wheezing.

Editorial comments: Cromolyn is used as an airway antiinflammatory agent for the prevention of asthma attacks. As such it is considered to be a steroid-sparing agent.

Cyclobenzaprine

Brand name: Flexeril.
Class of drug: Skeletal muscle relaxant.
Mechanism of action: Inhibits alpha and gamma motor neurons. Reduces tonic somatic motor activity.
Indications/dosage/route: Oral only.
• Muscle spasm associated with acute musculoskeletal conditions
  – Adults: 20–40 mg divided b.i.d. or q.i.d. Maximum: 60 mg/d. Maximum length of administration: 2–3 weeks.
Adjustment of dosage
• Kidney diseases: None.
• Liver diseases: None.
• Elderly: It may be necessary to reduce dose.
• Pediatric: Safety and efficacy in children <15 years have not been established.

Onset of Action	Duration
<1 h	12–14 h

Food: Avoid excessive intake of food and drink.
Pregnancy: Category B.
Lactation: Likely to appear in breast milk. Potentially toxic to infant. Avoid breastfeeding.
Contraindications: Recovery from MI, heart block, arrhythmias, congestive heart failure, hyperthyroidism. Not to be used along with or within 14 days of MAO inhibitor.

Warnings/precautions: Use with caution in patients with the following conditions: angle-closure glaucoma, increased intraocular pressure, BPH.

Advice to patient

• Avoid alcohol and other CNS depressants such as opiate analgesics and sedatives (eg, diazepam) when taking this drug.

• Do the following for symptomatic relief of dry mouth: Rinse mouth with warm water frequently, chew sugarless gum, suck on ice cube, use artificial saliva if necessary, carry out meticulous oral hygiene (floss teeth daily).

Adverse reactions

• Common: drowsiness, dizziness, dry mouth.

• Serious: arrhythmias, hypotension, hepatitis.

Clinically important drug interactions

• Drugs that increase effects/toxicity of cyclobenzaprine: CNS depressants, atropine-type drugs, MAO inhibitors, tricyclic antidepressants

• Cyclobenzaprine decreases effects/toxicity of guanethidine.

Parameters to monitor

• Liver enzymes.

• Efficacy of treatment: reduction in pain, tenderness, increased range of motion.

• Signs of urinary retention: overflow incontinence, abdominal distention.

• Signs and symptoms of pseudomembranous colitis.

Editorial comments: This agent is indicated only for short-term use (≤3 weeks). It is ineffective in the treatment of spasticity caused by spinal cord disease, cerebral disorders, and cerebral palsy.

Cyclophosphamide

Brand name: Cytoxan.
Class of drug: Alkylating anticancer drug.

Mechanism of action: Forms covalent bond with elements in DNA preventing separation of strands of DNA during cell division.
Indications/dosage/route: Oral, IV.
• Treatment of malignant diseases
  – Adults, children: IV 40–50 mg/kg in divided doses over 2–5 days. PO 1–5 mg/kg/d, initial and maintenance doses.
• Treatment of nonmalignant diseases: biopsy-proven "minimal change", nephrotic syndrome in children
  – PO 2.5–3 mg/kg/d for 60–90 days.

Onset of Action
1–2 wk

Pregnancy: Category D.
Lactation: Appears in breast milk. Potentially toxic to infant. Considered contraindicated by American Academy of Pediatrics.
Contraindications: Failure to respond to previously administered drug, hypersensitivity to cyclophosphamide, severe bone marrow depression.
Editorial comments: For additional information, see *busulfan*, p. 120.

Cycloserine

Brand name: Seromycin.
Class of drug: Antituberculous agent.
Mechanism of action: Inhibits bacterial cell wall synthesis.
Indications/dosage/route: Oral only.
• Adjunct in treatment of pulmonary or extrapulmonary tuberculosis
  – Adults: PO 15–20 mg/kg/d, 2 divided doses. Maximum: 1 g/d.
  – Children: 10–15 mg/kg/d. Maximum: 1 g/d.

• UTI
  – Adults: PO 250 mg q12h, 2 weeks.
Editorial commments: This drug is seldom used.

Cyclosporine

Brand names: Neoral, Sandimmune.
Class of drug: Antibiotic immunosuppressant.
Mechanism of action: Inhibits synthesis and release of inter-leukin II and activation of T lymphocytes.
Indications/dosage/route: Oral, IV. IV form should be used only for those patients who cannot tolerate oral administration.
• Prevention of organ rejection in kidney, liver, heart, bone marrow transplantation
  – Adults, children, PO: Initial: 10–14/kg as single dose 4–12 hours before transplantation. Postoperatively: 14–18 mg/kg as single daily dose; continue for 1–2 weeks, then taper over 6–8 weeks to maintenance dose of 5–10 mg/d.
  – Adults, children, IV: Initial, 5–6 mg/kg as single dose 4–12 hours before transplantation. Postoperatively: 5–6 mg/kg/d until patient can tolerate oral drug.
(A corticosteroid is generally administered along with IV cyclo-sporine. The following is suggested for prednisone: initial oral dose of 2 mg/kg for 4 days, tapered as follows: 1 mg/kg/d by day 7, 0.3 mg/kg/d by 30 days, 0.15 mg/kg/d after 2 months. Maintenance: 0.15 mg/kg/d after 2 months.)
Adjustment of dosage
• Kidney disease: Use with caution. Reduce dose if azotemia occurs.
• Liver disease: Reduce dose and monitor levels closely.
• Elderly: Same as adult dosage.
• Pediatric: Safety and efficacy have not been established although drug has been used in children as young as 6 months (see above).

Food: Can be taken with food, but *not* with grapefruit juice. Mix solution of cyclosporine with chocolate milk, milk, or orange juice to improve palatability. Stir well and drink immediately. Do not allow to stand after mixing.

Pregnancy: Category C.

Lactation: Appears in breast milk. Considered contraindicated in breastfeeding by American Academy of Pediatrics.

Contraindications: Hypersensitivity to cyclosporine or to excipient found in injectable form (Cremophor-EL, a castor oil derivative).

Warnings/precautions

- Can cause nephrotoxicity and hepatotoxicity.
- Use criteria to differentiate kidney rejection from cyclosporine nephrotoxicity.
- Advise patient of the necessity of repeated laboratory testing while on this drug.
- Do not use solutions of cyclosporine that contain particulate matter or are discolored.
- Because of its immunosuppressive action, cyclosporine may increase susceptibility to infections and development of lymphoma.
- For patients receiving cyclosporine intravenously: Observe carefully for at least 30 minutes after administration. In particular watch for possible severe allergic reaction including anaphylaxis. Appropriate measures must be available for treating anaphylactic shock.
- Warn patient to take cyclosporine exactly as directed in terms of time of day and eating schedule.
- Patients with hypoalbuminia, hypocholesterolemia, and hypomagnesemia are at higher risk for seizure from cyclosporine.

Advice to patient

- Do not stop taking this drug without consulting treating physician.
- Avoid vaccinations.
- Report persistent diarrhea to treating physician.

• Use two forms of birth control including hormonal and barrier methods.

Adverse reactions

• Common: tremor, hypertension, gum hyperplasia, hirsutism.
• Serious: **nephrotoxicity**, seizures, bone marrow depression, liver toxicity, anaphylactic shock, infections, pancreatitis, hypotension, hyperkalemia, sinusitis, respiratory distress.

Clinically important drug interactions

• Drugs that increase effects/toxicity of cyclosporine: gentamicin, tobramycin, vancomycin, amphotericin B, ketoconazole, melphalan, cimetidine, ranitidine, diclofenac, trimethoprim with sulfamethoxazole, diltiazem, verapamil, bromocriptine, erythromycin, methylprednisolone.
• Drugs that decrease effects/toxicity of cyclosporine: rifampin, phenytoin, phenobarbital, carbamazepine.
• Cyclosporine increases effects/toxicity of digoxin, prednisolone, lovastatin.

Parameters to monitor

• CBC with differential and platelets, baseline and subsequent serum BUN and creatinine, liver enzymes.
• Baseline and subsequent serum albumin and cholesterol levels.
• Signs of hepatotoxicity: elevated bilirubin, liver enzymes.
• Signs and symptoms of renal toxicity. Monitor closely for evidence of persistent high elevations of BUN and creatinine. Consider switching to another immunosuppressant.
• Plasma levels of cyclosporine. Posttransplant therapeutic levels: first 6 weeks, 300–400 ng/mL (by TOX); 6 weeks–6 months: 250–350 ng/mL; 6 months–1 year: 150–250 ng/mL; >1 year: 100–125 ng/mL. Toxic levels: generally >400 ng/mL.
• Signs of convulsions when cyclosporine is combined with high-dose methylprednisone.
• Signs and symptoms of CNS toxicity: headache, confusion, seizures, hallucinations, mania, encephalopathy.

Editorial comments

• Only physicians experienced in immunosuppressive therapy and management of organ transplant patients should administer cyclosporine. The physician responsible for follow-up care of the patient should have complete information about maintenance therapy with this drug.

• Rapidly rising BUN and creatinine levels are common to both renal toxicity and organ rejection. Accordingly, it is necessary to differentiate between them. If nephrotoxicity does not respond to reduction in cyclosporine dosage, further evaluation with possible addition of another immunosuppressant should be considered, eg, azathioprine plus prednisone. Commonly, oral cyclosporine is started after transplant, particularly using Neoral form. Newer uses include treatment of inflammatory bowel disease, rheumatoid arthritis, and psoriasis.

Cyproheptadine

Brand name: Periactin.
Class of drug: H_1 receptor blocker.
Mechanism of action: Antagonizes histamine effects on GI tract, respiratory tract, blood vessels.
Indications/dosage/route: Oral only.
• Allergic, vasomotor, seasonal rhinitis; mild urticaria; anaphylactic reactions (combined with other agents)
  – Adults: Initial: 4 mg q8h. Maintenance: 4–20 mg/d. Maximum: 0.5 mg/kg/d.
  – Children 2–6 years: 2 mg q8–12h. Maximum: 12 mg/d.
  – Children 6–14 years: 4 mg q8–12h. Maximum: 16 mg/d.
Adjustment of dosage
• Kidney disease: None.
• Liver disease: None.
• Elderly: Use with caution. At higher risk for side effects.
• Pediatric: See above. Avoid in neonates and premature infants. Children <2 years are at risk for overdosage.
Food: No restriction.
Pregnancy: Category B.
Lactation: No data available. Potentially toxic to infant. Avoid breastfeeding.

Contraindications: Hypersensitivity to antihistamines, acute asthma, narrow-angle glaucoma, concurrent use of MAO inhibitor, newborn premature infants, lactation.

Editorial Comments

• Cyproheptadine has antiserotonergic as well as antihistaminic properties. It has also been used as appetite stimulant and sedative (nonapproved).

• For additional information, see *brompheniramine*, p. 107.

Cytarabine

Brand name: Cytosar-U.

Class of drug: Antineoplastic antimetabolite.

Mechanism of action: Converted to active metabolite which is a competitive inhibitor of DNA polymerase.

Indications/dosage/route: IV, SC, IM, intrathecal.

• Acute leukemias (myelocytic, lymphocytic)
  – Adults, children, IV: Usual dose: 100 mg/m^2 q12h, continuous IV infusion, 5 days. Subsequently administered at various time intervals with a dose range of 100–200 mg/m^2/d for 5 days.
  – Adults, children, intrathecal: 5–75 mg/m^2/d every 4 days.
  – Adults: IM, SC 1–1.5 mg/kg every 1–4 weeks.

• Refractory leukemia, non-Hodgkin's lymphoma
  – High dose: IV 1–3 g/m^2 × q12h.

Adjustment of dosage: None.

Pregnancy: Category D.

Lactation: No data available. Potentially toxic to infant. Avoid breastfeeding.

Contraindications: Hypersensitivity to cytarabine.

Warnings/precautions

• Use with caution in patients with the following conditions: hepatic or kidney disease, reduced bone marrow reserve.

• Administer ophthalmic corticosteroids with high-dose therapy to avoid cytarabine-induced conjunctivitis.

Advice to patient
- Use two forms of birth control including hormonal and barrier methods.
- Use good oral hygiene to prevent adverse reactions in the mouth. Drink large amounts of fluids.
- Avoid taking NSAIDs together with this drug.
- Do not receive any vaccinations (particularly live attenuated viruses) without permission from treating physician.

Adverse reactions
- Common: oral ulceration, anal lesions, rash, nausea, vomiting, diarrhea.
- Serious: **myelosuppression, hepatic injury, cerebellar damage (high dose), seizures (intrathecal)**, "cytarabine syndrome" (bone pain, myalgia, fever, maculopapular rash, angina), anaphylaxis, peripheral neuropathy, pulmonary edema (high dose), cardiomegaly, pericarditis (high dose), sepsis, bleeding, respiratory failure.

Clinically important drug interactions
- Drugs that increase effects/toxicity of cytarabine: alkylating agents, methotrexate, purine-type agents, cyclophosphamide, radiation.
- Cytarabine decreases effects/toxicity of gentamicin, flucytosine, digoxin.

Parameters to monitor
- CBC with differential and platelets, liver enzymes.
- Signs and symptoms of bone marrow depression.
- Signs and symptoms of infection.
- Signs and symptoms of thrombocytopenia.
- Periodic eye examinations required.
- Intake of fluids and urinary and other fluid output to minimize renal toxicity. Closely monitor electrolyte levels.
- Signs and symptoms of stomatitis: mouth sores, painful swallowing, dry mouth, white patchy areas in oral mucosa. Treat with peroxide, tea, topical anesthetics such as benzocaine and lidocaine or antifungal drug.
- Signs of hyperuricemia: gouty arthritis, uric acid kidney stones.
- Signs and symptoms of anemia.
- Signs and symptoms of renal toxicity.

Editorial comments
- Use latex gloves and safety glasses when handling cytotoxic drugs. Avoid contact with skin as well as inhalation. If possible, prepare in biologic hood.
- This agent has potent bone marrow suppressant effects and patients on this drug require close supervision.
- During induction therapy, measurement of leukocyte and platelet counts should be performed daily. It is recommended that bone marrow examinations be performed after blasts disappear from peripheral blood.
- Also note other severe toxic effects of this agent, particularly those seen with high-dose therapy.
- Conjunctivitis, which is seen with high-dose therapy, and other ocular toxic effects may be prevented by the use of steroid eyedrops during therapy.

Dacarbazine

Brand name: DTIC-Dome.
Class of drug: Alkylating anticancer drug.
Mechanism of action: Forms covalent bond with elements in DNA, preventing separation of strands of DNA during cell division.
Indications/dosage/route: IV only.
• Malignant melanoma
 – Adults: 2–4.5 mg/kg/d, 10 days, repeat every 4 weeks.
• Hodgkin's disease
 – Adults: 150 µg/m^2/d, 5 days (combination and therapy); repeat every 4 weeks. Other dosage regimens have been used.
Adjustment of dosage: None.
Food: Restrict 4–6 hours prior to treatment.
Pregnancy: Category C.
Lactation: No data available. Potentially toxic to infant. Avoid breastfeeding.
Contraindications: Hypersensitivity to dacarbazine.
Warnings/precautions
• Use with caution in patients with diminished bone marrow reserve.
• Administer antiemetic drug 30–50 minutes before and after drug therapy and throughout thereafter.
Advice to patient
• Use good oral hygiene in order to avoid mucosal ulceration.
• Rinse mouth after eating or drinking.
• To minimize possible photosensitivity reactions, apply adequate sunscreen and use proper covering when exposed to strong sunlight.
• Receive vaccinations (particularly live attenuated viruses) only with permission from treating physician.
• Use two forms of birth control including hormonal and barrier methods.
• Report flulike symptoms to treating physician.

Adverse reactions
- Common: nausea and vomiting (90%).
- Serious: bone marrow depression (leukopenia, thrombocytopenia), anaphylaxis, hypocalcemia, tissue necrosis from extravasation, hepatic injury, hepatic vein thrombosis, hepatic necrosis, polyneuropathy, orthostatic hyptension, seizures.

Clinically important drug interactions: None.

Parameters to monitor
- CBC with differential and platelets, BUN and creatinine, liver enzymes.
- Signs and symptoms of bone marrow depression.
- Signs and symptoms of infection.
- Signs and symptoms of thrombocytopenia. Discontinue this medication if platelet count falls below 100,000/mm^3.
- Intake of fluids and urinary and other fluid output to minimize renal toxicity. Closely monitor electrolyte levels.
- Signs and symptoms of anemia.
- Signs and symptoms of hepatotoxicity.
- Signs and symptoms of renal toxicity.

Editorial comments: Use latex gloves and safety glasses when handling cytotoxic drugs. Avoid contact with skin as well as inhalation. If possible, prepare in biologic hood.

Dactinomycin

Brand name: Cosmegen.
Class of drug: Antineoplastic, antibiotic type.
Mechanism of action: Intercalates between DNA base pairs, resulting in inhibition of DNA synthesis and DNA-dependent RNA synthesis.
Indications/dosage/route: IV only.
- Uterine, testicular cancers; rhabdomyosarcoma; Wilms' tumor, Ewing's sarcoma

– Children >6 months, adults: 15 µg/kg/d or 400–500 µg/m^2/d for 5 days. May be repeated every 3–6 weeks.

Adjustment of dosage: None.

Pregnancy: Category C.

Lactation: No data available. Potentially toxic to infants. Avoid breastfeeding.

Contraindications: Patients with varicella or herpes zoster infection, infants <6 months.

Warnings and precautions

- Use with caution in patients who have had: radiation therapy, use within 2 weeks of radiation for treatment of right-sided Wilms' tumor.
- This drug may place patients at risk for secondary malignancies.

Advice to patients

- Inform patient of hair loss, which may occur 7–10 days after beginning therapy.
- Do not receive any vaccinations (particularly live attenuated viruses) without permission from treating physician.
- Avoid alcohol.
- Use two forms of birth control including hormonal and barrier methods.
- Do not take NSAIDs along with this drug.

Adverse reactions

- Common: Nausea and vomiting (90%), malaise, fatigue, fever, alopecia, skin pigmentation (irradiated areas), acne.
- Serious: **bone marrow suppression, hypocalcemia**, hepatitis, hepatocellular necrosis, hepatic vein thrombosis, anaphylactoid reactions, severe GI side effects.

Clinically important drug interactions: Dactinomycin increases effects/toxicity of radiation therapy.

Parameters to monitor

- CBC with differential and platelets, serum electrolytes (especially calcium), liver enzymes.
- Signs and symptoms of infection.
- Signs and symptoms of thrombocytopenia. Discontinue this medication if platelet count falls below 100,000/mm^3.
- Signs and symptoms of fluid extravasation from IV injection.

- Intake of fluids and urinary and other fluid output to minimize renal toxicity. Closely monitor electrolyte levels.
- Signs and symptoms of hepatotoxicity.
- Signs of hyperuricemia.

Editorial comments: Use latex gloves and safety glasses when handling cytotoxic drugs. Avoid contact with skin as well as inhalation. If possible, prepare in biologic hood.

Danazol

Brand name: Danocrin.
Class of drug: Antiestrogen, androgen, antiinflammatory.
Mechanism of action: Suppresses pituitary–ovarian axis; gonadal inhibitor. Inhibits ovarian output of FSH and LH; decreases growth of abnormal breast; increases level of C4 complement.
Indications/dosage/route: Oral only.
- Mild endometriosis
  – Initial: 100–200 mg b.i.d., usually 3–6 months.
- Moderate endometriosis
  – 400 mg b.i.d., maximum 9 months.
- Fibrocystic breast disease
  – 50–200 mg b.i.d., 2–6 months.
- Hereditary angioedema
  – 400–600 mg/day, 2–3 divided doses. Maximum: 800 mg/d.

Adjustment of dosage
- Kidney disease: Use with caution.
- Liver disease: Use with caution.
- Elderly: Use with caution.
- Pediatric: Safety and efficacy have not been established in children.

	Peak Effect
Fibrocystic disease	4 wk
Amerorrhea	6–8 wk

Pregnancy: Category X.

Lactation: Contraindicated.

Contraindications: Undiagnosed genital bleeding; porphyria; markedly impaired cardiac, renal, hepatic function; hypersensitivity to danazol.

Warnings/precautions

- Use with caution in patients with the following conditions: migraine headaches; seizure disorders; cardiac, hepatic, renal dysfunction; hereditary angioeclema.
- Perform pregnancy test (β–HCG) prior to initiating therapy.
- This drug is strongly associated with hepatotoxicity (females, patients >35 years are at higher risk).
- Perform mammography and breast cyst biopsy before and during treatment as clinically indicated.

Advice to patient

- Use two forms of birth control including hormonal and barrier methods.
- If taking oral contraceptives, use an alternative method of birth control.
- To minimize possible photosensitivity reaction, apply adequate sunscreen and use proper covering when exposed to strong sunlight.
- Examine breasts regularly. Notify treating physician if you notice enlargement of breast, nodules.

Adverse reactions

- Common: weight gain, vaginal bleeding, menstrual irregularities, emotional instability, hirsutism, decreased breast size, vaginal dryness, deepening voice.
- Serious: **hepatic dysfunction**, pericarditis, respiratory depression, cholestatic jaundice, hepatitis, hepatic adenoma, peliosis hepatis, benign intracranial hypertension.

Clinically important drug interactions

- Danazol increases effects/toxicity of oral anticoagulants. Danazol decreases effects/toxicity of carbamazepine, oral anticoagulants, insulin, cyclosporine.

Parameters to monitor

- Liver enzymes.

- Signs of virilization, menstrual irregularities, persistent erection, GI symptoms, eg, vomiting, nausea, visual disturbances.
- Signs and symptoms of hepatotoxicity.
- Signs of undiagnosed vaginal bleeding, noting frequency and precipitating factors.
- Symptoms of pseudotumor cerebri: headache, nausea, vomiting, visual disturbances.

Editorial comments: This agent is associated with several serious side effects including peliosis hepatis and hepatic adenoma, which can cause intraabdominal hemorrhage. Additionally, pseudotumor cerebri has been reported. The medication should be immediately discontinued if patients develop symptoms of these conditions.

Dantrolene

Brand name: Dantrium.
Class of drug: Skeletal muscle relaxant, antidote for NMS.
Mechanism of action: Interferes with release of calcium from sarcoplasmic reticulum in skeletal muscle.
Indications/dosage/route: Oral, IV.
- Upper motor neurospasicity
  - Adults: PO 25 mg/d, increasing gradually to maximum of 400 mg/d. Doses usually divided 3–4 times/d.
  - Children >5 years: PO 0.5 mg/kg increasing to maximum of 3 mg/kg 2–4 times/d up to 400 mg/kg d. Five to seven days between incremental dose increases.
- NMS: begin dantrolene as soon as possible
  - Adults, children: IV 1 mg/kg, increasing dosage to maximum cumulative dose of 10 mg/kg. Repeat dosage if fever, metabolic abnormalities recur. Follow up with 4–8 mg/kg/d in 3–4 divided doses, 1–3 days.

Adjustment of dosage
• Kidney disease: None.
• Liver disease: Contraindicated.
• Elderly: Use with caution.
• Pediatric: Long-term use in children <5 years is not recommended.

Food: Caution patient about eating because choking has been reported due to difficulty in swallowing. May be administered with food.

Pregnancy: Category C.

Lactation: No information available. Best to avoid.

Contraindications: Active liver disease (cirrhosis, hepatitis), upper motor neuron disorders, patients who use spasticity to maintain upright position and balance in moving or when spasticity is required to maintain increased body function.

Warnings/precautions
• Use caution in patients with preexisting cardiac disease or pulmonary disease, particularly COPD; in females; and in patients >35.
• Males may develop impotence.
• Long-term benefit should be evaluated because of potential hepatotoxicity.
• Should be administered as rapidly as possible when signs of malignant hyperthermia are observed. These include: cardiac arrhythmias, unstable blood pressure, rapidly rising temperature, shock.

Advice to patient
• To minimize possible photosensitivity reaction, apply adequate sunscreen and use proper covering when exposed to strong sunlight.
• Avoid driving and other activities requiring mental alertness or that are potentially dangerous until response to drug is known.
• Avoid alcohol and other CNS depressants such as opiate analgesics and sedatives (eg, diazepam) when taking this drug.

Adverse reactions
- Common: muscle weakness, drowsiness, lightheadedness, headache, diarrhea. These adverse reactions are generally transient.
- Serious: seizures, confusion, hepatitis, pleural effusion, pericarditis, respiratory depression, hemolysis.

Clinically important drug interactions: Drugs that increase effects/toxicity of dantrolene: alcohol, antianxiety drugs, neuroleptics, narcotics, tricyclic antidepressants, MAO inhibitors, clindamycin, verapamil, warfarin, clofibrate, tolbutamide, estrogens.

Parameters to monitor
- Liver enzymes (baseline and periodic).
- Efficacy of treatment: improvement of neuromuscular function or muscle weakness, ability to walk without losing balance.
- Signs and symptoms of hepatotoxicity.
- Bowel function. Severe or persistent diarrhea may necessitate discontinuing drug.
- With IV dosage, use cardiac and BP monitors.
- Signs and symptoms of pulmonary dysfunction.

Editorial comments
- Dantrolene has the potential to cause mammary tumors. Accordingly, women with a family history of breast tumors (malignant or benign) should undergo frequent mammography.
- Evaluate family history to determine if there had been a reaction to an anesthetic that caused the NMS.
- This drug is not indicated as treatment for spasticity associated with rheumatologic diseases.

Daunorubicin

Brand name: Cerubidine.
Class of drug: Antineoplastic antibiotic.

Mechanism of action: Inhibits DNA synthesis and DNA-dependent RNA synthesis by intercalating between DNA base pairs.

Indications/dosage/route: IV only.

- Acute nonlymphocytic leukemia: induction of remission
  - Adults <60 years: 45 mg/m^2, days 1–3, followed by subsequent courses days 1–2 (combined with cytosine arabinoside).
  - Adults ≥60 years: 30 mg/m^2, days 1–3, followed by courses days 1–2 (combined with cytosine arabinoside).
- Acute lymphocytic leukemia: induction of remission
  - Adults: 45 m^2, days 1–3.
  - Children ≥2 years: 25 mg/m^2, day 1, weekly up to 6 weeks.
  - Children <2 years: Dose should be calculated on mg/kg basis of body weight, not body surface area.

Adjustment of dosage

- Liver disease: Serum bilirubin >3.1–5 mg/dL: reduce dose by 50%; serum bilirubin >5 mg/dL: do not use.
- Kidney disease: Creatinine clearance 10 mL/min: reduce dose by 25–50%.
- Elderly: Use with caution; greater risk for bone marrow depression and cardiotoxicity.
- Pediatric: See above.

Pregnancy: Category D.

Lactation: No data available. Potentially toxic to infants. Avoid breastfeeding.

Contraindications: Hypersensitivity to daunorubicin.

Warnings/precautions

- Use with caution in patients with the following conditions: CHF, arrhythmias, cardiomyopathy to daunorubicin; if granulocyte count <750/µL, IM or SC administration.
- Patients receiving >400 mg/m^2 cumulative doses and radiation therapy that involves the heart are at high risk for cardiotoxicity.
- Infants and children are also at increased risk.

Advice to patient

- Use two forms of birth control including hormonal and barrier methods.

• Inform patient that urine may show red color for 1–2 days and that this is not due to bleeding.
• Avoid alcohol.
• Do not receive any vaccinations (particularly live attenuated viruses) without permission from treating physician.
• Avoid foods high in purines (organ meats).

Adverse reaction
• Common: nausea and vomiting (50%), fatigue, alopecia, stomatitis, red discoloration of urine.
• Serious: **myelosuppression, especially leukopenia; irreversible cardiomyopathy**, myocarditis, pericarditis, severe cellulitis, opportunistic infections, tissue necrosis from extravasation, hepatitis, neuropathy.

Clinically important drug interactions: Other hepatotoxic drugs, other myelosuppressive agents increase effects/toxicity of daunorubicin.

Parameters to monitor
• CBC with platelets.
• Left ventricular ejection fraction when high doses are administered (300–500 mg/m^2).
• Signs and symptoms of infection.
• Signs and symptoms of thrombocytopenia. Discontinue this medication if platelet count falls below 100,000/mm^3.
• Signs and symptoms of fluid extravasation from IV injection.
• Signs of hyperuricemia: gouty arthritis, uric acid kidney stones.
• Signs and symptoms of stomatitis. Treat with peroxide, tea, topical anesthetics such as benzocaine, and lidocaine or antifungal drug.
• Intake of fluids and urinary and other fluid output to minimize renal toxicity. Closely monitor electrolyte levels.
• Symptoms of CHF.

Editorial comments
• Use latex gloves and safety glasses when handling cytotoxic drugs. Avoid contact with skin as well as inhalation. If possible, prepare in biologic hood.
• This agent, particularly in combination with other antineoplastics

or radiation therapy, may place patients at risk for secondary malignancies.

Demeclocycline

Brand name: Declomycin.
Class of drug: Antibiotic.
Mechanism of action: Inhibits bacterial protein synthesis after specific ribosomal binding.
Susceptible organisms *in vivo*: *Borrelia burgdorferi, Borrelia recurrentis, Brucella* species, *Calymmatobacterium granulomatis, Chlamydia pneumoniae, Chlamydia psittaci, Chlamydia trchomatis, Ehrlichia* species, *Helicobacter pylori, Rickettsia* species, *Vibrio* species.
Indications/dosage/route: Oral only.
  – Adults: Usual daily dose: 4 divided doses of 150 mg each or 2 divided doses of 300 mg each.
  – Children >8 years: Usual daily dose: 3–6 mg/lb (6–12 mg/kg), depending on the severity of the disease, divided into 3–4 doses.
Adjustment of dosage
• Kidney disease: None.
• Liver disease: None.
• Elderly: None.
• Pediatric: Not to be used in children <8 years unless all other drugs are either ineffective or contraindicated.
Food: Take 1 hour before or 2 hours after meals. Dairy products interfere with tetracycline absorption.
Pregnancy: Category D.
Lactation: Appears in breast milk. Considered compatible by American Academy of Pediatrics.
Contraindications: Hypersensitivity to any tetracycline, patients with esophageal obstruction, children ≤8.
Editorial comments: For more information, see *tetracycline*, p. 885.

Desipramine

Brand name: Norpramin.
Class of drug: Tricyclic antidepressant.
Mechanism of action: Inhibits reuptake of CNS neurotransmitters, primarily serotonin and norepinephrine.
Indications/dosage/route: Oral only.
• Depression
  – Adults: Initial: 100–200 mg/d in single or divided doses. Maintenance: 50–100 mg/d. Maximum: 300 mg/d.
  – Elderly, adolescents: 25–50 mg/d in divided doses up to a maximum of 150 mg.
Adjustment of dosage
• Kidney disease: None.
• Liver disease: None.
• Elderly: Lower doses recommended.
• Pediatric: Not recommended for children <12 years.
Food: No restriction.
Pregnancy: Category C.
Lactation: Appears in breast milk. American Academy of Pediatrics expresses concern over use when breastfeeding.
Contraindications: Hypersensitivity to tricyclic antidepressants, acute recovery from MI, concurrent MAO inhibitor.
Editorial comments: For additional information, see *amitriptyline*, p. 39.

Dexamethasone

Brand name: Decadron.
Class of drug: Corticosteroid: systemic, ophthalmic, topical, intraarticular.
Mechanism of action: Inhibits migration of polymorphonuclear leukocytes; stabilizes lysosomal membranes; inhibits production of products of arachidonic acid cascade.

Indications/dosage/route: IV, IM, intraarticular, topical.

• Most uses
  – Adults: IM, IV 5–9 mg/d.
• Cerebral edema
  – Adults: Initial: IV 10 mg, then 4 mg q6h until maximum response is obtained.
• Shock
  – Adults: IV 1–6 mg/kg or 40 mg; repeat dose q2–6h as needed.
• Rheumatoid arthritis
  – Adults: Intraarticular, 4–16 mg, depending on size of joint. May repeat in 1–3 weeks.
• Bronchial asthma
  – Adults: Initial: 3 inhalations t.i.d. to q.i.d. Maximum: 12 inhalations/d.
  – Children: Initial: 2 inhalations t.i.d. to q.i.d. Maximum: 2 inhalations/dose, 8 inhalations/d.
• Allergies, intranasal polyps
  – Adults: 2 sprays in each nostril b.i.d. to t.i.d. Maximum: 12 sprays/d.
  – Children 6–12 years: 1–2 sprays in each nostril b.i.d. Maximum: 8 sprays/d.
• Ophthalmic use
  – Adults: Initial: 1–2 drops into conjunctival sac every hour during the day and q2h at night.

Adjustment of dosage

• Kidney disease: None.
• Liver disease: None.
• Elderly: None.
• Pediatric: Children on long-term therapy must be monitored carefully for growth and development.

Food: Not applicable.

Pregnancy: Category B.

Lactation: Steroids appear in breast milk. American Academy of Pediatrics considers prednisone to be compatible with breast-feeding.

Contraindications: Systemic fungal, viral, or bacterial infections.

Editorial comments: For additional information, see *prednisone*, p. 760.

Diazepam

Brand names: Valium, Dizac.
Class of drug: Antianxiety agent, hypnotic.
Mechanism of action: Potentiates effects of GABA in limbic system and reticular formation.
Indications/dosage/route: Oral, IV, IM.
- Anxiety, anticonvulsant, adjunct to skeletal muscle relaxants
  – Adults: PO 2–10 mg b.i.d. to q.i.d.
  – Elderly, debilitated patients: PO 2–2.5 mg 1–2 times/d.
  – Children >6 months: Initial: PO 1–2.5 mg t.i.d. to q.i.d.
- Alcohol withdrawal
  – Adults: Initial: PO 10 mg t.i.d. to q.i.d. Maintenance: 5 mg t.i.d. to q.i.d. as needed.
- Preoperative sedation
  – Adults: IV, IM 10 mg 5–30 min before procedure.
- Skeletal muscle spasm
  – Adults, initial: IV, IM 5–10 mg, repeat q3–4h if needed.
- Moderate anxiety
  – Adults: IV, IM 2–5 mg q3–4h as needed.
- Severe anxiety, muscle spasm
  – Adults: IV, IM 5–10 mg q3–4h as needed.
- Acute alcohol withdrawal
  – Initial: IV, IM 10 mg, then 5–10 mg q3–4h.
- Endoscopy
  – Adults: IV 10–20 mg, IM 5–10 mg 30 min prior to procedure.
- Cardioversion
  – Adults: IV 5–15 mg 5–10 min prior to procedure.
- Tetanus
  – Children >1 month: IV, IM 1–2 mg, repeat q3–4h as necessary.
  – Children ≥5 years: IV 5–10 mg q3–4h.

- Status epilepticus
  - Adults: Initial: IV 5–10 mg, repeat at 10- to 15-min intervals, repeat after 2–4 hours if needed. Maximum: 30 mg.
  - Children 1 month–5 years: IV 0.2–0.5 mg q2–5 min, repeat after 2–4 hours. Maximum: 5 mg.
  - Children ≥5 years: IV 1 mg q2–5 min, repeat after 2–4 hours if needed. Maximum: 10 mg.
  - Elderly or debilitated: IV, IM 5 mg. Maximum at any one time.

Adjustment of dosage
- Kidney disease: Use with caution.
- Liver disease: Use with caution.
- Elderly: See above.
- Pediatric: See above.

Food: No restrictions.

Pregnancy: Category D.

Lactation: Appears in breast milk. Potentially toxic to infant. American Academy of Pediatrics expresses concern about breastfeeding while taking benzodiazepines. Avoid breastfeeding.

Contraindications: Hypersensitivity to benzodiazepines, pregnancy.

Warnings/precautions
- Use with caution in patients with the following conditions: history of drug abuse, severe renal and hepatic impairment, suicidal tendencies and in elderly, neonates, infants.
- Benzodiazepines may cause psychologic and physical dependence.
- Benzodiazepines may cause paradoxical rage.
- It is best not to prescribe this drug for more than 6 months. If there is a need for long-term therapy, evaluate patient frequently.
- Use only for patients who have significant anxiety without medication, do not respond to other treatment, and are not drug abusers.

Advice to patient
- Avoid driving and other activities requiring mental alertness or that are potentially dangerous until response to drug is known.

- Avoid alcohol and other CNS depressants such as narcotic analgesics, alcohol, antidepressants, antihistamines, barbiturates, when taking this drug.
- Avoid use of OTC medications without first informing the treating physician.
- Cigarette smoking will decrease drug effect. Do not smoke when taking this drug.
- Do not stop drug abruptly if taken for more than one month. If suddenly withdrawn, there may be recurrence of the original anxiety or insomnia. A full-blown withdrawal symptom may occur consisting of vomiting, insomnia, tremor, sweating, muscle spasms. After chronic use, decrease drug dosage slowly, ie, over a period of several weeks at the rate of 25% per week.
- Avoid excessive use of xanthine-containing food (regular coffee, tea, chocolate) as these may counteract the action of the drug.

Adverse reactions
- Common: drowsiness, fatigue.
- Serious: respiratory depression, bone marrow depression, hypotension, drug dependence, rigidity, hostile behavior, hepatitis.

Clinically important drug interactions
- Drugs that increase effects/toxicity of benzodiazepines: CNS depressants (alcohol, antihistamines, narcotic analgesics, tricyclic antidepressants, SSRIs, MAO inhibitors), cimetidine, disulfiram.
- Drugs that decrease effects/toxicity of benzodiazepines: flumazenil (antidote for overdose), carbamazepine.

Parameters to monitor
- CBC with differential and platelets, liver enzymes.
- Signs of chronic toxicity: ataxia, vertigo, slurred speech.
- Dosing to make sure amount taken is as prescribed particularly if patient has suicidal tendencies.
- Efficacy of treatment: reduced symptoms of anxiety and tension, improved sleep.
- Signs of physical/psychologic dependence, particularly if patient is addiction-prone and requests frequent renewal of

prescription or is experiencing a diminished response to the drug.

- Neurologic status including memory (anterograde amnesia), disturbing thoughts, unusual behavior.
- Possibility of blood dyscrasias: fever, sore throat, upper respiratory infection. Perform total and differential WBC counts.

Editorial comments

- Overdose from a benzodiazepine is characterized by hyptension, respiratory depression, cardiac arrhythmias, coma.
- Treatment is supportive generally without mechanical ventilation.
- Flumazenil, a benzodiazepine antagonist, has been used successfully to reverse the CNS depression but its effectiveness in reversing respiratory depression is in doubt. The physician should be thoroughly familiar with the risks involved in using flumazenil including the possibility of drug-induced seizures.
- See entry for *flumazenil*, p. 369, or package insert before using this drug.
- The *Physician's Desk Reference*, 54th edition, 2000, lists no drug interactions for chlordiazepoxide or other benzodiazepines.

Diazoxide

Brand names: Hyperstat IV, Proglycem.
Class of drug: Vasodilator, antihypertensive, antihypoglycemic.
Mechanism of action: Antihypertensive action: relaxes arterial smooth muscle with resultant vasodilation. Antihypoglycemic action: inhibits secretion of insulin from the pancreas; inhibits peripheral utilization of glucose.
Indications/dosage/route: IV, oral.

- Hypertensive crisis
  – Adults, children: IV 1–3 mg/kg. Maximum: 150 mg. Repeat

dose q15min, until BP is controlled. Administer further doses every 4–24 hours.
- Hypoglycemia from excessive insulin, paraneoplastic source
  – Adults, children: PO 3–8 mg/kg/d, divided into 2 or 3 equal doses.
  – Infants, newborns: PO 8–15 mg/kg/d, divided into 2 or 3 equal doses. Use lowest doses initially; increase as tolerated.

	Onset of Action	Peak Effect	Duration
PO	1 h	8–12 h	8 h
IV	Immediate	5 min	3–12 h

Adjustment of dosage: None.
Pregnancy: Category C.
Lactation: No data available. Best to avoid.
Contraindications: Hypersensitivity to diazoxide or other sulfonamide-derived drugs (such as thiazide diuretics), coarctation of the aorta, arteriovenous shunts, dissecting aortic aneurysm.

Warnings/precautions
- Use with caution in patients with the following conditions: diabetes mellitus, kidney or liver disease, coronary artery disease, cerebrovascular insufficiency.
- This agent may produce rapid decreases in BP. Vascular events including MI and cerebral infarction have been associated with these instances.
- Administer only into a peripheral vein. Avoid extravascular injection or leakage.
- Use only to treat hypoglycemia to excessive insulin, not for other causes.

Advice to patient
- Notify dentist or treating physician prior to surgery if taking this medication.
- Report unusual bleeding or bruising to treating physicians.

Adverse reactions
- Common: hypotension, nausea, vomiting, hyperuricemia, hyperglycemia, dizziness.

- Serious: hypotension, seizures, cerebral ischemia, arrhythmias, MI, shock, leukopenia, thrombocytopenia, ketoacidosis, extra-pyramidal symptoms.

Clinically important drug interactions

- Drugs that increase effects/toxicity of diazoxide: nitrites, peripheral vasodilators, thiazide diuretics (cause increased hyperglycemia).
- Diazoxide increases effects/toxicity of oral anticoagulants.
- Diazoxide decreases effects/toxicity of phenytoin.

Parameters to monitor

- CBC with differential and platelets, chemistries (glucose, uric acid, albumen, potassium, creatinine, urine osmolality).
- Signs and symptoms of ocular toxicity: reduced visual acuity, floaters, eye pain.
- Symptoms of CHF.
- Monitor patient who develops hyperglycemia for up to 8 days because of the long half-life of dizoxide.
- BP and cardiac function for patient receiving IV form. Use cardiac and BP monitors.
- Signs and symptoms of hyperuricemia.

Editorial comments: Diazoxide was initially popularized for IV administration in hypertensive crisis. This drug is now rarely used due to the improved efficacy of nitroprusside, labetalol and hydralazine in producing vasodilation.

Diclofenac

Brand names: Cataflam, Voltaren.
Class of drug: NSAID.
Mechanism of action: Inhibits cyclooxygenase, resulting in inhibition of synthesis of prostaglandins and other inflammatory mediators.
Indications/dosage/route: Oral, topical (ophthalmic).
Immediate-release tablets, delayed-release tablets
- Analgesia, primary dysmenorrhea

   – Adults: PO 50 mg t.i.d. Maximum: 150 mg/d.
* Rheumatoid arthritis
   – Adults: PO 50 mg t.i.d. or q.i.d. Chronic therapy: use extended-release tablets, 100 mg q.d. or b.i.d. Maximum: 225 mg/d.
* Osteoarthritis
   – Adults: PO 50 mg b.i.d. or t.i.d. Chronic therapy: use extended-release tablets, 100 mg/d. Maximum: 200 mg/d.
* Ankylosing spondylitis
   – Adults: PO 25 mg q.i.d. Maximum: 125 mg/d.

Ophthalmic Solution
* Following cataract surgery
   – 0.1%, 1 drop in affected eye q.i.d. 24 hours after cataract surgery.

Adjustment of dosage
* Kidney disease: None.
* Liver disease: None.
* Elderly: May be necessary to reduce dose for patients >65 years.
* Pediatric: Safety and efficacy have not been established.

Food: Take with food or large quantities of water or milk.

Pregnancy: Category B. Category D in third trimester or near delivery.

Lactation: May appear in breast milk. Breastfeeding considered to be low risk by some authors.

Contraindications: Hypersensitivity and cross-sensitivity with other NSAIDs and aspirin, pregnancy.

Editorial comments: For additional information, see *ibuprofen*, p. 445.

Dicloxacillin

Brand names: Dycill, Pathocil, Dynapen.
Class of drug: Antibiotic, penicillin family.
Mechanism of action: Inhibits bacterial cell wall synthesis.

Susceptible organisms *in vivo*: MSSA, streptococci.
Indications/dosage/route: Oral only.
• Skin and soft tissue infections, mild to moderate UTIs
  – Adults, children >40 kg: 125 mg q6h.
  – Children <40 kg: 12.5 mg/kg/d in 4 equal doses.
• More severe lower respiratory tract infections or disseminated infections
  – Adults, children >40 kg: 250 mg q6h. Maximum: 4 g/d.
  – Children <40 kg: 25 mg/kg/d in 4 equal doses.
Adjustment of dosage: None.
Food: Take on empty stomach, 1 hour before or 2 hours after eating.
Pregnancy: Category B.
Lactation: No data available. Best to avoid.
Contraindications: Hypersensitivity to penicillin or cephalosporins.
Editorial comments: Dicloxacillin is an oral antistaphylococcal drug. It is not inactivated by the penicillinase of MSSA. It is used mainly to treat staphylococcal infections of the skin, soft tissues, and bones.
• This drug is not listed in the *Physician's Desk Reference*, 54th edition, 2000.
• For additional information, see penicillin G, p. 708.

Dicyclomine

Brand names: Antispas, A-Spas, Bentyl, Bentylol, Byclomine, Dibent, Di-Cyclonex, Dilomine, Di-Spaz, Formulex, Or-Tyl.
Class of drug: Cholinergic blocking agent.
Mechanism of action: Blocks acetylcholine effects at muscarinic receptors throughout the body.
Indications/dosage/route: Oral, IM.
• Hypermotility and spasms of GI tract
  – Adults: PO 10–20 mg t.i.d. to q.i.d.; increase to total dose 160 mg/d as needed.

- Children ≥6 years: PO 10 mg t.i.d. to q.i.d.
- Children 6 months–2 years: PO 5–10 mg t.i.d. to q.i.d.
- Children 2–6 years: PO 10 mg t.i.d. to q.i.d.
- Hypermotility and spasms of GI tract
  - Adults: IM 20 mg q4–6h.

Adjustment of dosage
- Kidney disease: None.
- Liver disease: None.
- Elderly: None.
- Pediatric: See above.

Pregnancy: Category C.

Lactation: Appears in breast milk. Potentially toxic to infant. Avoid breastfeeding.

Contraindications: Myasthenia gravis, narrow-angle glaucoma, GI obstruction, megacolon, active ulcerative colitis, obstructive uropathy, hypersensitivity to atropine-type compounds (belladonna alkaloids).

Warnings/precautions
- Use with caution in patients with the following conditions: GI infections, chronic biliary disease, CHF, arrhythmias, pulmonary disease, BPH, hyperthyroidism, coronary artery disease, hypertension, seizures, psychosis, spastic paralysis.
- Anticholinergic psychosis can occur in sensitive individuals.
- Elderly may react with agitation and excitement even to small doses of anticholinergic drugs.

Advice to patient
- Take medication exactly as directed. If dose is missed, do not double subsequent dose when it is remembered.
- Avoid driving and other activities requiring mental alertness or that are potentially dangerous until response to drug is known.
- Use caution when exercising in hot weather as this might cause heat prostration.
- Avoid alcohol and other CNS depressants such as opiate analgesics and sedatives (eg, diazepam) when taking this drug.
- If mouth is dry, rinse with warm water frequently, chew sugarless gum, suck on an ice cube, or use artificial saliva. Carry out meticulous oral hygiene (floss teeth daily).

Adverse reactions
- Common: dry mouth, dry skin, constipation, decreased sweating.
- Serious: disorientation, hallucinations, acute narrow-angle glaucoma, seizure, coma, urinary retention, asphyxia, hypotonia.

Clinically important drug interactions
- Drugs that increase effects/toxicity of systemic anticholinergics: phenothiazines, amantadine, other antipsychotic agentics, thiazide diuretics, tricyclic antidepressants, MAO inhibitors, quinidine, procainamide.
- Drugs that decrease effects/toxicity of systemic anticholinergics: antacids, cholinergic agents.

Parameters to monitor
- Signs and symptoms of severe toxicity: tachycardia, supraventricular arrythmias, delirium, seizures, agitation, hyperthermia. Discontinue if patient experiences dizziness, palpitations, rapid pulse. Use physostigmine (Eserine) as antidote only for life-threatening toxicity.
- Intake of fluids and urinary and other fluid output. Increase fluid intake if inadequate.
- Signs of urinary retention: pelvic pain and distention, decreased urine output. This is particularly important in elderly with BPH. Determine whether there is a need for catherization.
- Ophthalmic status: intraocular pressure before and during treatment, accommodation, pupillary response to light, visual acuity (blurred vision). Discontinue administration if the following occur: eye pain, conjunctivitis.

Editorial comments
- This drug is not to be used intravenously.
- This drug is listed without details in the *Physician's Desk Reference*, 54th edition, 2000.

Didanosine

Brand name: Videx.
Class of drug: Antiviral antimetabolite.

Mechanism of action: Converted to active metabolite which inhibits replication of HIV via blockage of HIV reverse transcriptase. This results in inhibition of DNA synthesis.

Indications/dosage/route: Oral only.

• Treatment of HIV infection

  – Adults ≥60 kg: 200 mg q12h.

  – Adults <60 kg: 125 mg q12h.

  – Children: 90–150 mg/m^2 q12h. Chewable tablets available.

  – Neonates: 50 mg/m^2 q12h. (*Note:* Dosages generally administered as at least two tablets/dose to achieve adequate buffering.)

Food: Should be taken on empty stomach (1 hour before or 2 hours after meals) with at least 4 oz of water with each dose. Not to be taken with fruit juice or other acidic beverages.

Pregnancy: Category B.

Lactation: Crosses into breast milk. Centers for Disease Control and Prevention recommends avoidance of breastfeeding in HIV-infected mothers.

Adjustment of dosage

• Kidney disease: Reduced dosage recommended.

• Liver disease: Monitor carefully.

• Elderly: No information available.

• Pediatric: See above.

Contraindications: Hypersensitivity to didanosine.

Warnings/precautions

• Use with caution in patients with the following conditions: pancreatitis, peripheral neuropathy, hyperuricemia, renal or hepatic disease.

• Didanosine is indicated only for treatment of HIV patients who are intolerant of zidovudine or have not responded to zidovudine.

• If another pancreatoxic drug such as pentamidine is administered, consider stopping didanosine unless pancreatitis is ruled out.

Advice to patient

• Avoid driving and other activities requiring mental alertness or that are potentially dangerous until response to drug is known.

- Avoid crowds as well as patients who may have a contagious disease.
- Male patients should use condoms if engaging in sexual intercourse while using this medication.
- Notify treating physician if experiencing severe nausea and vomiting and abdominal pain.

Adverse reactions

- Common: abdominal pain, nausea, vomiting, diarrhea, anxiety, insomnia.
- Serious: **peripheral neuropathy**, seizures, pancreatitis, thrombocytopenia, hepatitis, liver failure, retinal depigmentation.

Clinically important drug interactions

- Drugs that increase effects/toxicity of didanosine: aluminum, magnesium antacids.
- Drugs that decrease effects/toxicity of didanosine: H_2 blocking drugs, proton pump inhibitors.
- Didanosine decreases effects/toxicity of following drugs: quinolone antibiotics, dapsone, tetracyclines, fluoroquinolones, indinavir, ritonavir, ranitidine. Separate doses of didanosine from these agents (give these 1 hour before or 2 hours after didanosine).

Parameters to monitor

- Signs of visual disturbances. Children should receive a retinal examination at least every 6 months if they show visual problems.
- Symptoms of pancreatitis. Periodic measurement of serum amylase and lipase is suggested. If amalyase increases 1.5 to 2-fold and patient has symptoms of pancreatitis, discontinue drug.
- Signs and symptoms of neuropathy.

Editorial comments: The frequent occurrence of pancreatitis caused by didanosine has limited its usefulness as an antiretroviral agent.

Digoxin

Brand names: Lanoxin, Lanoxicaps.
Class of drugs: Cardiac glycoside.

Mechanism of action: Positive inotropic effects: Inhibits Na/K/ATPase, resulting in increased intracellular calcium and increased ventricular contractility. Antiarrythmic: Increases AV node refractory period.

Indications/dosage/route: Oral, IV.

• CHF, atrial fibrillation or flutter, paroxsymal atrial tachycardia
  – Adults: IV or PO loading dose: 0.013 mg/kg, rounded to nearest 0.25-mg dose, given over the first 24 hours. Maintenance: PO 0.125–0.5 mg/d.
  – Children: Loading dose: 2–5 years: IV 0.025–0.035 mg/kg, oral 0.030–0.040 mg/kg; 5–10 years: IV 0.015–0.030 mg/kg, oral 0.020–0.035 mg/kg; >10 years: IV 0.008–0.012 mg/kg, oral 0.010–0.015 mg/kg. Maintenance dose: 25–35% of digoxin loading dose.

Adjustment of dosage

• Kidney disease: Creatinine clearance 10–50 mL/min: decrease dose by 25–75%, consider q36h dosing; creatinine clearance <10 mL/min: decrease dose by 75–90%, consider 48-hour dosing.
• Liver disease: None.
• Elderly (>65 years): Daily dose 0.125 mg. Use with caution and adjust dosage according to serum levels to prevent accumulation and toxicity.
• Pediatric: Infants display considerable differences in metabolism of digoxin. Individualization of dosages required.

Food: Can be taken with or without food. Avoid high-fiber foods with administration. Try to take drug at same time daily.

Pregnancy: Category C.

Lactation: Appears in breast milk. Considered compatible by American Academy of Pediatrics.

Contraindications: Second- or third-degree heart block, hypokalemia (potassium <3 mmol/L), idiopathic hypertrophic subaortic stenosis, previous toxic reaction to digitalis-type drugs, beriberi heart disease, constrictive pericarditis, ventricular fibrillation, hypersensitivity to digitalis.

Warnings/precautions

• Use with caution in patients with the following conditions: acute MI, incomplete AV block, PVCs, renal insufficiency, hypothyroidism, acute myocarditis, Wolff–Parkinson–White syndrome, sick sinus syndrome, amyloid heart disease, severe pulmonary disease.

• Digoxin toxicity, if suspected, must be ruled out prior to administration.

Advice to patient: Carry identification card at all times describing disease, treatment regimen, name, address and telephone number of treating physician.

Adverse reactions

• Common: none (when serum levels are in therapeutic range).

• Serious: bradycardia, AV block, SA block, ventricular arrythmias, atrial or nodal ectopy, atrial tachycardia with AV block, disorientation.

Clinically important drug interactions

• Drugs that increase effects/toxicity of digoxin: amiodarone, amphotericin, anticholinergics, calcium products, corticosteroids, cyclosporine, diltiazem, erythromycin, furosemide, glucagon, isoproteronol, procainamide, propantheline, quinidine, quinine, spironolactone, succinylcholine, thiazide diuretics, verapamil.

• Drugs that decrease effects/toxicity of digoxin: cholestyramine, colestipol, kaolin–pectin, magnesium-containing antacids, metoclopramide, neomycin, *p*-aminosalicylic acid, rifampin, sulfasalazine.

Parameters to monitor

• Heart rate and rhythm, serum electrolytes (in particular potassium), and BP, before giving first dose and frequently thereafter.

• Serum digoxin levels. Therapeutic level ranges from 0.5 to 2 mg/mL. It is especially important to measure levels before loading (24 hours after IV dose, >6 hours after oral dose). Trough levels should be monitored in patients on maintenance therapy regimen involving agents that interact with digoxin. Levels should also be determined if changes are made in drug dosage.

• Signs of toxicity: visual disturbances (halos, red–green colorblindness, hazy vision), nausea, vomiting, anorexia. If patient

develops toxicity, consider administering the antidote, eg, digoxin immune FAB (Digibind), particularly if arrhythmias develop. Amount of Digibind should be 0.6 mg/40 mg digoxin.
• Intake of fluids and urinary and other fluid output to minimize renal toxicity. Increase fluid intake if inadequate. Closely monitor electrolyte levels.

Editorial comments
• Most patients receiving digoxin for CHF require a diuretic and all require ACE inhibitors. Reduce parenteral dosage by 20–40% for oral dosage. Various tables are available for adjustment of dosages based on lean body mass and creatinine clearance.
• Digoxin has been a mainstay of treatment for CHF of systolic dysfunction. Removal of digoxin from the regimen after chronic use has led to decompensation of CHF. The addition of β blockade to drug therapy for heart failure has enhanced survival and quality of life. Digoxin and β blockers must be used with care; focus on potential interactions, especially on the conduction system.
• Regarding supraventricular tachycardia, digoxin was previously considered to be a first-line drug of choice. It has now been proven to be less effective. Adenosine is now the initial drug of choice.

Dihydroergotamine

Brand name: D.H.E. 45, migranal nasal spray.
Class of drug: Ergot alkaloid, vasoconstrictor.
Mechanism of action: 5-HT agonist, α-adrenergic agonist, inhibits reuptake of catecholamines. May decrease local release of inflammatory mediators in the CNS.
Indications/dosage/route: IV, IM, SC, inhalation.
• Migraine headache, cluster, or vascular headaches
  – Adults: IV, IM, SC 1 mg (1 mg/mL dosage ampoules). Nasal spray 4 mg/mL, each nostril, single treatment.

Adjustment of dosage
- Kidney disease: Dosage guidelines are not available. Avoid if severely impaired.
- Liver disease: Dosage guidelines are not available. Avoid if severely impaired.
- Elderly: Use with caution because such patients are more susceptible to the adverse effects of the drug.
- Pediatric: Safety and efficacy in children have not been established.

	Onset of Action	Duration
IM	15–30 min	3–4 hr
IV	<5 min	No data

Pregnancy: Category X. Contraindicated.

Lactation: Appears in breast milk. Potentially toxic to infant. Avoid breastfeeding.

Contraindications: Pregnancy, ischemic heart disease, uncontrolled hypertension, hemiplegic or basilar migraine, peripheral arterial disease, sepsis, recent vascular surgery, Raynaud's disease, severe liver or kidney disease, ischemic bowel, hypersensitivity to ergot, high-dose aspirin therapy, known alcohol intolerance.

Warnings/precautions
- Serious cardiac adverse events have been described.
- Do not prescribed over prolonged period because of danger of ergotism or gangrene.
- Cerebrovascular accidents and subarachnoid hemorrhage have been associated with this drug. May precipitate vasospastic events.

Advice to patient
- Use two forms of birth control including hormonal and barrier methods.
- Lie down and relax after drug is administered.
- Avoid prolonged exposure to very cold temperatures.
- Do not smoke when taking dihydroergotamine. Nicotine intake may cause ischemia in some patients.

Adverse reactions
- Common: None.
- Serious: MI, myocardial ischemia, ventricular tachycardia, ventricular fibrillation, CVA, pleural and retroperitoneal fibrosis, cyanosis.

Clinically important drug interactions
- Drugs that increase effects/toxicity of dihydroergotamine: methysergide, β blockers, dopamine, macrolide antibiotics, heavy cigarette smoking, sumatriptan, SSRIs (fluoxetine, fluvoamine, paroxetine, sertraline).
- Dihydroergotamine decreases effects/toxicity of nitrates.

Parameters to monitor
- Signs of ergotism: nausea, vomiting, numbness, tingling of fingers or toes, confusion, weakness.
- Symptoms of myocardial ischemia.

Editorial comments: This drug should be used only when other measures, including analgesics, have failed. It should be administered only by physicians who are knowledgeable regarding potentially serious side effects and contraindications of the drug. Dihydroergotamine has a better record for lower frequency of recurrence of migraine than sumatriptan.

Diltiazem

Brand names: Cardizem, Dilacor, Tiazal.
Class of drug: Calcium channel blocker.
Mechanism of action: Inhibits calcium movement across cell membranes.
Indications/dosage/route: Oral, IV.
- Angina
  - Adults: Initial: PO 30 mg q.i.d. Maintenance: 180–360 mg, 3–4 divided doses. Sustained–release: Initial: 120 or 480 mg once daily.
- Hypertension

- Cardizem CD: Adults, Initial: 180–240 mg once daily. Maintenance: 240–360 mg once daily.
- Cardizem SR: Adults: initial: 60–120 mg b.i.d. Maintenance: 240–360 mg/d.
- Dilacor XR: Adults, initial: 180–240 once daily. Maintenance: 180–540 once daily.
- Atrial fibrillation/flutter, paroxysmal supraventricular tachycardia
  - Adults, initial: IV bolus: 0.15–0.25 mg/kg given over 2 min, second dose after 15 min if needed.
- Atrial fibrillation/flutter
  - Adults: IV infusion 5–15 mg/h.

Adjustment of dosage
- Kidney disease: Use with caution.
- Liver disease: Use with caution.
- Elderly: Use with caution.
- Pediatric: Safety and efficacy have not been established.

	Onset of Action	Peak Effect	Duration
Oral	0.5–1 h	2–3 h	4–8 h

Food: No restriction.

Pregnancy: Category C.

Lactation: Probably appears in breast milk. Potentially toxic to infant. Avoid breastfeeding.

Contraindications: Hypersensitivity to calcium blockers, sick sinus syndrome, 2nd or 3rd degree AV block w/o ventricular pacemaker, severe hypotension, acute MI with pulmonary congestion.

Warnings/precautions
- Use with caution in patients with CHF or severe left ventricular dysfunction and concomitantly with β blockers or digoxin.
- Do not withdraw drug abruptly, as this may result in increased frequency and intensity of angina.
- For the diabetic patient, the drug may interfere with insulin release and therefore produce hyperglycemia.

• Patient should be tapered off β blockers before beginning calcium channel blockers to avoid exacerbation of angina as a result of abrupt withdrawal of β blocker.

Advice to patient

• Use two forms of birth control including hormonal and barrier methods.

• Change position slowly, in particular from recumbent to upright, to minimize orthostatic hypotension. Sit at the edge of the bed for several minutes before standing, and lie down if feeling faint or dizzy. Avoid hot showers or baths and standing for long periods. Male patients should sit on the toilet while urinating rather than standing.

• Avoid driving and other activities requiring mental alertness or that are potentially dangerous until response to drug is known.

• Avoid use of OTC medications without first informing the treating physician.

• Determine BP and heart rate aproximately at the same time each day and at least twice a week, particularly at the beginning of therapy.

• Be aware of the fact that this drug may also block or reduce anginal pain, thereby giving a false sense of security on severe exertion.

• Include high-fiber foods to minimize constipation.

• Limit consumption of xanthine-containing drinks: regular coffee (more than 5 cups/d), tea, cocoa.

Adverse reactions

• Common: headache, edema.

• Serious: CHF, arrhythmias, hypotension, depression.

Clinically important drug interactions

• Drugs that increase effects/toxicity of calcium blockers: cimetidine, β blockers, cyclosporine.

• Drugs that decrease effects of calcium blockers: Barbiturates.

Parameters to monitor

• BP during initial administration and frequently thereafter. Ideally, check BP close to the end of dosage interval or before next administration.

- Liver and kidney function. Impaired renal function prolongs duration of action and increases tendency for toxicity.
- Intake of fluids and urinary and other fluid output to minimize renal toxicity. Increase fluid intake if inadequate. Closely monitor electrolyte levels.
- Efficacy of treatment for angina: decrease in frequency of angina attacks, need for nitroglycerin, episodes of PST segment deviation, anginal pain.
- If anginal pain is not reduced at rest or during effort, reassess patient as to medication.
- GI side effects; use alternative.
- ECG for development of heart block.
- Symptoms of CHF.

Diphenhydramine

Brand name: Benadryl.
Class of drug: H_1 receptor blocker.
Mechanism of action: Antagonizes histamine effects on GI tract, respiratory tract, blood vessels.
Indications/dosage/route: Oral, IV, IM.
- Allergies, emesis, motion sickness, parkinsonism
  - Adults: PO 25–50 mg t.i.d.to q.i.d.
  - Children >10 kg: PO 12.5–25 mg t.i.d. to q.i.d. Maximum: 300 mg/d.
- Hypnotic
  - Adults, children >12 years: PO 50 mg h.s.
- Antitussive
  - Adults: PO 25 mg q4h. Maximum: 100 mg/d.
  - Children 6–12 years: PO 12.5–25 mg q4h. Maximum: 25 mg/d.
- Parkinsonism, drug-induced extrapyramidal symptoms
  - Adults: IV, IM 10–100 mg. Maximum: 400 mg/d.
  - Children: IV, IM 1.25 mg/kg. Maximum: 300 mg/d.

Adjustment of dosage
- Kidney disease: None.
- Liver disease: None.
- Elderly: Use caution. At higher risk for side effects.
- Pediatric: See above.

Food: No restriction.

Pregnancy: Category B.

Lactation: Excreted in breast milk. Potentially toxic to infants. Avoid breastfeeding.

Contraindications: Hypersensitivity to antihistamines, acute asthma, narrow-angle glaucoma, concurrent use of MAO inhibitor.

Warnings/precautions
- Use with extreme caution in patients with active peptic ulcer, severe coronary artery disease, symptomatic prostatic hypertrophy.
- Use with caution in patients with hypertension, hyperthyroidism, asthma, heart disease, diabetes, increased intraocular pressure.
- Do not use in neonates or premature infants.
- Infants and young children are at risk for overdosage.

Advice to patient
- Avoid driving and other activities requiring mental alertness or that are potentially dangerous until response to drug is known.
- Use caution if used along with alcohol and other CNS depressants such as narcotic analgesics or sedatives (eg, diazepam).
- Drink large quantities of water to minimize drying of secretions.
- If mouth is dry, rinse with warm water frequently, chew sugarless gum, suck on an ice cube, or use artificial saliva. Carry out meticulous oral hygiene (floss teeth daily).
- Discontinue drug at least 4 days before skin testing (for allergies) to avoid the possibility of false-negative results.

Adverse reactions
- Common: drowsiness, dry mouth and throat, nervousness, thickened secretions.

- Serious: bone marrow depression, hypotension, hallucinations, confusion, urinary retention.

Clinically important drug interactions

- Drugs that increase effects/toxicity of antihistamines: CNS depressants (barbiturates, benzodiazepines, narcotic analgesics), MAO inhibitors (combination contraindication).
- Antihistamines decrease effects of sulfonylureas.

Parameters to monitor

- CBC with differential and platelets.
- Signs of dry mouth, eg, thickened secretions. Increase fluid intake to decrease viscosity of secretions.
- Signs and symptoms of severe CNS depression: dilated pupils or flushing. Administer syrup of ipecac if necessary.
- For topical preparations: signs and symptoms of allergic reaction (contact dermatitis or photosensitivity) or reaction of the skin: pruritus, inflammation, eczema.

Editorial comments

- Antihistamines are more effective in preventing allergic reactions than counteracting them once they have occurred.
- Parenteral form of diphenhydramine may cause skin necrosis if injected subcutaneously.
- Diphenhydramine has antiserotonergic as well as antihistaminic properties. It has also been used as an appetite stimulant and sedative (nonapproved) .

Dipyridamole

Brand name: Persantine.
Class of drug: Coronary vasodilator, inhibitor of platelet aggregation.
Mechanism of action: Inhibits platelet aggregation by blocking the enzyme phosphodiesterase. Produces coronary vasodilation by inhibiting uptake of adenosine into blood vessels.

Indications/dosage/route: PO, IV.
• Inhibitor of platelet adhesion in patients with prosthetic heart valve
  – Adults: PO 75–100 mg q.i.d.
• Thallium myocardial perfusion imaging as alternative to exercise
  – Adults: IV 0.1 or 2 mg/kg/min, infused over 4 minutes
• Prevention of thromboembolic complications in patients with thromboembolic disorders
  – Adults: PO 75–400 mg/d; should be combined with aspirin or warfarin.

Adjustment of dosage
• Kidney disease: None.
• Liver disease: None.
• Elderly: None.
• Pediatric: Safety and efficacy have not been established in children <12 years.

Food: Should be taken at least 1 hour before or 2 hours after meals.

Pregnancy: Category B.

Lactation: Appears in breast milk. Best to avoid.

Contraindications: Hypersensitivity to dipyridamole.

Warnings/precautions: Use with caution in patients with the following conditions: hypotension from peripheral vasodilation, hemostatic disorders.

Advice to patient: Notify physician if taking other drugs that affect coagulation (such as aspirin).

Adverse reactions
• Common: dizziness.
• Serious: exacerbation of angina, hypotension, dyspnea, hepatitis, tachycardia .

Clinically important drug interactions: None.

Parameters to monitor: Thromboembolic events.

Editorial comments: Dipyridamole is rarely used chronically as a single agent. It is generally combined with an oral anticoagulant or inhibitor of platelet aggregation.

Disopyramide

Brand name: Norpace.
Class of drug: Class 1A antiarrhythmic agent.
Mechanism of action: Decreases myocardial excitability and conduction rate; suppresses automaticity in His-Purkinje fibers. Sodium channel blocker with anticholinergic properties.
Indications/dosage/route: Oral only.

- Suppression and prevention of documented life-threatening ventricular arrhythmias
  - Adults >50 kg: 150 mg q6h or 300-mg extended-release (CR) capsule q12h.
  - Adults <50 kg: 100 mg q6h or 200-mg extended-release (CR) capsule q12h.
  - Children <1 years: 10–30 mg/kg/d.
  - Children 1–4 years: 10–20 mg/kg/d.
  - Children 4–12 years: 10–15 mg/kg/d.
  - Children 12–18 years: 6–15 mg/kg/d.

Adjustment of dosage

- Kidney disease: Creatinine clearance 15–30 mL/min: reduce dose by 50%; creatinine clearance <15 mL/min: reduce dose by 75%.
- Liver disease: Decrease dose by 25–50% as needed or increase dosing interval.
- Elderly: None.
- Pediatric: See above.

Food: Should be taken 1 hour before or 2 hours after meals. If patient experiences stomach irritation, try taking with food.
Pregnancy: Category C.
Lactation: Excreted in breast milk. Considered compatible by American Academy of Pediatrics.
Contraindications: Second- or third-degree heart block, cardiogenic shock, Torsade de pointes, hypersensitivity, congenital QT prolongation, hypersensitivity to disopyramide.

Warnings/precautions: Use with caution in patients with the following conditions: cardiomyopathy, myocarditis, atrial tachyarrhythmia, urinary retention, BPH, angle-closure glaucoma, myasthenia gravis, electrolyte abnormalities (particularly hyperkalemia), conduction abnormalities, sick sinus syndrome, Wolff–Parkinson–White syndrome, bundle branch blocks.

Advice to patient
- Report symptoms of worsening cardiac condition to treating physician.
- Notify physician of difficulty in urinating.
- Avoid extreme heat as disopyramide may increase the risk of heat stroke.

Adverse reactions
- Common: urinary hesitancy, dry mouth, constipation.
- Serious: urinary retention, chest pain, hypotension, heart failure, syncope, AV block, widening QRS complex, or QT interval, psychosis, depression, hypoglycemia, hepatitis, confusion.

Clinically important drug interactions
- Drugs that increase effects/toxicity of disopyramide: anticholinergics, oral hypoglycemic agents, insulin, erythromycin.
- Drugs that decrease effects/toxicity of disopyramide: rifampin, phenytoin, phenobarbital, other inducers of hepatic microsomal enzymes.
- Disopyramide increases effects of warfarin.

Parameters to monitor
- Signs of developing heart block, ie, QRS complex widening by more than 25%. If second- or third-degree heart block develops, discontinue drug.
- Glucose blood levels to avoid the possibility of hypoglycemia.
- Serum drug levels, particularly when therapy is initiated (strongly recommended in pediatric patients).
- Signs and symptoms of anticholinergic effects and CNS effects (confusion, hallucinations).
- Serum potassium levels. Disopyramide may be ineffective in hypokalemia, whereas its toxicity is increased in hyperkalemia.
- Intake of fluids and urinary and other fluid output to minimize renal toxicity. Closely monitor electrolyte levels.

Editorial comments
- Disopyramide has moderate clinical use as an antiarrhythmic. Typically, it is not well tolerated because of the anticholinergic effects. Efficacy in atrial fibrillation is about 50% and must be weighed against the potential proarrhythmia of the drug. Its negative ionotropic effects have led to its minimal use in patients with ventricular arrhythmias and depressed LV function.
- Clinically, very symptomatic atrial fibrillation and hypertrophic cardiomyopathy patients with atrial fibrillation or ventricular tachycardia may benefit most from its use.
- Disopyramide should not be used without consulting a cardiac electrophysiologist or cardiologist. The drug is not recommended for arrhythmias of lesser severity. Treatment of asymptomatic PVCs is not recommended.

Disulfiram

Brand name: Antabuse.
Class of drug: Deterrent of alcohol consumption.

Mechanism of action: Disulfiram inhibits the enzyme acetaldehyde dehydrogenase, which converts acetaldehyde to the inactive metabolite, actetate. The result is an accumulation of acetaldehyde causing uncomfortable symptoms that, it is hoped, deter the alcoholic from alcohol intake.

Indications/dosage/route: Oral only.
- Adjunct in treating chronic alcoholism
  - Adults: 250–500 mg/d, am, 1–2 weeks. Maintenance dose: 125–500 mg/d is given until self-control is established; this may take months or years.

Adjustment of dosage
- Kidney disease: None.
- Liver disease: Contraindicated in active hepatitis and portal hypertension.
- Elderly: None.

• Pediatric: No information available.

Pregnancy: Category C. Safety in pregnancy has not been established.

Lactation: No data available. Potentially toxic to infant. Best to avoid.

Contraindications: Recent use of alcohol or alcohol-containing substances (eg, cough syrups, tonics, aftershave lotion, alcohol-containing liniments), active hepatitis, portal hypertension, current or recent use of metronidazole or paraldehyde, severe cardiac disease, uncontrolled angina, hypersensitivity to disulfiram or thiuram (used in pesticides, rubber vulcanization), psychosis.

Warnings/precautions

• Use with caution in patients with the following conditions: concurrent phenytoin or oral anticoagulants, diabetes mellitus, epileptic disorders, brain damage, hypothyroidism, chronic and acute nephritis, cirrhosis of the liver, hepatic insufficiency, multiple drug dependence, cerebral damage.

• Warn patient that an adverse reaction can occur up to 2 weeks after a single dose of disulfiram.

• Patients on chronic disulfiram become increasingly sensitive to alcohol.

Advice to patient

• Do not use skin products containing alcohol for at least 3 days and perhaps as many as 14 days after stopping this medication.

• Carry identification card at all times describing disease, treatment regimen, and name, address, and telephone number of treating physician.

• Be aware that the antabuse reaction may start 5–10 minutes after ingesting alcohol.

• Avoid exposure to ethylene dibromide or ethylene bromide vapors.

Adverse reactions

• Common: None.

• Serious: Respiratory depression, arrhythmias, MI, seizures, heart failure, coma, death when combined with alcohol, hepatitis, liver failure, optic neuritis, peripheral neuropathy, polyneuritis, psychosis.

Clinically important drug reactions
• Disulfiram increases effects/toxicity of following drugs: alcohol, benzodiazepines, barbiturates, oral anticoagulants, phenytoin, isoniazid, cisplatin, isoniazid, theophylline.
• The following drugs taken with disulfiram may result in the Antabuse reaction: cyclosporine, omeprazole, paraldehyde, metronidazole.

Parameters to monitor
• Baseline liver enzymes, serum BUN and creatinine.
• CBC with differential and platelets, serum electrolytes every 6 months.

Editorial comments
• Following initiation of treatment (1–2 weeks), a 15-mL (0.5-oz) test dose of 100-proof whiskey is slowly consumed in a monitored setting by some clinicians.
• This drug requires close medical supervision. Patients must be warned to avoid alcohol in any form at least 12 hours before using this drug. That includes alcohol contained in various medications including many OTC products. It is to be used only in patients who are cooperative, well motivated, and receiving psychiatric therapy or counseling. Inform the patient and relatives about the dangers of using this drug. The patient should completely understand the nature of the Antabuse reaction.

Dobutamine

Brand name: Dobutrex.
Class of drug: Inotropic agent.
Mechanism of action: Selectively stimulates β_1-adrenergic receptors, increasing heart rate and contractility.
Indications/dosage/route: IV only.
• Short-term management of heart failure as a result of depressed contractility.

 – Adults: IV infusion 2–20 µg/kg/min. Dose adjusted to expected effect.
 – Children: IV infusion 2–20 µg/kg/min. Maximum: 40 µg/kg/min.

Adjustment of dosage
• Kidney disease: None.
• Liver disease: None.
• Elderly: None.
• Pediatric: Dosage similar to that of adults.

Onset of Action	Peak Effect	Duration
1–2 min	10 min	Few minutes

Food: Not applicable.
Pregnancy: Category C.
Lactation: No data available. Potentially toxic to infants. Best to avoid.
Contraindications: Idiopathic hypertrophic subaortic stenosis, sulfite hypersensitivity.

Warnings/precautions
• Use with caution in patients with the following conditions: MI, atrial fibrillation, hypertension.
• Before administration of dobutamine it is necessary to correct hypokalemia with plasma expanders.
• If patient has atrial fibrillation, consider administration of a cardiac glycoside before dobutamine. May precipitate ectopic beats.

Adverse reactions: Serious: **ectopy, tachycardia, ventricular tachycardia**, arrythmias, hypertension, chest pain, angina, dyspnea, worsening atrial fibrillation with rapid ventricular response.

Clinically important drug interactions
• Drugs that decrease effects/toxicity of dobutamine: β-adrenergic blockers.
• Drugs that increase effects/toxicity of dobutamine: general anesthetics (halothane, cycloprorane), MAO inhibitors, tricyclic antidepressants, nitroprusside, halothane, phenytoin, α adrenergic blockers.

• Dobutamine increases effects of guanethidine.

Parameters to monitor

• Monitor BP, heart rate. ECG must be continuously monitored. CVP, Swan–Ganz catheter (PCWP, SVR) often required.

• Dosage reduction will reverse marked increases in heart rate or BP which occur in about 10% of treated patients.

• Efficacy of treatment: increased cardiac and urine output.

Editorial comments

• Dobutamine is well tolerated and is a highly effective treatment for increasing cardiac output. Low cardiac output states respond well to decreasing vascular resistance and enhanced ventricular contractility; both are properties of dobutamine.

• Dobutamine increases intracellular cyclic AMP. This makes its use in conjunction with phosphodiesterase inhibitors ideal.

• Clinicians must maintain special attention to sustained effects of the drug even after infusion has ceased.

• Dobutamine infusion carries the risk of causing sudden death because of its adrenergic properties.

Dolasetron

Brand name: Anzemet.

Class of drug: Antinauseant/antiemetic.

Mechanism of action: Selective serotonin 5-HT$_3$ receptor antagonist. Binds to receptors that initiate vomiting reflex present on vagal efferent neurons.

Indications/dosage/route: IV, oral.

• Prevention of nausea and vomiting during chemotherapy
  – Adults, children 2–16 years: IV 1.8 mg/kg 30 minutes before chemotherapy. Maximum: 100 mg (in pediatric patients).

• Prevention of postoperative nausea and vomiting
  – Adults: IV 12.5 mg, single dose.
  – Adults: PO 100 mg 2 hours before surgery.

– Children 2–16 years: PO 1.2 mg/kg 2 hours before surgery. Maximum: 100 mg. IV 0.35 mg/kg 15 minutes before cessation of anesthesia. Maximum: 12.5 mg.

Adjustment of dosage
- Kidney disease: None.
- Liver disease: None.
- Elderly: None.
- Pediatric: Safety and efficacy have not been established in children <2 years.

Food: Not applicable.

Pregnancy: Category B.

Lactation: No data available. Best to avoid.

Contraindications: Hypersensitivity to dolasetron.

Editorial comments
- This drug has properties similar to those of ondansetron and granisetron. However, it may cause prolongation of the QT interval and other cardiac toxicities.
- For additional information, see *ondansetron*, p. 683.

Dopamine

Brand names: Intropin, Dopastate.

Class of drug: Dopamine receptor agonist, vasopressor, inotropic agent.

Mechanism of action: Adrenergic and dopamine receptor agonist. Renal and mesenteric vasodilator, α-adrenergic agonist.

Indications/dosage/route: IV only.
- Hypotension, CHF, cardiogenic shock
  - Adults: 1–5 µg/kg/min. Maximum: 20–50 µg/kg/min. Titrate dose by 1–4 µg/kg/min every 10–30 minutes until optimum response is obtained. Severe illness: 0.5 µg/kg/min. Increase by 5–10 µg/mg/min to maximum: 20–50 µg/kg/min.
  - Pediatric: 1–20 µg/kg/min. Increase to maximum: 50 µg/kg/min.

Adjustment of dosage
• Kidney disease: None.
• Liver disease: None.
• Elderly: Lower dosages recommended only if there is occlusive vascular disease.
• Pediatric: See above. Safety not fully established.

Onset of Action	Peak Effect	Duration
>5 min	5–7 min	<10 min

Pregnancy: Category C.
Lactation: No data available. Potentially toxic to infant. Avoid breastfeeding.
Contraindications: Hypersensitivity to sulfites, pheochromocytoma, uncorrected tachyarrhythmias or ventricular fibrillation.
Warnings/precautions
• Use with caution in patients with the following conditions: occlusive vascular disease, diabetic endarteritis, acidosis, pulmonary hypertension, hypoxemia, atrial embolism.
• Correct hypovolemia, hypoxia, hypercapnia, and acidosis before using dopamine.
• Vascular disease and arrhythmias may be exacerbated by dopamine.
• Patients that are not tolerant to other sympathomimetics may be intolerant to dopamine.
• Abrupt withdrawal may result in severe hypertension.
• Do not mix other drugs in dopamine solutions when giving IV.
Adverse reactions
• Common: headache, nausea, vomiting.
• Serious: **tachycardia, vasoconstriction, hypotension, conduction abnormalities, ventricular arrythmia, widened QRS complex, ectopy**, dyspnea, bradycardia, gangrene, decreased urine output.
Clinically important drug interactions
• Drugs that increase effects/toxicity of dopamine: MAO inhibitors, general anesthetics.
• Drugs that decrease effects/toxicity of dopamine: β blockers, α blockers.

• Dopamine increases effects/toxicity of diuretics.

Parameters to monitor

• BP, heart rate, ECG must be continuously monitored. Swan–Ganz catheter (PCVP, SVR), pulmonary wedge pressure often required.
• Intake of fluids and urinary and other fluid output.
• Signs of decreased circulation to the extremities (change in color, pain) particularly in patients with Raynaud's disease, diabetic endarteriatis, Berger's disease. Decrease rate of dopamine administration or discontinue.

Editorial comments: IV dopamine administration should be accomplished via a central line, particularly when used as maintenance therapy because of its potential to cause skin and soft tissue necrosis if infiltration occurs. In cases of skin infiltration, immediate SC injection of phentolamine should be given to minimize necrosis.

• This drug is listed without details in the *Physician's Desk Reference,* 54th edition, 2000.

Doxacurium

Brand name: Neuromax.
Class of drug: Nondepolarizing neuromuscular blocker.
Mechanism of action: Blocks nicotinic acetylcholine receptors at neuromuscular junction resulting in skeletal muscle relaxation and paralysis.
Indications/dosage/route: IV only.

• Muscle relaxation during anesthesia
  – Adults: Initial: 0.05 mg/kg.
• Tracheal intubation with succinylcholine
  – Initial: 0.025 mg/kg. Maintenance: 0.005–0.01 mg/kg.

Adjustment of dosage: None.

Onset of Action	Peak Effect	Duration
—	3.5–9.3 min	55–160 min

Food: Not applicable.
Pregnancy: Category C.
Lactation: No data available. Best to avoid.
Contraindications: Hypersensitivity to doxacurium, chemically related drugs, and benzyl alcohol.
Editorial comments: For additional information see *rocuronium*, p. 824.

Doxazosin

Brand name: Cardura.
Class of drug: α-Adrenergic blocker, antihypertensive agent.
Mechanism of action: Hypotensive effect: Blocks α_1-adrenergic receptors, resulting in decreased BP. Also blocks adrenergic receptors in neck of bladder and prostate resulting in smooth muscle relaxation and improved urine flow.
Indications/dosage/route(s): Oral only.
• Hypertension
  – Adults: Initial: 1 mg once daily in am or pm. Depending on response, the dose may be increased by 1–2 mg/d. Maintenance: 2–16 mg once daily.
• Concomitant therapy with a diuretic or other antihypertensive drug
  – Reduce dose initially and titrate up until desired effect is produced.
• BPH
  – Adults: Initial: 1 mg/d. Maintenance: 4–8 mg, once daily.
Adjustment of dosage
• Kidney disease: None.
• Liver disease: Reduce dose. Use with caution.
• Elderly: None.
• Pediatric: Safety and efficacy have not been established in children <18 years.

Onset of Action	Peak Effect	Duration
No data	2–6 h	No data

Food: Take with meals or milk to minimize GI upset.

Pregnancy: Category C.

Lactation: Present in breast milk. Best to avoid.

Contraindications: Hypersensitivity to doxazosin and other quinazoline drugs (prazosin and terazosin).

Warnings/precautions

- Use with caution in patients with the following conditions: liver disease, pulmonary embolism, aortic and mitral valve stenosis.
- Syncope may occur with first dose because of orthostatic hypotension.
- Use with caution when adding another antihypertensive agent to this drug or adding this drug to another antihypertensive regimen, to avoid rapid fall in BP.
- Symptoms of prostate cancer may mimic BPH.

Advice to patient

- Avoid driving and other activities requiring mental alertness or that are potentially dangerous until response to drug is known.
- Limit alcohol intake.
- Avoid standing for long periods, especially during hot weather.
- Take first dose at bedtime; lie down shortly after first dose.
- Use caution when going from lying down or seated position to standing, especially when dosage is being adjusted.
- Avoid excessive intake of caffeine (regular coffee), theobromine (cocoa, chocolates), and theophylline (regular tea).
- Report significant weight gain or ankle edema to treating physician.
- Notify physician if prolonged penile erection occurs.

Adverse reactions

- Common: dizziness, fatigue, headache.
- Serious: hypotension, orthostatic hypotension, depression, priapism, angina, arrhythmias, peripheral ischemia.

Clinically important drug interactions
- Drugs that increase effects/toxicity of α blockers: β blockers, diuretics, verapamil.
- Drugs that decrease effects/toxicity of α blockers: NSAIDs.
- α Blockers decrease effects of clonidine.

Parameters to monitor
- BP for possible first-dose orthostatic hypotension and syncope, particularly when increasing dose.
- Efficacy of treatment for patient with BPH: decreased nocturia, urgency, and frequency of urination.
- Prostate examination to rule out carcinoma prior to and during therapy.

Doxepin

Brand names: Adapin, Sinequan.
Class of drug: Tricyclic antidepressant.
Mechanism of action: Inhibits reuptake of CNS neurotransmitters, primarily serotonin and norepinephrine.
Indications/dosage/route: Oral only.
- Mild to moderate anxiety or depression
  - Adults: 25 mg t.i.d. or up to 150 mg at bedtime. Maintenance: 75–100 mg/d.
  - Elderly: 25–50 mg/d.
- Severe anxiety or depression
  - Adults: Initial: 50 mg t.i.d. Increase to maximum 300 mg/d if needed.

Adjustment of dosage
- Kidney disease: None.
- Liver disease: None.
- Elderly: See above.
- Pediatric: Safety and efficacy have not been established in children <12 years.

Food: No restriction.

Pregnancy: Safety has not been established.

Lactation: Appears in breast milk. American Academy of Pediatrics expresses concern over use when breastfeeding.

Contraindications: Hypersensitivity to doxepin or other dibenzoxepines, concomitant use of MAO inhibitor, glaucoma, urinary retention.

Editorial comments

• Side effect profile for this drug differs from those of other tricyclics in that doxepin does not cause arrhythmias (other than tachycardia).

• For additional information, see *amitriptyline*, p. 39.

Doxycycline

Brand names: Monodox, Vibramycin, Doryx, Monodox.

Class of drug: Antibiotic.

Mechanism of action: Inhibits bacterial protein synthesis after specific ribosomal binding.

Susceptible organisms *in vivo*: *Borrelia burgdorferi, Borrelia recurrentis, Brucella* species, *Calymmatobacterium granulomatis, Chlamydia pneumoniae, Chlamydia psittaci, Chlamydia trachomatis, Ehrlichia* species, *Helicobacter pylori,* Q fever, *Rickettsia* species, *Vibrio* species.

Indications/dosage/route: Oral.

– Adults: Usual dose: 200 mg on the first day of treatment (100 mg q12h). Follow with a maintenance dose of 100 mg/d. Maintenance dose may be administered as a single dose or as 50 mg q12h. More severe infections, 100 mg every 12 hours.

– Children >8 years: 100 lbs or less (<45 kg), 2 mg/lb (4.4 mg/kg) divided into 2 doses on the first day of treatment; follow with 1 mg/lb (2.2 mg/kg) given as a single daily dose or divided into 2 doses on subsequent days. More severe infections: ≤2 mg/lb (4.4 mg/kg) may be used. For children >100 lb (45 kg), use the usual adult dose.

• Uncomplicated urethral, endocervical, or rectal infections in adults caused by *C. trachomatis*
  – 100 mg twice daily for at least 7 days.

Adjustment of dosage
• Kidney disease: None.
• Liver disease: None.
• Elderly: None.
• Pediatric: Not to be used in children <8 years unless all other drugs are either ineffective or contraindicated.

Food: Take 1 hour before or 2 hours after meals. Dairy products interfere with tetracycline absorption.

Pregnancy: Category D.

Lactation: Appears in breast milk. Considered compatible by the American Academy of Pediatrics.

Contraindications: Hypersensitivity to any tetracycline, patients with esophageal obstruction, children <8 years.

Editorial comments: For more information, see *tetracycline*, p. 885.

Dronabinol

Brand names: Marinol, THC.
Class of drug: Antiemetic, appetite stimulant.
Mechanism of action: Inhibits chemoreceptor trigger zone in the medulla.
Indications/dosage/route: Oral only.
• Nausea, chemotherapy
  – Adults, children: Initial: 5 mg/m^2 1–3 hours before chemotherapy; then 5 mg/m^2 every 2–4 hours. Dose titrated to response. Maximum dose: 15 mg/m^2/dose.
• Anorexia in HIV-infected patients
  – Adults: Initial: 2.5 mg b.i.d. before lunch and supper. Reduce dose to 2.5 mg/d if not tolerated. Increase dose by 2.5-mg increments for desired effects. Maximum: 20 mg/d in divided doses.

Adjustment of dosage
• Kidney disease: None.
• Liver disease: None.
• Elderly: Reduce dose because elderly are most susceptible to CNS effects.
• Pediatric: Not recommended for HIV-associated anorexia.

Onset of Action	Peak Effect	Duration
30–60 min	1–3 h	2–4 h

Food: May be taken with food or on an empty stomach.
Pregnancy: Category C.
Lactation: Present in breast milk. Potentially toxic to infant. Avoid breastfeeding.
Contraindications: Hypersensitivity to cannabinoids, sesame oil.
Warnings/precautions
• Use with caution in patients with the following conditions: heart disease, hypertension, history of drug abuse, mania, depression, schizophrenia, concurrent psychoactive drugs.
• In general, amount prescribed limited to that required for a single cycle of chemotherapy.
Advice to patient
• Warn patient and family members that the drug may have mood-altering effects.
• Be aware that physical and/or psychologic dependence may occur in patients receiving high doses for extended periods. Withdrawal syndrome may occur, including "hot flashes," insomnia, loose stools, anorexia, and restlessness if drug is stopped abruptly.
• Weigh yourself on the same scale at approximately the same time each day wearing the same amount of clothing.
• Avoid driving and other activities requiring mental alertness or that are potentially dangerous until response to drug is known.
• Take 1–3 hours before chemotherapy.

Adverse reactions
• Common: euphoria and heightened awareness (8–24%), anxiety, dizziness, depersonalization.
• Serious: tachycardia, syncope, paranoia.

Clinically important drug interactions: Drugs that increase effects/toxicity of dronabinol: alcohol, cocaine, amphetamine, anticholinergics, tricyclic antidepressants, CNS depressants (opioids, antihistamines), lithium, muscle relaxants.

Parameters to monitor
• Frequency and degree of vomiting.
• Body weight and nutritional parameters.
• BP and pulse.
• Signs of CNS side effects including confusion, hallucinations, drowsiness.

Editorial comments: Dronabinol is used for the listed indications only when other agents prove to be ineffective. Patient should be supervised during treatment, particularly for adverse CNS effects.

Droperidol

Brand name: Inapsine.
Class of drug: Tranquilizer, butyrophenone derivative.
Mechanism of action: Antagonizes dopamine at dopaminergic receptors in CNS neurons.
Indications/dosage/route: IV, IM.
• Anesthetic premedication
  – Adults: IM 2.5–10 mg 30–60 minutes before surgery.
  – Children 2–12 years: IM 88–165 µg/kg.
• Diagnostic procedures
  – Adults: IM 2.5–10 mg 30–60 minutes before procedure. If necessary, IV 1.25–5 mg.
• Adjunct to general anesthesia

– Adults: IV 0.28 mg/kg with analgesic or anesthetic. Maintenance: 1.25–2.5 mg total dose.
• Adjunct to regional anesthesia
  – Adults: 2.5–5 mg.

Adjustment of dosage
• Kidney disease: Use with caution. Guidelines not available.
• Liver disease: Use with caution. Guidelines not available.
• Elderly: Use lower doses. Increase dosage more gradually.
• Prediatric: See above.

Food: No restrictions. Oral concentrate should be diluted in 2–4 oz of liquid or pudding.

Pregnancy: Category C.

Lactation: No data Available. Avoid breastfeeding.

Contraindications: Hypersensitivity to phenothiazines, concurrent use of high-dose CNS depressants (alcohol, barbituates, benzodiazepines, narcotics), CNS depression, comatose state.

Editorial comments
• This drug is listed without details in the *Physicians' Desk Reference*, 54th edition, 2000.
• For additional information, see *chlorpromazine*, p. 206.

Edrophonium

Brand name: Tensilon.
Class of drug: Cholinesterase inhibitor.
Mechanism of action: Inhibits acetylcholinesterase thereby increasing acetylcholine at cholinergic receptor sites.
Indications/dosage/route: IV, IM.
• Tensilon test in differential diagnosis of myasthenia gravis
  – Adults: Initial: IV 2 mg injected over 15–30 minutes with tuberculin syringe and needle *in situ*. Inject additional 8 mg if no response after 45 seconds. If a cholinergic response is obtained (eg, muscarinic side effects, skeletal muscle fasciculations, increased muscle weakness), discontinue test and administer atropine, 0.4–0.5 mg IV. Test may be repeated after 30 minutes.
  – Children ≤75 lb: IV 2 mg. If no response after 45 seconds, titrate up to 5 mg, and in heavier children, titrate up to 10 mg.
  – Infants: IV 0.5 mg.
  – Adults: IM 10 mg. If hyperreactivity occurs, administer 2 mg to rule out false negative.
• Tensilon test for evaluation of treatment requirements in myasthenia gravis
  – Adults: IV 1–2 mg 1 hour after oral intake of drug used for treatment. Undertreated patient will demonstrate myasthenic response; overtreated patient, a cholinergic response.
• Reversal of nondepolarizing blocking agent (curare-type drug) post-anesthesia:
  – Adults: IV 10 mg injected over 30–45 seconds. Repeat as necessary. Maximum: 40 mg.
Adjustment of dosage
• Kidney disease: None.
• Liver disease: None.
• Elderly: None.
• Pediatric: See above.

	Onset of Action	Duration
IM	2–10 min	5–30 min
IV	< 1 min	10 min

Food: Not applicable.
Pregnancy: Category C.
Lactation: It is not expected that edrophonium is excreted in milk. Probably safe to breastfeed.
Contraindications: Hypersensitivity to edrophonium, mechanical obstruction of intestinal or urinary tract.
Editorial comments: For additional information, see *neostigmine,* p. 652.

Efavirenz

Brand name: Sustiva.
Class of drug: Antiretroviral drug.
Mechanism of action: Inhibits reverse transcriptase of HIV-1 (nonnucleoside).
Indications/dosage/route: Oral only.
• HIV-1 infection
  – Adults: 600 mg once per day, combined with a protease inhibitor or nucleoside analog reverse transcriptase inhibitor.
  – Children ≥3 years, once daily dose: 10 to <15 kg: 200 mg; 15 to <20 kg: 250 mg; 20 to <25 kg: 300 mg; 25 to <32.5 kg: 350 mg; 32.5 to <40 kg: 400 mg; ≥40 kg 600 mg.
Adjustment of dosage:
• Kidney disease: None.
• Liver disease: None.
• Elderly: None.
• Pediatric: None.
Food: Avoid high-fat meals.

Pregnancy: Category C

Lactation: Centers for Disease Control and Prevention recommend avoidance of breastfeeding by HIV-infected mothers.

Contraindications: Hypersensitivity to efavirenz.

Warnings/precautions

- Do not use as monotherapy for HIV infection.
- This drug has potentially serious side effects including hepatoxicity, severe allergic reactions, and CNS toxicity.

Advice to patient

- Use two forms of birth control including hormonal and barrier methods.
- Avoid driving and other activities requiring mental alertness or that are potentially dangerous until response to drug is known.
- Avoid alcohol.
- Do not take any OTC product without consulting treating physician.
- Take this drug at bedtime to minimize dizziness, drowsiness, and impaired concentration.

Adverse reactions

- Common: CNS symptoms (dizziness, insomnia, hallucinations, agitation, decreased concentration), skin rash, nausea, diarrhea, fever.
- Serious: erythema multiforme, Stevens–Johnson syndrome, skin necrosis, seizures, neuropathy, pancreatitis, hepatitis, psychosis.

Clinically important drug interactions

- Drug that increases effects/toxicity of efavirenz: clarithromycin.
- Drug that decreases effects/toxicity of efavirenz: rifampin.
- Efavirenz decreases effects of oral contraceptives.

Parameters to monitor: Signs and symptoms of hypersensitivity reaction mainly in the form of rash. This will generally resolve after a few weeks of therapy.

Editorial comments: In patients that have failed other antiretroviral regimens, treatment with efavirenz should be initiated in conjunction with another agent that the patient has not previously received.

Enalapril

Brand names: Vasotec, Lexxel.
Class of drug: ACE inhibitor.
Mechanism of action: Inhibits ACE, thereby preventing conversion of angiotensin I to angiotensin II, resulting in decreased peripheral arterial resistance.
Indications/dosage/route: Oral, IV.
• Hypertension
  – Adults: Initial PO 5 mg/d.
• CHF
  – Adults: Initial PO 2.5 mg/d or b.i.d. Maintenance: 5 mg/d.
  – Adults: IV 0.625–1.25 mg q6h
Adjustment of dosage
• Kidney disease: Creatinine clearance >30mL/min: none;creatinine clearance <30mL/min: Initial 2.5 mg/d, maximum 40 mg/d.
• Liver disease: None.
• Elderly: None.
• Pediatric: Safety and efficacy have not been established.

Onset of Action	Peak Effect	Duration
PO:1 h	4–6 h	24 h
IV:15 min	1–4 h	6 h

Food: Administer without regard to meals.
Pregnancy: Category C for first trimester. Category D for second and third trimesters.
Lactation: Appears in breast milk. Considered compatible by American Academy of Pediatrics.
Contraindications: Hypersensitivity to ACE inhibitors, hereditary or ideopathic angioedema, second and third trimesters of pregnancy.

Warnings/precautions

- Use with caution in patients with the following conditions: kidney disease especially renal artery stenosis, drugs that cause bone marrow depression, hypovolemia, hyponatremia, cardiac or cerebral insufficiency, collagen vascular disease, lupus erythematosus, scleroderma, patients undergoing dialysis.
- ACE inhibitors have been associated with anaphylaxis and angioedema.
- Use extreme caution in combination with potassium-sparing diuretics (high risk of hyperkalemia).
- Sodium or volume-depleted patients may experience severe hypotension. Lower initial doses are advised.
- During surgery/anesthesia, the drug may increase hypotension. Volume expansion may be required.
- There may be a profound drop in BP after the first dose is taken. Close medical supervision is necessary once therapy is begun.

Advice to patient

- Do not use salt substitutes containing potassium.
- Use two forms of birth control including hormonal and barrier methods.
- Avoid NSAIDs; may be present in OTC preparations.
- Take BP periodically and report to treating physician if significant changes occur.
- Stop drug if the following occurs: prolonged vomiting or diarrhea. These symptoms may indicate plasma volume reduction.
- Discontinue drug immediately if signs of angioedema (swelling of face, lips, extremities, breathing or swallowing difficulty) become prominent, and notify physician immediately if this occurs.
- If chronic cough develops, notify treating physician.

Adverse reactions

- Common: none.
- Serious: bone marrow depression (neutropenia, agranulocytosis), hypotension, angioedema, hyperkalemia, oliguria, chest pain, angina, tachycardia, asthma, bronchospasm, autoimmune symptom complex (see Editorial Comments), hepatitis, liver failure.

Clinically important drug interactions

- Enalapril increases toxicity of the following drugs: lithium, azothioprine, allopurinol, potassium-sparing diuretics, digoxin.
- Drugs that increase toxicity of enalapril: potassium-sparing drugs, phenothiazines (eg, chlorpromazine).
- Drugs that decrease effectiveness of enalapril: NSAIDs, antacids, cyclosporine.

Parameters to monitor

- Electrolytes, CBC with differential and platelets, BUN and creatinine.
- Signs and symptoms of angioedema: swelling of face, lips, tongue, extremities, glottis, larynx. Observe in particular for obstruction of airway, difficulty in breathing. If symptoms are not relieved by an antihistamine, discontinue drug.
- Patient's BP closely, particularly at beginning of therapy. Observe for evidence of severe hypotension. Patients who are hypovolemic as a result of GI fluid loss or diuretics may exhibit severe hypotension. Also monitor for orthostatic changes.
- Signs of persistent, nonproductive cough; this may be drug-induced.
- Changes in weight in patients with CHF. Gain of more than 2 kg/wk may indicate development of edema.
- Signs and symptoms of infection.
- Possible antinuclear antibody development.
- Monitor WBC count monthly (first 3–6 months) and at frequent intervals thereafter for patients with collagen vascular disease or renal insufficiency. Discontinue therapy if neutrophil count drops below 1000.
- Signs and symptoms of bone marrow depression.
- Intake of fluids and urinary and other fluid output to minimize renal toxicity. Increase fluid intake if inadequate. Closely monitor electrolyte levels.
- Signs and symptoms of renal toxicity.

Editorial comments

- Unlabeled uses of ACE inhibitors include hypertensive crisis, diagnosis of renal artery stenosis, hyperaldosteronism, Raynaud's phenomenon, angina, diabetic nephropathy.

- ACE inhibitors have been associated with an autoimmune-type symptom complex including fever, positive antinuclear antibody, myositis, vasculitis, and arthritis.
- Typically twice-a-day administration is favorable but it may be used once daily even at higher doses.
- The ACE inhibitors have been highly efficacious and well-tolerated class of drug. Nearly every large randomized clinical trial examining their use has been favorable. First, the Consensus Trial proved that enalapril decreased mortality and increased quality of life in Class II and III CHF patients. Then the Solve trial and others proved their benefits in remodeling myocardium post MI. The DCCT trial of diabetic patients demonstrated the ability of ACE inhibitors to decrease the small vessel damage to retinas and glomeruli. Clinical trials looking into primary prevention of cardiac effects are ongoing. Treatment with this class of drug is the gold standard in patients with left ventricular systolic dysfunction. The two most common adverse effects of ACE inhibitors are cough and angioedema. Transient and persistent rises in antinuclear antibodies have been noted. As this class of drug is a vasodilator, orthostasis is another potential problem.

Enoxacin

Brand name: Penetrex.

Class of drug: Broad-spectrum quinolone antibiotic.

Mechanism of action: Inhibits DNA gyrase thereby blocking bacterial DNA replication.

Susceptible organisms *in vivo*: *Citrobacter* sp, *Enterobacter* sp, *Escherichia coli, Klebsiella pneumoniae, Neisseria gonorrhoeae, Proteus mirabilis, Proteus vulgaris, Pseudomonas aeruginosa* (variable), *Serratia, Marcescens, Staphylococcus aureus* (less than ciprofloxacin), *Staphylococcus epidermidis, Staphylococcus hemolyticus, Staphylococcus saprophyticus, Staphylococcus agalactiae, Streptococcus faecalis* .

Indications/dosage/route: Oral only.
- Uncomplicated gonorrhea
  - Adults: 400 mg for one dose.
- Uncomplicated UTIs, cystitis (use only for UTI)
  - Adults: 200 mg q12h for 7 days.
- Complicated UTIs
  - Adults: 400 mg q12h for 14 days.

Adjustment of dosage
- Kidney disease: Creatinine clearance > 30 mL/min: usual dose; creatinine clearance <30 mL/min: one half recommended dose q12h.
- Liver disease: None.
- Elderly: None.
- Pediatric: Safety and efficacy have not been established in children <18 years.

Food: Take 1 hour before or 2 hours after meals with a glass of water.

Pregnancy: Category C.

Lactation: No data available. Potentially toxic to infant. Avoid breastfeeding.

Contraindications: Hypersensitivity to fluoroquinolone antibiotics or quinolone antibiotics, eg, cinoxacin, nalidixic acid, acute liver disease.

Editorial comments
- Note urogenital indications only.
- For additional information, see *norfloxacin*, p. 675.

Ephedrine

Brand name: Ephedrine.
Class of drug: Adrenergic amine, bronchodilator, pressor agent.
Mechanism of action: Relaxes smooth muscles of the bronchioles by stimulating β_2 adrenergic receptors.
Indications/dosage/route: Oral, IV, IM, SC.
Oral bronchodilation, nasal decongestion

– Adults: 25–50 mg q3–4h.
– Pediatric: 3 mg/kg/d in four to six divided doses.
• Bronchodilation
 – Adults: SC or IV 12.5–25 mg.
 – Pediatric: 3 mg/kg in 4 to 6 doses.
• Vasopressor
 – Adults: IM, SC 25–50 mg or 5–25 mg by slow IV push; repeat at 5 to 10-minute intervals, if necessary.
 – Pediatric: IM 16.7 mg/m^2 q4–6h.

Adjustment of dosage
• Kidney disease: None.
• Liver disease: None.
• Elderly: Lower doses may be required.
• Pediatric: See above.

Food: Not applicable.

Pregnancy: Category C.

Lactation: Appears in breast milk. Potentially toxic to infant. Avoid breastfeeding.

Contraindications: Cardiac arrhythmias, heart block (from digitalis intoxication), narrow-angle glaucoma, concomitant use of other sympathomimetics, hypersensitivity to ephedrine, thyrotoxicity, diabetes.

Warnings/precautions
• Use with caution in patients with the following conditions: the elderly, diabetes mellitus, hyperthyroidism, history of seizures, BPH, cardiac diseases (angina, arrhythmia), hypertension, vasomotor disorders.
• Long-term use of ephedrine may cause anxiety, paranoia, schizophrenic symptoms.
• Correct dehydration or decreased blood volume prior to use of ephedrine.
• Tolerance may develop with prolonged use.

Adverse reactions
• Common: nervousness, CNS stimulation, tachycardia.
• Serious: hypertension, chest pain, arrhythmia, paranoia, dyspnea, cerebral hemorrhage, urinary retention.

Clinically important drug interactions
- Drugs that increase effects/toxicity of ephedrine: sympath-omimetics, theophylline, MAO inhibitors, atropine, digitalis and other cardiac glycosides, general anesthetics.
- Drugs that decrease the effects/toxicity of ephedrine: α blockers, β blockers.

Parameters to monitor: BP, pulse, urinary output, CNS status.

Editorial comments
- Ephedrine has very little utility as bronchodilator as newer, safer agents have been developed.
- This drug is not listed in the *Physician's Desk Reference*, 54th edition, 2000.

Epinephrine

Brand names: Adrenalin Chloride, Bronkaid Mist.

Class of drug: Adrenergic amine, bronchodilator, pressor agent, antiglaucoma agent.

Mechanism of action: As bronchodilator: Relaxes smooth muscles of the bronchioles by stimulating β_2-adrenergic receptors. As pressor agent: stimulates heart, causes vasoconstriction by stimulating α adrenergic receptors. As antiglaucoma agent: decreases production of aqueous humor.

Indications/dosage/route: IV, IM, SC, inhalant, intranasal, topical.
- Bronchodilation: metered dose inhaler
  - Adults, children >4 years: 0.2–0.275 mg (one inhalation of the aerosol) or 0.16 mg (one inhalation of Bitartrate Aerosol); repeat after 1–2 minutes if needed.
  - Children <4 years: Dosage not established.
- Bronchodilation: inhalation solution
  - Adults, children >6 years : 1 inhalation of the 1% solution; repeat after 1–2 minutes if needed.
- Bronchodilation: 1:1000 solution

– Adults, SC or IM 0.3–0.5 mg. Repeat in 20 minutes to 4 hours as needed.
– Infants, children (except premature infants and full-term newborns): SC 0.01 mg/kg. Maximum: 0.5 mg/dose. Repeat q15 min for two doses and q4h as needed.
- Bronchodilation using sterile suspension (1:200)
  – Adults: SC 0.5–1.5 mg.
  – Infants, Children 1 month–12 years: SC 0.025 mg/kg.
  – Children <30 kg: 0.75 mg as single dose.
- Anaphylaxis
  – Adults: SC 0.2–0.5 mg q10–15 min as needed. Maximum: 1 mg/dose if needed.
  – Children: 0.01 mg/kg. Maximum: 0.5 mg/dose. Repeat q15 min for two doses and then q4h as needed.
- Anaphylaxis: autoinjector
  – Adults: IM 0.3 or 0.15 mg (for children). Repeat injections may be necessary.
- Vasopressor
  – Adults: Initial: IM or SC 0.5 mg repeated q5 min if needed; then 0.015–0.050 mg IV q5–15 minutes. Initial: IV, 0.1–0.25 mg repeated q5–15min as needed. Or IV infusion 0.001 mg/min, increase to 0.004 mg/min if needed.
  – Children: SC 0.01 mg/kg. Maximum: 0.3 mg. Repeat q5min if needed. IV 0.01 mg/kg q5–15min.
- Cardiac stimulant
  – Adults, Intracardiac or IV 0.1–1 mg repeated q5min if needed.
  – Children: Intracardiac or IV 0.005–0.01 mg/kg repeated q5min if needed.
- Adjunct to local anesthesia
  – Adults, children: 0.1–0.2mg in a 1:200,000–1:20,000 solution.
- Antihemorrhagic, mydriatic
  – Adults, children: Intracameral or subconjunctival 0.01–0.1% solution, 1 drop twice daily into affected eye.
- Antihemorrhagic: topical
  – Adults, children: 0.002–0.1% solution, 1 drop twice daily into affected eye.

• Nasal decongestant
  – Adults, children >6 years: 0.1% solution as drops or spray.

Adjustment of dosage

• Kidney disease: None.
• Liver disease: None.
• Elderly: Lower doses may be required.
• Pediatric: See above

	Onset of Action	Peak Effect	Duration
PO	>60 min	—	3–5 h
SC	>20 min	—	≤ 1 h
IM	10–20 min	—	≤ 1 h

Food: Not applicable.

Pregnancy: Category C.

Lactation: No data available. Best to avoid.

Contraindications: hypersensitivity to adrenergic compounds, tachycardia (idiopathic or from digitalis), cardiac arrhythmias, cardiac dilation, heart block (from digitalis intoxication), shock (except anaphylactic shock), narrow-angle glaucoma, organic brain damage, cerebral arteriosclerosis, intra-arterial administration.

Warnings/precautions

• Use with caution in patients with the following conditions: hyperthyroidism, diabetes, coronary insufficiency, ischemic heart disease, MI, arrhythmia, history of stroke, CHF, hypertension, history of seizures, Parkinson's disease, angina, cerebrovascular disease.
• Some preparations contain bisulfite, which may cause an allergic reaction in sensitive individuals.
• Instruct patient in proper technique for using nebulizer and/or inhaler.
• Do not administer for acute asthmatic attack. If given along with short-acting β agonist, advise patient to discontinue the latter and use it only along with salmeterol for relief of symptoms.

- Drug overdose is characterized by CNS stimulation (nervousness, insomnia) bronchial irritation.
- Discontinue if acute symptoms do not subside or decrease significantly in 20 minutes.
- Tolerance may develop with prolonged use.

Advice to patient

- Use OTC products only with approval of treating physician.
- Do not use solutions that contain a precipitate or are discolored.
- Wait at least 1 minute after 1 or 2 inhalations before taking a third dose.
- Keep inhalant away from eyes.
- Maintain adequate fluid intake (2000–3000 mL/d) to facilitate clearing of secretions.
- Rinse mouth with water after each inhalation to minimize dry mouth and throat irritation.
- Administer inhalant when arising in the morning and before meals.
- Notify treating physician if more than 3 aerosol inhalations are required to achieve relief within a 24-hour period. Do not increase dose in an attempt to obtain relief.

Adverse reactions

- Common: tachycardia, palpitations, GI upset, nervousness.
- Serious: hypertension, increased myocardial oxygen consumption, arrythmias, sudden death, urinary retention, paradoxical bronchospasm, precipitation of narrow-angle glaucoma.

Clinically important drug interactions

- Drugs that increase effects/toxicity of epinephrine: ipratropium, MAO inhibitors, tricyclic antidepressants, sympathomimetic drugs (nasal decongestants, weight loss drugs, eg, phenylpropanolamine), anticholinergic drugs.
- Drugs that decrease activity of epinephrine: phenothiazines.

Parameters to monitor

- Heart rate, BP.
- Possible development of tolerance with prolonged use. Discontinue drug temporarily and effectiveness will be restored.

- Signs of paradoxical bronchospasm.
- Pulmonary function on initiation and during bronchodilator therapy. Assess respiratory rate, sputum character (color, quantity), peak airway flow, O_2 saturation and blood gases.
- Efficacy of treatment: improved breathing, prevention of bronchospasm, reduction of asthmatic attacks, prevention of exercise-induced asthma. If no relief is obtained from 3–5 aerosol inhalations within 6–12 hours, reevaluate effectiveness of treatment.
- FEV_1 to determine effectiveness of the drug to reverse bronchostriction. Efficacy is indicated by an increase in FEV_1 of 10–20%. In addition such patients, as well as those who have chronic disease, should be given a peak flow gauge and told to determine peak expiratory flow rate at least twice daily.
- Determine arterial blood gases if applicable.

Editorial comments: For patients with acute asthma or acute exacerbation of COPD, reduce dose to minimum necessary to control condition after initial relief is achieved. For chronic conditions, the patient should be reassessed every 1–6 months following control of symptoms.

Eptifibatide

Brand name: Integrillin.
Class of drug: Antiplatelet drug for angioplasty and acute coronary syndrome.
Mechanism of action: Inhibits platelet aggregation by binding fibrinogen and von Willebrand factor and other platelet surface receptors.
Indications/dosage/route: IV only.
- Acute coronary syndrome
  - Adults: Initial: IV bolus 180 µg/kg, followed by continuous infusion of 2 µg/kg/min up to 72 hours.

- Percutaneous coronary intervention without acute coronary syndrome
  - Adults: Initial: IV bolus 135 μg/kg before procedure, followed by continuous infusion of 0.5 μg/kg/min for 20–24 hours afterward.

Adjustment of dosage: None.

Food: Not applicable.

Pregnancy: Category B.

Lactation: No data available. Best to avoid.

Contraindications: History of abnormal bleeding within past 30 days, severe uncontrolled hypertension (systolic greater than 200 mm Hg or diastolic greater than 110 mm Hg), major surgery within past 6 weeks, history of stroke or hemorrhagic stroke, platelet count <100,000/mL^3, creatinine >4.0 mg/dL.

Editorial comments:

- Eptifibatide is another platelet inhibitor used in conjunction with angioplasty.

Ergotamine

Brand names: Ergomar, Wigraine.

Class of drug: Ergot alkaloid, vasoconstrictor.

Mechanism of action: 5-HT agonist, α-adrenergic agonist, inhibits reuptake of catecholamines. May decrease local release of inflammatory mediators in the CNS.

Indications/dosage/route: Oral, sublingual, inhalation.

- Migraine or cluster headaches
  - Adults: Initial: PO or sublingual 2 mg; then PO or sublingual 1–2 mg q30min. Maximum: 6 mg/attack. Maximum: 10 mg/24 hours.
  - Adults: Alternative: One inhalation at beginning of attack. Repeat at 5-minute intervals to maximum of 6 inhalations per 24 hours.

Adjustment of dosage
- Kidney disease: Dosage guidelines are not available. Avoid if severely impaired.
- Liver disease: Dosage guidelines are not available. Avoid if severely impaired.
- Elderly: Use with caution because such patients are more susceptible to the adverse effects of the drug.
- Pediatric: Safety and efficacy in children have not been established.

Pregnancy: Category X. Contraindicated.

Lactation: Appears in breast milk. Potentially toxic to infant. Avoid breastfeeding.

Contraindications: Pregnancy, ischemic heart disease, uncontrolled hypertension, hemiplegic or basilar migraine, peripheral arterial disease, sepsis, recent vascular surgery, Raynaud's disease, severe liver or kidney disease, ischemic bowel, hypersensitivity to ergot, high-dose aspirin therapy, known alcohol intolerance.

Editorial comments: For additional information, see *dihydroergotamine,* p. 287.

Erythromycin

Brand names: Erythromycin Base Filmtabs (erythromycin), Ilosone (erythromycin esolate), E.E.S., EryPed, Pediazole (erythromycin ethylsuccinate), Ilotycin Gluceptate (erythromycin gluceptate) Erythrocin Lactobionate, Erythromycin Stearate Filmtab, Wyamycin S (erythromycin stearate), ErythraDerm, Erycette (erythromycin topical).

Class of drug: Antibiotic, macrolide.

Mechanism of action: Inhibits RNA-dependent protein synthesis at the level of the 50S ribosome.

Susceptible organisms *in vivo*
- Gram-positive organisms: Group A *Streptococcus* and *Streptococcus pneumoniae* (increasing resistance especially outside the United States); MSSA (not MRSA) with limited activity, viridans streptococci, *Corynebacterium diphtheriae*, *Listeria monocytogenes*.
- Gram-negative organisms: *Neisseria gonorrhoeae* (some resistant strains), *Neisseria meningitidis*, *Bordetella pertussis*, *Campylobacter jejuni*, *Treponema pallidum*, *Mycoplasma pneumoniae*, *Chlamydia pneumoniae*, *Chlamydia trachomatis*, *Bartonella* sp. Less active against *Hemophilus influenzae*.

Indications/dosage/route: Oral, IV.
- Streptococcal upper respiratory tract infections (pharyngitis, tonsillitis)
  - Adults: 250 mg q.i.d. 10 or more days. Maximum: 4 g/d.
  - Children: 30–50 mg/kg/d, equally divided doses, ≥10 days. Maximum: 4 g/d.
- Prophylaxis of recurring attacks of rheumatic fever in patients allergic to penicillin and sulfonamides
  - Adults: 250 mg b.i.d.
- Prophylaxis against bacterial endocarditis in patients allergic to penicillin
  - Adults: 1 g 1 hour prior to procedure, then 500 mg 6 hours later.
- Conjunctivitis caused by *C. trachomatis*
  - Newborn: 50 mg/kg/d, 4 divided doses, ≥2 weeks.
- Pneumonia of infancy caused by *C. trachomatis*
  - Infants: 50 mg/kg/d, 4 divided doses, ≥3 weeks.
- GU infections during pregnancy
  - Adults: 500 mg/d q.i.d., ≥7 days.
- Uncomplicated urethral, endocervical, or rectal infections caused by *C. trachomatis* and other nongonococcal urethritis (*Ureaplasma* and *Mycoplasma genitalium*) when a tetracycline cannot be tolerated
  - Adults: 500 mg q.i.d., ≥ 7 days.
- Primary syphilis
  - Adults: 30–40 g in divided doses, 10–15 days.

- Acute pelvic inflammatory disease (in combination therapy)
  - Adults: IV 500 mg (Erythrocin Lactobionate) q4h, 3 days. Then 500 mg Erythromycin Base PO q12h, 7 days.
- Pertussis
  - Children: PO 40–50 mg/kg/d, divided doses, 5–14 days.
- Legionnaires' disease
  - Adults: 2–4 g/d, divided doses.
- Respiratory tract infections caused by *M. pneumoniae* and *C. pneumoniae*:
  - 500 PO mg q6h 5–10 days (up to 3 weeks if severe).
- Upper respiratory tract infections (mild to moderate) caused by *S. pyogenes* and *S. pneumoniae*
  - Adults: PO 250–500 mg q.i.d. 10 days.
  - Children: PO 20–50 mg/kg/d, in divided doses, 10 days.
- Lower respiratory tract infections (mild to moderate) caused by *S. pyogenes* and *S. pneumoniae*
  - 250–500 PO mg q.i.d. (or 20–50 mg/kg/d in divided doses), 10 days.

Adjustment of dosage: None.

Food: Take on empty stomach.

Pregnancy: Category B.

Lactation: Appears in breast milk. Considered compatible by American Academy of Pediatrics.

Contraindications: Hypersensitivity to macrolide antibiotics, concomitant administration of pimozide.

Warnings/precautions: Use with caution in patients with liver and kidney disease, long QT syndrome or prolonged QT interval.

Adverse reactions

- Common: nausea, diarrhea, abdominal pain.
- Severe: pseudomembranous colitis, ventricular arrhythmias, nephritis, cholestatic jaundice, angioedema.

Clinically important drug interactions

- Drugs that decrease effects/toxicity of macrolides: rifampin, aluminum or magnesium containing antacids.
- Macrolides increase effects/toxicity of following drugs: oral anticoagulants, astemizole, benzodiazepines, bromocriptine, buspirone, carbamazepine, cisapride, cyclosporine, digoxin,

ergot alkaloids, felodipine, grepafloxacin, statins, pimozide, sparfloxacin, tacrolimus.

Parameters to monitor

- Signs and symptoms of superinfection, in particular pseudomembranous colitis.
- Signs and symptoms of renal toxicity.
- Signs and symptoms of hearing impairment. Patients with kidney or liver disease are at highest risk.

Editorial comments

- Erythromycin is used in penicillin-allergic patients to treat streptococcal tonsillitis (resistance is increasing outside the United States.
- It is used to treat *S. pneumoniae*, *M. catarrhalis* and *H. influenzae* infections (acute otitis media, sinusitis).
- It is the drug of choice in atypical pneumonia caused by *Legionella*, *M. pneumoniae,* and *C. trachomatis*.
- It is first choice for diphtheria and whooping cough.
- It is often used to treat acne.

Esmolol

Brand name: Brevibloc.
Class of drug: β-Adrenergic receptor blocker.
Mechanism of action: Competitive blocker of β-adrenergic receptors in heart and blood vessels.
Indications/dosage/route: IV only.

- Supraventricular tachycardia
  - Adults, initial: 500 µg/kg/min for 1min; then 50 µg/kg/min for 4 min. Repeat dosage to achieve desired effect.
- Intraoperative and postoperative tachycardia/hypertension
  - Adults: 1 mg/kg bolus over 30 seconds, then 150 µg/kg/min infusion. May increase to 300 µg/kg/min.

Adjustment of dosage

- Kidney disease: None.
- Liver disease: None.

• Elderly: None.
• Pediatric: Safety and efficacy have not been established.
Food: No restriction:
Pregnancy: Category C.
Lactation: As this drug is used only acutely, breastfeeding is unlikely to be relevant.
Contraindications: Cardiogenic shock, asthma, CHF unless it is secondary to tachyarrhythmia treated with a β blocker, sinus bradycardia and AV block greater than first degree, severe COPD.
Editorial Comments
• Alternative drugs for treating supraventricular tachycardia: propranolol, IV 10–20 mg q4–6 h; diazoxin IV, PO 0.125–0.5 mg q6h; verapamil IV 80 mg q6h.
• *Warning*: The 2500-mg ampoule is not to be administered by direct IV. It must be diluted prior to use.
• For additional information, see *propranolol*, p. 790.

Estrogen/Progestin Combination Oral Contrceptive

Brand name: See table in Appendix.
Class of drug: Oral contraceptive.
Mechanism of action: Inhibits ovulation by negative feedback inhibition of LH and FSH release from hypothalamus.
Indications/dosage/route: Oral only.
• Oral contraception: See table in Appendix for individual dosages and preparations.
Adjustment of dosage
• Kidney disease: None.
• Liver disease: None.
Food: No restriction.
Pregnancy: Category X.
Lactation: Norethindrone suppresses lactation. Use lowest dose and monitor weight of infant. Considered compatible with breastfeeding by American Academy of Pediatrics.

Contraindications
• Thrombophlebitis, thromboembolic disorders, history of deep vein thrombophlebitis, angina pectoris, cerebrovascular or coronary artery disease, known or suspected breast carcinoma or estrogen-dependent neoplasm, endometrial carcinoma, undiagnosed abnormal vaginal bleeding, known or suspected pregnancy, jaundice with prior contraceptive use, hepatic adenoma.

Warnings/precautions
• Do not use preparations containing more than 50 μg estrogen unless medically indicated.
• Inform patient of risks involved in taking oral contraceptive. Give patient a copy of the patient information booklet for this drug.
• Perform complete physical examination including Pap smear if used for >1 year.
• Determine whether there is a family history of breast or uterine cancer. These may preclude administration of an oral contraceptive.
• Advise patient to use a different form of contraception if taking the following drugs which may decrease effectiveness of the contraceptive and cause pregnancy: rifampin, anticonvulsants, tetracyclines, ampicillin.
• If the oral contraceptive is to be used following unprotected intercourse, perform a pregnancy test prior to administering the drug.

Advice to patient
• Do not smoke.
• Inform treating physician if you experience any of the following symptoms suggestive of thrombotic disorder: sudden or severe headache, pain in leg or chest, respiratory distress, disturbed vision or speech, vomiting, numbness of extremity, dizziness, fainting, cough, chest heaviness, abdominal pain, presence of abdominal mass. If these occur, stop taking drug immediately.
• Use barrier form of contraception to avoid possible sexually transmitted disease.
• If you miss two consecutive menstrual periods, stop taking drug and have a pregnancy test.
• Take drug at the same time each day for maximum effectiveness.

- Be aware that pregnancy may not be achieved for several months after stopping the drug.

Adverse reactions

- Common: abdominal pain, back pain, headache, breast pain.
- Serious: hypertension, thromboembolism, MI, CVA, depression, breast tumor, cholestatic jaundice.

Clinically important drug interactions

- Drugs that decrease effects of oral contraceptives: erythromycins, penicillins, barbiturates, phenytoin, rifampin, tetracyclines, carbamazepine.
- Oral contraceptives increase effects/toxicity of following drugs: tricyclic antidepressants, corticosteroids, β blockers, theophylline, dantrolene.

Parameters to monitor

- Pretreatment examinations and periodic monitoring: BP. Pap smear, breasts, abdominal organs.
- Signs and symptoms of depression. If observed, it is recommended to reduce amount of progesterone.
- Signs and symptoms of edema. If this persists beyond 4 cycles, adjust dose or use a different combination of drugs.
- Sexually transmitted diseases, including HIV infection.
- Signs and symptoms of thrombolic disorders.
- Signs of ocular changes, including changes in ocular contour and quality of tears. If these occur, it may necessitate changes in contact lenses.

Editorial comments

- A variety of estrogen/progestin combinations are available in the United States (see table in Appendix). These vary according to formulation and dosages of base compounds. They are divided into monophasic therapy (single dosage of estrogen/progestin for specific time), biphasic (increased progestin dose for "second phase"), and triphasic (three dosage regimens per month with variance of either estrogen or progestin dosage). These dosages and sequences are specified by the manufacturers.
- These agents have been used as a treatment for chronic GI bleeding.

• The following are considered to be the best choices for an adolescent desiring an oral contraceptive: adolescent with acne (moderate or severe), candidiasis, scanty menstrual flow: estrogen-dominant contraceptive; Fibrocystic breast disease, hyper- or dysmenorrhea: progestin-dominant contraceptive.

Ethacrynic Acid

Brand name: Edecrin.
Class of drug: Loop diuretic.
Mechanism of action: Inhibits sodium and chloride reabsorption in proximal part of ascending loop of Henle.
Indications/dosage/route: Oral, IV.
• Diuresis
  – Adults: Initial: PO 50–200 mg/d in single or divided doses. Increase by 25–50 mg/d if needed. Maintenance: 50–400 mg/d. IV 50–100 PO mg. Repeat in 2–4 hours if needed.
  – Children: Initial: 25 mg/d. Increase by 25 mg/d if needed. Maintenance: adjust dose as needed.
Adjustment of dosage
• Kidney disease: None.
• Liver disease: Use with caution. At higher risk for toxicity.
• Elderly: Use with caution. At higher risk for toxicity.
• Pediatric: Safety and efficacy in infants (oral) and children (IV) have not been established.

	Onset of Action	Peak Effect	Duration
Oral	Within 30 min	120 min	6–8 h
IV	Within 5 min	15–30 min	2 h

Food: Take with food or milk.
Pregnancy: Category D.

Lactation: No data available. Considered contraindicated by the manufacturer.

Contraindications: Hypersensitivity to sulfonamides, anuria, severe progressive renal disease, hepatic coma, severe electrolyte depletion.

Editorial Comments: For additional information, see *furosemide*, p. 394.

Ethambutol

Brand name: Myambutol.

Class of drug: Antituberculosis agent.

Mechanism of action: Inhibits cell wall synthesis by inhibiting RNA synthesis.

Indications/dosage/route: Oral only.

• Adjunct in treatment of pulmonary tuberculosis
  – Adults, children ≥13 years: Initial: 15 mg/kg/d.
  – Adults who have received previous antitubercular therapy: 25 mg/kg for 60 days, then 15 mg/kg daily for retreatment if initial treatment fails.

• Combined with other antitubercular drugs
  – Adults: 50 mg/kg/d, 3 times/wk.

Note. Ethambutol is administered in combination with the following antituberculosis drugs: isoniazid, rifampin, pyrazinamide. Streptomycin is an alternative to ethambutol in this four-drug regimen.

Adjustment of dosage

• Kidney disease: Creatinine clearance 30–60 mL/min: decrease dosage by 50%; creatinine clearance 10–30 mL/min: decrease dosage by 75%; creatinine clearance <10 mL/min: dose 3 times/wk.

• Liver disease: None.

• Pediatric: Use with extreme caution in children <6 because of inability to perform visual examinations. May be necessary if infection with multiresistant organism occurs.

Food: Take with food to prevent gastric upset.

Pregnancy: Category B.

Lactation: Excreted in breast milk. Considered compatible by American Academy of Pediatrics.

Contraindications: Optic neuritis (relative contraindication), hypersensitivity to ethambutol.

Warnings/precautions

- Use with caution in patients with the following conditions: cataracts, inflammatory conditions of the eye, renal disease, gout, diabetic retinopathy.
- In patients with renal insufficiency disease, adjustment is necessary to prevent irreversible eye damage.

Advice to patient: Do not discontinue drug without approval.

Adverse reactions

- Common: headache, hyperuricemia, nausea.
- Serious: thrombocytopenia, anaphylactic reactions, disorientation, optic neuritis, peripheral neuritis, increased liver enzymes, pulmonary infiltrates, eosinophilia.

Clinically important drug interactions: Ethambutol increases effects/toxicity of drugs that produce neurotoxicity.

Parameters to monitor

- CBC with differential and platelets, liver enzymes.
- Culture organisms for sensitivity testing before and periodically during therapy. Be aware that drug resistance may develop.
- Symptoms of visual disturbances: changes in color discrimination (red/green color blindness), blurred vision. Discontinue if these occur, particularly when there are changes in color perception. If visual impairment occurs and is not identified, continued treatment with ethambutol may lead to permanent blindness.
- Signs and symptoms of hepatotoxicity.
- Signs of hyperuricemia.

Editorial comments

- Ethambutol is not to be used as the sole therapy for tuberculosis as resistance can develop rapidly.
- Frequent testing of visual acuity for each eye is required during therapy with ethambutol. Employment of Snellen charts for all

patients is suggested. Visual acuity changes are noted with these tests. Ethambutol should be discontinued and patient reevaluated at frequent intervals.

Etidocaine

Brand name: Duranest.
Class of drug: Local and regional anesthetic.
Mechanism of action: Reversibly inhibits initiation and conduction of nerve impulses near site of injection.
Indications/dosage/route: Local injection only.
• Caudal, epidural anesthesia, peripheral nerve block
  – Adults: Initial: Maximum dose 400 mg etidocaine plus epinephrine 1:200,000 or 300 mg without epinephrine. Repeat after 2–3 hours.
• Maxillary infiltration and/or inferior nerve block (etidocaine-plus epinephrine)
  – Adults: 1–5 mL or 1.5% solution. Total:15–75 mL.
Adjustment of dosage
• Kidney disease: None.
• Liver disease: Use with extreme caution in severe liver disease.
• Elderly: None.
• Pediatric: No information is available for appropriate dose in children.
Food: Not applicable.
Pregnancy: Category C.
Lactation: No data available. Use with caution.
Contraindications: Hypersensitivity for amide-type local anesthetic (eg, lidocaine), sensitivity to sodium metabisulfate (in preparations containing epinephrine).
Warnings/precautions
• Use local anethetics plus vasoconstrictor (eg, epinephrine, norepinephrine) with caution in patients with the following

conditions: peripheral vascular disease, hypertension, administration of general anesthetics, liver disease.

- Use local anesthetics with or without vasoconstrictor with caution in patients with severe liver disease.
- Use with extreme caution for lumbar and caudal epidural anesthesia in patients with the following conditions: spinal deformities, existing neurologic disease, severe uncontrolled hypotention, septicemia.
- Epidural anesthesia: A test dose of the local anesthetic should first be given before the full dose is administered to ensure that the catheter is not within a blood vessel. The test dose should include 10–15 µg epinephrine. Any increase in heart rate and systolic pressure within 45 seconds (the epinephrine response) would indicate that the injection is intravascular.
- Local anesthetics can trigger familial malignant hyperthermia. Symptoms of this condition include tachycardia, labile BP, tachypnea, muscle rigidity. The necessary means must be available to manage this condition (dantrolene, oxygen, supportive measures).
- A local anesthetic containing a vasoconstrictor should be injected with great caution into areas of the body supplied by end-organ arteries (nose, ears, penis, digits).

Editorial comments
- Etidocaine is not recommended for obstetric or non-obstetric paracervical block.
- For additional information, see *bupivacaine*, p. 113.

Etodolac

Brand name: Lodine.
Class of drug: NSAID.
Mechanism of action: Inhibits cyclooxygenase, resulting in inhibition of synthesis of prostaglandins and other inflammatory mediators.

Indication/dosage/route: Oral only.
• Rheumatoid arthritis, osteoarthritis
 – Adults: Initial: 300 mg b.i.d. or t.i.d.
Extended release tablets: 400–1000 mg once daily
• Acute pain
 – Adults: 200–1000 mg q6–8h.
Adjustment of dosage
• Kidney disease: None.
• Liver disease: None.
• Elderly: May be necessary to reduce dose for patients >65 years.
• Pediatric: Safety and efficacy have not been established.
Food: Take with food or large quantities of water or milk.
Pregnancy: Category C. Category D in third trimester or near delivery.
Lactation: No data available. Best to avoid.
Contraindications: Hypersensitivity to etedolac and cross-sensitivity with other NSAIDs and aspirin.
Editorial comments
• Anaphlactoid reactions have occurred with this drug in patients who have shown hypersensitivity to other NSAIDs and aspirin.
• For additional information, see *ibuprofen*, p. 445.

Etoposide

Brand names: VePesid, Etopophos.
Class of drug: Antineoplastic.
Mechanism of action: Inhibits topoisomerase, causing breaks in DNA strands.
Indications/dosage/route: Oral, IV.
• Small cell carcinoma of the lung
 – Adults: PO 35 mg/m^2/d, daily for 4 days; repeat q3–4wk.
  Alternative: 50–100 mg/m^2/d for 7–10 days; repeat q3–4wk.
• Testicular carcinoma

– Adults: IV 50–100 mg/m^2/d, on days 1,3,5; repeat 3 or 4 weeks for 3 or 4 courses.

Adjustment of dosage

- Kidney disease: Creatinine clearance 10–50 mL/min: reduce dose by 25%; creatinine clearance $\leq$10 mL min: reduce dose by 50%.
- Liver disease: Reduce dosage if liver enzymes or bilirubin is elevated by 50–75%.
- Pediatric: Safety and efficacy have not been established.

Food: May be taken with food.

Pregnancy: Category D.

Lactation: Appears in breast milk. Potentially toxic to infant.

Contraindications: Hypersensitivity to etoposide; intrapleural or intrathecal route.

Warnings/precautions: Use with caution in patients with low serum albumin, liver and kidney disease.

Advice to patient

- Use two forms of birth control including hormonal and barrier methods.
- Avoid crowds as well as patients who may have a contagious disease.
- Receive vaccinations (particularly live attenuated viruses) only with permission from treating physician.

Adverse reactions

- Common: nausea and vomiting (30–40%), diarrhea (10%), anorexia (10–16%), reversible alopecia, mucositis.
- Serious: **Myelosuppression (thrombocytopenia, leukopenia)**, anaphylaxis, hypotension, hypersensitivity reactions, neuropathy, hepatitis.

Clinically important drug interactions

- Drugs that increase effects/toxicity of etoposide: calcium channel blockers.
- Etoposide increases effects/toxicity of cisplatin, warfarin, methotrexate, carmustine, cyclosporine, cyclophosphamide, cytarabine.

Parameters to monitor
- CBC with differential and platelets, liver enzymes. Tests should be carried out twice weekly during the course of therapy. Discontinue drug administration if platelets <50,000/mm^3 or neutrophil count <500/mm^3.
- Signs of emesis. Administer antiemetic drug to reduce frequency and duration of vomiting.
- BP before infusion and frequently thereafter (30-minute intervals). If systolic pressure falls below 90 mm Hg, stop infusion.
- Signs and symptoms of fluid extravasation from IV injection.
- Signs and symptoms of hypersensitivity reactions.
- Intake of fluids and urinary and other fluid output to minimize renal toxicity. Closely monitor electrolyte levels.

Editorial comments
- Use latex gloves and safety glasses when handling cytotoxic drugs. Avoid contact with skin as well as inhalation. If possible, prepare in biologic hood.
- Myelosuppression is dose-limiting toxic effect. The nadir for WBC count occurs after 5–15 days, and for platelets, 9–16 days. Recovery takes 21–28 days.
- This drug is to be used only under direct supervision of a physician who is experienced in dealing with anticipated toxicity with cytotoxic drugs. It is indicated only when the potential benefits outweigh the risks involved.
- Hypotension generally occurs only with rapid infusion. Best to administer drug over 1 hour or longer.

Famciclovir

Brand name: Famvir.
Class of drug: Synthetic antiviral drug.
Mechanism of action: Inhibits herpes simplex virus (HSV1, HSV2) and varicella zoster by reducing viral DNA synthesis.
Indications/dosage/route: Oral only.
• Management of acute herpes zoster (shingles)
 – Adults: 500 mg q8h, 7 days.
• Recurrent genital herpes
 – Adults: 125 mg b.i.d., 5 days. Start therapy at first evidence of recurrence.

Adjustment of dosage
• Kidney disease: Creatinine clearance 40–59 mL/min: dose q12h; creatinine clearance 20–30 mL/min: dose q24h; creatinine clearance <20 mL/min: dose q48h.
• Liver disease: None.
• Elderly: Monitor closely and adjust dosage accordingly.
• Pediatric: Safety and efficacy have not been established in children <18 years.

Food: May be taken with or without meals.
Pregnancy: Category B.
Lactation: Not known if excreted in milk. Potentially toxic to infant. Best to avoid breastfeeding.
Contraindications: Hypersensitivity to famciclovir.
Warnings/precautions: Use with caution in patients with kidney disease.

Advice to patient
• Inform patient how to recognize early symptoms of herpes zoster infection, eg, itching, pain.
• Start taking famciclovir within 48 hours if a rash occurs.
• During active infection, do not have sexual intercourse without condom or while lesions are still present.
• Women who have genital herpes should have annual Pap smears.

Adverse reactions
- Common: headache (25%), nausea (13%).
- Serious: urticaria, hallucinations, confusion (CNS symptoms predominantly in elderly).

Clinically important drug interactions: None.

Parameters to monitor: Signs and symptoms of infection.

Famotidine

Brand name: Pepcid AC.

Class of drug: H_2 receptor blocker.

Mechanism of action: Competitively blocks H_2 receptors on parietal cells, thereby blocking gastric acid secretion.

Indications/dosage/route: Oral, IV, IM.
- Duodenal ulcer, acute therapy
  - Adults: PO 40 mg once daily h.s. or 20 mg b.i.d.
- Duodenal ulcer, maintenance therapy
  - Adults: PO 20 mg once daily h.s.
- Benign gastric ulcer, acute therapy
  - Adults: PO 40 mg h.s.
- Hypersecretory conditions
  - Adults: Initial: PO 20–160 mg q6h.
- Gastroesophageal reflux disease
  - Adults: PO 20–40 mg b.i.d. for 6–12 weeks.
- Prophylaxis of upper GI bleeding
  - Adults: PO 20 mg b.i.d.
- Prophylaxis of stress ulcers
  - Adults: PO 40 mg/d.
- Heartburn, acid indigestion, sour stomach
  - Adults, children >12 years: PO 10 mg 1 hour before eating. Maximum: 20 mg/24 h.
- Hospitalized patients with hypersecretory conditions, duodenal ulcers, gastric ulcers
  - Adults: IV 20 mg q12h.

• Before anesthesia to prevent aspiration of gastric acid
  – Adults: IM or PO 40 mg.

Adjustment of dosage

• Kidney: Creatinine clearance <30 mL/min: 20 mg h.s.
• Liver disease: None.
• Elderly: None.
• Pediatric: Safety and efficacy have not been established in children.

	Onset of Action	Peak Effect	Duration
Oral	60 min	—	10–12 h

Food: Take with food.
Pregnancy: Category B.
Lactation: Appears in breast milk. Cimetidine (another H_2 blocker) is considered compatible by American Academy of Pediatrics.
Contraindications: Hypersensitivity to H_2 blockers.
Editorial comments: For additional information see *ranitidine*, p. 810.

Felodipine

Brand name: Plendil.
Class of drug: Calcium channel blocker.
Mechanism of action: Inhibits calcium movement across cell membranes.
Indications/dosage/route: Oral only.

• Hypertension
  – Initial: 5 mg once daily. Maintenance: 2.5–10 mg daily. Maximum: 10 mg/d.

Adjustment of dosage

• Kidney disease: None.

- Liver disease: Initial dose 2.5 mg/d.
- Elderly: Initial dose 2.5 mg/d.
- Pediatric: Safety and efficacy have not been established.

Onset of Action	Peak Effect	Duration
1–2 h	2–5 h	24 h

Food: No restriction.
Pregnancy: Category C.
Lactation: Probably appears in breast milk. Potentially toxic to infant. Avoid breastfeeding.
Contraindications: Hypersensitivity to calcium blockers.
Warnings/precautions
- Use with caution in patients with the following conditions: CHF, severe left ventricular dysfunction, concomitant use with β blockers or digoxin, liver disease, elderly.
- Do not withdraw drug abruptly, as this may result in increased frequency and intensity of angina.
- For the diabetic patient, the drug may interfere with insulin release and therefore produce hyperglycemia.
- Patient should be tapered off β blockers before beginning calcium channel blockers to avoid exacerbation of angina caused by abrupt withdrawal of the β blocker.
Advice to patient
- Change position slowly, in particular from recumbent to upright, to minimize orthostatic hypotension. Sit at the edge of the bed for several minutes before standing, and lie down if feeling faint or dizzy. Avoid hot showers or baths and standing for long periods. Male patients should sit on the toilet while urinating rather than standing.
- Avoid driving and other activities requiring mental alertness or that are potentially dangerous until response to drug is known.

- Avoid use of OTC medications without first informing the treating physician.
- Determine BP and heart rate aproximately at the same time each day and at least twice a week, particularly at the beginning of therapy.
- Be aware of the fact that this drug may also block or reduce anginal pain, thereby giving a false sense of security on severe exertion.
- Include high-fiber foods to minimize constipation.
- Limit consumption of xanthine-containing drinks: regular coffee (>5 cups/d), tea, cocoa.

Adverse reactions
- Common: headache, edema.
- Serious: CHF, arrhythmias, hypotension, depression.

Clinically important drug interactions
- Drugs that increase effects/toxicity of calcium blockers: cimetidine, β blockers, cyclosporine.
- Drugs that decrease effects of calcium blockers: barbiturates.

Parameters to monitor
- BP during initial administration and frequently thereafter. Ideally, check BP close to the end of dosage interval or before next administration.
- Status of liver and kidney function. Impaired renal function prolongs duration of action and increases tendency for toxicity.
- Intake of fluids and urinary and other fluid output to minimize renal toxicity. Increase fluid intake if inadequate. Closely monitor electrolyte levels.
- Efficacy of treatment for angina: decrease in frequency of angina attacks, need for nitroglycerin, episodes of PST segment deviation, anginal pain.
- If anginal pain is not reduced at rest or during effort reassess patient as to medication.
- GI side effects: Use alternative.
- Monitor ECG for development of heart block.
- Symptoms of CHF.

Fenoldapam

Brand name: Corlopam.
Class of drug: Dopamine-receptor agonist, antihypertensivedrug.
Mechanism of action: Stimulates Dopamine A_1 receptor causing vasodilation.
Indications/dosage/route: IV only.
- Short-term (48 hours) treatment of hypertensive emergency
  – Continuous IV infusion: 0.1–1.6 µg/kg/min. Increase dose prn in increments of 0.05–0.1 µg/kg/min, q15 min.

Adjustment of dosage
- Kidney disease: None.
- Liver disease: None.
- Elderly: None.
- Pediatric: Safety and efficacy have not been established.

Onset of Action	Steady-State Levels
5 min	20 min

Food: Not applicable.
Pregnancy: Category B.
Lactation: No data available. Best to avoid.
Contraindications: None.
Warnings/precautions
- Use with caution in patient with glaucoma.
- Do not give as a bolus dose.
- Use calibrated mechanical infusion pump to administer proper dose accurately.
- Close monitoring of BP and pulse required during administration.
- This drug has the potential to cause severe hypotension with associated end-organ damage.
- Do not use solutions >24 hours after diluting for infusion.
- Contains sulfite; this has the potential to cause a hypersensitivity reaction in sensitive individuals.

Advice to patient: Not applicable.
Adverse reactions
• Common: none.
• Serious: severe hypotension, heart failure, MI, cardiac ischemia, tachycardia, bradycardia, dyspnea, bleeding.
Clinically important drug interactions: Other antihypertensive agents increase effects/toxicity of fenoldapam.
Parameters to monitor
• BP, heart rate, ECG.
• Serum BUN and creatinine, liver enzymes.
• Intraocular pressure.
Editorial comments: Fenoldapam has advantages over nitroprusside because of its beneficial effects on renal function, particularly in patients with renal impairment. Increase in urine output will be maintained in patients on fenoldapam who are recovering from surgery (cardiac or noncardiac).

Fenoprofen

Brand name: Nalfon.
Class of drug: NSAID.
Mechanism of action: Inhibits cyclooxygenase, resulting in inhibition of synthesis of prostaglandins and other inflammatory mediators.
Indications/dosage/route: Oral only.
• Rheumatoid arthritis, osteoarthritis
  – Adults: 300–600 mg t.i.d. to q.i.d. Maximum: 3200 mg/d.
• Mild to moderate pain
  – Adults: 200 mg q4–6h.
Adjustment of dosage
• Kidney disease: None.
• Liver disease: None.
• Elderly: May be necessary to reduce dose for patients >65 years.

• Pediatric: Safety and efficacy have not been established.

Food: Take with food or large quantities of water or milk.

Pregnancy: Category B. Category D in third trimester or near delivery.

Lactation: Appears in breast milk. Breastfeeding considered to be low risk by some authors.

Contraindications: Hypersensitivity to fenoprofen and cross-sensitivity with other NSAIDs and aspirin.

Editorial comments: For additional information, see *ibuprofen*, p. 445.

Fentanyl

Brand names: Duragesic Transdermal, Actiq.

Class of drug: Narcotic analgesic agonist.

Mechanism of action: Binds to opiate receptors and blocks ascending pain pathways. Reduces patient's perception of pain without altering cause of the pain.

Indications/dosage/route: IM, IV, transdermal.

• Breakthrough cancer pain
  – Adults: PO 200 µg. Repeat after 15 minutes if necessary. Maximum: 80 µg/d.
• Preanesthetic medication
  – Adults: IV, IM 0.05–0.1 mg 30–60 min before surgery.
• Adjunct to anesthesia
  – Adults: IV 0.002–0.05 mg/kg. Maintenance: 0.025–0.1 mg/kg when indicated.
• Adjunct to regional anesthesia
  – Adults: IM, IV 0.05–0.1 mg over 1–2 minutes.
• Postoperative analgesia
  – Adults: IM 0.05–0.1 mg q1–2h.
• Induction and maintenance of anesthesia in children
  – Children 2–12 years: IM 2–3 µg/kg.
• General anesthetic

– Children: IM 0.05–0.1 mg/kg with oxygen.
- Chronic pain control
  – Initial: Transdermal 25 μg/h system. If receiving concomitant opiates, convert to fentanyl equivalent. Titrate every 3 days after initial application and every 6 days thereafter. Patch is applied every 72 hours.

Adjustment of dosage
- Kidney disease: Creatinine clearance 10–50 mL/min: give 75% of normal dose; creatinine clearance <10 mL/min: give 50% of normal dose.
- Liver disease: Use with caution.
- Elderly: None.
- Pediatric: See above.

Onset of Action	Peak Effect	Duration
IV, IM 7–8 min	No data	1–2 h

Food: May be taken with food to lessen GI upset.

Pregnancy: Category B. Category D if prolonged use or if given in high doses at term.

Lactation: Appears in breast milk. Potentially toxic to infant. Considered compatible with breastfeeding by American Academy of Pediatrics.

Contraindications: Hypersensitivity to narcotics of the same chemical class, management of acute or postoperative pain, use in outpatient surgeries.

Warnings/precautions
- Use with caution in patients with the following conditions: head injury with increased intracranial pressure, serious alcoholism, prostatic hypertrophy, chronic pulmonary disease, severe liver or kidney disease, postoperative patients with pulmonary disease, disorders of biliary tract.
- Administer drug before patient experiences severe pain for fullest efficacy.

- Have the following available when treating patient with this drug: naloxone (Narcan) or other antagonist, means of administering oxygen, and support of respiration.
- Nausea, vomiting, and orthostatic hypotension occur most prominently in ambulatory patients. If nausea and vomiting persist, it may be necessary to administer an antiemetic, eg, droperidol or prochlorperazine. This drug can cause severe hypotension in a patient who is volume depleted or if given along with a phenothiazine or general anesthetic.
- Careful diagnosis must be made of acute abdominal condition before this drug is administered.

Editorial comments
- Transdermal fentanyl has become an important therapy for severe chronic pain.
- Fentanyl should not be administered to children <12 years or those <18 who weigh <50 kg.
- Patients who have experienced adverse effects should be monitored for a least 12 hours after the fentanyl patch has been removed.
- Concomitant use of other CNS depressants (other narcotics, sedatives, hypnotics, phenothiazines, skeletal muscle relaxants, sedating antihistamines, alcohol) may produce additive CNS toxicity. When such combination therapy is contemplated, the dose of one or the other drugs should be reduced by 50% or more.
- For additional information, see *morphine*, p. 633.

Ferrous Sulfate

Brand name: Feosol.
Class of drug: Oral iron supplement.
Mechanism of action: Iron in ferrous sulfate replaces ferrous iron in formation of hemoglobin which is reduced in anemia.

Indications/dosage/route: Oral (all forms) of ferrous sulfate.
• Prevention and treatment of iron deficiency anemia
  – Adults: 50–100 mg iron, t.i.d.
  – Pregnant women: 30 mg iron/d.
  – Children, 6 months to 3 years: 10 mg iron/d.
  – Children >10 years: 2–5 mg iron/d.
  – Infants: 10–25 mg/kg/d, 3 or 4 divided doses.

Adjustment of dosage
• Kidney disease: None.
• Liver disease: None.
• Elderly: None.
• Pediatric: See above.

Food: Take with food to lessen gastric intolerance. Eggs, coffee, tea, milk inhibit iron absorption and should be avoided when taking ferrous sulfate.

Pregnancy: Category A.

Lactation: Safe to breastfeed.

Contraindications: Primary hemochromatosis. Generally avoid using >6 months unless ongoing bleeding or repeated pregnancy.

Advice to patient
• Diet should be high in iron.
• If experiencing constipation, increase intake of fluids and consume high-fiber foods (bran, whole-grain bread, raw vegetables and fruits).

Adverse reactions
• Common: constipation, black stools, epigastric pain (15%), heartburn.
• Serious: none.

Clinically important drug interactions
• Drugs that increase effects/toxicity of ferrous sulfate: ascorbic acid (vitamin C).
• Drugs that decrease effects/toxicity of ferrous sulfate: antacids, cholestyramine, tetracyclines, chloramphenicol.

Parameters to monitor
• CBC, serum iron, total iron binding capacity, and ferritin.
• Signs of symptoms of overdose, particularly after parenteral administration: Initial symptoms: lethargy, abdominal pain, rapid

pulse, hypotension, coma. Later symptoms: pulmonary edema, shock, anuria, seizures, death.

Editorial comments: Intolerance of ferrous sulfate frequently occurs because of GI side effects. Consider switching patient to newer forms of iron such as ferrous gluconate and ferrous fumarate which have less GI toxicity.

Fexofenadine

Brand name: Allegra.
Class of drug: H_1 receptor blocker, nonsedating.
Mechanism of action: Antagonizes histamine effects on GI tract, respiratory tract, blood vessels.
Indications/dosage/route: Oral only.
• Seasonal allergic rhinitis
  – Adults, children >12 years: 60 mg b.i.d.
Adjustment of dosage
• Kidney disease: Reduce initial dose to 60 mg/d.
• Liver disease: None.
• Elderly: None.
• Pediatric: See above. Safety and efficacy have not been established in children <12 years.
Food: No restriction.
Pregnancy: Category C.
Lactation: No data available. Best to avoid.
Contraindications: Hypersensitivity to fexofenadine.
Warnings/precautions: Do not use in neonates or premature infants. Infants and young children are at risk for overdosage, kidney disease.
Advice to patient
• Avoid driving and other activities requiring mental alertness or that are potentially dangerous until response to drug is known.
• Use caution if used along with alcohol and other CNS depressants such as narcotic analgesics and sedatives (eg, diazepam).

- Drink large quantities of water to minimize drying of secretions.
- Discontinue drug at least 4 days before skin testing (for allergies) to avoid the possibility of false-negative results.

Adverse Reactions
- Common: none.
- Serious: none.

Clinically important drug interactions: None.

Parameters to monitor: Efficacy of treatment: improvement of symptoms of rhinitis including sneezing, rhinorrhea, itchy/watery eyes.

Editorial comments: Fexofenadine has an exellent safety profile. It does not cause prolongation of the QT interval seen with other non-sedating antihistamines. Interactions with erythromycin, cimetidine, and ketoconazole do not appear to be clinically significant.

Finasteride

Brand names: Propecia, Proscar.
Class of drug: Inhibitor of androgen synthesis.
Mechanism of action: Inhibits steroid 5α-reductase, thereby blocking the conversion of testosterone to 5α-hydroxytestosterone.

Indications/dosage/route: Oral.
- Treatment of symptomatic BPH
  - Adults: 5 mg/d; 6–12 months of therapy may be required to achieve desired effect.
- Male pattern baldness
  - 1mg b.i.d.

Adjustment of dosage
- Kidney disease: None.
- Liver disease: Use with caution.
- Elderly: None.
- Pediatric: Contraindicated.

Food: May be taken with or without meals.
Pregnancy: Category X.
Lactation: Contraindicated.
Contraindications: Hypersensitivity to finasteride, women of childbearing age, children.
Warnings/precautions: Women who may become pregnant should not come in contact with crushed tablet.
Advice to patient: Use two forms of birth control including hormonal and barrier methods.
Adverse reactions
• Common: none.
• Serious: hypersensitivity reactions.
Clinically important drug interactions: None.
Parameters to monitor
• Efficacy of action: decreased size of enlarged prostate, decreased hesitancy, improvement in size and force of urinary stream, decreased dribbling.
• PSA levels.
Editorial comments
• Patients must be closely evaluated for conditions that might resemble BPH before therapy is instituted. Among these are prostate cancer, infection, hypotonic bladder, stricture, various neurologic conditions.
• Long-term effects of this drug are not known.
• Physician should perform follow-up evaluations to determine response to finasteride and to rule out other abnormalities.
• This drug is generally well tolerated. Improvement in sexual dysfunction is seen in the majority of patients with long-term use.
• PSA level may decrease even if prostate cancer is present.

Flecainide

Brand name: Tambocor.
Class of drug: Antiarrhythmic, type IC.

Mechanism of action: Reduces automaticity of SA node; prolongs refractory period in conduction pathways in atria, AV node, His-Purkinje system.

Indications/dosage/route: Oral only.

• Ventricular tachycardia and PVCs, life threatening
  – Adults: 100 mg q12h; increase if necessary to maximum 400 mg daily.
• Ventricular tachycardia, atrial fibrillation, or flutter
  – Adults: 50 mg q12h; increase if necessary to maximum 400 mg daily.

Adjustment of dosage

• Kidney disease: Creatinine clearance <10 mL/min: decrease dose by 25–50%.
• Liver disease: This drug should be used only when benefits outweigh risks. Adjustment of dosage in hepatic disease has not been fully evaluated; it is recommended to monitor flecainide plasma levels because of significantly increased half-life.
• Elderly: Use with caution and monitor patient carefully.
• Pediatric: Safety and efficacy have not been established in children <18 years.

Onset of Action	Duration
1–6 h	12–30 h

Food: Foods that increase urinary pH may cause increased levels of flecainide in patients on a strict vegetarian diet. Foods or beverages such as acidic juices that lower urinary pH may decrease effectiveness of flecainide.

Pregnancy: Category C.

Lactation: Excreted in breast milk. Considered compatible by American Academy of Pediatrics.

Contraindications: Second- or third-degree AV block, right bundle branch block with left hemiblock (bifasicular block), trifasicular block, cardiogenic shock, marked decrease in LV function, hypersensitivity to flecainide, recent MI.

Warnings/precautions

- Use with caution in patients with the following conditions: heart failure, severe kidney or liver disease, prolonged QT interval, increased PR interval, sick sinus syndrome, blood dyscrasias, second- or third-degree AV block, pacemakers.
- Stop all antiarrhythmic drugs before beginning flecainide.
- Flecainide is not recommended for chronic atrial fibrillation.
- Correct electrolyte disturbances (especially hypokalemia or hyperkalemia) prior to treatment.

Advice to patient

- Notify dentist or treating physician prior to surgery if taking this medication.
- Carry identification card at all times describing disease, treatment regimen, name, address, and telephone number of treating physician.

Adverse reactions

- Common: dizziness, visual disturbances.
- Serious: **dyspnea**, heart failure, cardiac arrest, worsening of arrthymias, new arrthymias, bradycardia, heart block, prolonged PR interval, increased QRS duration, hepatitis, blood dyscrasias, urticaria.

Clinically important drug interactions

- Drugs that increase effects/toxicity of flecainide: β blockers, amiodarone, disopyramide, verapamil, cimetidine, high-dose antacids, carbonic anhydrase inhibitors.
- Flecainide increases effects/toxicity of digoxin.

Parameters to monitor

- Determine serum levels of flecainide, particularly in patients with kidney or liver impairment. Trough levels are particularly important; the probability of adverse reactions increases greatly if this level is >1 μg/mL.
- Intake of fluids and urinary and other fluid output to minimize renal toxicity. Closely monitor electrolyte levels.
- Symptoms of CHF.
- Signs and symptoms of hepatotoxicity.
- Efficacy of treatment: resolution of symptoms of arrhythmia such as palpitations, chest pain, syncope, shortness of breath.

• Electrocardiogram for evidence of new arrhythmia or worsening of existing arrhythmia. ECG should be repeated 1 week after initiation of therapy to determine whether there is prolongation of the PR interval (>0.2 seconds) or QRS complex (>25% increase). In such circumstances, flecainide should be discontinued.

Editorial comments

• Flecainide is suited for patients with symptomatic and persistent atrial fibrillation and atrial tachycardias that are refractory to radiofrequency ablation. Patients must have a structually normal heart and be monitored closely for side effects and efficacy.

• Therapy with flecainide should be initiated in a hospital setting to monitor for possible proarrthymic effect.

• A baseline evaluation of left ventricular function is considered important prior to starting flecainide. The CAST study has shown that there is increased mortality in patients with asymptomatic ventricular arrhythmias given flecainide post-MI.

Floxuridine

Brand name: FUDR.
Class of drug: Antineoplastic antimetabolite.
Mechanism of action: Inhibits synthesis of DNA and RNA in rapidly dividing cells.
Indication/dosage/route: IV, intraarterial.
• GI adenocarcinoma/metastatic to liver
  – Adults: 0.1–0.6 mg/kg/d continuous intraarterial infusion via implanted pump for 1–6 weeks.
  – Adults: Alternative: IV 0.5–1 mg/kg/d, 6–15 days.

Adjustment of dosage

• Kidney disease: None.
• Liver disease: None.

- Elderly: None.
- Pediatric: Safety and efficacy have not been established.

Pregnancy: Category D.

Lactation: No data available. Potentially toxic to infant. Avoid breastfeeding.

Contraindications: Leukopenia (WBC <5000/mm^3), thrombocytopenia, active infection, moderate to severe malnutrition.

Warnings/precautions

- Use with caution in patients with the following conditions: kidney, liver disease, high dose pelvic radiation, akylating antineoplastic drugs.
- Give concomitant acid-blocking agent to prevent ulcer formation.
- This drug is associated with severe toxicity.

Advice to patients

- Use good mouth care to avoid adverse reactions in the oral cavity.
- Use two forms of birth control including hormonal and barrier methods.

Adverse reactions

- Common: anorexia, nausea, vomiting, localized erythema.
- Serious: **severe diarrhea, esophagopharyngitis, GI hemorrhage, bone marrow suppression, elevated liver enzymes, severe stomatitis, pharyngitis**, pancytopenia, anaphylaxis, angina, myocardial ischemia, acute cerebellar dysfunction, confusion, hepatic injury.

Clinically important drug interactions: None.

Parameters to monitor

- CBC with platelets, serum BUN and creatinine, liver enzymes.
- Severe GI reactions, eg, diarrhea, stomatitis, intractable vomiting, GI bleeding, ulceration. Stop drug.
- Signs of hypersensitivity reactions.
- Signs and symptoms of thrombocytopenia. Discontinue this medication if platelet count falls below 100,000/mm^3.
- Signs and symptoms of bone marrow depression.
- Signs and symptoms of infection.

• Liver function. Severe hepatic enzyme elevation may indicate biliary sclerosis.

Editorial comments

• Use latex gloves and safety glasses when handling cytotoxic drugs. Avoid contact with skin as well as inhalation. If possible, prepare in biologic hood.

• Floxuridine should be administered by a physician who is experienced in cancer chemotherapy and drug administration by the intraarterial route.

• This is a highly toxic agent with a narrow margin of safety.

• All patients should be hospitalized prior to the first treatment with floxuridine because of potential for severe toxic reactions.

• Patients receiving combination therapy with other agents that may affect bone marrow function or nutritional status are at higher risk for toxicity from this agent.

• Significant toxic effects include hematologic, GI hemorrhage and even death.

• This agent should be discontinued immediately if signs of any of the following toxic effects develop: myocardial ischemia, severe esophagitis, pharyngitis or stomatitis, WBC count below 3500 or other evidence of bone marrow suppression, intractable vomiting, severe diarrhea, GI bleeding, thromobocytopenia (platelet count <100,000), or hemorrhage from other sites.

Fluconazole

Brand name: Diflucan.

Class of drug: Triazole antifungal agent.

Mechanism of action: Inhibits fungal cytochrome P450 synthesis of ergosterol, resulting in decreased cell wall integrity and leakage of essential cellular components.

Susceptible organisms *in vitro*: *Cryptococcus neoformans. Candida krusei* is resistant; *Torulopsis glabrata* is less susceptible.

Indications/dosage/route: Oral, IV (Same dose for both routes).
• Vaginal candidiasis
  – Adults: 150 mg as single oral dose.
• Orpharyngeal or esophageal candidiasis
  – Adults: 200 mg, then 100 mg/d for minimum of 14 days.
  – Children: 6 mg/kg first day, then 3 mg/kg once daily for minimum of 14 days.
• Candidal UTI and peritonitis
  – Adults: 50–200 mg/d.
• Systemic candidiasis
  – Adults: Optimal dosage and duration have not been determined although doses up to 400 mg/d have been used.
  – Children: 6–12 mg/kg/d.
• Cryptococcal meningitis
  – Adults: 400 mg first day, then 200–400 mg/d for 10–12 weeks after CSF culture is negative.
  – Children: 12 mg/kg first day, then 6 mg/kg once daily for 10–12 weeks after CSF culture is negative.
• Prevention of relapse of cryptococcal meningitis in AIDS patients
  – Adults: 200 mg once daily.
  – Children: 6 mg/kg once daily.
• Prevention of candidiasis in bone marrow transplant patients
  – Adults: 400 mg once daily in patients expected to have severe granulocytopenia <500 neutrophils/mm^3. Start fluconazole several days before the anticipated onset of neutropenia and continue for 7 days after the neutrophil count rises about 1000 cells/ mm^3.

Adjustment of dosage
• Kidney disease: Creatinine clearance 10–50 mL/min: administer 50% of usual dose.
• Liver disease: None.
• Elderly: None.
• Pediatric: See above.
Food: No restrictions.
Pregnancy: Category C.
Lactation: Appears in breast milk. Use with caution.

Contraindications: Hypersensitivity to fluconazole.

Warnings/precautions

• Use with caution in patients with hypersensitivity to other azoles, kidney disease.

• Review drugs that patient is currently taking to avoid possible dangerous drug interactions.

• There have been several reports of fatal exfoliative skin reactions, particularly in patients with serious diseases.

Advice to patient

• Report symptoms of possible liver dysfunction: jaundice, anorexia, dark urine, pale stools, nausea, vomiting.

• Avoid driving and other activities requiring mental alertness or that are potentially dangerous until response to drug is known.

• Avoid alcohol.

• To minimize possible photosensitivity reaction, apply adequate sunscreen and use proper covering when exposed to strong sunlight.

Adverse reactions

• Common: nausea, vomiting, diarrhea, abdominal pain, rash.

• Serious: hepatotoxicity (rare), exfoliative skin disorders (rare).

Clinically important drug interactions

• Fluconazole increases effects/toxicity of following drugs: cyclosporine, glipizide, glyburide, phenytoin, theophylline, tolbutamide, warfarin, zidovudine, cisapride.

• The following drugs decrease effects/toxicity of fluconazole: cimetidine, rifampin.

Parameters to monitor

• Signs and symptoms of liver toxicity.

• For AIDS patients: Signs and symptoms of rash which might indicate serious exfoliative skin disorder. Discontinue if lesions do not subside.

Editorial comments

• Fluconazole is very well absorbed after oral dosing, even in neutropenic patients, patients with AIDS, and patients on antacids.

• High drug levels achieved in CSF.

- Fluconazole is used in cryptococcal meningitis (usually after initial treatment with amphotericin B ± flucytosine × 2 weeks) and coccidiomycosis meningitis.
- Also useful in infections such as esophagitis, mucocutaneous candidiasis, and *Candida* vaginitis.

Flucytosine

Brand names: Ancobon, 5-FC, 5-Fluorocytosine.
Class of drug: Antifungal.
Mechanism of action: Flucytosine is converted to fluorouracil, which interferes with DNA synthesis. Interferes with fungal RNA and protein synthesis.
Indications/dosage/route: Oral only.
- Severe infections, endocarditis, meningitis, septicemia, UTI, pulmonary infections caused by susceptible strains of *Candida* and *Cryptococcus*
  – Adults, children >110 lb: 50–150 mg/kg/d, divided doses q6h.
  – Adults, children <110 lb: 1.5–4.5 g/m^2/d, 4 divided doses.
Adjustment of dosage
- Kidney disease: Creatinine clearance 20–40 mL/min: administer q12h; creatinine clearance 10–20 mL/min: increase dosage interval to q24h; creatinine clearance <10 mL/min: increase dosage interval to q24–48h.
- Liver disease: None.
- Pediatric: See above.
Food: Should be taken with food.
Pregnancy: Category C.
Lactation: No data available. Potentially toxic to fetus. Avoid breastfeeding.
Contraindications: Hypersensitivity to flucytosine.
Warnings/precautions: Use with caution in patients with kidney disease, bone marrow depression (extreme caution).

Advice to patient: None.
Adverse reactions
• Common: nausea, vomiting, diarrhea, skin rash, anorexia.
• Serious: bone marrow depression, cardiac arrest, renal failure, hepatitis, confusion, parkinsonism, psychosis, hypoglycemia, hypokalemia, respiratory arrest.

Clinically important drug interactions: Flucytosine increases effects/toxicity of amphotericin B.

Parameters to monitor
• CBC with differential and platelets, serum BUN and creatinine, liver enzymes before and frequently after instituting therapy.
• Serum flucytosine levels. Therapeutic concentrations are 25–100 µg/mL with peak plasma concentrations between 40 and 60 µg/mL. Concentrations >100 µg/mL may cause serious toxicity.
• Signs and symptoms of antibiotic-induced bacterial or fungal superinfection. Use of yogurt (4 oz/d) may be helpful in prevention of superinfection.

Editorial comments
• Flucytosine is generally administered with amphotericin B to improve its efficacy. This combination is required for severe infections and/or CNS involvement.
• Patients receiving flucytosine must be under close medical supervision.

Fludarabine Phosphate

Brand name: Fludara.
Class of drug: Antineoplastic antimetabolite.
Mechanism of action: Metabolized to derivative that inhibits DNA polymerase and ribonucleotide reductase, resulting in inhibition of DNA synthesis.
Indications/dosage/route: IV only.
• Chronic lymphocytic leukemia in patients who have not responded to a standard alkylating agent

– Adults: 15–40 mg/m^2 over 30 minutes, 5 consecutive days; repeat every 28 days for 3 additional courses and then discontinue drug.
– Children: 20–25 mg/m^2/d over 30 min. Continue as for adults.
• Acute leukemia
– Children: 10 mg/m^2 over 15 min followed by 30 mg/m^2 over 5 days.

Adjustment of dosage
• Kidney disease: Guidelines are not available for adjustment of dosage in patients with kidney disease; monitor closely for possible increased toxicity.
• Liver disease: None
• Elderly: Increased potential for toxicity; adjustment of dosage may be necessary.
• Pediatric: See above.

Pregnancy: Category D.

Lactation: No data available. Potentially toxic to infant. Avoid breastfeeding.

Contraindications: Hypersensitivity to fludarabine, acute infections.

Warnings/precautions: Use with caution in patients with the following conditions: renal insufficiency, fever, infection, bone marrow depression, epilepsy, spasicity, peripheral neuropathy.

Advice to patient
• Use two forms of birth control including hormonal and barrier methods.
• Avoid alcohol.
• Do not receive any vaccinations (particularly live attenuated viruses) without permission from treating physician.

Adverse reactions
• Common: fatigue, weakness, paresthesia, muscle pain, edema (19%), visual disturbances, nausea and vomiting (36%), cough (44%), rash, fever (69%), chills, infection (44%), stomatitis.
• Serious: **bone marrow depression (75%), GI bleeding, UTI (15%), pneumonitis**, CHF, renal failure, anaphylaxis, hemolytic anemia, acidosis, CNS demyelinaton (blindness, coma, neuropathy), hearing loss, tumor lysis syndrome, hepatotoxicity.

Clinically important drug interactions: Other drugs that cause bone marrow depression increase effects/toxicity of fludarabine.

Parameters to monitor

• CBC with differential and platelets, serum BUN and creatinine, serum electrolytes, liver enzymes.
• Signs and symptoms of infection.
• Signs and symptoms of hepatotoxicity.
• Signs and symptoms of renal toxicity.
• Signs and symptoms of bone marrow depression.
• Signs and symptoms of pulmonary toxicity: basilar rales, tachypnea, cough, fever, exertional dyspnea.
• Signs of hyperuricemia: gouty arthritis, uric acid kidney stones.
• Signs and symptoms of stomatitis: mouth sores, painful swallowing, dry mouth, white patchy areas in oral mucosa. Treat with peroxide, tea, topical anesthetics such as benzocaine, lidocaine or antifungal drug.
• Signs and symptoms of ocular toxicity: reduced visual acuity, floaters, eye pain.
• Intake of fluids and urinary and other fluid output to minimize renal toxicity. Increase fluid intake if inadequate.
• Signs and symptoms of anemia: shortness of breath, dizziness, angina, pale conjunctiva, skin and nailbeds.

Editorial comments

• Use latex gloves and safety glasses when handling cytotoxic drugs. Avoid contact with skin as well as inhalation. If possible, prepare in biologic hood.
• Fludarabine should be administered under direct supervision of a physician experienced in chemotherapeutic drug administration.

Fludrocortisone

Brand name: Florinef.
Drug classification: glucocorticoid, antiinflammatory.
Mechanism of action: Inhibits migration of polymorphonuclear leukocytes; stabilizes lysosomal membranes; inhibits production of products of arachidonic acid cascade.

Indications/dosage/route: Oral only.

• Addison's disease
  – Initial: 0.1–0.2 mg/d. Maintenance: 0.1 mg 3 times/wk, usually in conjunction with hydrocortisone or cortisone.
• Salt-losing adrenogenital syndrome
  – 0.1–0.2 mg/d.

Adjustment of dosage

• Kidney disease: None.
• Liver disease: None.
• Elderly: None.
• Pediatric: Children on long-term therapy must be monitored carefully for growth and development.

Food: Administer with food to minimize GI upset.

Pregnancy: Category C.

Lactation: Appears in breast milk. Avoid.

Contraindications: Systemic fungal, viral, or bacterial infections, myasthenia gravis, severe cardiovascular disease.

Editorial comments

• Fludrocortisone induces pronounced fluid retention. Increased potassium excretion and retention of sodium and water occur with therapy. Monitoring of serum electrolytes, especially potassium, is required for patients on this medication. Potassium supplementation and salt restriction may be required.
• Usage should be restricted to patients with proper indications.
• In general, patients with Addison's disease will be treated with fludrocortisone in combination with a glucocorticoid.
• For additional information, see *prednisone*, p. 760.
• This drug is not listed in the *Physician's Desk Reference*, 54th edition, 2000.

Flumazenil

Brand name: Romazicon.

Class of drug: Benzodiazepine antagonist.

Mechanism of action: Competitive inhibitor of benzodiazepines on GABA/benzodiazepine receptor.

Indications/dosage/route: IV only.

- Reversal of CNS depressant effects of benzodiazepine used for conscious sedation
  - Adults: Initial: 0.2 mg over 15 seconds. Repeat dose every 1 minute as needed to achieve arousal.
  - Children: 0.01 mg given over 15 seconds. Repeat after 45 seconds and thereafter at 60-second intervals if necessary for a maximum of 4 additional times after initial dosing. Maximum: 1 mg. May repeat dosage after 20 minutes; maximum: 3 mg/h.
- Suspected benzodiazepine overdose
  - Adults: 0.2 mg over 15 seconds. Repeat dose of 0.3 mg over 30 seconds at 1-minute intervals. Maximum cumulative dose: 3–5 mg. If no response 5 minutes after 5 mg total drug is administered, it is unlikely that a benzodiazepine is the cause of toxicity and additional drug should not be administered.
- Reversal of sedative effects of benzodiazepines given for sedation
  - Children: 0.01 mg/kg given over 15 seconds. Repeat after 45 seconds and at 60-second intervals if necessary to a maximum of 4 additional times.

Adjustment of dosage

- Kidney disease: None.
- Liver disease: Severe liver dysfunction: reduce dose by 40–60%.
- Elderly: None.
- Pediatric: Safety and efficacy in reversing conscious sedation by benzodiazepines have not been established in children <1 year.

Onset of Action	Peak Effect
1–2 min	6–10 min

Food: Not applicable.
Pregnancy: Category C.

Lactation: No data available. Best to avoid.

Contraindications: Hypersensitivity to flumazenil or benzodiazepines, patients receiving a benzodiazepine for life-threatening indications (status epilepticus, controlling intracranial pressure), patient exhibiting severe overdose from tricyclic antidepressant, treatment of benzodiazepine dependence, management of withdrawal syndrome from benzodiazepines.

Warnings/precautions

- Use with caution in patients with the following conditions: seizure disorder or myoclonic jerking, concurrent sedative–hypnotic withdrawal, recent administration of repeated benzodiazepine, concurrent tricyclic antidepressant overdose, alcohol-dependent patient, head injuries, psychiatric patient, severe liver disease.

- It has not been established that the drug can reverse the respiratory depression caused by benzodiazepines. Make sure respiratory assistance is not required. Flumazenil is only considered as an adjunct to reversing the effects of benzodiazepine overdose. Take steps to enable patient to emerge slowly from benzodiazepine overdose to avoid withdrawal reaction.

Advice to patient: Avoid alcohol and other CNS depressants such as opiate analgesics and sedatives (eg, diazepam) when taking this drug.

Adverse reactions

- Common: nausea and vomiting (11%), dizziness (10%).
- Serious: severe bradycardia, tachycardia, chest pain, hypertension, ventricular arrhythmia.

Clinically important drug interactions: Drugs that increase toxicity of flumazenil: mixed drug overdoses, tricyclic antidepressant overdose.

Parameters to monitor

- Status of sedation after dosing. Carefully administer additional flumazenil as necessary.
- Signs of resedation: Observe patient for at least 2 hours following flumazenil administration for respiratory depression and other signs of benzodiazepine overdose. If resedation occurs, administer additional doses at 20-minute intervals.

- Signs of seizures during administration. Treat with a barbiturate or phenytoin.
- Monitor ECG if chest pain or arrhythmia develops.

Editorial comments

- Flumazenil does not reverse the amnesic effect of benzodiazepine overdose. Accordingly, the physician should advise patient's family or caregiver of the need to follow the patient carefully following recovery.
- Patient and family should be provided written post-procedure care. Flumazenil should be used cautiously in outpatients and hospitalized patients because of the possibility that patients may have frequent benzodiazepines use or dependence.
- Deaths after flumazemil use have generally occurred in patients with overdoses of benzodiazepines combined with other agents or with serious underlying illnesses.
- Seizures caused by flumazenil have occurred most often in patients who have been on long-term benzodiazepine therapy or have experienced overdose with tricyclic antidepressants or other drugs with convulsant activity, eg, cyclosporine, isoniazid, MAO inhibitors, cocaine, buproprion. Such seizures may be treated with a benzodiazepine, barbituate, or phenytoin.
- This drug is not intended to be used as a diagnostic tool for benzodiazepine overdose.

Flunisolide

Brand names: Aerobid, Nasalide.
Drug classification: Inhalation corticosteroid.
Mechanism of action: Inhibits elaboration of many of the mediators of allergic inflammation, eg, leukotrienes and other products of the arachidonic acid cascade.
Indications/dosage/route: Inhalation, intranasal.
- Inhalation: Bronchial asthma

- Adults: 2 inhalations in a.m. and p.m. Maximum: 4 inhalations b.i.d.
- Children 6–15 years: 2 inhalations in a.m. and p.m. Maximum: 1 mg.
• Intranasal: Rhinitis
- Adults: Initial: 2 sprays in each nostril b.i.d.; increase to 8 sprays in each nostril as needed.
- Children 6–14 years: Initial: spray in each nostril t.i.d. Maximum: 4 sprays in each nostril per day.
- Maintenance, adults and children: 1–2 sprays in each nostril daily.

Adjustment of dosage
• Kidney disease: None.
• Liver disease: None.
• Elderly: None.
• Pediatric: Safety and efficacy have not been established in children <6 years.

Pregnancy: Category C.

Lactation: Present in breast milk. Safe to use.

Contraindications: Untreated fungal, bacterial, or viral infections, ocular herpes simplex, septic ulcers, nasal surgery or trauma, untreated infections of nasal mucosa, hypersensitivity to corticosteroids.

Warnings/precautions: Use with caution in patients with tuberculosis of the respiratory tract (active or quiescent), exposure to measles or chicken pox.

Editorial comments
• Each dose of aerosoli delivers 250 µg of active drug. Each intranasal dose is 25 µg.
• For additional information, see *budesonide*, p. 109.

Fluocinolone

Brand names: Synalar, Synemol, Lidex.
Class of drug: Topical antiinflammatory corticosteroid.

Mechanism of action: Inhibits migration of polymorphonuclear leukocytes; stabilizes lysosomal membranes; inhibits production of products of arachidonic acid cascade.

Indications/dosage/route: Topical only. Dosages of corticosteroids are variable. These should be individualized according to the disease being treated and the response of the patient. Apply as a thin film to affected area two to four times daily.

Adjustment of dosage: None.

Pregnancy: Category C. This drug should not be used in large amounts or for prolonged periods during pregnancy.

Lactation: No data available. Fluocinolone is considered compatible by American Academy of Pediatrics.

Contraindications: Hypersensitivity to corticosteroids, marked impaired circulation, occlusive dressing if primary skin infection; monotherapy in primary bacterial infections (eg, impetigo, cellulitis, rosacea), ophthalmic use, plaque psoriasis (widespread).

Warnings/precautions

- Use with caution in patients with primary skin infection and in those receiving other immunosuppressant drugs.
- Occlusive dressing may cause atrophy, stria, monilia, or secondary infections when applied over topical steroids. They are used at times for psoriasis or other refractory skin conditions. Advise patient to use such dressing only if approved by treating physician.
- Choice of vehicle for topical drug depends on the following: Dry scaly lesions: use ointment; oozing area: use cream; hairy areas: use gel, lotion, solution, or aerosol.

Advice to patient

- Avoid long-term application to the following areas of the body: eyes, face, rectum, genitals, skinfolds. These are areas most susceptible to development of skin atrophy and decoloration.
- Do not use bandages, cosmetics, or other skin products over area where steroid has been applied.

• Parents should not use tight-fitting diapers or plastic pants if steroid is applied to diaper area.

Adverse reactions

• Common: itching, burning, skin dryness, erythema, folliculitis, hypertrichosis, allergic contact dermatitis, skin maceration, secondary infection, striae, millaria, skin atrophy.
• Serious: HPA axis suppression, Cushing's syndrome.

Parameters to monitor

• Signs of infection: increased pain, purulent exudate, erythema. Treat with appropriate antibiotics. Organisms most likely to produce intercurrent infection include *Candida, Mycobacterium, Toxoplasma, pneumocystis, Nocardi, Ameba.*
• Signs of skin atrophy. This condition may become clinically significant after 3–4 weeks of drug application.
• Signs and symptoms of systemic absorption, particularly in patients receiving high-potency steroid for long periods. Monitor for Cushing's syndrome, HPA suppression, glycosuria, hyperglycemia. Children and infants are most susceptible to HPA suppression. Patients using topical steroids over large areas of the body for prolonged periods are also at risk.

Editorial comments: Only 5% strength is suggested for topical treatment of superficial basal cell carcinoma.

Fluorouracil (5-Fluorouracil [5-FU])

Brand names: Adrucil, Efudex, Fluroplex.
Class of drug: Antineoplastic antimetabolite.
Mechanism of action: Blocks methylation of deoxyuridylic acid by inhibiting thymidylate synthetase.
Indications/dosage/route: IV, topical.

• Management of colon, rectal, breast, pancreatic, gastric cancers
  – Adults, children: IV 12 mg/kg, 4–5 days (400 mg/m^2/d) continuous or IV push daily, followed by 6 mg/kg IV

days 6, 8, 10, 12. Repeat cycle each 30 days. Maximum: 800 mg/d.
- Actinic or solar keratosis
  - Adults: Cover lesions with cream b.i.d, 2–4 weeks.
- Superficial basal cell carcinomas
  - Adults: Cover lesion with 5% solution or cream b.i.d, up to 12 weeks.

Adjustment of dosage
- Kidney disease: None.
- Liver disease: Do not use if bilirubin >5 mg/dL.
- Elderly: None.
- Pediatric: Safety and efficacy of topical preparation have not been determined.

Pregnancy: Category X.

Lactation: No data available. Potentially toxic to fetus. Avoid breastfeeding.

Contraindications: Hypersensitivity to fluorouracil, poor nutritional state, bone marrow depression (WBC count <5000/mm^2 or platelet count <100,000/mm^2), patients who have had major surgery within 1 month, active serious infection, pregnancy.

Warnings/precautions
- Use with caution in patients with kidney or liver disease, high-dose pelvic radiation or who are concomitantly using other neoplastic drugs, in particular alkylating agents.
- Solution should not be used if it is cloudy.
- An antemetic should be administered 1 hour before fluorouracil.

Advice to patient
- Use two forms of birth control including hormonal and barrier methods.
- Use plastic gloves when applying topical drug.
- Do not apply topically to a large ulcerated area as this may result in systemic absorption and potential toxicity.
- To minimize possible photosensitivity reaction, apply adequate sunscreen and use proper covering when exposed to strong sunlight.

- Avoid crowds as well as persons who may have a contagious disease.
- Receive vaccinations (particularly live attenuated viruses) only with permission from treating physician.
- Drink large amounts of fluids (2–3 L/d) when taking the drug.

Adverse reactions
- Common: dermatitis, alopecia (reversible), stomatitis, nausea, vomiting, diarrhea, anorexia, mucositis.
- Serious: myelosuppression, GI ulceration, hypotension, chest pain, ischemic ECG changes, coronary spasm, ataxia, coagulopathy, hepatitis, dyspnea, palmar–plantar syndrome .

Clinically important drug interactions: Allopurinol, cimetidine increase effects/toxicity of fluorouracil.

Parameters to monitor
- CBC with differential and platelets, serum BUN and creatinine, liver enzymes.
- Hematologic status for bone marrow suppression.
- Signs of intractable or severe vomiting. Discontinue drug.
- Symptoms of cerebellar dysfunction: ataxia, dizziness, weakness. Supervise ambulation.
- Signs and symptoms of infection.
- Signs and symptoms of fluid extravasation from IV injection.
- Signs and symptoms of stomatitis. Treat with peroxide, tea, topical anesthetics such as benzocaine, lidocaine or antifungal drug.
- Symptoms of severe GI disturbances: diarrhea, hemorrhage. Discontinue immediately.

Editorial comments
- Fluorouracil is used alone or in combination with other modalities of treatment, eg, radiation therapy, surgery, other chemotherapeutic agents.
- If used along with methotrexate, fluorouracil must be given after, not before, methotrexate.
- Granulocytopenia occurs at 9–14 days and thrombocytopenia at 7–17 days after dose. Function returns 22 days after stopping drug.
- The IV form of fluorouracil is not listed in the *Physician's Desk Reference*, 54th edition, 2000.

Fluoxetine

Brand name: Prozac.
Class of drug: SSRI.
Mechanism of action: Inhibits reuptake of serotonin into CNS neurons.
Indications/dosage/route: Oral only.
• Depression
  – Adults: Initial: 20 mg/d in a.m. Maintenance: 20–40 mg/d. Maximum: 80 mg/d.
• Obsessive–compulsive disorder
  – Initial: 20 mg/d in a.m. Maintenance: 20–60 mg/d. Maximum: 80 mg/d.
• Bulimia nervosa
  – 20–60 mg/d in the morning.

Adjustment of dosage
• Kidney disease: None.
• Liver disease: Decrease dose and/or interval in cirrhosis.
• Elderly: Consider lower dose.
• Pediatric: Safety and efficacy have not been established.

Food: May be taken with meals.
Pregnancy: Category B.
Lactation: Appears in breast milk. Best to avoid. American Academy of Pediatrics expresses concern with use during breast-feeding.
Contraindications: MAO inhibitor taken within 14 days, hypersensitivity to fluoxetine.

Warnings/precautions
• Use with caution in patients with the following conditions: diabetes mellitus, seizures, liver or kidney disease.
• Advise patient that effectiveness of the drug may not be apparent until 4 weeks of treatment.
• A withdrawal syndrome has been described after abrupt withdrawal of this drug. Symptoms include blurred vision, diaphoresis, agitation, and hypomania.
• Mania or hypomania may be unmasked by SSRIs.

Advice to patient
- Avoid driving and other activities requiring mental alertness or that are potentially dangerous until response to drug is known.
- Avoid alcohol and other CNS depressants such as opiate analgesics and sedatives (eg, diazepam) when taking this drug.
- Report excessive weight loss to treating physician.
- Take this drug in the morning as it may cause insomnia.
- Patients on glucose-lowering agents should carry sugar or sugar-containing candy. Patients should wear a bracelet identifying the condition and possibility of developing hypoglycemia.

Adverse reactions
- Common: anorexia, body pain, nausea, insomnia, anxiety, tremor, dry mouth.
- Serious: hypoglycemia, hyponatremia, anaphylaxis, suicidal tendency, extrapyramidal reactions, SIADH.

Clinically important drug interactions
- Drugs that increase effects/toxicity of SSRIs: MAO inhibitors (combination contraindicated), clarithromycin, tryptophan.
- SSRIs increase effects/toxicity of following drugs: tricyclic antidepressants, diazepam, dextromethorphan, encainide, haloperidol, perphenazine, propafenone, thioridizine, trazadone, warfarin, carbamazepine, lithium.
- Drug that decreases effects/toxicity of SSRIs: buspirone.

Parameters to monitor
- Progressive weight loss. Recommend dietary management to maintain weight. This may be particularly important in underweight patients.
- Signs of hypersensitivity reactions.
- Signs and symptoms of hypoglycemia.

Editorial comments
- SSRIs are recommended for patients who are at risk for medication overdose because they are safer than tricyclic antidepressants. There have been no reported deaths from overdose with this drug.
- SSRIs may be a better choice than tricyclic antidepressants for the following patients: those who cannot tolerate the

anticholinergic effects or excessive daytime sedation of tricyclic antide-pressants; and those who experience psychomotor retardation or weight gain. SSRIs are generally very well tolerated.

- If coadministered with tricyclic antidepressant, dosage of the latter may need to be reduced and blood levels monitored. Do not administer for at least 14 days after discontinuing a MAO inhibitor. Do not initiate MAO inhibitor until at least 5 weeks after discontinuing this agent.
- SSRIs have generally replaced tricyclics, MAO inhibitors as drugs of choice for depression.
- Sexual dysfunction appears to be less of a problem with fluoxetine than other SSRIs.

Fluoxymesterone

Brand name: Halotestin.
Class of drug: Androgenic hormone.
Mechanism of action: Stimulates receptors in androgen-responsive organs, thereby promoting growth and development of male sex organs. Maintains secondary male characteristics in deficit states.
Indications/dosage/route: Oral only.
- Hypogonadism
  - Males: 5–20 mg daily.
- Delayed puberty
  - Males: 2.5–20 mg daily, 4–6 months.
- Inoperable breast carcinoma
  - Females: 10–40 mg daily in divided doses.
- Prevention of postpartum breast pain and engorgement
  - Females: 2.5 mg shortly after delivery, then 5–10 mg daily in divided doses for 4–5 days.

Adjustment of dosage
- Kidney disease: None.
- Liver disease: None.

- Elderly: Use with caution because of possibility of developing prostatic hypertrophy.
- Pediatric: Use with great caution. Drug should be administered only by physician who is aware of possible adverse effects of drug on bone maturation. Head and wrist should be examined radiologically every 6 months.

Food: Information not available.
Pregnancy: Category X. Contraindicated.
Lactation: No data available. Best to avoid.
Contraindications: Hypersensitivity, males with carcinoma of the breast, known or suspected carcinoma of the prostate, serious cardiac, renal, or hepatic decompensation.

Editorial comments
- Men should inform physician if they develop priapism.
- Women should inform physician if they develop menstrual irregularities.
- All patients should report if they experience the following: diarrhea, persistent gastric upset, jaundice.
- For additional information, see *methyltestosterone*, p. 596.
- This drug is not listed in the *Physician's Desk Reference*, 54th edition, 2000.

Fluphenazine

Brand names: Prolixin decanoate.
Class of drug: Phenothiazine antipsychotic (neuroleptic).
Mechanism of action: Antagonist of dopamine at dopaminergic receptors in CNS neurons.
Indications/dosage/route: Oral, IM, SC.
- Psychotic disorders
  - Adults, adolescents: Initial: PO 2.5–10 mg/d, divided doses q6–8h. Maintenance 1–5 mg/d. Maximum: 40 mg/d.
  - Elderly: Initial: PO 1–2.5 mg/d. Maximum: 20 mg/d.

- Children: PO 0.25–0.75 mg 1–4 times/d.
- Adults: Initial: IM, SC 12.5–25 mg. Maintenance: 50 mg. Maximum: 100 mg/dose.
- Children ≥12 years: IM, SC 6.25–18.75 mg/wk.
- Children 5–12 years: IM, SC 3.125–12.5 mg/wk.

Adjustment of dosage
- Kidney disease: Use with caution. Guidelines not available.
- Liver disease: Use with caution. Guidelines not available.
- Elderly: See above.
- Pediatric: See above.

Food: No data available.
Pregnancy: Category C.
Lactation: No data available. Considered to be an agent of concern by American Academy of Pediatrics. Avoid breastfeeding.
Contraindications: Hypersensitivity to phenothiazines, concurrent use of high-dose CNS depressants (alcohol, barbituates, benzodiazepines, narcotics), CNS depression, comatose state.

Editorial comments
- This drug is listed without details in the *Physician's Desk Reference*, 54th edition, 2000.
- For additional information, see *chlorpromazine*, p. 206.

Flurbiprofen

Brand name: Ansaid.
Class of drug: NSAID, ophthalmic.
Mechanism of action: Inhibits cyclooxygenase, resulting in inhibition of synthesis of prostaglandins and other inflammatory mediators.
Indications/dosage/route: Oral, topical (ophthalmic).
- Rheumatoid arthritis, osteoarthritis
  - Adults: PO 200–300 mg/d in divided doses. Maximum: 300 mg/d.
- Prevention of intraoperative miosis

– 1 drop q30min starting 2 hours before surgery.

Adjustment of dosage
• Kidney disease: None.
• Liver disease: None.
• Elderly: May be necessary to reduce dose for patients >65 years.
• Pediatric: Safety and efficacy have not been established.

Food: Take with food or large quantities of water or milk.

Pregnancy: Category B. Category D in third trimester or near delivery.

Lactation: Appears in breast milk. Breastfeeding considered to be low risk by some authors.

Contraindications: Hypersensitivity and cross-sensitivity with other NSAIDs and aspirin, dendritric keratitis.

Editorial comments: For additional information, see *ibuprofen*, p. 445.
• This drug is listed without details in the *Physician's Desk Reference*, 54th edition, 2000.

Flutamide

Brand name: Eulexin.

Class of drug: Antiandrogen antineoplastic.

Mechanism of action: Prevents uptake of androgens and blocks nuclear binding of androgens in prostatic tissue.

Indications/dosage/route: Oral only.
• Treatment of locally confined (stage B_2–C) and metastatic prostatic carcinoma (stage D2) in combination with a gonadotropin such as leuprolide
  – Adults: 250 mg q8h.

Adjustment of dosage
• Kidney disease: None.
• Liver disease: No data available.
• Elderly: None.
• Pediatric: Safety in children has not been established.

Food: No restrictions.

Pregnancy: Not applicable; not used in women.

Lactation: Not applicable: not used in women.

Contraindications: Hypersensitivity to flutamide.

Warnings/precautions

• Warn patient not to discontinue therapy without consulting with physician.

• Perform periodic liver function test because of danger of hepatotoxicity.

Advice to patient

• To cut down on diarrhea, reduce intake of dairy products, use antidiarrheal agents, and eat foods high in fiber.

• To minimize possible photosensitivity reaction, apply adequate sunscreen and use proper covering when exposed to strong sunlight.

Adverse reactions

• Common (seen with combination therapy): diarrhea, skin rash, hot flashes, loss of libido, impotence, nausea, vomiting, gynecomastia.

• Serious: confusion, depression, anemia, leukopenia, severe photosensitivity reactions, methemoglobinemia, hepatitis.

Clinically important drug interactions: Flutamide may increase effects/toxicity of warfarin.

Parameters to monitor

• CBC with differential and platelets, liver enzymes.

• Signs and symptoms of hepatotoxicity. Discontinue if present.

• Efficacy of treatment: decrease in PSA, decrease in testosterone production, decreased spread of prostatic cancer.

• Periodic testing of PSA.

Editorial comments

• Use of flutamide at doses higher than those recommended has resulted in production of testicular interstitial cell adenoma.

• Common treatment regimens are as follows: For stage B_2–C prostatic cancer: Begin flutamide plus leuprolide 8 weeks before radiation therapy and continue throughout radiation treatment. For stage D2 metastatic prostate cancer: Begin treatment with both drugs and continue until disease progression is halted.

Fluticasone

Brand names: Cutivate, Flonase, Flovent.
Class of drug: Inhalation, topical corticosteroid
Mechanism of action: Inhalant: Inhibits elaboration of many of the mediators of allergic inflammation, eg, leukotrienes and other products of the arachidonic acid cascade. **Topical drug**: Inhibits migration of polymorphonuclear leukocytes; stabilizes lysosomal membranes; inhibits production of products of arachidonic acid cascade.

Indications/dosage/route: Inhalation, oral, topical. Dosages of corticosteroids are variable. These should be individualized according to the disease being treated and the response of the patient.

Metered dose inhaler
- Asthma
  - Adults, children >4 years: Initial: 100 µg b.i.d.
  - Steroid sparing: PO 1,000 µg b.i.d.

Rotadisk inhaler
- Prevention of asthma
  - Children >4 years: 50–100 µg, b.i.d.

Nasal spray
- Allergic rhinitis
  - Adults, children >4 years: Initial: One 50-µg spray in each nostril once a day. Maximum: 2 sprays (200 µg) in each nostril once a day.

Cream, ointment
- Eczema and other corticosteroid-responsive dermatoses
  - Apply thin film to affected area once or twice daily. Rub in gently.

Adjustment of dosage
- Kidney disease: None.
- Liver disease: None.
- Elderly: None.
- Pediatric: Safety and effectiveness of the topical preparation have not been established.

Food: No restriction.

Pregnancy: Category C.

Lactation: No data available. Best to avoid.

Contraindications: Inhalant: untreated fungal, bacterial, or viral infections. Topical: use with occlusive dressings, hypersensitivity to corticosteroids.

Warnings/precautions

- Inhalant: Use with caution in patients with tuberculosis of the respiratory tract (active or quiescent), diabetes mellitus, cardiovascular disease, hypertension, thrombophlebitis, renal or hepatic insufficiency.
- Topical agent: Use with caution in patients with primary skin infection and those receiving other immunosuppressant drugs.

Advice to patient

- Rinse mouth and gargle with warm water after each inhalation. This may minimize the development of dry mouth, hoarseness, and oral fungal infection.
- This drug should be inhaled 5 minutes after a previously inhaled bronchodilator, eg, albuterol.
- Do not exceed recommended dosage of the drug. Excessive doses have been associated with adrenal insufficiency.
- Notify physician if worsening symptoms occur.
- Carry a card indicating your condition, drugs you are taking, and need for supplemental steroid in the event of a severe asthmatic attack. Attempt to decrease dose once the desired clinical effect is achieved.
- Decrease dose gradually every 2–4 weeks. Return to initial starting dose if symptoms recur.
- Stop smoking.
- Do not overuse the inhaler.

Adverse reactions

Inhalant

- Common: nasal irritation.
- Serious: hypersensitivity reactions, hypercorticism, growth retardation, depression, eosinophilic vasculitis.

Topical

- Common: itching, burning.
- Serious: secondary infections, skin atrophy.

Editorial comments: For additional information, see *prednisone*, p. 760.

Fluvastatin

Brand name: Lescol.
Class of drug: Antilipidemic agent.
Mechanism of action: Inhibits HMG-CoA reductase. Reduces total LDL cholesterol, serum triglyceride levels. There is little if any effect on serum HDL levels.
Indications/dosage/route: Oral only.
  – Adults: 20–40 mg. Maintenance: 20–40 mg/d in the evening.
Adjustment of dosage
• Kidney disease (severe): Lower doses recommended. Guidelines not available.
• Liver disease: None.
• Elderly: None.
• Pediatric: Safety and efficacy have not been established in children <18 years.
Food: Take with meals.
Pregnancy: Category X. Contraindicated.
Lactation: Appears in breast milk. Contraindicated.
Contraindications: Hypersensitivity to statins, active liver disease or unexplained persistent elevations of serum transaminase, pregnancy, lactation.
Editorial comments: For additional information, see *lovastatin*, p. 543.

Fluvoxamine Maleate

Brand name: Luvox.
Class of drug: SSRI.

Mechanism of action: Inhibits reuptake of serotonin into CNS neurons.
Indications/dosage/route: Oral.
• Obsessive–compulsive disorder
  – Adults: Initial: 50 mg h.s. Maintenance: Increase in 50-mg increments until maximum benefit is reached. Maximum: 300 mg/d.
  – Children/adolescents 8–17 years: 25 mg h.s. Maintenance: Increase dose in 25-mg increments until maximum benefit is reached. Maximum: 200 mg/d.
Adjustment of dosage
• Kidney disease: Use with caution.
• Liver disease: Tritrate dose slowly.
• Elderly: Tritrate dose slowly.
• Pediatric: See above.
Food: May be taken with meals.
Pregnancy: Category C.
Lactation: Appears in breast milk. Best to avoid. American Academy of Pediatrics expresses concern with use during breastfeeding.
Contraindications: MAO inhibitor taken within 14 days, hypersensitivity to fluvoxamine.
Editorial comments: For additional information, see *fluoxetine*, p. 378.

Foscarnet

Brand name: Foscavir.
Class of drug: Antiviral agent, pyrophosphate analog.
Mechanism of action: Inhibits viral RNA and DNA polymerase. Inhibits HIV reverse transcriptase.
Indications/dosage/route: IV only.
• Cytomegalovirus, retinitis in AIDS patients
  – Adults: Initial: 60 mg/kg infusion over 1 hour, q8h, or 100 mg/kg q12h. Maintenance: 90–120 mg/kg/d.

– Adults: Alternative: 90–120 mg/kg/daily over 2 hours.
- Acyclovir-resistant herpes simplex virus infection
  – Adults: 40 mg/kg infusion over 1 hour, q8–12h, 2 or 3 weeks, or 40–60 mg/kg, q12h up to 3 weeks.

Adjustment of dosage
- Kidney disease: Creatinine clearance 0.7 mL/kg/min: reduce dose by 50%; creatinine clearance 0.4–0.6 mL/kg/min: reduce maintenance dose by 60%; creatinine clearance <0.4 mL/kg/min: discontinue.
- Liver disease: None.
- Elderly: Information about adjustment of dosage is not available. More likely to develop toxicity. Use cautiously; reduce dosage.
- Pediatric: Safety and efficacy have not been established in children <18 years.

Pregnancy: Category C.

Lactation: Appears in breast milk of laboratory animals. Potentially toxic to infant. Avoid breastfeeding.

Contraindications: Hypersensitivity to foscarnet, creatinine clearance <0.4 mL/kg/min.

Warnings/precautions
- Use with caution in patients with kidney disease.
- Do not administer by rapid IV injection.

Adverse reactions
- Common: headache (25%), nausea (47%), diarrhea (30%), vomiting (25%), fever (65%).
- Serious: seizures, acute renal failure, seizures, bone marrow suppression, malignant hyperpyrexia, hypocalcemia, hypokalemia, cardiomyopathy, cardiac arrest, cardiac failure, pulmonary embolism, pulmonary hemorrhage, depression, neuropathy, visual disturbances, sepsis, cerebral edema, hypothermia, hepatitis, vocal chord paralysis.

Clinically important drug interactions: Drugs that increase effects/toxicity of foscarnet: pentamidine, amphotericin B, aminoglycosides, other nephrotoxic drugs, zidovudine, didanosine, ciprofloxacin, cyclosporine.

Parameters to monitor
- Levels of serum electrolytes, in particular calcium, potassium, magnesium, phosphate. Values should be obtained 2–3 weeks

after start of treatment and then weekly during maintenance therapy. In particular, monitor for signs of hypocalcemia, paresthesia, numbness of extremities. If systemic electrolyte disturbances occur, correct and hold dosage.
- Ophthalmic status, at the end of drug induction and q4wk during maintenance therapy.
- Renal function. In particular, creatinine clearance must be determined 2–3 times per week during induction and weekly during maintenance period.
- CNS status, seizures.

Editorial comment
- Foscarnet causes renal impairment in virtually all patients. Thus, it is absolutely essential to assess the patient's risk and perform determinations of serum creatinine levels 2–3 times per week at induction and at least once q1–2wk during maintenance, particularly in the elderly. Adjustment of dosage is imperative if there are changes in renal function.
- One of the consequences of alteration in serum electrolytes is the production of seizures. Because of the significant number of serious side effects, foscarnet should be prescribed only by physicians experienced with its use and familiar with monitoring for these side effects.

Fosinopril

Brand name: Monopril.
Class of drug: ACE inhibitor.
Mechanism of action: Inhibits ACE, thereby preventing conversion of angiotensin I to angiotensin II, resulting in decreased peripheral arterial resistance.
Indications/dosage/route: Oral only.
- Hypertension
  – Adults Initial: 10 mg/d. May be increased as required (range, 20–40 mg/d).

- CHF
  - 10 mg/d (5 mg in patients who have moderate/severe renal impairment or who have been vigorously diuresed). May be increased over several weeks up to 40 mg/d (usual range, 20–40 mg/d).

Adjustment of dosage
- Kidney disease: None.
- Liver disease: None.
- Elderly: None.
- Pediatric: Safety and efficacy have not been established.

Food: Administer without regard to meals.

Pregnancy: Category C first trimester. Category D for second and third trimesters.

Lactation: No information available. Likely to be present in breast milk. Other similar agents considered safe.

Contraindications: Hypersensitivity to ACE inhibitors, hereditary or ideopathic angioedema, second and third trimesters of pregnancy.

Warnings/precautions
- Use with caution in patients with the following conditions: kidney disease especially renal artery stenosis, drugs that cause bone marrow depression, hypovolemia, hyponatremia, cardiac or cerebral insufficiency, collagen vascular disease, lupus erythematosus, scleroderma, patients undergoing dialysis.
- ACE inhibitors have been associated with anaphylaxis and angioedema.
- Use extreme caution in combination with potassium-sparing diuretics (high risk of hyperkalemia).
- Sodium- or volume-depleted patients may experience severe hypotension. Lower initial doses are advised.
- During surgery/anesthesia, the drug may increase hypotension. Volume expansion may be required.
- There may be a profound drop in BP after the first dose is taken. Close medical supervision is necessary once therapy is begun.

Advice to patient
- Do not use salt substitutes containing potassium.

- Use two forms of birth control including hormonal and barrier methods.
- Avoid NSAIDs, may be present in OTC preparations.
- Take BP periodically and report to treating physician if significant changes occur.
- Stop drug if prolonged vomiting or diarrhea occurs. These symptoms may indicate plasma volume reduction.
- Discontinue drug immediately if signs of angioedema (swelling of face, lips, extremities, breathing or swallowing difficulty) become prominent, and notify physician immediately.
- If chronic cough develops, notify treating physician.

Adverse reactions
- Common: none.
  Serious: bone marrow depression (neutropenia, agranulocytosis), hypotension, angioedema, hyperkalemia, oliguria, chest pain, angina, tachycardia, asthma, bronchospasm, autoimmune symptom complex (see Editorial Comments), hepatitis, liver failure.

Clinically important drug interactions
- Fosinopril increases toxicity of following drugs: lithium, azothioprine, allopurinol, potassium-sparing diuretics, digoxin.
- Drugs that increase toxicity of fosinopril: potassium-sparing drugs, phenothiazines (eg, chlorpromazine).
- Drugs that decrease effectiveness of fosinopril: NSAIDs, antacids, cyclosporine.

Parameters to monitor
- Electrolytes, CBC with differential and platelets, BUN and creatinine.
- Signs and symptoms of angioedema: swelling of face, lips, tongue, extremities, glottis, larynx. Observe in particular for obstruction of airway, difficulty in breathing. If symptoms are not relieved by an antihistamine, discontinue drug.
- BP closely, particularly at beginning of therapy. Observe for evidence of severe hypotension. Patients who are hypovolemic as a result of GI fluid loss or diuretics may exhibit severe hypotension. Also monitor for orthostatic changes.

- Signs of persistent, nonproductive cough; this may be drug-induced.
- Changes in weight in patients with CHF. Gain of more than 2 kg/wk may indicate edema development.
- Signs and symptoms of infection.
- Possible antinuclear antibody development.
- WBC count monthly for first 3–6 months and at frequent intervals thereafter for patients with collagen vascular disease or renal insufficiency. Discontinue therapy if neutrophil count drops below 1000.
- Signs and symptoms of bone marrow depression.
- Intake of fluids and urinary and other fluid output to minimize renal toxicity. Increase fluid intake if inadequate. Closely monitor electrolyte levels.
- Signs and symptoms of renal toxicity.

Editorial comments

- Unlabeled uses of ACE inhibitors include hypertensive crisis, diagnosis of renal artery stenosis, hyperaldosteronism, Raynaud's phenomenon, angina, diabetic nephropathy.
- ACE inhibitors have been associated with an autoimmune type symptom complex including fever, positive antinuclear antibody myositis, vasculitis, and arthritis.
- The ACE inhibitors have been a highly efficacious and well-tolerated class of drugs. Nearly every large randomized clinical trial examining their use has been favorable. First, the Consensus trial proved that enalapril decreased mortality and increased quality of life in class II–III CHF patients. Then the SOLVE trial and others proved their benefits in remodeling myocardium post-MI. The DCCT trial of diabetic patients demonstrated the ability of ACE inhibitors to decrease the small vessel damage to retina and glomeruli. Clinical trials looking into primary prevention of cardiac effects are ongoing. Treatment with this class of drug is the gold standard in patients with left ventricular systolic dysfunction. The two most common adverse effects of ACE inhibitors are cough and angioedema. Transient and persistent rises in antinuclear antibody have

been noted. Because these drugs are vasodilators, orthostasis is another potential problem.

Furosemide

Brand name: Lasix.
Class of drug: Loop diuretic.
Mechanism of action: Inhibits sodium and chloride reabsorption in proximal part of ascending loop of Henle.
Indications/dosage/route: Oral, IV, IM.
Oral
• Edema
  – Adult: Initial: PO 20–80 mg/d as single dose. Increase by 20–40 mg q6–8h prn. Maximum: 600 mg/d.
  – Children: Initial: PO 2 mg/kg as single dose. Increase by 1–2 mg/kg q6–8h prn. Maximum: 6 mg/kg.
• Hypertension
  – Adults: Initial: PO 40 mg b.i.d.
• CHF, chronic renal failure
  – Adults: PO 2–2.5 g/d.
• Hypercalcemia
  – Adults: PO 120 mg/d in 1–3 doses.
IV, IM
• Edema
  – Adults: Initial: IV, IM 20–40 mg. Increase dose in 20-mg increments if needed.
  – Children: Initial: IV, IM 1 mg/kg. After 2 hours, increase dose by 1 mg/kg if needed. Maximum: 6 mg/kg.
• Hypercalcemia
  – Adults: IV, IM 80–100 mg. Repeat q1–2h.
• Acute pulmonary edema
  – Adults: IV 40 mg over 1–2 min if needed. Give 80 mg over 1–2 min after 1 hour.
• CHF, chronic renal failure

– Adults: IV 2–2.5 g/d. Maximum: 1 g/d over 30 min.
• Hypertensive crisis, normal renal function
  – Adults: IV 40–80 mg.
• Hypertensive crisis with pulmonary edema or acute renal failure
  – Adults: IV 100–200 mg.

Adjustment of dosage
• Kidney disease: May require higher dosage. See Warnings/Precautions.
• Liver disease: Use with caution. At higher risk for toxicity.
• Elderly: Use with caution. At higher risk for toxicity.
• Pediatric: See above.

	Onset of Action	Peak Effect	Duration
Oral	Within 60 min	60–120 min	6–8 h
IV	Within 5 min	30 min	2 h

Food: Take with food or milk.
Pregnancy: Category C.
Lactation: Appears in breast milk. Potentially toxic to infants. Best to avoid.
Contraindications: Hypersensitivity to sulfonamides, anuria, hepatic coma, severe electrolyte depletion.

Warnings/precautions
• Use with caution in patients with the following conditions: hepatic cirrhosis, depressed renal function, elderly.
• Generally requires concomitant potassium supplementation. May require addition of aldosterone antagonist.
• Systemic lupus erythematosis may be exacerbated by the drug.
• May cause ototoxicity, especially in setting of renal insufficiency, if recommended doses are exceeded or when given with other ototoxic agents.
• Administer drug in the morning so as to promote diuresis before bedtime.
  Consider magnesium supplement for all patients receiving large doses of the drug IV for acute CHF.

- Hepatic encephalopathy and coma may be precipitated in patients with cirrhosis.
- Hypokalemia may be particularly serious in patients who are taking digitalis or have potassium-losing nephropathy or history of ventricular arrthymias.
- If serum potassium is <3.5 meq/L, consider addition of potassium-sparing diuretic.

Advice to patient

- Change position slowly, in particular from recumbent to upright, to minimize orthostatic hypotension. Sit at the edge of the bed for several minutes before standing, and lie down if feeling faint or dizzy. Avoid hot showers or baths and standing for long periods. Male patients should sit on the toilet while urinating rather than standing.
- To minimize possible photosensitivity reaction, apply adequate sunscreen and use proper covering when exposed to strong sunlight.
- Do not stand in one position for a prolonged period.
- Use caution when taking hot baths or showers and when performing strenuous exercise in hot weather.
- Supplement diet with potassium-rich foods: bananas, citrus fruit, peaches, dates.

Adverse reactions

- Common: dizziness.
- Serious: orthostatic hypotension, hypokalemia, hyponatremia, alkalosis, renal insufficiency, pancreatitis, hepatitis, bone marrow suppression, hearing loss, kidney stones.

Clinically important drug interactions

- Drugs that increase effects/toxicity of loop diuretics: other nephrotoxic or ototoxic drugs, amphotericin B, steroids.
- Drugs that decrease effects/toxicity of loop diuretics: probenecid, indomethacin, potassium-sparing diuretics.
- Loop diuretics increase levels/toxicity of the following: lithium.
- Loop diuretics potentiate hypotensive effects of other diuretics, most antihypertensive drugs.

Parameters to monitor

- Serum electrolytes (K, Na, Cl, bicarbonate, Ca, Mg, uric acid).

- CBC with differential and platelets.
- Efficacy of treatment: ideal weight loss of 0.3-1 kg/d, urine output >300–1000 mL/d over normal daily output.
- Signs of severe hypotension for patients with severe mitral or aortic stenosis. Ischemia may result.
- Liver function for patients in hepatic failure.
- Signs of oliguria. Consider discontinuation of therapy if persistent >24 hours.
- Symptoms of dehydration.
- Signs and symptoms of ototoxicity: tinnitus, vertigo, hearing loss, initially in range of 4000–8000 Hz. Irreversible deafness may occur in this setting.
- Signs and symptoms of renal toxicity.
- Signs and symptoms of bone marrow depression.
- Signs and symptoms of too vigorous diuresis: rapid weight loss, acute fall in BP. In elderly the following symptoms may occur: lightheadedness, dizziness, vomiting, muscle cramps, bladder spasm, urinary frequency.
- Signs of hyperglycemia particularly in diabetics.
- Intake of fluids and urinary and other fluid output. Increase fluid intake if inadequate to minimize renal toxicity.

Editorial comments

- Oral furosemide is the drug of first choice for therapy for fluid overload states caused by mild to moderate heart failure.
- Furosemide is considered to be a secondary drug for treatment of ascites associated with hepatic cirrhosis if spironolactone has not controlled the edema.

Gabapentin

Brand name: Neurontin.
Class of drug: Anticonvulsant.
Mechanism of action: Unknown.
Indications/dosage/route: Oral only.
- Adjunct for treating partial and secondary generalized seizures that do not respond to other drugs
  - Adults, children >12 years: Initial: 300 mg t.i.d. Maintenance: 900–1800 mg/d, 3 divided doses. Maximum: 3600 mg/d.

Adjustment of dosage
- Kidney disease: Creatinine clearance 30–60 mL/min: 300 mg b.i.d.; creatinine clearance 15–30 mL/min: 300 mg/d; creatinine clearance 15 mL/min: 300 mg q.o.d.
- Liver disease: None.
- Elderly: Use with caution because of age-related decrease in renal function.
- Pediatric: Safety and effectiveness have not been established in children <12 years.

Food: No restrictions.
Pregnancy: Category C.
Lactation: No data available. Best to avoid.
Contraindications: Hypersensitivity to gabapentin.
Warnings/precautions
- Use with caution in patient with renal insufficiency, elderly.
- Do not withdraw gabapentin suddenly because there is a risk of precipitating seizures. Withdraw over a period of about 1 week.

Advice to patient
- Take first dose h.s.
- Do not take gabapentin within 2 hours of an antacid.
- Notify dentist or treating physician prior to surgery if taking this medication.

- Carry identification card at all times describing disease, treatment regimen, name, address, and telephone number of treating physician.
- Avoid alcohol.
- Avoid driving and other activities requiring mental alertness or that are potentially dangerous until response to drug is known.

Adverse reactions
- Common: dizziness (15%), ataxia (12%), fatigue, somnolence.
- Serious: depression, leukopenia, bronchospasm, nystagmus, diplopia, pancreatitis, thyroid abnormalities, personality changes, poor coordination.

Clinically important drug interactions
- Drugs that decrease effect/toxicity of gabapentin: antacids.
- Drug that increases effect/toxicity of gabapentin: cimetidine.

Parameters to monitor
- CBC with differential and platelets, serum BUN and creatinine.
- CNS side effects.

Editorial comments
- Gabapentin is used as an adjunct in the treatment of partial and secondary generalized seizures in adults.
- Off-label indications include treatment of chronic pain syndromes.

Gallium Nitrate

Brand name: Ganite.
Class of drug: Antihypercalcemic.
Mechanism of action: Inhibition of calcium resorption from bone.
Indications/dosage/route: IV only.
- Treatment of cancer-related hypercalcemia not adequately managed by conventional treatment

– Adults: 200 mg/m^2/d, 5 consecutive days. Discontinue once optimum serum calcium level has been achieved.

Adjustment of dosage
- Kidney disease: Creatinine clearance <30 mL/min, serum creatinine >2.5 mg/dL: avoid use.
- Liver disease: None.
- Elderly: No data available.
- Pediatric: Safety and efficacy have not been established in children <18 years.

Pregnancy: Category C.

Lactation: No data available. Best to avoid.

Contraindications: Severe renal impairment (serum creatinine >2.5 mg/dL).

Warnings/precautions
- Use with caution in patients with impaired cardiovascular function, kidney disease.
- Administer gallium only after adequate hydration has been established with IV saline.

Adverse reactions
- Common: hypophosphatemia.
- Serious: **hypocalcemia**, acute renal failure.

Clinically important drug interactions: Aminoglycosides, amphotericin B increase effects/toxicity of gallium nitrate.

Parameters to monitor
- Renal function including BUN and serum creatinine before and q2–3d during administration of gallium. Discontinue if serum creatinine >2.5 mg/dL.
- Serum calcium levels daily and serum phosphate levels twice a week. If serum calcium level returns to normal within 5 days, discontinue drug treatment.
- Symptoms of hypercalcemia: nausea, anorexia, lethargy, thirst, arrhythmias.
- Symptoms of hypocalcemia: muscle twitching, laryngospasm, Chvostek's or Trousseau's sign.
- Serum albumin levels before and during the course of therapy.
- Urine output. This should be maintained at 2000 mL/d.

Editorial comments
- Nephrotoxicity is the most frequent adverse effect of gallium; increased levels of BUN and serum creatinine may be observed after only a single dose.
- This drug is not listed in the *Physician's Desk Reference*, 54th edition, 2000.

Ganciclovir

Brand name: Cytovene.
Class of drug: Synthetic antiviral drug.
Mechanism of action: Inhibits herpes simplex virus (HSV1, HSV2) and varicella zoster by reducing viral DNA synthesis.
Indications/dosage/route: Oral, IV.
- Treatment of cytomegalovirus retinitis
  - Adults: Initial:, IV 5 mg/kg at constant rate over 1 hour q12h for 14–21 days. Maintenance: IV 5 mg/kg at constant rate over 1 hour daily, 7 d/wk, or 6 mg/kg daily, 5 d/wk.
  - Adults: PO maintenance after initial IV treatment: 100 mg t.i.d. with food.
- Prevention of cytomegalovirus disease in patients with advanced HIV infection
  - Adults: PO 1000 mg t.i.d. with food.
- Prevention of cytomegalovirus disease in transplant recipients
  - Adults: IV 5 mg/kg at constant rate over 1 hour q12h for 7–14 days. Followed by 5 mg/kg once daily 7 d/wk or 6 mg/kg once daily 5 d/wk.
  - Adults: PO 1000 g t.i.d. with food.
Adjustment of dosage
- Kidney disease: Creatinine clearance >60 mL/min: usual dose q8h; creatinine clearance 40–59 mL/min: usual dose q12h; creatinine clearance 20–39 mL/min: usual dose q24h; creatinine clearance >20 mL/min: half dose q48h.

- Liver disease: None
- Elderly: Monitor closely and adjust dosage accordingly.
- Pediatric: Safety and efficacy have not been established in children <18 years.

Food: Should be taken with meals.

Pregnancy: Category C.

Lactation: No data available. Potentially toxic to infant. Avoid breastfeeding.

Contraindications: Hypersensitivity to ganciclovir, acyclovir, famciclovir.

Editorial comments: For additional information, see *famciclovir*, p. 344.

Gentamicin

Brand name: Garamycin.

Class of drug: Antibiotic, aminoglycoside.

Mechanism of action: Binds to ribosomal units in bacteria, inhibits protein synthesis.

Susceptible organisms *in vivo*: Staphylococci (penicillinase and nonpenicillinase), Staphylococcus *epidermidis, Acinetobacter* sp, *Citrobacter* sp, *Enterobacter* sp, *Escherichia coli, Klebsiella* sp, *Proteus* sp, *Providencia* sp, *Pseudomonas* sp, *Serratia* sp.

Indications/dosage/route: IV, IM.

- Serious infections caused by susceptible microorganisms
  - Adults: 3 mg/kg/d, in 3 equal doses q8h.
  - Children: 2.0–2.5 mg/kg q8h.
  - Infants, neonates: 2.5 mg/kg q8h.
  - Prematures, full-term neonates (≤ week): 2.5 mg/kg q12h.
- Life-threatening infections
  - Adults: ≤5 mg/kg/d in 3 or 4 equal doses.

Adjustment of dosage

- Kidney disease: Creatinine clearance 55–70 mL/min: 65% of usual dose; creatinine clearance 40–45 mL/min: 50% of usual dose; creatinine clearance 25–30 mL/min: 30% of usual dose; creatinine clearance <10 mL/min: 10% of usual dose.

• Liver disease: None.
• Elderly: As higher risk for toxicity.
• Pediatric: See above.

Food: No restrictions.

Pregnancy: Category D.

Contraindications: Hypersensitivity to aminoglycoside antibiotics.

Editorial comments

• The usual duration of treatment with gentamicin is 7–10 days. There is a low risk of toxicity in patients who have normal renal function and do not receive high-dose gentamicin longer than the recommended period.
• Once daily dosing has been advocated by some authorities to increase efficacy and reduce toxicity.

Editorial comments: For additional information, see *amikacin*, p. 33.

Glimepiride

Brand name: Amaryl.

Class of drug: Oral hypoglycemic agent, second generation.

Mechanism of action: Stimulates release of insulin from pancreatic beta cells; decreases glucose production in liver; increases sensitivity of receptors for insulin, thereby promoting effectiveness of insulin.

Indications/dosage/route: Oral only.

• Diabetes, type II (non-insulin-dependent diabetes mellitus)
  – Adults: Initial: 1–2 mg/d with breakfast. Maintenance: 1–4 mg once daily.

Adjustment of dosage

• Kidney disease: None.
• Liver disease: None.

• Elderly: Administer conservatively. Guidelines not available.
• Pediatric: Not recommended.

Onset of Action	Duration
1–1.5 h	10–16 h

Food: No restriction. Patient should be told to eat regularly and not to skip meals. Sugar supply should be kept handy at all times. If stomach is upset Tums should be taken with meal. Dose is best administered before breakfast or, if taken twice a day, before the evening meal.

Pregnancy: Category C.

Lactation: Probably appears in breast milk. Potentially toxic to infant. Avoid breastfeeding.

Contraindications: Hypersensitivity to glimepiride, diabetes complicated by ketoacidosis.

Editorial comment: For additional information, see *glyburide*, p. 409.

Glipizide

Brand name: Glucotrol.

Class of drug: Oral hypoglycemic agent, second generation.

Mechanism of action: Stimulates release of insulin from pancreatic beta cells; decreases glucose production in liver; increases sensitivity of receptors for insulin, thereby promoting effectiveness of insulin.

Indications/dosage/route: Oral only.

• Diabetes, type II (non-insulin-dependent diabetes mellitus)
  – Adults: Initial: 5 mg 30 min before breakfast. Adjust dosage by 2.5–5 mg every few days. Maintenance: 15–40 mg/day mg/d.
  – Elderly: 2.5 mg.
• Extended release tablets: 5–10 mg/d.

Adjustment of dosage
- Kidney disease: None.
- Liver disease: None.
- Elderly: See above.
- Pediatric: Not recommended.

Onset of Action	Duration
1–1.5 h	10–16 h

Food: No restriction. Patient should be told to eat regularly and not to skip meals. Sugar supply should be kept handy at all times. If stomach is upset Tums should be taken with meal. Dose is best administered before breakfast or, if taken twice a day, before the evening meal.

Pregnancy: Category C.

Lactation: No data available. Potentially toxic to infant. Avoid breastfeeding.

Contraindications: Hypersensitivity to glipizide, diabetes complicated by ketoacidosis.

Warnings/precautions
- Current data suggest that there is an increased risk of cardiovascular mortality with oral hypoglycemic drugs.
- All sulfonylureas are capable of causing severe hypoglycemia. Patients should be educated concerning the signs and symptoms of hypoglycemia and how it can be prevented or reversed.
- When this drug is used to replace insulin, instruct patient to test urine for glucose and acetone at least 3 times a day and check results with treating physician.
- If the patient is experiencing stressful situations (surgery, infection, trauma), it may be necessary to administer insulin temporarily.
- A long-term prospective study performed by the University Group Diabetes Program showed that patients on tolbutamide (a sulfonylurea) had 2.5 times the risk of patients treated with diet alone.

Advice to patient

- Do not undereat because skipping meals may result in loss of glucose control.
- Avoid even moderate amounts of alcohol, eg, more than 2 oz of 100-proof whiskey. The combination with the drug you are taking may result in a disulfiram reaction: flushing, sweating, palpitation, nausea, vomiting, abdominal cramps.
- To minimize possible photosensitivity reactions, apply adequate sunscreen and use proper covering when exposed to strong sunlight.
- Carry identification card at all times describing disease, treatment regimen, name, address, and telephone number of treating physician.
- Carry hard candy or candy bar at all times.

Adverse reactions

- Common: GI upset.
- Serious: **hypoglycemia**, aplastic anemia, agranulocytosis, thrombocytopenia, hypersensitivity reaction, cholestatic jaundice.

Clinically important drug interactions

- Drugs that increase effects/toxicity of sulfonylureas: NSAIDs, β blockers, MAO inhibitors, cimetidine, glucocorticoids, alcohol (disulfiram effect).
- Drugs that decrease effects/toxicity of sulfonylureas: phenytoin, rifampin, cholestyramine.

Parameters to monitor

- Serum glucose, liver enzymes.
- Signs and symptoms of hyperglycemia.
- Signs and symptoms of hypokalemia: muscle cramps or weakness, anorexia, thirst, hypoactive reflexes, polyuria, paresthesias, arrhythmias, dyspnea, confusion, paralytic ileus. If severe, hospitalize patient and administer 50 mL of 50% glucose solution by rapid IV injection followed by 10% glucose infusion to maintain blood glucose at 90–180 mg/dL. Monitor patient for 24–48 hours for possible recurrence of hypoglycemia. For moderate hypoglycemia, administer fruit juices (1/2 cup orange juice), honey, sugar cubes (2), or corn syrup. Follow this with milk or sandwich which are sources of longer-acting carbohydrate.

- Monitor therapeutic response carefully for the first 7 days after beginning treatment and for the first 3–5 days after transferring patient from insulin or another sulfonylurea. Continue monitoring to detect secondary failure after initial success; failure rate of oral hypoglycemic agent is 5–15% per year after 5 years of therapy.
- Determine glycosolated hemoglobin fraction (HbAlc or HbA$_1$) levels 2–4 times a year. These are the best indices of glycemic control as they are indications of blood glucose over the previous 6–10 weeks.
- Possible causes of hypoglycemia.
- Signs and symptoms of bone marrow depression.
- Signs and symptoms of hepatotoxicity.

Editorial comments

- In most cases, institute drug therapy only if a trial of 6–8 weeks of appropriate dietary control has not been successful in achieving satisfactory glycemic control. Begin drug at lowest dose and titrate upward q1–2wk.
- Patients at risk for hypoglycemia include those >60 years, alcoholics, malnourished patients, and those with severe or prolonged exertion, adrenal insufficiency, renal or hepatic dysfunction.
- Oral hypoglycemic agents should be prescribed only by physicians who are familiar with the proper criteria for patient selection and who know the risks versus benefits associated with these drugs.

Glucagon

Brand name: Glucagon.
Class of drug: Antihypoglycemic agent.
Mechanism of action: Stimulates production of glucose from liver glycogen stores (glycogenolysis).
Indications/dosage/route: IV, IM, SC.

- Coma caused by insulin shock therapy
  - Adults: SC, IM or IV 0.5–1 mg 1 hour after coma develops. Repeat in 25 minutes if necessary.
- Insulin-induced hypoglycemia during diabetic therapy
  - Adults, children >20 kg: SC, IM IV 0.5–1 mg. Repeat q20 minutes if necessary.
  - Children <20 kg: SC, IM, IV 0.025–0.2 mg/kg 1 hour after coma develops. Repeat within 25 minutes if necessary.
- To facilitate radiographic examination of GI tract
  - Adults: IV or IM 2 mg 10 minutes before procedure is started.

Adjustment of dosage: None.

Onset of Action	Peak Effect	Duration
5–20 min	20–30 min	60–120 min

Pregnancy: Category B.
Lactation: Safe to use.
Contraindications: Hypersensitivity to beef or porcine protein, known pheochromocytoma.
Warnings/precautions
- Use with caution in patients with history of pheochromocytoma or insulinoma, kidney or liver disease or in emaciated or undernourished patients.
- If possible, IV glucose should be administered first to treat severe hypoglycemia.
- Instruct patient and family about the signs of hypoglycemia.
- Instruct patient how to prepare and administer glucagon in the event of insulin shock.

Advice to patient
- Carry identification card at all times describing disease, treatment regimen, name, address, and telephone number of treating physician.
- Notify physician if a hypoglycemic episode occurs so that the dosage of insulin may be adjusted accordingly.
- Carry sugar or sugar-containing candy at all times.

Adverse reactions
- Common: none.
- Serious: hypersensitivity reaction including bronchospasm, rash; hypotension.

Clinically important drug interactions
- Drug that decreases effects/toxicity of glucagon: phenytoin.
- Glucagon increases effects/toxicity of following drugs: oral anticoagulants, epinephrine, corticosteroid, estrogens.

Parameters to monitor
- BP, blood glucose.
- Signs and symptoms of hypoglycemia: nervousness, involuntary shaking, abnormal sleep pattern, abdominal discomfort, hypotension, coma. If symptoms of hypoglycemia occur at home, advise patient to take a glass of fruit juice, honey (2–3 teaspoons), 1 or 2 sugar tablets, or corn syrup dissolved in water.
- Nausea and vomiting. If necessary, administer antiemetic drug.

Editorial comments
- Glucagon should not be used to treat hypoglycemia in newborn or premature infants.
- It is necessary to determine the reason for hypoglycemia, if it occurs, as this may be a result of chronic starvation or adrenal insufficiency. In such circumstances, administration of glucose rather than glucagon is indicated.

Glyburide

Brand names: DiaBeta, Micronase, Glynase Pres Tab.
Class of drug: Oral hypoglycemic agent, second generation.
Mechanism of action: Stimulates release of insulin from pancreatic beta cells; decreases glucose production in liver; increases sensitivity of receptors for insulin, thereby promoting effectiveness of insulin.
Indications/dosage/route: Oral only.

Nonmicronized (DiaBeta/Micronase)
• Diabetes, type II (non-insulin-dependent diabetes mellitus)
  – Adults: Initial: 2.5–5 mg mg/d with breakfast. Increase by 2.5 mg/wk to achieve desired response. Maintenance: 1.25–20 mg/d. Maximum: 20 mg/d.

Micronized (Glynase)
  – Adults: Initial: 1.5–3 mg/d with breakfast. Increase by 1.5 mg/wk to achieve desired response. Maintenance: 0.75–12 mg/d.

Adjustment of dosage
• Kidney disease: None.
• Liver disease: None.
• Elderly: See above.
• Pediatric: Not recommended.

Onset of Action	Duration
2–4 h	24 h

Food: No restriction. Patient should be told to eat regularly and not to skip meals. Sugar supply should be kept handy at all times. If stomach is upset Tums should be taken with meal. Dose is best administered before breakfast or, if taken twice a day, before the evening meal.

Pregnancy: Category C.

Lactation: No data available. Potentially toxic to infant. Avoid breastfeeding.

Contraindications: Hypersensitivity to glyburide, diabetes complicated by ketoacidosis.

Warnings/precautions
• Current data suggests that there is an increased risk of cardiovascular mortality with oral hypoglycemic drugs.
• All sulfonylureas are capable of causing severe hypoglycemia. Patients should be educated concerning the signs and symptoms of hypoglycemia and how it can be prevented or reversed.
• When this drug is used to replace insulin, instruct patient to test urine for glucose and acetone at least 3 times a day and check results with treating physician.

- If the patient is experiencing stressful situations (surgery, infection, trauma), it may be necessary to administer insulin temporarily.
- A long-term prospective study performed by the University Group Diabetes Program showed that patients on tolbutamide (a sulfonylurea) had 2.5 times the risk of patients treated with diet alone.

Advice to patient

- Do not undereat because skipping meals may result in loss of glucose control.
- Avoid even moderate amounts of alcohol, eg, more than 2 oz of 100-proof whiskey. The combination with the drug you are taking may result in a disulfiram reaction: flushing, sweating, palpitation, nausea, vomiting, abdominal cramps.
- To minimize possible photosensitivity reactions, apply adequate sunscreen and use proper covering when exposed to strong sunlight.
- Carry identification card at all times describing disease, treatment regimen, name, address, and telephone number of treating physician.
- Carry hard candy or candy bar at all times.

Adverse reactions

- Common: GI upset.
- Serious: **hypoglycemia**, aplastic anemia, agranulocytosis, thrombocytopenia, hypersensitivity reaction, cholestatic jaundice.

Clinically important drug interactions

- Drugs that increase effects/toxicity of sulfonylureas: NSAIDs, β blockers, MAO inhibitors, cimetidine, glucocorticoids, alcohol (disulfiram effect).
- Drugs that decrease effects/toxicity of sulfonylureas: phenytoin, rifampin, cholestyramine.

Parameters to monitor

- Serum glucose, liver enzymes.
- Signs and symptoms of hyperglycemia.
- Signs and symptoms of hypokalemia: muscle cramps or weakness, anorexia, thirst, hypoactive reflexes, polyuria, paresthesias, arrhythmias, dyspnea, confusion, paralytic ileus. If severe, hospitalize patient and administer 50 mL of 50% glucose solution

by rapid IV injection followed by 10% glucose infusion to maintain blood glucose at 90–180 mg/dL. Monitor patient for 24–48 hours for possible recurrence of hypoglycemia. For moderate hypoglycemia, administer fruit juices (1/2 cup orange juice), honey, sugar cubes (2), or corn syrup. Follow this with milk or sandwich, which are sources of longer-acting carbohydrate.

- Monitor therapeutic response carefully for the first 7 days after beginning treatment and for the first 3–5 days after transferring patient from insulin or another sulfonylurea. Continue monitoring to detect secondary failure after initial success; failure rate of oral hypoglycemic agent is 5–15% per year after 5 years of therapy.
- Determine glycosolated hemoglobin fraction (HbAlc or HbA$_1$) levels 2–4 times a year. These are the best indices of glycemic control as they are indications of blood glucose over the previous 6–10 weeks.
- Possible causes of hypoglycemia.
- Signs and symptoms of bone marrow depression.
- Signs and symptoms of hepatotoxicity.

Editorial comments
- In most cases, institute drug therapy only after a trial of 6–8 weeks of appropriate dietary control has not been successful in achieving satisfactory glycemic control. Begin drug at lowest dose and titrate upward q1–2wk.
- Patients at risk for hypoglycemia include those >60 years, alcoholics, malnourished patients, and those with severe or prolonged exertion, adrenal insufficiency, renal or hepatic dysfunction.
- Oral hypoglycemic agents should be prescribed only by physicians who are familiar with the proper criteria for patient selection and who know the risks versus benefits associated with these drugs.

Griseofluvin

Brand names: Fulvicin-U/F (microsize), Fulvicin-P/G (ultramicrosize), Grifulvin-V (microsize), Gris-PEG (ultramicrosize).

Class of drug: Antifungal.

Mechanism of action: Disrupts fungal mitotic spindle structure, arresting cell division in metaphase.

Susceptible organisms *in vivo*: Species of *Trichophyton, Microsporum,* and *Epidermophyton*.

Indications/dosage/route: Oral only.

• Tinea corporis, tinea cruris, tinea capitis
  – Adults: Microsize: 0.5 g/d, single or divided doses. Ultramicrosize: 330–375 mg/d.
• Tinea pedis, tinea unguium
  – Adults: Microsize: 0.75–1 g/d.
  – Children 13.6–22.7 kg: Microsize: 125–250 mg/d. Ultramicrosize: 82.5–165 mg/d.
  – Children >22.7 kg: Microsize: 250–500 mg/d. Ultramicrosize: 165–330 mg/d.

Adjustment of dosage

• Kidney disease: None.
• Liver disease: None.
• Elderly: None.
• Pediatric: Safety has not been determined in children <2 years.

Food: Should be taken with high-fat food (ice cream, fried chicken, etc).

Pregnancy: Category C.

Lactation: No data available. Best to avoid.

Contraindications: Pregnancy, history of porphyria, hepatocellular failure, hypersensitivity to griseofulvin.

Warnings/precautions

• Use with caution in patients with penicillin sensitivity.
• This drug should not be used for minor or trivial infections that can respond to topical drugs.

Advice to patient

• Avoid alcohol.
• Use protective clothing and sunscreen to avoid photosensitivity reactions if exposed to strong sunlight.

Adverse reactions

• Common: Headache, skin rash.

• Serious: **urticaria**, granulocytopenia, hepatotoxicity, protein-uria, renal toxicity.

Clinically important drug interactions

• Barbiturates decrease effects/toxicity of griseofulvin.
• Griseofuvin increases effects/toxicity of alcohol.
• Griseofuvin decreases effects/toxicity of oral anticoagulants and oral contraceptions.

Parameters to monitor

• CBC with differential and platelets, serum BUN and creatinine, liver enzymes, urinalysis (long-term therapy).
• Signs and symptoms of granulocytopenia. Discontinue drug.

Editorial comments: Griseofuvin administration must be con-tinued until the infecting organism is completely eradicated. Suggested times of treatment are the following: tinea capitis, 4–6 weeks; tinea corporis, 2–4 weeks; tinea pedis, 4–8 weeks; tinea unguium of fingernails, at least 4 months; of toes, at least 6 months.

Haloperidol

Brand names: Haldol Decanoate (IM form).

Class of drug: Butyrophenone, antipsychotic.

Mechanism of action: Antipsychotic effect is believed to result from blockade of dopamine receptors in CNS. Mechanism of action in Tourette's syndrome is unknown.

Indications/dosage/route: Oral, IM.

• Management of psychotic disorders: Moderate symptoms
  – Adults: PO 0.5–2 mg, 2 or 3 times/d.
  – Children 3–12 years: PO 0.5 mg/d, 2 or 3 divided doses.

• Management of psychotic disorders: Severe symptoms
  – Adults: PO 3–5 mg, 2 or 3 times/d. IM 2–5 mg q4–8h maximum 100 mg/d.

• Tourette's syndrome
  – Adults: Same as above.
  – Children 3–12 years: 0.05–0.75 mg/kg/d, 2 or 3 divided doses.

Adjustment of dosage

• Kidney disease: None.

• Liver disease: None

• Elderly: May require initial lower doses and more gradual dosage increase.

• Pediatric: Not recommended for children <3 years.

Food: Should be taken with food to decrease GI side effects.

Pregnancy: Category C.

Lactation: Appears in breast milk. Potentially toxic to infant. Considered by American Academy of Pediatrics on be an agent whose effect on the breastfeeding infant is unknown but of possible concern.

Contraindications: Parkinson's disease, severe CNS depression, hypersensitivity to haloperidol.

Warnings/precautions

• Use with caution in patients with seizures, cardiovascular disease, history of seizures, concurrent anticonvulsant therapy, EEG abnormalities, history of allergies.

- Because the drug is a potent antiemetic, it may mask signs and symptoms of nausea and vomiting caused by other drugs in overdose or mask symptoms of a number of diseases including brain tumor, Reyes' syndrome, intestinal obstruction.
- Some preparations contain tartrazine (FD&C Yellow No.5). This dye can cause a severe allergic reaction, even an asthmatic attack, in susceptible patients, particularly those who are allergic to aspirin. Prescribe drug preparation that does not contain dye for these individuals.

Advice to patient
- Do not drive or operate machinery that requires alertness.
- Wear protective clothing and sunscreen if exposed to sunlight to minimize photosensitivity reaction.
- Avoid alcohol.
- Do not stop taking drug abruptly because this may precipitate withdrawal reaction, particularly extrapyramidal symptoms. Other symptoms of withdrawal include abdominal disconfort, dizziness, headache, tachycardia, insomnia. Reduce dosage gradually over a period of several weeks, eg, 10–25% q2wk.
- Patient should change position slowly, particularly when rising from supine position or standing, to avoid orthostatic hypotension. Patient should be cautioned about taking hot baths or showers and long exposure to high environmental temperatures.

Adverse reactions
- Common: dry mouth, sedation, anxiety.
- Serious: **Extrapyramidal reactions, tardive dyskinesia, dystonic reactions**, neuroleptic malignant syndrome (rare), arrhythmias, orthostatic hypotension, hallucinations, bone marrow suppression, jaundice, cholestasis, laryngospasm, seizures, altered central temperature regulation, malignant hyperthermy, priapism, urinary retention, retinopathy, cataracts.

Clinically important drug interactions
- Drugs that increase effects/toxicity of haloperidol: CNS depressants (barbiturates, opiates, general anesthetics) quinidine, procainamide, anticholinergic drugs, MAO inhibitors, phenothiazines, antihistamines, nitrates, β blockers.

- Drugs that decrease effects/toxicity of haloperidol: barbiturates, aluminum- and magnesium-containing antacids, heavy smoking, caffeine.
- Haloperidol increases effects/toxicity of following drugs: anticonvulsants, β blockers, quinidine, procainamide, antidepressants, MAO inhibitors.
- Haloperidol decreases effects/toxicity of following drugs: centrally acting antihypertensive drugs (guanethidine, clonidine, methyldopa), bromocriptine, levodopa.

Parameters to monitor

- CBC with differential and platelets, liver enzymes.
- Abnormal body movements periodically. This may reflect extrapyramidal syndrome. If it occurs, give anticholinergic drug. Considered discontinuation if tardive dyskinesia is suspected.
- GI complications including fecal impaction and constipation. Urge patient to increase fluid intake and bulk-containing food.
- Signs and symptoms of bronchial pneumonia due to suppression of cough reflex. This may be a particular problem in the elderly and severely depressed patient.
- Signs and symptoms of extrapyramidal symptoms. Be aware that maximum risk for developing these symptoms is as follows: 1–5 days for acute dystonia, 50–60 days for dyskinesia.
- Signs and symptoms of tardive dyskinesia: uncontrolled rhythmic movements of face, mouth, tongue, jaw, protrusion of tongue, uncontrolled rapid or wormlike movements of tongue, chewing movements. At first indication of tardive dyskinesia—vermicular movements of tongue—withdraw drug immediately. Tardive dyskinesia generally develops several months after treatment with a phenothiazine. Patient should be monitored every 6 months for possible development of tardive dyskinesia.
- Monitor blood and urine glucose in diabetic or prediabetic patients on high drug dose for loss of diabetes control. If control is lost, it may be necessary to discontinue the drug and substitute another.
- Hematologic evaluation for signs of agranulocytosis.

- Signs and symptoms of cholestatic jaundice. This may occur between the second and fourth weeks of treatment.
- Signs and symptoms of overdose: somnolence, coma. Treat by gastric lavage and patent airway. Do not induce vomiting.
- Ocular status.
- Hypersensitivity reaction.
- Signs and symptoms of cholestasis, jaundice, pruritus.
- Efficacy of treatment: improvement in mental status, including orientation, mood, general behavior, improved sleep, reduction in auditory and visual hallucinations, disorganized thinking, blunted affect, agitation.
- Signs and symptoms of NMS: fever, tachycardia, convulsions, respiratory distress, irregular BP, severe muscle spasms. Use supportive measures and administer dantrolene.

Editorial comments
- Haloperidol is a high-potency neuroleptic with low anticholinergic properties. It is the drug of choice in elderly patients or in patients with preexisting cardiovascular or seizure disorders.
- In the noncompliant patient, the depot form is the drug of choice.

Heparin

Brand name: Hep-Lock.
Class of drug: Anticoagulant, parenteral.
Mechanism of action: Heparin enhances the rate of formation of antithrombin III–thrombin complexes. Inhibits thrombin and activated coagulation factors (IX, X, XI, XII), promotes conversion of fibrinogen to fibrin.
Indications/dosage/route: IV, SC.
- DVT, pulmonary embolism, other intravascular coagulation disorders
  - Adults: Initial: IV push; 5000–10,000 units (alternate 80 units/kg). Maintenance: intermittent: IV 4000–5000 units

q4hs; continuous: 15–25 units/kg/h. Adjust dose to maintain APTT 1.5–2.0 times baseline APTT.
- Embolism prophylaxis
  – Adults: SC 5000 units q8–12h.
- Open heart surgery
  – Adults: continuous IV infusion 150–400 units/kg.
- To maintain patency of catheters (line flush)
  – Adults: 1–10 units/mL. May add 1 unit/mL to TPN solutions. 0.5–2 mL for arterial lines.

Adjustment of dosage
- Kidney disease: None.
- Liver disease: Dosage should be adjusted based on PTT determination.
- Elderly: Women >60 years are thought to be at greatest risk for developing hemorrhage with heparin.
- Pediatric: Follow recommended pediatric texts. Initial: 50 units/kg (IV). Maintenance: 100 units/kg (IV) q4h.

	Onset of action
IV	Immediate
SC	20–30 min

Food: Not applicable.

Pregnancy: Category C. Heparin is preferred over warfarin as an anticoagulant during pregnancy.

Lactation: Not excreted in breast milk. Safe to use during breast-feeding.

Contraindications: Hypersensitivity to heparin, beef or porcine proteins, known antiheparin antibodies, high-dose heparin in patients with severe thrombocytopenia, patients in whom blood coagulation tests cannot be performed, uncontrolled bleeding except when caused by disseminated intravascular clotting, hemophilia, thrombocytopenia, blood dyscrasias, hypoprothrombinemia secondary to hepatic disease, suspected intra- cranial hemorrhage, ulcerative conditions of GI tract or skin, acute or subacute bacterial endocarditis, shock, severe renal disease, severe hypotension, dissecting aneurysm, threatened abortion.

Warnings/precautions
- Use with caution in patients with the following conditions: recent surgery of the eye, brain, or spinal cord, severe hypertension, severe hepatic or renal disease, history of GI ulcer, higher risk of bleeding (menstruating women, postpartum patients), hemorrhagic stroke, history of heparin-related thrombocytopenia, "White clot" syndrome.
- Do not use by the IM route.

Advice to patient
- Notify dentist or treating physician prior to surgery if taking this medication.
- Avoid taking NSAIDs together with this drug.
- Use electric razor for shaving and soft-bristle toothbrush to avoid bleeding gums.
- Report excessive menstrual flow to treating physician.

Adverse reactions
- Common: see serious.
- Serious: **hemorrhage (hematuria, GI bleeding, gum bleeding), thrombocytopenia (up to 30%)**, anemia, cutaneous necrosis (from local irritation), osteoporosis, heparin-associated thrombocytopenia and thrombosis syndrome, neuropathy, hepatitis, skin necrosis with injection (deep SC).

Clinically important drug interactions
- Drugs that increase effects/toxicity of heparin: platelet inhibitors, warfarin and other oral anticoagulants, dipyridamole, dextran, quinidine, cephalosporins, thrombolytic agents, aspirin, NSAIDs.
- Drugs that decrease effects of heparin: tetracyclines, nicotine, antihistamines, cardiac glycosides, digitalis.
- Protamine is used to neutralize heparin in the event of severe hemorrhage from heparin overdose with evidence of internal bleeding.

Parameters to monitor
- INR, PT, PTT. PTT should be measured 4–6 hours after IV dose, 12–24 hours after SC dose. Value of PTT should be 1.5–2 times that of control values.

- Signs of hypersensitivity reactions.
- Hematologic status regularly. Check for excessive bleeding in gums, as well as for nosebleeds, bruising on arms or legs, tarry stools, hematuria. If severe hemorrhage occurs, administer protamine sulfate immediately.
- Platelet counts weekly after the first week. Terminate heparin immediately if thrombocytopenia occurs (platelet count falls below 100,000/mm^3) and give another anticoagulant, eg, warfarin, or a low-molecular-weight heparin. Monitor patient's heparin antibodies.
- Monitor for signs of venous embolism on a daily basis. Examine for changes in limb circumference, tenderness, swelling perfusion.

Editorial comments

- There is no need to monitor blood coagulation in low-dose heparin therapy.
- Heparin should not be stopped abruptly as this may cause a significant increase in coagulability of the blood. Heparin therapy should be followed by oral anticoagulant therapy for prophylactic purposes.
- Warfarin administration should be started simultaneously with heparin when treating DVT or pulmonary embolism.
- All patients having experienced a MI should receive heparin to prevent thromboembolism.
- Heparin should be used to prevent coronary reocclusion following coronary artery bypass surgery or angioplasty.
- Some preparations of heparin contain benzyl alcohol. Benzyl alcohol, when administered to neonates, has been associated with fatal toxicity (gasping syndrome). It is recommended that heparin without preservatives be used in neonates.
- It may be advisable to administer a test dose of heparin (1000 units, SC) to patients with a history of asthma or multiple allergies.
- If cutaneous necrosis develops with SC injections, discontinue immediately.
- Monitoring for antiheparin antibodies should be considered if thrombocytopenia or skin necrosis occurs.

Hyaluronidase

Brand name: Wydase.
Class of drug: Antidote for extravasation.
Mechanism of action: Modifies permeability of connective tissue by hydrolyzing hyaluronic acid, thereby promoting diffusion of injected solution.
Indication/dosage/route: SC only.
- Hypodermoclysis
  – 150 USP units for each liter of clysis solution administered.
- To promote absorption and dispersion of injected drug
  – 150 USP units added to the solution containing the other drug.
Adjustment of dosage: None.

Onset of Action	Duration
Immediate	24–48 h

Food: Not applicable.
Pregnancy: Category C.
Lactation: Not applicable.
Contraindications: Hypersensitivity to hyaluronidase. Drug must not be injected in or around inflamed, infected, or cancer-containing areas. Do not use for infiltration of dopamine or α–adrenergic agents.
Warnings/precautions
- Before using, skin test for sensitivity with an intradermal injection of a small volume of hyaluronidase solution (0.02 mL). The following is a positive reaction to the drug: wheal with pseudopods that appear within 5 minutes and last 20–30 minutes. This is accompanied by itch.
- Discolored solutions or those that contain a precipitate should not be used.
- Hyaluronidase is not compatible with epinephrine or heparin.
Advice to patients: Solution must not come in contact with eyes.

Adverse reactions: Rare: tachycardia, urticaria, chills, hypotension.
Clinically important drug interactions: Hyaluronidase increases effects/toxicity of local anesthetics, dopamine, α-adrenergic agonists.
Parameters to monitor: Signs of hypersensitivity reaction.
Editorial comments
• Before using hyaluronidase with other drugs, it must be determined that such combinations are compatible.
• A detailed description of hyaluronidase is not given in the *Physician's Desk Reference*, 54th edition, 2000.

Hydralazine

Brand name: Apresoline.
Class of drug: Peripheral vasodilator; antihypertensive agent.
Mechanism of action: Reduces total peripheral resistance by direct action on vascular smooth muscle. It has greatest effect on arterioles and causes only minor venous dilation.
Indications/dosage/route: Oral, IM, IV.
• Moderate to severe hypertension.
  – Adults: Initial: PO 10 mg q.i.d., 2–4 days. Increase dosage by 10–25 mg every 2–5 days to 50 mg q.i.d. Maximum: 300–400 mg/d.
  – Children: Initial: PO 0.75 mg/kg/d, 4 divided doses. Maximum: 100 mg/d. Increase gradually over 3–4 weeks to 7.5 mg/kg/d if needed. Alternative dosing: IM or IV 0.1–0.5 mg/kg every 4–6 hours. Increase to 1.7–3.5 mg/kg/d.
• Severe hypertensive crisis
  – Adults: IV, IM 20–40 mg. Repeat every 4–6 hours as needed.
  – Children: IV, IM 0.1–0.2 mg/kg q4–6h as needed.
• Hypertensive crisis of pregnancy (preclampsia, eclampsia)
  – Adults: Initial: IV 5–10 mg, followed by IV 5–10 mg q20–30min. Alternative dosing: 0.5–10 mg/h.

Adjustment of dosage

- Kidney disease: The interval between doses should be increased. Creatinine clearance: 10–50 mL/min; administer q8h; creatinine clearance: <10 mL/min: administer q8–16h. In fast acetylators, q12–24h.
- Liver disease: In severe liver disease the dose interval should be increased.
- Slow acetylators: Maximum 200 mg/d.
- Elderly: Lower dosage and slower increases in dose are desirable. Oral: Initial: 10 mg b.i.d. or t.i.d.; increase by 10–25 mg/d every 2–5 days.
- Pediatric: See above.

	Onset of Action	Peak Effect	Duration
Oral	20–30 min	—	3–8 h
IV	10–30 min	10–80 min	2–4 h
IM	10–30 min	—	2–4 h

Food: Oral dose should be taken with meals to minimize GI problems.

Pregnancy: Category C. Avoid in third trimester unless there is no alternative.

Lactation: American Academy of Pediatrics states that hydralazine is compatible with breastfeeding.

Contraindications: Rheumatic heart disease (mitral valular), coronary artery disease, angina, dissecting aortic aneurysm, hypersensitivity to hydralazine, advanced renal disease (chronic renal hypertension, glomerulonephritis).

Warnings/precautions

- Use with caution in patients with the following conditions: stroke, pulmonary hypertension, patients receiving other antihypertensive drugs, liver and kidney disease, elderly.
- Use IM or IV route only when the drug cannot be given orally.
- Tartrazine is present in solutions of hydralazine and can cause severe allergic reactions in sensitive individuals. Often those sensitive to aspirin are also sensitive to tartrazine.

- Hydralazine should be withdrawn slowly to avoid sudden increases in BP.

Advice to patient

- Change position slowly, in particular from recumbent to upright, to minimize orthostatic hypotension. Sit at the edge of the bed for several minutes before standing and lie down if feeling faint or dizzy. Avoid hot showers or baths and standing for long periods. Male patients with orthostatic hypotension may be safer urinating while seated on the toilet rather than standing.
- Avoid alcohol.
- Take last dose of drug at bedtime.
- Use of OTC medications only after first informing the treating physician.

Adverse reactions

- Common: headache, palpitation, tachycardia, nausea, vomiting, diarrhea, anorexia.
- Serious: angina, MI, hypotension, orthostasis, lupuslike syndrome, agranulocytosis, peripheral neuritis, positive serum antinuclear antibody.

Clinically important drug interactions

- Hydralazine increases effects/toxicity of the following: diuretics, other antihypertensives, in particular diazoxide, β blockers, procainamide, quinidine, sympathomimetics.
- Antihypertensive effects of hydralazine are decreased by MAO inhibitors, NSAIDs.

Parameters to monitor

- Monitor BP every 5 minutes during IV infusion, until stable, then every 15 minutes during crisis.
- Determine antinuclear antibody titer before initiating therapy and at regular intervals thereafter, eg, every 6 months.
- Symptoms of lupus erythematosus: fever, chest pain, joint pain. If these occur together with an increase in antinuclear antibody titer, drug should be discontinued.
- Changes in weight at least weekly following initiation of therapy. An increase of 5 lb/wk may indicate accumulation of edema fluid.

- Pulmonary function.
- Signs and symptoms of neuropathy. Administer pyridoxine to reverse this toxicity.

Editorial comments
- Hydralazine may cause systemic lupus erythematosus syndrome, particularly in doses greater than 200 mg/d for prolonged periods. Patients who are slow acetylators (20% of the US population) are at higher risk.
- Hydralazine is most often used in combination with a diuretic as well as a sympatholytic agent.
- The routine use of hydralazine for chronic management of hypertension is discouraged because of the availability of newer agents with safer side effect profiles.
- This drug is listed without detail in the *Physician's Desk Reference*, 54th edition, 2000.

Hydrochlorothiazide

Brand name: HydroDiuril.
Class of drug: Thiazide diuretic.
Mechanism of action: Inhibits sodium resorption in distal tubule, resulting in increased urinary excretion of sodium, potasssium, and water.
Indications/dosage/route: Oral only.
- Edema (adjunct for edema associated with CHF, hepatic cirrhosis, corticosteroid or estrogen therapy)
  – Adults: 25–100 mg/d as single or divided doses.
- Hypertension:
  – Adults: Initial: 25 mg/d as single dose. Increase 50 mg/d in single or 2 divided doses. Maximum: 50 mg.
  – Children 2–12 years: 37.5–100 mg/d in 2 divided doses.
  – Children ≤2 years: 12.5–37.5 mg/d in 2 divided doses.

Adjustment of dosage
- Kidney disease: Use with caution. Ineffective in severe renal failure.

- Liver disease: Use with caution. May cause electrolyte imbalance.
- Elderly: Use with caution because of age-related impairment of kidney function.
- Pediatric: See above.

	Onset of Action	Peak Effect	Duration
Diuretic	<2 h	4 h	16–12 h

Food: Should be taken with food.

Pregnancy: Category D.

Lactation: Excreted in breast milk. Considered compatible by American Academy of Pediatrics. Thiazide diuretics may suppress lactation.

Contraindications: Anuria, hypersensitivity to thiazides or sulfonamide-derived drugs.

Warnings/precautions

- Use with caution in patients with the following conditions: severe renal or liver disease, systemic lupus erythematosus, patients receiving lithium concurrently, and in jaundiced infants (risk of hyperbilirubinemia).
- Consider reducing dose of other antihypertensive drug if a thiazide is added to the regimen.
- A potassium supplement should be administered only when diet alone is inadequate. Provide patient with list of potassium-rich foods: citrus juices, grape, apple or cranberry juices, bananas, tomatoes, apricots, dates, fish, cereals. If a potassium supplement is needed, the liquid preparation should be used rather than tablets.
- Discontinue drug prior to parathyroid function tests as thiazides raise serum calcium.
- Be aware that elderly patients may experience significant orthostatic hypotension, in particular after a meal.
- Consider using an alternative drug if the patient has significant hyperlipidemia.

- Hypersensitivity reactions may occur even if there is no previous history of allergy or bronchial asthma.
- A thiazide may exacerbate or activate systemic lupus erythematosus.

Advice to patient

- Take this drug in the morning to avoid nocturia.
- Change position slowly, in particular from recumbent to upright, to minimize orthostatic hypotension. Sit at the edge of the bed for several minutes before standing and lie down if feeling faint or dizzy. Avoid hot showers or baths and standing for long periods. Male patients should sit on the toilet while urinating rather than standing.
- Avoid drinking alcoholic beverages as these may exacerbate orthostatic hypotension.
- Do not engage in unaccustomed strenuous exercise without consulting treating physician.
- Do not drink large quantities of xanthine-containing liquids: regular coffee, tea, or cocoa.
- Eat limited quantities of foods containing large amounts of sodium: beer, pretzels, luncheon meats, snack foods, bacon, Chinese foods, tomato juice, prepared soups.
- Use salt substitute rather than regular salt.
- Take OTC drugs only after consulting with physician as many of these contain large amounts of sodium.

Adverse reactions

- Common: none.
- Serious: hypokalemia, bone marrow suppression, hypotension, hyponatremia, orthostatic hypotension, hypocalcemia, hypomagnesemia, aplastic anemia, hemolytic anemia, uremia, hypersensitivity reactions.

Clinically important drug interactions

- Drugs that increase effects/toxicity of thiazides: alcohol, barbiturates, narcotics, other antihypertensive drugs, glucocorticoids.
- Drugs that decrease effects/toxicity of thiazides: cholestyramine, colestipol, NSAIDs.
- Thiazides increase effects/toxicity of digitalis glycosides,

lithium, corticosteroids, nondepolarizing muscle relaxants (curare-type drugs).
• Thiazides decrease effects/toxicity of sulfonylureas, insulin.

Parameters to monitor

• Serum electrolytes including sodium, potassium, glucose, BUN, creatinine, uric acid, bicarbonate.
• Feet, legs, and sacral area for edema; this should be done on a daily basis.
• If the patient is also taking digitalis, monitor serum digoxin levels and signs of digitalis toxicity (vomiting, muscle cramps, confusion).
• BP before and periodically after administration.
• Signs and symptoms of hypokalemia, particularly in the elderly, the debilitated, and those with edema: dry mouth, anorexia, nausea, vomiting, thirst, mental confusion, paralytic ileus, muscle cramps, cardiac arrhythmias, depressed reflexes. If hypokalemia develops, administer potassium-sparing diuretic or potassium supplement.
• Kidney function. Serum electrolytes, BUN, creatinine, uric acid, blood sugar, should be determined weekly at beginning of therapy. For patients on long-term therapy, these determinations should be made q6–8mon.
• Intake of fluids and urinary and other fluid output to minimize renal toxicity. Increase fluid intake if inadequate. Closely monitor electrolyte levels.
• Monitor electrolyte imbalance as a result of excessive diuresis or oliguria.
• Evaluate patient for orthostasis with BP measurements in the sitting, lying, and standing positions repeatedly before and after initiating therapy.
• Therapeutic efficacy. Weigh patient before breakfast and immediately before voiding. This should be done at the same time each day and with the same clothing. Other indications of efficacy: increased urine output, reduction of edema with weight loss, control of hypertension, adequate tissue perfusion (warm, dry skin).
• Skin and mucous membranes for signs of petechiae for those receiving large doses of the drug or for extended periods.

- For diabetic or diabetic-prone patients: Monitor blood glucose for hyperglycemia and adjust dose if necessary. Hyperglycemia is usually not a problem unless high doses of drug are used.
- Signs of hyperuricemia.
- Symptoms of CHF.

Editorial comments
- Hydrochlorothiazide is the diuretic of choice for patients with the following conditions: mild to moderate hypertension, asthma, COPD, hypertension in patients with urinary calcium calculi, CHF in patients with hypertension.
- Thiazides are often used in combination therapy with many other antihypertensive drugs including β blockers, ACE inhibitors, angiotensin receptor blockers, and potassium-sparing diuretics.

Hydrocortisone

Brand names: Cortef, Hydrocortone.
Class of drug: Topical, systemic antiinflammatory glucocorticoid.
Mechanism of action: Inhibits migration of polymorphonuclear leukocytes; stabilizes lysomal membranes; inhibits production of products of arachidonic acid cascade.
Indications/dosage/route: Oral, IM, rectal, topical. Dosages of corticosteroids are variable. These should be individualized according to the disease being treated and the response of the patient.
- Adrenal insufficiency
  - Adults: PO 20–240 mg/d.
  - Adults: Initial: IV 100 mg, then 100 mg q8h in an IV fluid.

- Children >1 year: Initial: IV bolus 1–2 mg/kg, then IV 150–250 mg/kg/d in divided doses.
  - Infants: initial: IV bolus 1–2 mg/kg, then 25–150 mg/kg/d in divided doses.
  - Adults: IM, one-third to one-half the PO dose q12h.
- Rectal
  - 100 mg in retention enema nightly for 21 days.
- Inflammation
  - Ointment, cream, gel, lotion, solution, spray: Apply sparingly to affected area and rub in lightly t.i.d. to q.i.d.
  - Intralesional, intraarticular, soft tissue: 5–50 mg, depending on condition

Adjustment of dosage
- Kidney disease: None.
- Liver disease: None.
- Elderly: None.
- Pediatric: For systemic use, children on long-term therapy must be monitored carefully for growth and development.

Food: Administer with food to minimize GI upset.

Pregnancy: Category C.

Lactation: No data available. Best to avoid.

Contraindications: Systemic fungal, viral, or bacterial infections, Cushing's syndrome. Topical use: Hypersensitivity to corticosteroids, markedly impaired circulation, occlusive dressing if primary skin infection is present, monotherapy in primary bacterial infections, eg, impetigo, cellulitis, roscea, ophthalmic use, plaque psoriasis (widespread).

Warnings/precautions
- Use with caution in patients with diabetes mellitus, cardiovascular disease, hypertension, thrombophlebitis, renal or hepatic insufficiency.
- Skin test patient for tuberculosis before beginning treatment if patient is at high risk.
- For long-term treatment consider alternative-day dosing. However, if the disease flares, may need to return to initial daily dose.

- Observe neonates for signs of adrenal insufficiency if mother has taken steroids during pregnancy.
- Tapering is always required when administration of a steroid is stopped. A variety of procedures for tapering after long-term therapy have been suggested. For example, taper dose by 5 mg/wk until 10 mg/d is reached. Then 2.5 mg/wk until therapy is discontinued or lowest dosage giving relief is reached. Longer tapering periods may be required for some patients. Adrenal insufficiency may persist for up to 1 year.
- Attempt dose reduction periodically to determine if disease can be controlled at a lower dose. When every-other-day therapy is initiated, twice the daily dose should be administered on alternate days in the morning.
- Check whether patient is allergic to tartrazine, which is present in some of these drugs.

Advice to patient
- It is best to take steroid medication before 9 a.m.
- Adhere to dosing schedule and do not increase dose or interval between recommended doses without consulting physician.
- Maintain a salt-restricted diet high in potassium. Consume citrus fruits and bananas for extra potassium.
- Pay attention to foot care and report easy bruising and skin abrasions.
- Use caution when excessive physical activity if being treated for arthritis. Because the drug may decrease joint pain, you may feel an exaggerated sense of security concerning the effects of too-vigorous exercise. Permanent damage could result.
- Use OTC medications only after first informing the treating physician.
- Increase intake of calcium and vitamin D to minimize bone loss. Recommended intake of 1500 mg/d calcium and 400 IU vitamin D twice a day.
- Carry identification card at all times describing disease, treatment regimen, name, address, and telephone number of treating physician.

- Receive vaccinations (particularly live attenuated viruses) only with permission from treating physician.

Adverse reactions
- Common: dyspepsia, appetite stimulation, insomnia, anxiety, fluid retension, cushinoid facies.
- Serious: Cushing-like syndrome, adrenocortical insufficiency, muscle wasting, osteoporosis, immunosuppression with increased susceptibility to infection, potassium loss, glaucoma, cataracts (nuclear, posterior, subcapsular), hyperglycemia, hypercorticism, peptic ulcer, psychosis, insomnia, skin atrophy, thrombosis, seizures, angioneuritic edema. Children: Growth suppression, pseudotumor cerebri (reversible papilledema, visual loss, nerve paralysis [abducens or oculomotor]), vascular bone necrosis, pancreatitis.

Clinically important drug interactions
- Drugs that increase effects/toxicity of corticosteroids: broad-spectrum antibiotics, anticholinergics, oral contraceptives, cyclosporine, loop diuretics, thiazide diuretics, NSAIDs, tricyclic antidepressants.
- Drugs that decrease effects of corticosteroids: barbiturates, cholestyramine, ketoconazole, phenotoin, rifampin.
- Corticosteroids increase effects/toxicity of digitalis glycosides, neuromuscular blocking drugs.
- Cortiocosteroids decrease effects of vaccines and toxoids.

Parameters to monitor
- Serum electrolytes, glucose.
- BP. Check at least twice daily during period of dose adjustment.
- Signs and symptoms of hypokalemia: cardiac arrythmias, flaccid paralysis, tetany, polydipsia.
- Periodic ophthalmoscopic examinations. Long-term use may cause cataracts, glaucoma, secondary fungal or viral infections.
- Signs of infection.
- Fluid and electrolyte balance. Check for salt and water retention. Weigh patient on regular basis.
- Symptoms of peptic ulcer.
- Signs and symptoms of Cushing's syndrome: moon face, obesity, hirsutism, ecchymoses, hypertension, muscle atrophy,

diabetes, cataracts, peptic ulcer, fluid and electrolyte imbalance.
• Rheumatoid arthritis patients: Assess patient's symptoms and x rays each month for the first 2 months, every 3 months for 6 months after the disease is under control, and every 6 months thereafter.
• Signs and symptoms of drug-induced psychologic disturbances: changes in mood (eg, depression), behavior (aggression) or disorientation, agitation, hallucinations, suicidal tendencies, sleep disturbances, lethargy.

Editorial comments: Corticoid treatment remains challenging for clinicians because of commonly occurring short-term and long-term side effects. With chronic use, adrenal suppression may persist for up to 1 year. The agents produce accelerated bone resorption as well as decreased bone formation, resulting in overall bone loss with chronic use. Individuals <40 years on high-dose therapy are at highest risk for bone loss. Ongoing monitoring is suggested and treatment with bisphosphonates or calcitonin is suggested when decreased bone mineral density occurs.

Hydroflumethiazide

Brand name: Diucardin.
Class of drug: Thiazide diurectic.
Mechanism of action: Inhibits sodium resorption in distal tubule, resulting in increased urinary excretion of sodium, potasssium, and water.
Indications/dosage/route: Oral only.
• Diuretic
  – Adults: Initial: 25–100 mg, 1–2 times daily, once every other day, or once a day 3–5 d/wk.
  – Children: Initial: 1 mg/kg/d.

- Hypertension
  - Adults: 50–100 mg/d as single dose or 2 divided doses. Maximum: 200 mg/d in divided doses.
  - Children: 1 mg/kg/d.

Adjustment of dosage
- Kidney disease: Use with caution. Ineffective in severe renal failure.
- Liver disease: Use with caution. May cause electrolyte imbalance.
- Elderly: Use with caution because of age-related impairment of kidney function.
- Pediatric: See above.

Onset of Action	Peak Effect	Duration
1–2 h	3–4 h	18–24 h

Food: Should be taken with food.
Pregnancy: Category D.
Lactation: No data available. Hydrochlorathiazide (another thiazide diuretic) is considered compatible with breastfeeding by American Academy of Pediatrics. Thiazide diuretics may suppress lacation.
Contraindications: Anuria, hypersensitivity to thiazides or sulfonamide-derived drugs.
Editorial comments: For additional information, see *hydrochlorothiazide*, p. 426.

Hydromorphone

Brand names: Dilaudid, Dilaudid HP.
Class of drug: Narcotic analgesic, agonist.

Mechanism of action: Binds to opiate receptors and blocks ascending pain pathways. Reduces patient's perception of pain without altering cause of the pain.

Indications/dosage/route: Oral, SC, IM, IV.

• Analgesia: Dilaudid
  – Adults: PO 2 mg q4–6h. For severe pain, 4 mg q4–6h.
• Analgesia: Dilaudid HP
  – Adults: SC, IM, IV 1–2 mg q4–6h. For severe pain, 3–4 mg q4–6h.

Adjustment of dosage

• Kidney disease: None.
• Liver disease: None.
• Elderly: None.
• Pediatric: Safety and efficacy have not been established.

Onset of Action	Peak Effect	Duration
15–30 min	0.5–1 h	4–5 h

Food: May be taken with food to lessen GI upset.

Pregnancy: Category B. Category D if prolonged use or if given in high doses at term.

Lactation: Appears in breast milk. Potentially toxic to infant. Considered compatible with breastfeeding by American Academy of Pediatrics.

Contraindications: Dilaudid HP: use in patients who are not receiving large amounts of parenteral narcotics, hypersensitivity to opiates of the same chemical class, severe respiratory depression, status epilepticus, abdominal pain of undetermined origin, obstetric analgesia. Dilaudid: hypersensitivity to opiates of the same chemical class, status asthmaticus, obstetric analgesia, severe respiratory depression, abdominal pain of undetermined origin, increased intracranial pressure.

Warnings/precautions

• Use with caution in patients with the following conditions: head injury with increased intracranial pressure, serious alcoholism, prostatic hypertrophy, chronic preliminary disease, severe liver

or kidney disease, postoperative patients with pulmonary disease, disorders of biliary tract.
- Dilaudid-HP (high potency) is a highly concentrated solution of hydromorphone. It is intended only for narcotic-tolerant patients. This preparation should be given only to those patients already receiving large doses of narcotics.
- Administer drug before patient experiences severe pain for fullest efficacy of the drug.
- Have the following available when treating patient with this drug: naloxone (Narcan) or other antagonist, means of administering oxygen, and support of respiration.
- Nausea, vomiting, and orthostatic hypotension occur most prominently in ambulatory patients. If nausea and vomiting persist, it may be necessary to administer an antiemetic, eg, droperidol or prochlorperazine.
- This drug can cause severe hypotension in a patient who is volume-depleted or if given along with a phenothiazine or general anesthesia.
- Careful diagnosis must be made of acute abdominal condition before this drug is administered.
- For additional information, see *morphine,* p. 633.

Hydroxyprogesterone

Brand name: Hylutin.
Class of drug: Progestational hormone, contraceptive.
Mechanism of action: Inhibits secretion of pituitary gonadotropins (FSH, LH) by positive feedback.
Indications/dosage/route: Oral only.
- Secndary amenorrhea, dysfunctional uterine bleeding.
  – Adults: 375 mg.
- Production of secretory endometrium and desquamation.
  – Adults: 125–250 mg given on tenth day of cycle; repeat q7d until suppression is no longer desired.

• Uterine cancer
  – 1 g daily. Continue treatment up to 12 weeks.
Food: No restrictions.
Adjustment of dosage
• Kidney disease: None.
• Liver disease: Contraindicated.
• Elderly: None.
• Pediatric: Safety and efficacy have not been determined.
Food: No restrictions.
Pregnancy: Category X.
Lactation: Another drug from this class (medroxyprogesterone) is considered compatible by American Academy of Pediatrics.
Contraindications: Hypersensitivity to progestins, history of thrombophlebitis, active thromboembolic disease, cerebral hemorrhage, liver disease, missed abortion, use as diagnostic for pregnancy, known or suspected pregnancy (first 4 months), undiagnosed vaginal bleeding, carcinoma of the breast, known or suspected genital malignancy.
Editorial comments
• This drug is not listed in the *Physician's Desk Reference*, 54th edition, 2000.
• For additional information, see *medroxyprogesterone*, p. 553.

Hydroxyurea

Brand names: Hydrea, Droxia.
Class of drug: Antimetabolite, antineoplastic agent.
Mechanism of action: Inhibits DNA synthesis, specific for S phase of dividing cells.
Indications/dosage/route: Oral only. Doses are adjusted according to clinical response, toxicity, and local protocols.
• Solid tumors, intermittent therapy or when used with radiation
  – Adults: 80 mg/kg/d q3d, beginning 7 days prior to radiation therapy.

- Solid tumors, continuous therapy
  - 20–30 mg/kg, single or divided doses.
- Chronic myelocytic leukemia (chronic phase)
  - Adults: 20–30 mg/kg/d, single or two divided doses.
- Sickle cell disease (reduction of pain crisis, decrease transfusions)
  - 15 mg/kg/d. Increase by 5 mg/kg/d q12wk as needed. Maximum: 35 mg/kg/d.

Adjustment of dosage
- Kidney disease: No specific guidelines are available.
- Liver disease: No specific guidelines are available.
- Elderly: Lower dosage may be required.
- Pediatric: Safety and effectiveness have not been determined.

Food: May be taken with food.

Pregnancy: Category D.

Lactation: Appears in breast milk. Potentially toxic to fetus. Avoid breastfeeding.

Contraindications: Severe bone marrow depression (leukopenia <2500 WBCs/mm^3), thrombocytopenia (<100,000/mm^3), severe anemia, hypersensitivity to previously administered hydroxyurea, pregnancy.

Warnings/precautions
- Use with caution in patients with kidney disease, active infections, bone marrow depression, previous radiation therapy, other cytotoxic drugs.
- Avoid IM injections if platelet count falls below 100,000/mm^3.

Advice to patient
- Receive vaccinations (particularly live attenuated viruses) only with permission from treating physician.
- Drink large amounts of fluids to facilitate excretion of uric acid.
- Avoid crowds as well as persons who may have a contagious disease.
- Avoid driving and other activities requiring mental alertness or that are potentially dangerous until response to drug is known.
- Use two forms of birth control including hormonal and barrier methods.
- Wear sunglasses in bright light.

• Avoid taking NSAIDs together with this drug.

Adverse reactions

• Common: anorexia, nausea, vomiting, diarrhea, mucositis, drowsiness, dermatitis, increased liver enzymes.

• Serious: **bone marrow suppression**, seizures, kidney damage, procarcinogenic effect, hyperuricemia, pulmonary infiltrates, elevated liver enzymes.

Clinically important drug interactions

• The following drugs increase effects/toxicity of hydroxyurea: zidorudine (AZT), zalcitabine (ddC), didanosine (DDI).

• Hydroxyurea increases effects/toxicity of fluorouracil, cytarabine.

Parameters to monitor

• CBC with differential and platelets, liver enzymes.

• Signs and symptoms of thrombocytopenia: excessive bleeding and easy bruising. Discontinue this medication if platelet count falls below 80,000/mm^3.

• Signs and symptoms of anemia: shortness of breath, dizziness, angina, pale conjunctiva, skin and nailbeds. Discontinue medication if hemoglobin falls below 4.59g/dL.

• Monitor patient's liver function prior to and periodically during therapy.

• Patients with sickle cell anemia: Monitor blood count every 2 weeks.

• Signs of muscle weakness. Knee and ankle reflexes should be tested every 6 months. If there is evidence of muscle weakness, drug should be discontinued.

Editorial comments

• Hydroxyurea must be used only when patient is under close supervision of a physician who has experience with this type of cytotoxic agent.

• Bone marrow suppression is generally seen in the first week of use.

• Cytotoxic drug. Use latex gloves and safety glasses when handling this medication; avoid contact with skin and inhalation. If possible prepare in biologic hood.

• Hydroxyurea is considered a drug of choice for treatment of chronic myelogenous leukemia for patients who are not candidates for allogenic bone marrow transplant.

- Dosage as well as indications may vary from patient to patient. The current literature should be consulted for recommended protocols. Local protocols vary.
- Almost all patients need a drug holiday to permit blood counts to return to acceptable levels.
- This drug is commonly used to treat myeloproliferative disorders with elevated platelet counts, eg, essential thrombocythemia, polycythemia vera, and is used as a radiosensitizing agent in patients with cervical, head, or neck cancer.

Hydroxyzine

Brand names: Vistaril, Atarax.
Class of drug: Antihistamine, sedative–hypnotic.
Mechanism of action: Competitive antagonist of histamine (H_1) receptors. Mechanism of anxiolytic and sedative actions: inhibits subcortical neuronal activity.
Indications/dosage/route: Oral, IM.
- Anxiety, sedative–hypnotic
  - Adults: 50–100 mg PO q.i.d. Maximum: 600 mg/d.
  - Children <6 years: PO 50 mg/d in divided doses.
  - Children >6 years: PO 50–100 mg/d in divided doses.
- Antiemetic, antipruritic
  - Adults: PO or IM 25–100 mg t.i.d. or q.i.d.
  - Children <6 years: PO or IM 50 mg/d in divided doses.
  - Children >6 years: PO or IM 50–100 mg/d in divided doses.
- Sedation before and after general anesthesia.
  - Adults: PO or IM 25–100 mg.
  - Children: PO or IM 0.5 mg/kg.
- Pre/postoperative adjunct for nausea and vomiting
  - Adults: IM 25–100 mg.
  - Children: IM 0.5 mg/kg.
- Alcohol withdrawal, acute anxiety

– Adults: IM 50–100 mg q4–6 h, prn.

Adjustment of dosage
• Kidney disease: None.
• Liver disease: Increase interval (q24h in primary biliary cirrhosis).
• Elderly: Dosage reduction may be required.
• Pediatric: See above.

	Onset of Action	Peak Effect	Duration
Oral	15–30 min	2–4 h	4–6 h

Food: May be taken with food.
Pregnancy: Category C.
Lactation: Probably appears in breast milk. Avoid breastfeeding.
Contraindications: Hypersensitivity to hydroxyzine or related compounds. Early pregnancy is listed in the *Physician's Desk Reference*.

Warnings/precautions
• Use with caution in patients with hypertension, thyroid disease, asthma, heart disease, diabetes, prostatic hyperplasia, angle-closure glaucoma.
• Parenteral form is for IM injection only.

Advice to patient
• Avoid alcohol and other CNS depressants such as opiate analgesics, barbituates, sedatives (eg, diazepam) when taking this drug.
• Avoid driving and other activities requiring mental alertness or that are potentially dangerous until response to drug is known.
• Use two forms of birth control including hormonal and barrier methods.
• For symptomatic relief of dry mouth: rinse mouth with warm water frequently, chew sugarless gum, suck on ice cube, use artificial saliva if necessary, carry out meticulous oral hygiene (floss teeth daily).
• Obtain approval from treating physician before taking OTC cold or allergy preparations that may contain an antihistamine.

Adverse reactions
- Common: drowsiness, dry mouth.
- Serious: involuntary movements, seizures.

Clinically important drug interactions
- Hydroxyzine increases effects/toxicity of CNS depressants, including opiates, barbiturates, other sedative hypnotic drugs, anticholinergic drugs, antihistamines, haloperidol, phenothiazines, tricyclic antidepressants; quinidine.
- Hydroxyzine decreases effects/toxicity of epinephrine.

Parameters to monitor: Signs of excessive sedation.

Editorial comment: Parenteral hydroxyzine is given by deep IM injection only. It is not for IV, intraarterial, or SC use. May cause vascular thrombosis and/or gangrene if used by these routes.

Hyoscyamine

Brand names: Levsin, Cytospaz
Class of drug: Anticholinergic.
Mechanism of action: Blocks acetylcholine effects at muscarinic receptors throughout the body.
Indications/dosage/route: Oral, IV, IM, SC.
- GI tract disorders (spasms), adjunctive therapy for peptic ulcers
  - Adults: PO 0.125–0.25 mg, before meals and h.s.
  - Adults: PO, extended-release form, 0.375–0.75 mg q12h.
  - Adults: IM, IV, SC 0.25–0.5 mg b.i.d. or q.i.d.
  - Children 2–12 years: 0.033–0.125 mg/d.
  - Children <2 years: 0.0125–0.05 mg/d.
- Diagnostic procedures
  - Adults: IV 0.25–0.5 mg 5–10 minutes before procedure.
- Preanesthetic medication
  - Adults, children >2 years: IV 0.005 mg/kg 30–60 minutes prior to anesthesia.

Adjustment of dosage
• Kidney disease: None.
• Liver disease: None.
• Elderly: None.
• Pediatric: See above.

Pregnancy: Category C.

Lactation: Limited data available. Potentially toxic to infant. Atropine is considered compatible by American Academy of Pediatrics.

Contraindications: Myasthenia gravis, narrow-angle glaucoma, GI obstruction, megacolon, active ulcerative colitis, obstructive uropathy, hypersensitivity to atropine-type compounds (belladonna alkaloids).

Editorial comments: For additional information, see *atropine*, p. 67.

Ibuprofen

Brand name: Motrin.
Class of drug: NSAID.
Mechanism of action: Inhibits cyclooxygenase, resulting in inhibition of synthesis of prostaglandins and other inflammatory mediators.
Indications/dosage/route: Oral only.
• Mild to moderate pain
  – Adults: 400 mg q4–6h, prn.
  – Children 6 months–12 years: 10 mg/kg q6–8h. Maximum: 40 mg/kg.
• Rheumatoid arthritis, osteoarthritis
  – Adults: 1200–3200 mg/d, 3–4 divided doses. Maximum: 3200 mg/d.
• Juvenile arthritis
  – 20–40 mg/kg/d, 3–4 divided doses.
• Fever reduction
  – Children 6 months–12 years: Temperature <102.5°F: 5 mg/d; temperature >102.5°F: 10 mg/d. Maximum: 40 mg/kg/d.
Adjustment of dosage
• Kidney disease: None.
• Liver disease: None.
• Elderly: May be necessary to reduce dose for patients over 65 years.
• Pediatric: Safety and efficacy have not been established in children <6 months.
Food: Take with food or large quantities of water or milk.
Pregnancy: Category B. Category D in third trimester or near delivery.
Lactation: Does not appear in breast milk. Considered compatible with breastfeeding by American Academy of Pediatrics.
Contraindications: Hypersensitivity and cross-sensitivity with other NSAIDs and aspirin.

Warnings/precautions
- Use with caution in patients with history of GI bleeding, decreased renal function, rhinitis, urticaria, hay fever, nasal polyps, asthma.
- Administer this drug with caution in patients having infections or other diseases as the drug may mask symptoms of the disease, eg, fever, inflammation.
- NSAIDs may cause severe allergic reactions including urticaria and vasomotor collapse. Cross-reactivity may occur in patients allergic to aspirin.

Advice to patient
- Avoid use of alcohol.
- Notify physician if your stool turns dark, if you develop abdominal pain, or if you vomit blood or dark material.
- Notify dentist or treating physician prior to surgery if taking this medication.
- Avoid taking OTC products that contain aspirin or other NSAIDs, eg, Alka-Seltzer.
- Take drug with full glass of water and sit up for 15–30 minutes to avoid lodging of tablet in esophagus.
- If pain occurs with physical activity, take drug 30 minutes before physical therapy or other planned exercise.

Adverse reactions
- Common: nausea, indigestion, dizziness, fatigue.
- Serious: GI bleeding (peptic ulcer, diverticular NSAID colitis), acute renal failure, bronchospasm, Stevens–Johnson syndrome, renal or hepatic toxicity, GI perforation.

Clinically important drug interactions
- Drugs that increase effects/toxicity of NSAIDs: alcohol, insulin, cimetidine.
- Drugs that decrease effects/toxicity of NSAIDs: barbiturates, corticosteroids, antacids.
- NSAIDs increase effects/toxicity of oral anticoagulants, cyclosporine, lithium, methotrexate, sulfonamides, streptokinase, valproic acid, oral hypoglycemics.
- NSAIDs decrease effects/toxicity of β blockers, calcium channel blockers, loop diuretics, probenecid, sulfinpyrazone.

Parameters to monitor
• CBC, liver enzymes, stool hemoccult, serum BUN and creatinine.
• Efficacy of treatment: pain reduction, decreased temperature, improved mobility. Assess pain reduction 1 or 2 hours after taking drug.
• Monitor patient for rhinitis, asthma, urticaria before beginning treatment. Such patients have increased risk for developing a hypersensitivity reaction to NSAID.
• Blood glucose of diabetic patients taking oral hypoglycemic drugs. An NSAID may potentiate the hypoglycemic effect of oral hypoglycemic drugs.
• Signs and symptoms of auditory toxicity, in particular tinnitus in elderly patients. Stop drug to avoid irreversible hearing loss. Restart at 50% of previous dose after reversal occurs.
• Symptoms of iron deficiency anemia, particularly in patients on long-term, high-dose drug. Perform hematocrit and guaiac tests periodically.
• Signs and symptoms of renal toxicity.
• Signs and symptoms of hepatotoxicity.
• Symptoms of GI toxicity: occult blood loss, symptoms of ulcer, hematochezia, melena, abdominal pain.
• Efficacy in treating rheumatoid arthritis. Increase dose if drug is not effective within 7 days. If maximum dose is not effective, change to another NSAID. If a second- or third-line drug is required, the NSAID should not be stopped.

Editorial comments
• Some rheumatologists consider aspirin to be the first-line drug for treatment of rheumatoid arthritis. Patient should be given 14-day trial at dose of 3.2 g/d; if ineffective, another drug should be used.
• It is recommended that misoprostol should be given prophylactically for the following patients requiring long-term treatment with an NSAID: those >60 years, those with a past history of peptic ulcer disease, those concurrently receiving anticoagulants or corticosteroids. Misoprostol has also been shown to reduce the incidence of NSAID-induced ulcers in younger patients.

- Concomitant acid-blocking agents (H_2 blockers and (Proton pump inhibitors) may reduce the incidence of duodenal ulcers but not gastric ulcers in patients on chronic NSAID therapy. They may also reduce NSAID-induced GI symptoms.
- Treat *Helicobacter plyori* if present in patients developing active ulcer on NSAID therapy; use proton pump inhibitor plus two additional antibiotics.
- Newer COX-2 inhibitors are potential alternatives for patients requiring chronic NSAID therapy.

Ibutilide

Brand name: Corvert.
Class of drug: antiarrhythmic agent, class III.
Mechanism of action: Prolongation of cardiac action potentials, K^+ channel blockade.
Indications/dosage/route: IV only.
- Rapid conversion of recent-onset atrial flutter or fibrillation to normal sinus rhythm
  - Adults >60 kg: IV infusion 1 mg over 10 minutes. Repeat 10 minutes after completion of first infusion if necessary.
  - Adults <60 kg: IV infusion 10 µg/kg. Repeat 10 minutes after completion of first infusion if necessary.
Adjustment of dosage: None.

Onset of Action	Duration
Within first 90 min of initiation of infusion	4 h

Food: Not applicable.
Pregnancy: Category C.
Lactation: No data available. Best to avoid.
Contraindications: Hypersensitivity to ibutilide, long QT syndrome.

Warnings/precautions: May cause fatal arrhythmias including Torsade de pointes.

Advice to patients: Not applicable.

Adverse reactions

• Common: none.

• Serious: Torsade de pointes (1.7–8%), nonsustained polymorphic ventricular tachycardia (2.7%), nonsustained monomorphic ventricular tachycardia (4.9%), AV block, bradycardia, QT prolongation, renal failure.

Clinically important drug interactions

• The following drugs increase effects/toxicity of ibutilide: class Ia antiarrhythmics (disopyramide, quinidine, procainamide), amiodarone, sotalol, phenothiazines, tricyclic antidepressants, astemizole, macrolide antibiotics.

• Ibutilide increases effects/toxicity of digoxin.

Parameters to monitor

• Serum BUN and creatinine, serum electrolytes including potassium, magnesium, calcium.

• Continuous ECG for at least 4 hours after dosing or at least until the corrected QT interval has returned to baseline.

Editorial comments

• This drug should be administered only by personnel skilled in treating ventricular arrhythmias in a setting of continuous ECG monitoring. Proper equipment must be available for treating sustained proarrhythmic ventricular tachycardia (eg, Torsades de pointes), including cardiac monitor, external defibrillator, and intracardiac pacing (the mechanism is often pause- dependent).

• Efficacy in treating arrhythmias of more than 90 days' duration has not been determined.

• The efficacy of this drug in ventricular arrhythmia suppression or termination has yet to be assessed.

• Monitoring should take place for at least 8–12 hours after infusion. This antiarrhythmic in relatively efficacious (60–85%) for acute spontaneous atrial arrhythmics (<24 hours in duration). The effects last about 12 hours. Ibutilide is being used with increased frequency in critical care and telemetry units as well as the electrophysiology laboratory.

Idoxuridine (IDU)

Brand name: Herplex Liquifilm.
Class of drug: Antiviral, ophthalmic agent.
Mechanism of action: Inhibits viral DNA synthesis, resulting in blockage of herpes simplex virus replication.
Indications/dosage/route: Topical (ophthalmic).
• Herpes simplex keratitis
  – Adults/children: Instill 1 drop of solution into conjunctival sac, q1h during day, q2h at night. Continue therapy for 5–7 days following complete healing. Maximum duration of therapy: 21 days.
Adjustment of dosage: Pediatric: Safety and efficacy have not been established.
Pregnancy: Category C.
Lactation: No data available. Best to avoid.
Contraindications: Hypersensitivity to idoxuridine, ulceration of stromal layers of cornea, concurrent corticosteroids in herpes simplex keratitis.
Warnings/precautions: Idoxuridine should not be mixed with other medications.
Advice to patient
• Old solutions should not be used because they may cause adverse ocular reactions and have little if any antiviral activity.
• To minimize possible photosensitivity reaction, apply adequate sunscreen and use proper covering when exposed to strong sunlight.
• Wear dark glasses to minimize photophobia.
• Report signs of vision loss to treating physician.

Adverse reactions
- Common: irritation of the eye, burning sensation, pain in eye, corneal clouding.
- Serious: none.

Clinically important drug interactions: Boric acid solutions increases effects/toxicity of idoxuridine.

Parameters to monitor
- Signs of hypersensitivity such as constant burning, itching of eyelids. Drug should be stopped immediately.
- Monitor patient for improvement, ie, control of infection, epithelialization of eye lesions.

Editorial comments
- Recurrence of the viral infection is common. To limit such recurrence, medication should be continued for at least 5–7 days after the lesion appears to be healed.
- Idoxuridine is not to be used long term, ie, longer than 21 days. It should not be used longer than 7 days after complete healing. These restrictions are designed to avoid damage to the corneal epithelium. If fluorescein staining does not show reduction of infection in 14 days, it is strongly advised to resort to alternate therapy. Some strains of herpes simplex may have become resistant to idoxuridine.
- This drug is not listed in the *Physician's Desk Reference*, 54th edition, 2000.

Ifosamide

Brand name: Ifex.
Class of drug: Antineoplastic alkylating agent, cyclophosphamide analogue.
Mechanism of action: Ifosamide is activated in the liver to a compound that crosslinks strands of DNA. This inhibits synthesis of DNA and proteins.

Indications/dosage/route: IV only and always in conjunction with the uroprotectant mesna.

• Testicular cancer: Adults
 – Adults: 1–2 g/m^2/d, consecutive 3–5 days. Repeat regimen q3wk.
• Other uses (off-label): lung cancer, breast cancer, Hodgkin's and non-Hodgkin's lymphoma, ovarian cancer
 – Adults: 1–2 g/d, 3–5 days; repeat q3–4wk.
 – Children: 1200–1800 mg/m^2/d, 3–5 days treatment. Repeat q3–4wk.

Adjustment of dosage

• Kidney disease: Serum creatinine <3.0 mg/dL: do not administer the drug.
• Liver disease: Higher doses may possibly be necessary although no guidelines are available.
• Elderly: Use with caution.
• Pediatric: Safety and efficacy have not been established.

Pregnancy: Category D.

Lactation: Appears in breast milk. Potentially toxic to infant. Avoid breastfeeding.

Contraindications: Severe bone marrow depression, hypersensitivity to ifosamide, pregnancy.

Warnings/precautions

• Use with caution in patients with the following conditions: kidney or liver disease, compromised bone marrow reserve, prior or concomitant radiation therapy, prior therapy with cytotropic drugs.
• Stop the drug if confusion or coma occurs.
• Ifosamide causes hemorrhagic cystitis; administer mesna for protection against this condition.
• Vigorous hydration and possible addition of mesna (cytoprotective agent) will reduce incidence of hematuria.
• Keep patient well hydrated during therapy.
• Ideally, patient should urinate every 2 hours during the day and twice during the night while receiving ifosamide.

Advice to patient

• Avoid crowds as well as persons who may have a contagious disease.

- Use method of birth control other than oral contraceptives.
- Male patients should use condoms if engaging in sexual intercourse while using this medication.
- Receive vaccinations (particularly live attenuated viruses) only with permission from treating physician.
- Drink at least 3000 mL of fluids/d to reduce the risk of hemorrhagic cystitis.

Adverse reactions
- Common: alopecia (83%), nausea and vomiting (58%).
- Serious: **hematuria (46%), CNS toxicity (12%)** including sleepiness, confusion, depression and psychosis, metabolic acidosis, pulmonary toxicity, renal toxicity, hepatitis, neuropathy, cranial nerve damage, cardiac toxicity, SIADH.

Parameters to monitor
- CBC with differential and platelets, urinalysis (for microhematuria).
- Signs and symptoms of bone marrow depression.
- Symptoms of bladder toxicity: hematuria, hemorrhagic cystitis, dysuria. Administer the drug mesna for protection against this toxicity.
- Symptoms of cardiotoxicity: edema, CHF.
- Signs and symptoms of renal toxicity.
- Symptoms of CNS toxicity: hallucinations, confusion, disorientation. If these occur, discontinue drug and institute supportive measures. Generally reversible within 1–3 days.
- Signs and symptoms of pulmonary toxicity: decreased breath sounds, crackles, decreased oxygenation. Methylene blue 50 mg IV has been reported to be useful treatment for this problem.

Editorial comments
- This drug should be administered by a physician who is experienced in the use of cancer therapeutic drugs.
- Cytotoxic drug: Use latex gloves and safety glasses when handling this medication; avoid contact with skin and inhalation. If possible prepare in biologic hood.
- It is essential to perform complete hematologic evaluation every 2 weeks for patients on this drug.

- Physician should check current literature for recommended protocols, in particular dosages and indications. There are many unlabeled uses for this drug.
- Drug should be administered by slow IV infusion over at least 30 minutes. It should be noted that the most effective dose or dose regimen have not been determined.
- Ifosamide is also an effective agent for treatment of sarcomas.
- Physicians should monitor closely for CNS symptoms which are reversible within 24–72 hours.

Imipramine

Brand name: Tofranil.
Class of drug: Tricyclic antidepressant.
Mechanism of action: Inhibits reuptake of CNS neurotransmitters, primarily serotonin and norepinephrine.
Indications/dosage/route: Oral, IM.
- Depression
  - Hospitalized patients: PO 50 mg b.i.d. to t.i.d.; may be increased by 25 mg every few days up to 200 mg/d. Maximum: 250–300 mg/d at bedtime.
  - Outpatients: PO 75–150 mg/d. Maintenance: PO 50–150 mg/d at bedtime.
  - Adolescents, elderly: PO 30–40 mg/d. Maximum: 100 mg/d.
  - Children: PO 1.5 mg/kg/d in three divided doses; may be increased to 1–1.5 mg/kg/d q3–5d. Maximum: 5 mg/kg/d.
- Enuresis
  - Children >5 years: PO 25 mg/d 1 hour before bedtime. Increase to maximum: 2.5 mg/kg/d as needed.
- Depression
  - Adults: IM up to 100 mg/d in divided doses.

Adjustment of dosage
- Kidney disease: None.
- Liver disease: None.

- Elderly: Lower doses recommended.
- Pediatric: Not recommended for children <12 years except for treatment of enuresis.

Food: No restriction.

Pregnancy: Category B.

Lactation: Appears in breast milk. American Academy of Pediatrics expresses concern over use when breastfeeding.

Contraindications: Hypersensitivity to tricyclic antidepressants, acute recovery from MI, concurrent MAO inhibitor.

Warnings/precautions

- Use with caution in patients with the following conditions: epilepsy, angle-closure glaucoma, cardiovascular disease, history of urinary retention, suicidal tendencies, BPH, concurrent anticholinergic drugs, hyperthyroid patients receiving thyroid drugs, alcoholism, schizophrenia.
- May cause psychosis in schizophrenic patients.
- May unmask mania or hypomania.

Advice to Patient

- Avoid alcohol and other CNS depressants such as opiate analgesics and sedatives (eg, diazepam) when taking this drug.
- Avoid driving and other activities requiring mental alertness or that are potentially dangerous until response to drug is known.
- Change position slowly, in particular from recumbent to upright, to minimize orthostatic hypotension. Sit at the edge of the bed for several minutes before standing, and lie down if feeling faint or dizzy. Avoid hot showers or baths and standing for long periods. Male patients should sit on the toilet while urinating rather than standing.
- If you are experiencing dry mouth rinse with warm water frequently, chew sugarless gum, suck on ice cube, or use artificial saliva. Carry out meticulous oral hygiene (floss teeth daily).
- To minimize possible photosensitivity reaction, apply adequate sunscreen and use proper covering when exposed to strong sunlight.
- If constipation develops, increase fiber and fluid intake. Notify physician if constipation is severe.

Adverse reactions
- Common: sedation, anticholinergic effects (dry mouth, constipation), nausea, dizziness, headache, taste disturbance, weight gain.
- Serious: Orthostatic hypotension, arrhythmias, extrapyramidal symptoms, seizures, bone marrow depression, hepatitis, increased intraocular pressure, allergic reactions.

Clinically important drug interactions
- Drugs that increase effects/toxicity of tricyclic antidepressants: MAO inhibitors, cimetidine, SSRIs, β blockers, estrogens.
- Drugs that decrease effects/toxicity of tricyclic antidepressants: barbiturates, cholestyramine.
- Tricyclic antidepressants increase effects/toxicity of CNS depressants (alcohol, sedatives, hypnotics), oral anticoagulants, carbamazepine, sympathomimetic amines (dobutamine, dopamine, epinephrine, ephedrine), opioids (morphine-type drugs), drugs with anticholinergic activity (atropine, anti-Parkinson drugs).
- Tricyclic antidepressants decrease effects/toxicity of clonidine, guanethidine.

Parameters to monitor
- CBC with differential and platelets, liver enzymes.
- Suicidal ideation. Advise patient's family to remove firearms from the home.
- Signs and symptoms of hepatotoxicity.
- Drug levels. Therapeutic level: 160–250 ng/mL; toxic level: >500 ng/mL.
- Neurologic and mental status: mood changes, agitation. May require dose reduction. Hypomania, mania, or delusions: stop medication.
- Signs and symptoms of angle-closure glaucoma and visual or other ophthalmic disturbances, eg, halos, eye pain, dilated pupils.
- Signs and symptoms of bone marrow depression.
- Patient with history of hyperthyroidism or cardiovascular disease: monitor for arrhythmias.
- Efficacy of treatment: increased appetite and energy level and sense of well-being, renewed interest in environment, improved sleep.

Editorial comments
- Patients with depression are at increased risk of suicide. To reduce this risk as well as the chance of overdose, prescribe limited amounts.
- Withdrawal symptoms have been reported after abrupt cessation of administration. These include nausea, headache, irritability, and sleep disturbances.
- It may take several months for maximum response to be realized.
- This drug is listed without details in the *Physician's Desk Reference*, 54th edition, 2000.

Indapamide

Brand name: Lozol.
Class of drug: Thiazide diurectic.
Mechanism of action: Inhibits sodium resorption in distal tubule, resulting in increased urinary excretion of sodium, potasssium, and water.
Indications/dosage/route: Oral only.
- Diuretic (edema of CHF)
  - Adults: Initial: 2.5 mg as single dose in a.m. Increase to 5 mg/d after 1 week if needed.
- Hypertension
  - Adults: Initial: 1.25 mg as single dose in a.m. Increase to 2.5 mg as single dose if response is not satisfactory after 4 weeks. Increase to 5 mg/d if response is not satisfactory after 4 weeks or consider giving another antihypertensive drug.

Adjustment of dosage
- Kidney disease: Use with caution. Ineffective in severe renal failure.
- Liver disease: Use with caution. May cause electrolyte imbalance.
- Elderly: Use with caution because of age-related impairment of kidney function.
- Pediatric: Safety and efficacy have not been established.

	Onset of Action	Peak Effect	Duration
Diuretic	1–2 h	2 h	36 h
Antihypertensive	1–2 wk	—	Up to 8 wk (multiple doses)

Food: Should be taken with food.
Pregnancy: Category D.
Lactation: No data available. Manufacturer recommends to discontinue nursing. Thiazide diuretics may suppress lactation.
Contraindications: Anuria, hypersensitivity to thiazides or sulfonamide-derived drugs.
Editorial comments: For additional information, see *hydrochlorothiazide*, p. 426.

Indomethacin

Brand name: Indocin.
Class of drug: NSAID.
Mechanism of action: Inhibits cyclooxygenase, resulting in inhibition of synthesis of prostaglandins and other inflammatory mediators.
Indications/dosage/route: Oral only.
• Rheumatoid arthritis, osteoarthritis, ankylosing spondylitis
  – Adults: Initial: PO 25 mg b.i.d., t.i.d.; increase by 25–50 mg/wk. Maximum: 150–200 mg/d.
• Acute gouty arthritis
  – Adults: Initial: 50 mg t.i.d.
• Bursitis/tendinitis
  – 75–100 mg/d in three to four divided doses for 1–2 weeks.
• Patent ductus arteriosus
  – Infants <2 days: Initial: 0.2 mg/kg, then 2 doses of 0.1 mg/kg each.
  – Infants 2–7 days: three doses of 0.2 mg/kg.

– Infants >7 days: Initial: 0.2 mg/kg, then two doses of 0.25 mg/kg.

Adjustment of dosage
• Kidney disease: None.
• Liver disease: None.
• Elderly: May be necessary to reduce dose for patients >65 years.
• Pediatric: See above.

Food: Take with food or large quantities of water or milk.

Pregnancy: Category B. Category D if used longer than 48 hours.

Lactation: Appears in breast milk. Considered compatible with breastfeeding by American Academy of Pediatrics.

Contraindications: Hypersensitivity and cross-sensitivity with other NSAIDs and aspirin, history of severe kidney disease.

Editorial comments: For additional information, see *ibuprofen*, p. 445.

Insulin (Injection)

Brand names: Regular insulin: Pork, Regular Iletin, Humulin R, Velosulin Human, Isophane Insulin Suspension (NPH). Insulin combined with protamine and zinc: NPH-Iletin, NPH Insulin. Insulin zinc suspension (lente): Humulin L, Novolin L. Generic extended zinc suspension (ultralente): Humulin U Ultralente.

Class of drug: Parenteral hypoglycemic agent.

Mechanism of action: Antidiabetic action: Insulin facilitates transport of glucose across cell membranes of fat and muscle, resulting in a reduction of blood glucose levels. In addition, it enhances the rate of conversion of glucose to glycogen. Hyperkalemia: Insulin causes a shift of potassium from serum into cells, thereby lowering serum potassium levels.

Indications/dosage/route: SC, IV.
• Diabetes mellitus I: insulin injection (crystaline zinc insulin, unmodified insulin, regular insulin)

- Adults: Usual, initial: 5–10 units 15–30 minutes before meals and at bedtime.
- Children: 2–4 units 15–30 minutes before meals and at bedtime.
- Insulin zinc suspension
  - Usual, intial: 7–26 units 30–60 minutes before breakfast. Increase dose by 2–10 units daily or weekly until satisfactory glucose level is established.
- Insulin zinc suspension extended (Ultralente)
  - Usual, initial: 7–26 units 30–60 minutes before breakfast.

Adjustment of dosage
- Kidney disease: Creatinine clearance 10–50 mL/min: 75% of normal dose; creatinine clearance <10 mL/min: 25–50% of normal dose.
- Liver disease: None.
- Elderly: May require lower doses.
- Pediatric: See above.

Type	Onset of Action	Peak Effect	Duration
Regular insulin	0.5–1 h	2–4 h	5–7 h
NPH	3–4 h	6–12 h	18–24 h
Semilente	1–3 h	2–8 h	12–16 h
Lente	1–3 h	8–12 h	18–28 h
Ultralente	4–6 h	18–24 h	36 h

Food: Patient should follow prescribed diet and exercise regularly.

Pregnancy: Insulin is drug of choice for hyperglycemia in pregnant women. It should be noted that during pregnancy insulin requirements may increase drastically, but then decline immediately postpartum.

Lactation: Not present it breast milk. Safe to use.

Contraindications: Hypoglycemia, hypersensitivity to specific type of insulin given.

Warnings/precautions

- Advise patient not to make any change in the insulin without consulting the treating physician.
- Some individuals may develop resistance to insulin, requiring large doses of the drug to control symptoms of diabetes.
- Blood glucose monitoring is essential to provide information concerning the correct dosage and to ensure therapeutic success.
- Advise patient that increased work or exercise may result in hypoglycemia and increased insulin requirements and that illness, emotional stress, or travel may require adjustment of dosage.
- Maintain daily contact with the patient to be certain that satisfactory control is achieved and that hypoglycemia is not occurring. This is particularly important when therapy is initiated.
- Determine the reason for hypoglycemia if it occurs. Hypoglycemia may result from decreased food intake, vomiting, excessive exercise, excessive alcohol consumption. If the patient experiences three hypoglycemic reactions in less than 6 months, insulin dosage should be reduced.
- Provide advice concerning the type of insulin product patient is taking by name, species, source, and manufacturer. Patient should be warned not to change brands without consulting physician.
- Educate family members concerning the symptoms and treatment of hypoglycemic reaction.
- Be sure that the patient is fully knowledgeable about instructions regarding the administration and care of such specialized delivery systems as insulin pumps.
- If changing from beef to pork insulin, be sure to take into account the need for adjustment of dosage.

Advice to patient

- Avoid alcohol.
- Carry identification card at all times describing disease, treatment regimen, name, address, and telephone number of treating physician.

- Always carry sufficient insulin and syringes as well as sugar and candy for symptoms of hypoglycemia.
- Use good personal hygiene in particular with the feet, to minimize the possibility of diabetic ulcers developing.
- Do not change the order of mixing insulins or the model or type of syringe/needle being used.
- Do not smoke within 30 minutes following insulin administration.
- Check the expiration date of each vial before it is used and discard outdated insulin.
- It is very important to recognize the symptoms of hypoglycemia, including tremulousness, tachycardia, lightheaded- ness, hunger, diaphoresis, hypotension. If severe, irreversible brain damage may result. Patient should be advised how to reverse mild hypoglycemia: drink fruit juice (orange), eat sugar or candy.
- Rotate injection site to avoid lipohypertrophy from repeated same-site injections.

Adverse reactions
- Common: palpitations, fatigue, subcutaneous lipid, atrophy or hypertrophy, blurred vision.
- Serious: hypoglycemia, anaphylaxis, coma, hyopothermia.

Clinically important drug interactions
- Drugs that decrease effects/toxicity of insulin: oral contraceptives, corticosteroids, dextrothyroxine, diltiazem, epinephrine, smoking, thiazide diuretics, thyroid hormone.
- Drugs that increase effects/toxicity of insulin: oral alcohol, α blockers, anabolic steroids, clofibrate, fenfluoramine, guanethidine, pentamidine, phenylbutazone, salicylates, sulfinpyrazone, tetracyclines.

Parameters to monitor
- Serum glucose level frequently. Glucose levels of 80–120 mg/dL are considered to be the target for good/optimum control. Monitor blood glucose frequently at times of stress because under such conditions there is an increased need for insulin.
- Determine HbA_{1C} level in serum at least every 6 months following onset of treatment. A HbA_{1C} value of 6–8% indicates good glucose control whereas values of 11–13% indicate poor glucose control.

- Ocular status. Order a retinal examination by an ophthalmologist at least once a year in all patients with a 5-year history of insulin-dependent diabetes.
- Perform urinalysis, with attention to urine protein and serum creatinine levels, once a year.
- Status of the patient's foot and leg should be determined for signs of ulcer at the time of diagnosis and at regular intervals after insulin therapy is begun.

Editorial comments

- Human insulin may have an advantage to patients who are allergic to porcine or beef forms of the drug.
- Human insulin is preferred over other forms in patients requiring short-term therapy such as pregnancy, infection, surgery to prevent antibody development as well as for patients who have developed insulin resistance or lipoatrophy.
- In general the patient should be scheduled for an office visit at least every 3 months while receiving insulin.
- Patient should be taught how to self-monitor blood glucose levels. Those patients with insulin-dependent diabetes who are receiving intensive therapy must test their blood glucose as often as 4–8 times a day to provide information necessary for maintaining the proper insulin dosage.

Interferon Alfa 2α Recombinant

Brand name: Roferon-A.
Class of drug: Antineoplastic biologic response modifier.
Mechanism of action: Interferon inhibits replication of viruses or tumor cells, enhances macrophage phagocytic activity, and activates natural killer cells.
Indications/dosage/route: IM, SC.

- Hairy cell leukemia
  - Adults: Induction: SC or IM 2–3×10^6 IU daily or 3 times/wk. Protocols vary from 16 to 24 weeks. Maintenance: SC or IM 3×10^6 IU 3 times weekly.

- AIDS-associated Karposi sarcoma
  - Adults: Induction: SC or IM 36×10^6 IU daily, 10–12 weeks; Maintenance: SC or IM 36×10^6 IU 3 times weekly.
- Chronic hepatitis C
  - Adults: SC or IM 3×10^6 IU three times weekly. Continue therapy for 12 months. Longer-duration therapies under investigation.
- Chronic hepatitis B
  - Adults: SC or IM $5–10 \times 10^6$ IU three times weekly. Reduce dose to minimize development of side effects. 16-week course. Also used for condyloma infection, experimental chemotherapy.

Adjustment of dosage
- Kidney disease: None.
- Liver disease: None.
- Elderly: Use with caution due to increased tendency for neurotoxicity and cardiotoxicity.
- Pediatric: No data available. Best to avoid.

Pregnancy: Category C.

Lactation: Appears in breast milk. Potentially toxic to infant. Avoid breastfeeding.

Contraindications: Hypersensitivity to interferon or to mouse immunoglobulin, decompensated liver disease, recipients of transplants receiving immunosuppressant drugs, sensitivity to benyzl alcohol.

Warnings/precautions
- Use with caution in patients with the following conditions: COPD, pulmonary embolism, diabetes mellitus (prone to ketoacidosis), severe bone marrow suppression, seizure disorders, cardiac disease (uncontrolled CHF, unstable angina), limited cardiac reserve, chicken pox (history), herpes zoster, brain metastasis, multiple sclerosis, severe kidney or hepatic disease, coagulation disorders, hemophilia, pulmonary embolism, thrombophlebitis.
- Warn patient that different brands of interferon may not be therapeutically equivalent and therefore are not interchangeable.
- The SC route is suggested for patients who are at risk for bleeding or who are thrombocytopenic.

• Instruct patient and family on the proper technique for preparation and administration of interferon, including proper technique for SC injection and care and disposal of solution and equipment.

Advice to patient

• Do not change brands of interferon without consulting treating physician.
• Avoid alcohol.
• Store interferon in the refrigerator not in the freezer.
• Receive vaccinations (particularly live attenuated viruses) only with permission from treating physician.
• Do not have close contact with individuals who may have taken an oral polio vaccine.
• Avoid driving and other activities requiring mental alertness or that are potentially dangerous until response to drug is known.
• Avoid crowds as well as patients who may have a contagious disease.
• Drink large amounts of fluids (2–3 L/d).
• Use two forms of birth control including hormonal and barrier methods.
• Use proper oral hygiene because there may be an increased tendency for oral infections as a result of bone marrow depression.
• Do not take OTC medications for colds, coughs, allergies without obtaining medical approval.
• Do not reuse syringes and needles.

Adverse reactions

• Common: confusion, dizziness, decreased mental status, dry mouth, inflammation of pharynx, anorexia, nausea, vomiting, abdominal pain, weight loss, cough, dyspnea, rash, flu-like syndrome.
• Serious: **bone marrow suppression**, neuropathy, liver toxicity, arrhythmias, CHF, psychiatric disturbance, hypothyroidism, renal toxicity.

Clinically important drug interactions

• Drugs that increase effects/toxicity of interferon: bone marrow depressant therapy, radiation therapy, vincristine, vinblastine, ziduvidine, ACE inhibitors, acyclovir.

- Interferon increases effects/toxicity of CNS depressants, live virus vaccine, theophylline, aminophylline.

Parameters to monitor

- Signs and symptoms of bone marrow depression.
- Signs and symptoms of thrombocytopenia. Discontinue this medication if platelet count falls below 100,000/mm^3.
- Cardiac status (ECG), particularly in those who have cardiac disease.
- For diabetic patients, baseline ophthalmologic evaluation.
- Signs of autoimmune disease. If these appear, interferon should be discontinued.
- Neuropsychiatric monitoring for depression, suicidal ideation, headaches, diplopia, seizures, sluggish affect, depression, coma.

Editorial comments

- Interferon should be administered only by a physician qualified and experienced in its use.
- Cytotoxic drug. Use latex gloves and safety glasses when handling this medication; avoid contact with skin and inhalation. If possible prepare in biologic hood. Solutions should be stored in a biologic containment cabinet. Before use, the vials should not be shaken.
- The following tests should be performed before initiating therapy with interferon to determine the outcome of the response to treatment in patients with hairy cell leukemia: CBC, hemoglobin, platelet count, granulocytes, bone marrow hairy cells. Treatment should be discontinued if there is not a good response in 6 months.

Isoniazid (Isonicotinic Acid Hydrazide)

Brand names: INH, Laniazid, Nidrazide, Rifamate.
Class of drug: Antituberculous drug.
Mechanism of action: Inhibits cell wall synthesis in mycobacterial organisms.

Indications/dosage/route: Oral, IM.

• Primary treatment for active tuberculosis; first-line drug for combination therapy
  – Adults: PO or IM 5–10 mg/kg daily. Maximum: 300 mg/d. Therapy should be continued for 9–24 months.
  – Infants/children: PO or IM 10 mg/kg daily. Maximum: 300 mg/kg/d. Therapy should be continued for 18–24 months.
• Prophylaxis against TB bacillus, prophylaxis following exposure: Drug of choice
  – Adults: 5 mg/kg/d Maximum: PO 300 mg/d. Treatment is continued for 6–12 months.
  – Infants/children: PO 10 mg/kg/d. Maximum: 300 mg/d. Treatment for 6–12 months.

Adjustment of dosage

• Kidney disease: Creatinine clearance <30 mL/min: decrease dosage by 50%.
• Liver disease: Dose should be reduced in severe liver disease.
• Elderly: Use with caution.
• Pediatric: See above.

Food: Ideally, should be taken on an empty stomach; may administer with food if gastric irritation occurs. There may be a severe reaction if isoniazid is taken along with foods that contain large amounts of tyramine (eg, aged cheese, Chianti wine, pickled herring).

Pregnancy: Category C.

Lactation: Appears in breast milk. Potentially toxic to infant. Considered compatible by American Academy of Pediatrics. Monitor infant closely for neurotoxicity.

Contraindications: Acute liver disease, prior liver toxicity associated with INH therapy, severe hypersensitivity reaction to isoniazid (drug fever, arthritis).

Warnings/precautions

• Use with caution in patients with the following conditions: chronic liver disease, seizures, severe renal disease, chronic alcoholism, malnutrition, predisposition to neuropathy, concurrent use of phenytoin.

- Administer pyridoxone (10–50 mg/d) to diabetics, alcoholics, malnourished patients to prevent development of peripheral neuropathy.
- Seizures should be controlled before beginning therapy with isoniazid.

Advice to patient

- Avoid alcohol.
- Drink 2–3 L of fluids/d.
- Report symptoms of drug side effects such as fatigue, anorexia, weakness (symptoms of hepatitis) to treating physician and stop drug.
- Continue therapy uninterrupted to prevent relapse and spread of infection.

Adverse reactions

- Common: anorexia, nausea, abdominal pain, weakness.
- Serious: **peripheral neuropathy, hepatitis**, bone marrow suppression, seizures, depression, optic neuritis, blindness.

Clinically important drug interactions

- Drugs that increase effects/toxicity of isoniazid: alcohol, rifampin, *para*-aminosalicylic acid, atropine.
- Drugs that decrease effects/toxicity of isoniazid: corticosteroids, aluminum-containing antacids.
- Isoniazid increases effects/toxicity of phenytoin, benzodiazepines (diazepam, triazolam), carbamazepine, disulfiram, cycloserine, meperidine.
- Isoniazid decrease effects/toxicity of oral anticoagulants, ketoconazole.

Parameters to monitor

- Symptoms of peripheral neuropathy, particularly in patients who are diabetic, malnourished, or alcoholics. Administer pyridoxine 10–50 mg/d prophylactically to reverse these effects.
- Hepatic function for hepatitis. This should be evaluated prior to and at least monthly throughout therapy. Discontinue drug immediately if normalization of liver enzymes does not occur despite continuing drug administration. Rapid acetylators are more likely to develop hepatitis.

- Signs and symptoms of ocular toxicity. Periodic fundic examination should be performed to check for optic neuritis. Patient should be examined for changes in visual acuity, eye pain, and blurred vision.
- Signs and symptoms of adverse CNS effects: dizziness, drowsiness, uncontrolled eye movements, headache, diplopia, seizures, sluggish affect, depression, coma.
- Signs of hypersensitivity reactions.
- Signs and symptoms of bone marrow depression.

Editorial comments

- Isoniazid is only used along with a variety of other drugs including rifampin, ethambutol, pyrazinamide. Such combinations are essential to reduce the possibility of resistance development by the TB bacillus.
- Patients who have close personal contact with persons with active TB should receive isoniazid for prophylaxis.
- In poorly compliant patients, isoniazid may be administered on a twice weekly basis at a dose of 15 mg/kg PO. Maximum dose is 900 mg/d.
- Individuals who are exposed to a potentially infectious case of TB should undergo tuberculin skin testing and have a chest x-ray. Such individuals should be given isoniazid as preventive therapy even if skin test is negative after clinical disease is excluded, as should those who have had x-ray evidence of a history of inactive TB or active TB that was not treated adequately.
- The agent is generally available in combination with rifampin.

Isoprotrenol

Brand names: Dispos-a-Med Isoproterenol HCl, Isuprel, Medi-haler-Iso.

Class of drug: β-Adrenergic agonist, bronchodilator, pressor agent.

Mechanism of action: Agonist at α- and β-adrenergic receptors, thereby producing bronchodilation and inotropic and chronotropic actions on heart.

Indications/dosage/route: IV, IM, SC, inhalation.

- Shock, cardiac standstill, cardiac arrhythmias
  - Adults: IV, infusion, 5 μg/min.
- Cardiac standstill, cardiac arrhythmias
  - Adults: IV 0.02–0.06 mg.
- Cardiac standstill and cardiac arrhythmias
  - Adults: IM, SC 1 mL of 1:5000 solution.
- Intracardiac (in extreme emergencies)
  - Adults: IM, SC 0.1 mL of 1:5000 solution.
- Acute bronchial asthma: handheld nebulizer
  - Adults/children: 5–15 deep inhalations of the 1:200 solution. If no relief after 5–10 minutes, repeat one more time up to 5 times/d if necessary.
- Bronchospasm in COPD
  - Adults/children: 5–15 deep inhalations of the 1:200 solution. 3–4 hours should elapse between uses.
- Acute bronchial asthma: metered-dose inhalation
  - Adults: 1–2 inhalations. If no relief within 2–5 minutes, second inhalation may be used. Maintenance: 1–2 inhalations 4–6 times/d. Maximum: 6 inhalations in 1 hour.
- Bronchospasm in COPD
  - Adults/children: 1–2 inhalations repeated at 3- to 4-hour intervals.
- Bronchospasms in COPD: intermittent positive-pressure breathing
  - Adults/children: 0.5 mL of a 1:200 solution diluted to 2–2.4 mL with water or isotonic saline.

Adjustment of dosage

- Kidney disease: None.
- Liver disease: None.
- Elderly: Lower doses may be required.
- Pediatric: See above

	Onset of Action	Peak Effect	Duration
SC	≈30 min	—	1–2 h
IV	Immediate	—	<1 h
Inhalation	2–5 min	—	0.5–2 h

Food: Not applicable.

Pregnancy: Category C.

Lactation: No data available. Potentially toxic to infant. Best to avoid.

Contraindications: Hypersensitivity to adrenergic compounds, tachycardia (idiopathic or from digitalis).

Warnings/precautions

- Use with caution in patients with the following conditions: hyperthyroidism, diabetes, coronary insufficiency, ischemic heart disease, cardiac arrhythmias, history of stroke, CHF, hypertension.
- Some preparations contain bisulfite, which may cause an allergic reaction in sensitive individuals.
- Instruct patient in proper technique for using nebulizer and/or inhaler.
- Overuse as bronchodilator is potentially toxic. May cause systemic adrenergic effects including tachycardia. Can produce paradoxical bronchospasm.

Advice to patient

- Avoid OTC products without consulting treating physician.
- Do not use solutions that contain a precipitate or are discolored.
- Wait at least 1 minute after 1 or 2 inhalations before taking a third dose.
- Keep inhalant away from eyes.
- Maintain adequate fluid intake (2000–3000 mL/d) to facilitate clearing of secretions.
- Rinse mouth with water after each inhalation to minimize dry mouth and throat irritation.
- Administer inhalant when arising in the morning and before meals.

• Notify treating physician if more than 3 aerosol inhalations are required to achieve relief within a 24-hour period. Do not increase dose in an attempt to obtain relief.

Adverse reactions

• Common: tremor, restlessness, tachycardia, nervousness, insomnia, discolored saliva, dry mouth.
• Serious: hypertension, ventricular arrhythmias, profound hypotension, bronchospasm.

Clinically important drug interactions

• Drugs that increase effects/toxicity of isoproterenol: ipratropium, MAO inhibitors, tricyclic antidepressants.
• Drugs that decrease activity of isoproterenol: sympathomimetic drugs (nasal decongestants, weight loss drugs, eg, phenylpropanolamine), anticholinergic drugs, phenothiazines.

Parameters to monitor

• Heart rate, BP.
• Observe for worsening bronchospasm after use.
• Possible development of tolerance with prolonged use. Discontinue drug temporarily and effectiveness will be restored.
• Signs of paradoxical bronchospasm.
• Pulmonary function on initiation and during bronchodilator therapy. Assess respiratory rate, sputum character (color, quantity), peak airway flow, O_2 saturation and blood gases.
• Efficacy of treatment: improved breathing, prevention of bronchospasm, reduction of asthmatic attacks, prevention of exercise-induced asthma. If no relief is obtained from 3–5 aerosol inhalations within 6–12 hours, reevaluate effectiveness of treatment.
• FEV_1 to determine effectiveness of the drug to reverse bronchostriction. Efficacy is indicated by an increase in FEV_1 of 10–20%. In addition such patients, as well as those who have chronic disease, should be given a peak flow gauge and told to determine peak expiratory flow rate at least twice daily.
• Determine arterial blood gases if applicable.

Editorial comments

• For patients with acute asthma or acute exacerbation of COPD,

reduce dose to minimum necessary to control condition after initial relief is achieved. For chronic conditions, the patient should be reassessed every 1–6 months following control of symptoms.
• This drug is listed without details in the *Physician's Desk Reference*, 54th edition, 2000.

Isosorbide Dinitrate

Brand names: Isordril, Sorbitrate.
Class of drug: Antianginal, vasodilator, oral nitrate.
Mechanism of action: Reduces peripheral resistance (arterial and venous) by vasodilation; decreases left ventricular pressure.
Indications/dosage/route: Oral, sublingual.
• Acute anginal attack
  – Initial: PO 5–20 mg q6h. Maintenance: 20–40 mg q6h. Sublingual: 2.5–5 mg q2–3h as needed.
• Prophylaxis or treatment of anginal attacks
  – PO, sublingual 5–10 mg q2–3h.
Adjustment of dosage
• Kidney disease: None.
• Liver disease: None.
• Elderly: Lower doses may be required.
• Pediatric: Safety and efficacy have not been established in children.

	Onset of Action	Duration
Sublingual	2–5 min	1–3 h
Oral	20–40 min	4–6 h

Food: Take 1 hour before or 2 hours after meals with full glass of water (oral preparations only).
Pregnancy: Category C.

Lactation: No data available. Best to avoid.

Contraindications: Hypersensitivity to nitrates or nitrites, very low BP, shock, acute MI with low ventricular filling pressure.

Warnings/precautions

- Use with caution in patients with the following conditions: depleted blood volume, increased intraocular pressure, severe obliterative vascular disease, low systolic BP (below 90 mm Hg), allergy to tartrazine dye, volume depletion, coronary artery disease, heart rate <50 beats/min.
- Tolerance cannot be overcome by increasing the dose. Fourteen-hour drug holidays are recommended to restore activity when tolerance develops.
- Withdrawal responses with associated chest pain and myocardial ischemia are a concern with chronic exposure to nitrates.
- Sustained-release forms may not be effective in patients with small intestinal malabsorption.
- May exacerbate angina in patients with hypertrophic cardiomyopathy.
- Be aware that this agent may produce marked hypotension, at times associated with bradycardia and/or worsening angina.
- Benefit of this drug in the setting of acute MI or CHF has not been established.

Advice to patient

- Be aware of disulfiram reaction after drinking alcohol. Symptoms include headache, facial flush, abdominal cramps, tachycardia. These symptoms generally occur within 2–3 minutes of alcohol ingestion and may last 1–4 hours. Contact treating physician.
- Change position slowly, in particular from recumbent to upright, to minimize orthostatic hypotension. Sit at the edge of the bed for several minutes before standing, and lie down if feeling faint or dizzy. Avoid hot showers or baths and standing for long periods. Male patients should sit on the toilet while urinating rather than standing.
- Avoid alcohol.
- Carry identification card at all times describing disease, treatment regimen, name, address, and telephone number of treating physician.

- Sit when taking a nitrate to avoid injury from dizziness or syncope.
- Headache may frequently accompany use of the drug. Use acetaminophen or aspirin to treat. Notify physician if headache is persistent or severe.
- Do not stop taking the drug abruptly as this may precipitate angina.
- Use OTC medications only after first informing the treating physician.
- Avoid abrupt withdrawal as this may precipitate angina.

Adverse reactions
- Common: headache.
- Serious: postural hypotension, cardiovascular collapse, arrhythmias, methemoglobinema.

Clinically important drug interactions
- Drugs that increase effects/toxicity of nitrates: alcohol, antihypertensive drugs, aspirin, β blockers, calcium channel blockers, vasodilators.
- Drugs that decrease effects/toxicity of nitrates: sympathomimetics.

Parameters to monitor
- Symptoms of angina, CHF.
- Frequency and severity of anginal attacks. Monitor for development of tolerance as shown by worsening coronary disease.
- Signs and symptoms of hypotension. BP should be monitored every 5 minutes when the drug is used for an acute angina attack and every 20–30 minutes thereafter. Maximal drug effect is achieved when systolic BP decreases by 15 mm Hg, diastolic BP decreases by 10 mm Hg, or pulse increases by 10 beats/min.
- Signs and symptoms of methemoglobinemia: blood becomes dark colored, mucosa and nails turn bluish; dyspnea, headache, vertigo. This condition requires immediate attention.
- Changes in intraocular pressure. Patient should be monitored periodically if long-term use is required.
- Monitor BP and pulse rate when changing dosage.

Editorial comments
- Nitrates, including nitroglycerin, are the drugs of choice for chronic stable angina. This includes patients with the following preexisting conditions: COPD, asthma, CHF, diabetes.

- This drug serum should not be administered in such a way as to cause constant levels over 24-hour period as this may result in tolerance to vasodilating effects.
- Isosorbide dinitrate and isosorbide mononitrate are useful for patients with angina who do not respond to nitroglycerin. These patients benefit from the longer duration of action of isosorbide dinitrate and isosorbide mononitrate.
- Methemoglobinema (occurring when hemoglobin is oxidized to methemoglobin) may occur in patients on prolonged IV nitrate therapy or following moderate overdosage. This is treated with intravenous methylene blue.

Isosorbide Mononitrate

Brand names: Monoket, Imdur, Ismo.
Class of drug: Antianginal, vasodilator, oral nitrate.
Mechanism of action: Reduces peripheral resistance (arterial and venous) by vasodilation; decreases left ventricular pressure.
Indications/dosage/route: Oral only.
- Prophylaxis of angina (Imdur)
  – Initial: 30 or 60 mg once daily. Maitenance: 120 mg once daily.
- Prophylaxis and treatment of angina (Ismo, Monoket)
  – 20 mg t.i.d.
Adjustment of dosage
- Kidney disease: None.
- Liver disease: None.
- Elderly: Lower doses may be required.
- Pediatric: Safety and efficacy have not been established in children.

Onset of Action	Duration
30–60 min	4–6 h

Food: Take 1 hour before or 2 hours after meals with full glass of water.
Pregnancy: Category B.
Lactation: No data available. Best to avoid.
Contraindications: Hypersensitivity to nitrates or nitrites.
Editorial comments: For additional information, see *isosorbide dinitrate*, p. 473.

Isotretinoin

Brand name: Accutane.
Class of drug: Antiacne agent, retinoic acid derivative.
Mechanism of action: Isotretinoin decreases the size of sebaceous glands, reduces production of sebum.
Indications/dosage/route: Oral only.
• Severe nodular acne only in patients who do not respond to conventional therapy. (This includes oral antibiotics.)
  – Adults, adolescents, children: Initial: 0.5–1 mg/kg/d. Maintentance: 0.5–2 mg/kg/d, 2 divided doses; 15–20 weeks or until cyst count decreases by 70%. The drug may be discontinued if the total cyst count is reduced by more than 70% before the 15- to 20-week period of treatment.
Adjustment of dosage: None.
Food: Should be taken with food.
Pregnancy: Category X. Contraindicated. Should be avoided in patients potentially capable of becoming pregnant. Women of childbearing age can use isotretinoin only if they can reliably understand risks and use proper contraceptive methods.
Lactation: Probably appears in breast milk. Potentially toxic to infant. Avoid breastfeeding.
Contraindications: Sensitivity to other retinoids, pregnancy, hypersensitivity to parabens (preservative used in the drug capsule).

Warnings/precautions
- Use with caution in patients with the following conditions: diabetes, hypertriglyceridemia.
- Effective contraception must be used for at least 1 month before isotretinoin is administered and for 1 month after therapy is discontinued.
- See Editorial Comments for detailed pregnancy warnings.

Advice to patient
- Use two forms of birth control including hormonal and barrier methods.
- Do not donate blood when taking this drug.
- Inform patient that the acne condition may worsen initially.
- Avoid alcohol and other CNS depressants such as opiate analgesics and sedatives (eg, diazepam) when taking this drug.
- Avoid driving and other activities requiring mental alertness or that are potentially dangerous until response to drug is known.
- Do not ingest vitamin supplements containing vitamin A when taking this drug.

Adverse reactions
- Common: cheilitis, dry skin, arthralgias, rash, nausea, vomiting, thinning hair, elevated plasma triglycerides, cholesterol, decreased HDL cholesterol.
- Serious: pseudotumor cerebri (benign intracranial hypertension), depression, psychosis, suicide, seizures, hepatitis, skeletal hyperostosis.

Clinically important drug interactions
- Drugs that increase effects/toxicity of isotretinoin: vitamin A products, tetracyclines, alcohol, benzoyl peroxide, tretinoin.
- Isotretinoin increases effects/toxicity of minocycline, tetracycline, vitamin A.
- Isotretinoin decreases effects/toxicity of carbamazepine.

Parameters to monitor
- Baseline sedimentation rate, serum triglycerides, CBC with differential and platelets.
- Skin condition. Note whether improvement is occurring.

- Symptoms of pseudotumor cerebri including headache, nausea, vomiting, visual disturbances, papilledema. Patient exhibiting these symptoms should discontinue drug immediately.
- Symptoms of visual difficulties including corneal opacities. If these are observed, drug should be discontinued and an ophthalmologic exam performed.
- Liver enzymes. If these are increased significantly, reduce dose. If the values do not return to baseline, discontinue drug.
- Evidence of psychiatric distrubances occurring during therapy. Discontinue medication if these occur.

Editorial comments
- An informed consent must be obtained from the patient or other authorized individuals before isotretinoin is administered. All parties concerned must be made fully aware of the consequences of exposure of the fetus to the drug.
- Contraindicated in adults or children capable of becoming pregnant unless the patient meets all the following criteria:
    1. Has severe disfiguring cystic acne that does not respond to standard therapy.
    2. Has been apprised and understands completely instructions concerning its use.
    3. Is fully aware of the problems of becoming pregnant and is capable of complying with contraceptives that are mandated.
    4. Has been given oral and written warnings and hazards of taking isotretinoin during pregnancy.
    5. Has had a serum pregnancy test (sensitivity of at least 50 mIU/mL) that is negative within 1 week of beginning therapy.
    6. Has agreed to begin therapy only on the second or third day of next normal menstrual cycle.
- This medication should be prescribed only by physicians with competence in treating severe, recalcitrant nodular acne and experienced in the use of retinoid therapy. They should also be knowledgeable of the potential teratogenic effects of isotretinoin.

Itraconazole

Brand name: Sporanox.
Class of drug: Antifungal agent.
Mechanism of action: Inhibits fungal cytochrome P450 synthesis of ergosterol, resulting in decreased cell wall integrity and leakage of essential cellular components.
Susceptible organisms *in vitro*: Not for cryptococcosis (fluconazole is preferred). *Blastomyces dermatidis, Candida, Histoplasma, Aspergillus flavus, Coccidioides immitis, Sporotrichosis.*
Indications/dosage/route: Oral only.
• Blastomycosis or histoplasmosis
  – Adults: 200 mg once daily. If there is no improvement or the disease is progressive, the dose may be increased in 100-mg increments. Maximum: 400 mg/d.
  – Children 3–16 years: 100 mg/d.
• Aspergillosis
  – Adults: 400 mg daily.
• Life-threatening infections
  – Adults: 200 mg t.i.d. for the first 3 days.
• Onychomycosis
  – Adults: 200 mg once a day for 12 consecutive weeks.
• Oral solution: oropharyngeal candidiasis
  – Adults: 200 mg/d for 1–2 weeks.
• Oral solution: esophageal candidiasis
  – Adults: 100 mg/d, minimum 3 weeks.
Adjustment of dosage
• Kidney disease: None.
• Liver disease: None.
• Elderly: None.
• Pediatric: Safety and efficacy have not been established in children <3 years.
Food: Should be taken with food.
Pregnancy: Category C.
Lactation: Appears in breast milk. Avoid breastfeeding.

Contraindications: Hypersensitivity to itraconazole and other azole antifungals, coadministration of astemizole, triazolam, midazolam; treatment of onchomycosis during pregnancy.

Warnings/precautions

• Review drugs that patient is currently taking to avoid possible dangerous drug–drug interactions.

Advice to patient

• Report symptoms of possible liver dysfunction: jaundice, anorexia, dark urine, pale stools, nausea, vomiting.

• Avoid driving and other activities requiring mental alertness or that are potentially dangerous until response to drug is known.

• Avoid alcohol.

• To minimize possible photosensitivity reaction, apply adequate sunscreen and use proper covering when exposed to strong sunlight.

Adverse reactions

• Common: nausea, vomiting, diarrhea, abdominal pain, rash.

• Serious: hepatotoxicity (rare), exfoliative skin disorders (rare).

Clinically important drug interactions

• Itraconazole increases effects/toxicity of the following: astemizole, calcium blockers, cisapride, cyclosporine, digoxin, midazolam, sulfonylureas, tacrolimus, triazolam, warfarin.

• The following drugs decrease effects/toxicity of the following: itraconzole: isoniazid, phenytoin, rifampin, phenobarbital.

Parameters to monitor

• Signs and symptoms of liver toxicity, particularly in patients receiving treatment longer than 1 month.

• Symptoms indicating reactivation of blastomycosis: rales, chest pain, cough, fever, rash, SOB, weight loss.

• Symptoms indicating reactivation of histoplasmosis: Chest pain, generalized pain, rales, SOB, weight loss.

Editorial comments

• Itraconazole is not used for cryptococcosis (fluconazole is preferred). It is a broad-spectrum antifungal agent and covers *Aspergillus* species.

• For severe infections, amphotericin B is preferred.

- Itraconazole is very effective against onycomycosis, *Candida* infections, *Blastomyces, Histoplasma*, coccidiomycosis, aspergillosis, and sporotrichosis. It is effective for CNS infections. In general, amphotericin B is used acutely, then itraconazole is given as long-term therapy.

Ketamine

Brand name: Ketalor.
Class of drug: Intravenous general anesthetic.
Mechanism of action: Direct CNS effect causing dissociative anesthesia.
Indications/dosage/route: IV, IM.
• Induction of general anesthesia
  – Adults/children: IV 1–4.5 mg/kg administered over 60 seconds. IM 6.5–13 mg/kg. *Note*: Repeat in increments of half to complete initial dose to maintain anesthesia.
Adjustment of dosage
• Kidney disease: None.
• Liver disease: None.
• Elderly: Must be used with caution, particularly in patients with hypertension, cardiac disease.
• Pediatric: See above.

	Onset of Action	Duration
IV	30 s	5–10 min
IM	3–4 min	12–25 min

Food: Not applicable.
Pregnancy: Category D.
Lactation: Avoid nursing for at least 11 hours after dosage.
Contraindications: Acute psychosis, schizophrenia, CHF, increased intracranial pressure, aneurysm, thyrotoxicosis, psychotic disorders, hypersensitivity to ketamine.
Warnings/precautions: Emergent reactions including hallucinations, delerium, and vivid dreams may occur up to 24 hours after administration.
Advice to patient: Not applicable.
Adverse reactions
• Common: hypertension, tachycardia, hallucinations.

• Serious: **emergent reactions, myocardial depression, increased intracranial pressure,** arrhythmias, respiratory depression or apnea (if administered too rapidly), bradycardia, increased intraocular pressure, depressed cough reflex.

Clinically important drug interactions

• Drugs that increase effects/toxicity of ketamine: barbiturates, opioids, thyroid hormone, halothane, hydroxyzine, muscle relaxants.
• Ketamine increases toxicity of nondepolarizing relaxants (curare-type drugs).

Parameters to monitor: Cardiac effects, pulse, BP, respirations, oxygen saturation.

Editorial comments

• Ketamine should be used only under the strict guidance and supervision of physicians who are experienced in the administration of general anesthetics. Such physicians must be knowledgeable in maintaining an airway and controlling respiration. It is essential that methods be available for resuscitation if necessary.
• This drug is not listed in the *Physician's Desk Reference*, 54th edition, 2000.

Ketoconazole

Brand name: Nizoral.
Class of drug: Antifungal agent.
Mechanism of action: Inhibits synthesis of steroids in fungal cell membranes, resulting in leakage of essential cellular components.
Susceptible organisms *in vitro*: *Candida* sp, *Cryptococcus, Coccidioides, Histoplasma, Blastomyces.*
Indications/dosage/route: Oral only.

• Systemic fungal infections
 – Adults: 200 mg once daily. Increase to 400 mg once daily if needed.

– Children >2 years: 3.3–6.6 mg/kg once daily.

Adjustment of dosage

• Kidney disease: None.
• Liver disease: None.
• Elderly: None.
• Pediatric: Safety and efficacy in children <2 years have not been established.

Food: Should be taken with food, especially citrus juices.

Pregnancy: Category C.

Lactation: Probably present in breast milk. Avoid breastfeeding.

Contraindications: Hypersensitivity to ketoconazole or other azole antifungals, concomitant astemizole, triazolam.

Warnings/precautions

• Treatment of candidiasis requires 1–2 weeks; for other systemic mycoses, 6 months.
• Do not administer along with astemizole or other azoles.

Advice to patient

• Take antacids, if needed, 2 hours after this drug. The same is true for other drugs that decrease gastric activity, eg, H_2 blockers.
• Report symptoms of possible liver dysfunction: jaundice, anorexia, dark urine, pale stools, nausea, vomiting.
• Avoid driving and other activities requiring mental alertness or that are potentially dangerous until response to drug is known.
• Avoid alcohol.
• To minimize possible photosensitivity reaction, apply adequate sunscreen and use proper covering when exposed to strong sunlight.

Adverse reactions

• Common: nausea, vomiting, diarrhea, abdominal pain.
• Serious: hepatotoxicity.

Clinically important drug interactions

• Ketoconazole increases effects/toxicity of hepatotoxic drugs, cisapride, oral anticoagulants, astemizole, cyclosporine, astemizole, corticosteroids, midazolam, triazolam.
• Ketoconazole decreases effects/toxicity of theophylline.

- The following drugs decrease effects/toxicity of ketoconazole: antacids (containing calcium, aluminum), anticholinergics, rifampin, isoniazid.

Parameters to monitor: Signs and symptoms of liver toxicity.

Editorial comments

- Ketoconazole is effective in non-CNS infections caused by *Candida,* blastomycosis, histoplasmosis, and coccidiomycosis.
- Problems with oral absorption occur, especially in patients with AIDS, neutropenic patients, or patients on antacids or other acid-blocking agents.
- This drug should not be used in cryptoccal infections. Fluconazole should be substituted.

Ketoprofen

Brand name: Orudis.

Class of drug: NSAID.

Mechanism of action: Inhibits cyclooxygenase, resulting in inhibition of synthesis of prostaglandins and other inflammatory mediators.

Indications/dosage/route: Oral only.

- Rheumatoid arthritis, osteoarthritis
  - Adults: 75 mg t.i.d. or 50 mg q.i.d. Maintenance: 150–300 mg in 3–4 divided doses. Maximum: 300 mg/d.
- Mild to moderate pain, dysmenorrhea
  - Adults: 25–50 mg q6–8h. Maximum: 300 mg/d.
  - Adults, children >16 years: 12.5–25 mg q4–6h. Maximum: 75 mg/d.

Adjustment of dosage:

- Kidney disease: Monitor carefully. Guidelines for drug administration are not available.
- Liver disease: Monitor carefully. Administer minimum doses.

• Elderly: May be necessary to reduce dose for patients >75 years.

• Pediatric: Safety and efficacy have not been established.

Food: Take with food or large quantities of water or milk.

Pregnancy: Category B. Category D in third trimester or near delivery.

Lactation: Appears in breast milk. Breastfeeding considered by some authors to be low risk.

Contraindications: Hypersensitivity and cross-sensitivity with other NSAIDs and aspirin.

Editorial comments: For additional information, see *ibuprofen*, p. 445.

Ketorolac

Brand names: Toradol, Acular (Ophthalmic).
Class of drug: NSAID.
Mechanism of Action: Inhibits cyclooxygenase, resulting in inhibition of synthesis of prostaglandins and other inflammatory mediators.
Indications/dosage/route: Oral, IV, IM, topical (ophthalmic).

• Analgesia, short term only (up to 5 days)
  – Adults ≤65 years: IM 60 mg or IM, IV 30 mg q6h. Maximum: 120 mg/d.
  – Adults <65 years: IM 30 mg or IM, IV 15 mg q6h. Maximum: 60 mg/d.
  – Adults <65 years: IM 60 or 30 mg q6h. Maximum: 120 mg.
  – Adults >65 years: IM 30 mg or IV, IM 15 mg q6h. Maximum: 60 mg/d.

• Seasonal allergic conjunctivitis, ophthalmic solution, 1 week only
  – 1 drop 0.25 mg q.i.d.

• Following cataract surgery, ophthalmic solution
  – 1 drop to the affected eye(s) q.i.d.

Adjustment of dosage
• Kidney disease: None.
• Liver disease: None.
• Elderly: Maximum: 60 mg daily.
• Pediatric: Safety and efficacy have not been established in children under 12 years.

Food: Take with food or large quantities of water or milk.

Pregnancy: Category C. Category D in third trimester or near delivery.

Lactation: Appears in breast milk. Considered compatible with breastfeeding by American Academy of Pediatrics.

Contraindications: Active peptic ulcer, history of peptic ulcer disease, severe kidney disease, patients at risk for renal failure due to volume depletion, cerebrovascular bleeding (suspected or confirmed), prophylactic analgesia before or during surgery, concurrent aspirin or NSAID, epidural or intrathecal administration of ketorolac, hypersensitivity and cross-sensitivity with other NSAIDs and aspirin. Ophthalmic solution: hypersensitivity to any ingredient in the formulations of patients wearing soft contact lenses.

Warnings/precautions
• Use with caution in patients with the following conditions: history of GI bleeding, decreased renal function, CHF, acute or chronic liver disease, rhinitis, urticaria, hay fever, nasal polyps, asthma, elderly.
• Administer this drug with caution in patients having infections or other diseases as the drug may mask symptoms of the disease, eg, fever, inflammation.
• Bleeding and perforation of GI ulcers are serious and common toxic effects of ketorolac.
• Combined duration of IV and oral use should not exceed 5 days.
• Elderly and debilitated patients and patients with a prior history of peptic ulcer disease are at high risk for GI toxicity.
• NSAIDs may cause severe allergic reactions including urticaria and vasomotor collapse. Cross-reactivity may occur in patients allergic to aspirin.

- Renal toxicity occurs most commonly in patients with hypovolemia or decreased renal blood flow.
- Ketorolac may cause fluid retention.
- Inhibition of platelet function by ketorolac lasts from 24 to 48 hours.

Advice to patient

- Avoid use of alcohol.
- Notify physician if your stool turns dark, if you develop abdominal pain, or if you vomit blood or dark material.
- Notify dentist or treating physician prior to surgery if taking this medication.
- Avoid taking OTC products that contain aspirin or other NSAIDs, eg, Alka-Seltzer.
- Take drug with full glass of water and sit up for 15–30 minutes to avoid lodging of tablet in esophagus.
- If pain occurs with physical activity, take drug 30 minutes before physical therapy or other planned exercise.

Adverse reactions

- Common: nausea, indigestion, dizziness, fatigue.
- Serious: depression, postoperative hematomas, dyspnea, GI bleeding (peptic ulcer, diverticular NSAID colitis), acute renal failure, bronchospasm, Stevens–Johnson syndrome, renal or hepatic toxicity, GI perforation.

Clinically important drug interactions

- Drugs that increase effects/toxicity of ketorolac: alcohol, corticosteroids, insulin, cimetidine, probenicid.
- Drugs that decrease effects/toxicity of ketorolac: barbiturates.
- Ketorolac increases effects/toxicity of oral anticoagulants, heparin, lithium, methotrexate, phenytoin, carbomazepines, SSRIs, sulfonamides, sufonlyureas, nondepolarizing neuromuscular relaxants.
- Ketorolac decreases effects/toxicity of β blockers, furosemide.

Parameters to monitor

- CBC, liver enzymes, stool hemoccult, serum BUN and creatinine.
- Efficacy of treatment: pain reduction, improved mobility. Assess pain reduction 1 or 2 hours after taking drug.

- Rhinitis, asthma, urticaria before beginning treatment. Such patients have increased risk for developing a hypersensitivity reaction to an NSAID.
- Blood glucose of diabetic patients taking oral hypoglycemic drugs. An NSAID may potentiate the hypoglycemic effect of oral hypoglycemic drugs.
- Signs and symptoms of auditory toxicity, in particular tinnitus in elderly patients. Stop drug to avoid irreversible hearing loss. Restart at 50% of previous dose after reversal occurs.
- Symptoms of iron deficiency anemia, particularly in patients on long-term, high-dose drug. Perform hematocrit and guaiac tests periodically.
- Signs of hypersensitivity reactions.
- Signs and symptoms of renal toxicity.
- Signs and symptoms of hepatotoxicity.
- Symptoms of GI toxicity: occult blood loss, symptoms of ulcer, hematochezia, melana, abdominal pain.

Editorial comments: Ketorolac is recommended only for short-term use (up to 5 days) for management of moderate to severe pain.

Labetolol

Brand name: Normodyne.
Class of drug: β Blocker.
Mechanism of action: Competitive blocker of β-adrenergic receptors in heart and blood vessels.
Indications/dosage/route: Oral, IV.
• Severe hypertension
  – Adults: Repeated IV injection: 20 mg injected over 2 minutes. Additional injections of 40–80 mg at 10-minute intervals as needed for supine BP control. Maximum: 300 mg.
  – Adults: Slow continuous infusion: Infuse 1 mg/mL at 2 mL/min (2 mg/min).
  – Adults: Initial: PO 200 mg when BP is under control. Follow in 6–12 hours with additional dose of 200 or 400 mg.
• Hypertension
  – Adults: Initial 100 mg b.i.d, maintenance 200–400 mg b.i.d.
Adjustment of dosage
• Kidney disease: Use caution.
• Liver disease: Use caution.
• Elderly: Use caution. Increased risk for CNS and cardiovascular side effects.
• Pediatric: See above. Intravenous administration not recommended.
Food: No restriction.
Pregnancy: Category C
Lactation: Appears in breast milk. Considered compatible by American Academy of Pediatrics.
Contraindications: Cardiogenic shock, asthma, CHF unless it is secondary to tachyarrhythmia treated with a β blocker, sinus bradycardia and AV block greater than first degree, severe COPD.
Editorial comments
• Labetolol injection is intended for use only in hospitalized patients.
• BP should be monitored carefully during IV administration and after completion of injection.

- Rapid or excessive changes in BP should be avoided.
- Patient should always be in supine position during IV administration.
- For additional information, see *propranolol*, p. 790.

Lamivudine

Brand names: Epivir, Epivir-HBV.
Class of drug: Antiviral nucleoside analogue.
Mechanism of action: Lamivudine inhibits HIV reverse transcriptase and DNA polymerase of HIV.
Indications/dosage/route: Oral only.
- HIV infection, together with zidovudine
  – Adults ≥110 lb, children ≥12: PO 150 mg b.i.d.
  – Adults <110 lb: 2 mg/kg b.i.d.
  – Children 3 months–12 years: 5 mg/kg b.i.d.
- Chronic hepatitis B infection
  – Adults: 100 mg qd.
- Post-HIV exposure in health care worker
  – 150 mg b.i.d. × 4 weeks with zidovudine 200 mg t.i.d. A protease inhibitor may be added for high-risk situations. Initiate therapy within 2 hours of exposure. *Note*: When used along with zidovudine, lamivudine dose is 150 mg b.i.d., zidovudine 200 mg t.i.d.

Adjustment of dosage
- Kidney disease: Creatinine clearance 30–59 mL/min: maintenance 150 mg/d; creatinine clearance 5–14 mL/min: initial 150 mg, maintenance 50 mg/d.
- Liver disease: None.
- Elderly: Dose reduction may be necessary.
- Pediatric: See above.

Food: Should be taken on an empty stomach.
Pregnancy: Category C.

Lactation: No data available. Centers for Disease Control and Prevention recommend that HIV-infected mothers should not breastfeed.

Contraindications: Hypersensitivity to lamivudine.

Warnings/precautions: Use with caution if there is prior history or risk of developing pancreatitis, particularly in children. Stop drug administration if there are clinical or laboratory abnormalities suggestive of pancreatitis, kidney disease, elderly.

Adverse reactions
- Common: headache, insomnia, fatigue, nausea, diarrhea, vomiting, cough, fever, chills, musculoskeletal pain.
- Serious: **pancreatitis (in pediatric patients),** thrombocytopenia, neutropenia, peripheral neuropathy, hepatitis.

Clinically important drug interactions
- The following drugs increase effects/toxicity of lamivudine: trimethoprim–sulfamethoxazole.
- Lamivudine increases effects/toxicity of zidovudine.

Parameters to monitor
- Signs of pancreatitis: abdominal pain, nausea, vomiting. Discontinue therapy if pancreatitis is diagnosed.
- Signs and symptoms of neuropathy.
- Signs and symptoms of hepatotoxicity.

Editorial comments: Lamivudine is not intended as the sole treatment for HIV infection. It is generally administered with zidovudine and/or a protease inhibitor. Epivir-HBV has recently been approved as treatment for chronic hepatitis B infection.

Lamotrigine

Brand name: Lamictal.

Class of drug: Anticonvulsant.

Mechanism of action: Inhibits release of glutamate and aspartate in the brain.

Indications/dosage/route: Oral only.

- Treatment of partial seizures (epilepsy)
  - Adults: 50 mg/d. Maintenance: 500 mg/d in 2 divided doses.
  - Adjustment of dosages required when used in combination with other anticonvulsants including valproic acid, phenytoin, phenobarbital, carbamazepine and primidone.

Adjustment of dosage

- Kidney disease: Limited data available. Use with caution. Reduced dose of maintenance therapy should be considered.
- Liver disease: Reduce dose by 50% for moderate dysfunction and by 75% in severe dysfunction. Increase dose as clinically indicated.
- Elderly: Safety and efficacy in patients >65 years have not been established.
- Pediatric: Safety and efficacy have not been established in children <16 years.

Food: May be taken with food.

Pregnancy: Category C.

Lactation: Appears in breast milk. Potentially toxic to infant. Avoid breastfeeding.

Contraindications: Hypersensitivity to lamotrigine.

Warnings/precautions

- Use with caution in patients with the following conditions: kidney, liver, cardiac diseases.
- Taper slowly (over 2 weeks) prior to discontinuation. Dose should be reduced by 50% per week.
- Serious rashes, including Stevens–Johnson syndrome, have been seen in approximately 0.3% of adults and 1% of pediatric patients treated with lamotrigine.

Advice to patient

- Avoid driving and other activities requiring mental alertness or that are potentially dangerous until response to drug is known.
- To minimize possible photosensitivity reaction, apply adequate sunscreen and use proper covering when exposed to strong sunlight.
- If you experience a loss in seizure control, notify treating physician immediately.

Adverse reactions
- Common: headache, ataxia, dizziness, diplopia, sleepiness, blurred vision, nausea, vomiting, rhinitis, rash.
- Serious: Stevens–Johnson syndrome, angioedema, toxic epidermal necrolysis.

Clinically important drug interactions
- Drug that increases effects/toxicity of lamotrigine: valproic acid.
- Drugs that decrease effects/toxicity of lamotrigine: carbamazepine, phenytoin, primidone, phenobarbital, acetaminophen.
- Lamotrigine increases effects/toxicity of co-trimoxazole, methotrexate.

Parameters to monitor
- Signs of hypersensitivity reactions.
- Signs and symptoms of Stevens–Johnson syndrome: urticaria, edema of mucous membranes (lips, genital organs), headache, high fever, conjunctivitis, rhinitis, stomatitis.
- Efficacy in reducing symptoms of seizure (frequency and duration).
- When the drug is given in adjunctive situations, measure serum levels of the second drug.

Editorial comments: Dosage of lamotrigine is complicated by the enhancement of its metabolism by several antiepileptic drugs (phenytoin, phenobarbital, primidone) and its half-life prolongation by valproic acid. Awareness of these interactions is vital to the proper administration of this drug.

Leflunomide

Brand name: Arava.
Class of drug: Antiarthritic drug, immunomodulator.
Mechanism of action: Inhibits dihydroorotate dehydrogenase, resulting in inhibition of pyrimidine synthesis; also has antiproliferative effect on T cells as well as antinflammatory actions.
Indications/dosage/route: Oral only.
- Rheumatoid arthritis

– Adults: Initial: 100 mg/d, 3 days. Maintenance: 20 mg/d; reduce to 10 mg/d if not well tolerated.

Adjustment of dosage

• Kidney disease: Use with caution. Guidelines not available.
• Liver disease: Contraindicated.
• Elderly: None.
• Pediatric: Contraindicated for children <18 years.

Food: May be taken with or without food.

Pregnancy: Category X. Contraindicated.

Lactation: No data available. Avoid breastfeeding.

Contraindications: Pregnancy, significant liver disease, serology positive for hepatitis B or C. Patients with bone marrow suppression, severe immunodeficiency, or severe infection.

Warnings/precautions

• Use with caution in patients with kidney, liver disease.

Advice to patient

• Use two forms of birth control including hormonal and barrier methods.
• Receive live virus vaccines only with permission from treating physician.
• Report to treating physician if diarrhea, nausea, headache, and rash persist or become intolerable.

Adverse reactions

• Common: hypertension, diarrhea, nausea, headache, rash, respiratory infection.
• Serious: **elevated liver enzymes**, angina, hyperthyroidism, diabetes, depression, asthma.

Clinically important drug interactions

• Drugs that increase effects/toxicity of leflunomide: folic acid, rifampin.
• Drugs that decrease effects/toxicity of leflunomide: charcoal, cholestyramine.
• Leflunomide increases effects/toxicity of methotrexate, other hepatoxic agents.

Parameters to monitor: Signs and symptoms of hepatotoxicity.

Editorial comments

• This is a newer agent for treating severe rheumatoid arthritis. The following method has been suggested to promote elimination of leflunomide in the event of severe toxicity: (1) discontinue leflunomide; (2) take 8 g of cholestyramine t.i.d. for 11 days (these do not have to be consecutive); (3) measure plasma levels and be certain that they are less than 0.02 mg/L; (4) determine plasma levels in two separate tests at least 14 days apart. If levels remain elevated, continue cholestyramine treatment. Full drug elimination may take up to 2 years. This process is recommended for females and males prior to attempt at conception.

• Because of its immunosuppressant properties, this drug has the potential to increase risk of malignancy; however, thus far, studies have not shown this effect.

Leucovorin

Brand names: Leucovorin, Wellcovorin.

Class of drug: Folic acid-derived antidote for folic acid antagonist toxicity.

Mechanism of action: Drug acts as a cofactor in the biosynthesis of purines and pyrimidines which is blocked by folic acid antagonists such as methotrexate, trimethoprim, and pyrimethamine.

Indication/dosage/route: Oral, IV, IM.

• Toxicity of folic acid antagonist overdose
  – PO 2–15 mg/d, 3 days or until blood counts normalize.
• Megaloblastic anemia (secondary to folate deficiency)
  – IM 1 mg/d.
• Rescue dose (within 24 hours of methotrexate treatment)
  – PO or IV 10 mg/m^2 q6h until serum methotrexate is 10^{-8} M.
• Elevated serum creatinine (>50%) after methotrexate
  – 100 mg/m^2 q3h until methotrexate is 10^{-8} M.
• **Adjustment of dosage:** None.

	Onset of Action	Duration
Oral	20–30 min	3–6 h
IV	<5 min	3–6 h
IM	10–20 min	3–6 h

Pregnancy: Category C.

Lactation: Folic acid is required for lactating females. Leucovorin is an active metabolite of folic acid and should therefore be compatible.

Contraindications: Pernicious anemia, megaloblastic anemia secondary to vitamin B_{12} deficiency.

Warnings/precautions

• Use with caution in children treated for seizures.

• Methotrexate rescue: Hydrate patient and alkalinize urine with sodium bicarbonate or acetazolamide.

• Folic acid deficiency: Advise diet high in meat, dried beans, green leafy vegetables.

Advice to patient: Drink 3 L of fluid per day.

Adverse reactions

• Common: none.

• Serious: anaphylactoid reaction, thrombocytosis.

Clinically important drug interactions

• Leucovorin decreases effects/toxicity of trimethoprim–sulfamethoxazole, barbiturates, phenytoin, primidone.

• Leucovorin increases effects/toxicity of 5-fluorouracil, other fluoropyrimidines.

Parameters to monitor

• Plasma methotrexate levels. Leucovorin level should be greater than or equal to that of methotrexate. Treatment should continue until methotrexate plasma level is less than 5×10^{-8} M.

• Signs of hypersensitivity reactions.

• Level of B_{12}, folic acid, hematologic status.

• Serum creatinine to detect possible renal toxicity; this should be done daily during high-dose methotrexate therapy because creatinine level >50% of pretreatment level after 24 hours indicates severe renal toxicity.

- Urinary pH every 6 hours. pH should be maintained >7 to decrease the nephrotoxic effects of methotrexate. Alkalinize urine with acetazolamide or sodium bicarbonate.

Editorial comments

- Parenteral leucovorin is advised for treatment of megaloblastic anemia due to folic acid deficiency when it is not feasible to use oral therapy.
- Leucovorin should be administered as soon as possible after it is determined that the folic acid antagonists have caused toxicity. Doses should be given within 24 hours of last dose of methotrexate. Most effective if given within 1 hour of overdose.
- Cytotoxic drug: Use latex gloves and safety glasses when handling this medication; avoid contact with skin as well as inhalation. If possible prepare in biologic hood.
- This drug is widely used in combination with 5-fluorouracil in the treatment of colorectal cancer, in both the adjuvant and advanced settings. Leucovorin potentiates the action of the fluoropyrimidine.
- This drug is not listed in the *Physician's Desk Reference*, 54th edition, 2000.

Leuprolide

Brand name: Lupron.
Class of drug: Antineoplastic agent, inhibitor of gonadotropin secretion.
Mechanism of action: Inhibits synthesis of estrogen and androgens in the ovaries and testicles, thus reducing serum and tissue levels of these hormones. Inhibits release of FSH and LH from pituitary gland. Decreases size and activity of endometrial implants.
Indications/dosage/route: IM, SC.

- Management of advanced prostate cancer
  - Adults: IM 7.5 mg depo injection once a month.

- Treatment of endometriosis
  - Adults: IM 3.75 mg depo injection/mo. Maximum: 6 months.
- Management of central precocious puberty
  - Children: SC 50 µg/kg/d; increase by 10 µg/kg/d to achieve desired effect.
  - Children <25 kg: IM 7.5 mg q4wk.

Adjustment of dosage

- Kidney disease: None.
- Liver disease: None.
- Elderly: Same as adult dose.
- Pediatric: See above.

Pregnancy: Category X.

Lactation: No data available. Avoid breastfeeding.

Contraindications: Hypersensitivity to GnRH or GnRH agonists, undiagnosed vaginal bleeding, pregnancy. Should not be given to women of childbearing potential who might become pregnant during leuprolide therapy.

Warnings/precautions

- Injection is done in the presence of physician.
- Use with caution in patients allergic to benzyl alcohol. Such patients may show induration and erythema at the site of injection. Treatment should be stopped.
- Determine pre- and posttreatment levels of serum estradiol in female patients.
- Use calcium supplements when taking this drug.
- Leuprolide is often given with an androgen receptor blocker, eg, flutamide or bicalutamide, when used as a treatment for prostate cancer.

Advice to patient

- Do not stop medication without first consulting with physician.
- Use two forms of birth control including hormonal and barrier methods.
- Report immediately to treating physician if you experience the following: respiratory difficulty, numbness, weakness, urination problems.

Adverse reactions

Common: headache, hot flashes, dizziness, vaginitis.

Serious: **depression**, myocardial ischemia and infarction, spontaneous abortion, fetal anomalies, urticaria, neuropathy.

Clinically important drug interactions: Leuprolide increases effects/toxicity of antineoplastic drugs: megestrol, flutamide.

Parameters to monitor

- Serum testosterone, PSA, and acid phosphatase before and during therapy. PSA levels should decrease and remain at low levels during therapy.
- Signs of bladder distention, particularly those with urinary tract obstruction.
- Presence of bone pain, particularly at start of treatment. Responds to analgesics.

Editorial comments

- Leuprolide is used as palliative treatment of advanced prostate cancer when alternatives such as orchiectomy and estrogen administration are unacceptable to the patient.
- Prior to administration of leuprolide for central precocious puberty, diagnosis of this condition should be confirmed by performing a complete physical and endocrine examination. This exam should include the following: height, weight, hand/wrist x-ray, sex steroid level (estradiol, testosterone), other hormones, CT scan of the head. Such parameters should be monitored periodically during therapy. Therapy should be discontinued before age 11 in girls and age 12 in boys.

Levalbuterol

Brand name: Xopenex.

Class of drug: Adrenergic agonist, asthma.

Mechanism of action: Relaxes bronchial smooth muscles of the bronchioles by stimulating β_2-adrenergic receptors.

Indications/dosage/route: Inhalation only.

- Acute bronchospasm
  - Initial: 0.63–1.25 mg t.i.d. by nebulization.

Adjustment of dosage: None.
Food: No restriction.
Pregnancy: Category C.
Lactation: Appears in breast milk. Best to avoid.
Contraindications: Hypersensitivity to adrenergic compounds.
Editorial comments
• This new drug is available only with a nebulizer. Properties are similar to those of albuterol, and levalbuterol offers no specific advantages according to *The Medical Letter*.
• For additional information, see *albuterol*, p. 12.

Levamisole

Brand name: Ergamisol.
Class of drug: Antineoplastic immunomodulator.
Mechanism of action: Restores depressed immune function: stimulates antibody formation, activates T cells and macrophages.
Indications/dosage/route: Oral only.
• Adjunct treatment with fluorouracil in Dukes' stage C colon cancer.
  – Adults: Initial: 50 mg q8h, 3 days, starting 7–30 days following surgery. Repeat regimen q14d for 1 year.
Note: Fluorouracil is always given with levamisole. Dosage of fluorouracil is 450 mg/m^2/d for 5 days, then 450 mg/m^2 weekly after with 4-week break, together with 3-day course of levamisole starting 21–34 days following surgery.
Adjustment of dosage
• Kidney disease: Lower dosage may be needed.
• Liver disease: Lower doses may be needed.
• Elderly: Lower dosage may be needed.
• Pediatric: Safety and efficacy have not been established in children.

Food: No recommendations; probably acceptable to take with food.

Pregnancy: Category C.

Lactation: No data available; potentially toxic to infant. Avoid breastfeeding.

Contraindications: Hypersensitivity to levamisole.

Advice to patients

• Inform treating physician if you experience flu-like symptoms.

• Avoid alcohol.

Adverse reactions

• Common: nausea, vomiting, diarrhea, constipation, dermatitis, alopecia, fatigue, fever, arthralgia, myalgia.

• Serious: acute neurologic syndrome, bone marrow suppression, agranulocytosis, thrombocytopenia, infections, depression.

Clinically important drug interactions

• Drugs that increase effects/toxicity of levamisole: alcohol (disulfiam-like reaction).

• Levamisole increases effects/toxicity of warfarin, phenytoin.

Parameters to monitor

• Stomatitis and diarrhea during the initial administration of fluorouracil. If these conditions develop, discontinue the regimen prior to giving full 5 doses.

• Flu-like symptoms including cough, fever, and sore throat because this may herald the onset of agranulocytosis.

• Hematologic status including CBC with differential and platelets at baseline and weekly with treatment.

• Serum electrolytes.

• Liver function: testing should be performed every 3 months.

• Assess patient for bleeding, easy bruising, petechiae, blood in urine and in vomit.

• WBC count: if 2500–3500/mm^3, discontinue both fluorouracil and levamisole.

Editorial comments

• Before instituting therapy with levamisole, the patient should be out of the hospital, ambulatory, and fully recovered from postsurgical complications.

• Before beginning treatment, physician should familiarize himself or herself with the labeling of fluorouracil. (see p. 375)

Levodopa/Carbidopa

Brand name: Sinemet.
Class of drug: Dopamine precursor plus decarboxylase inhibitor, treatment for Parkinson's disease.
Mechanism of action: Carbidopa blocks conversion of levodopa to dopamine in the periphery. Levodopa increases dopamine levels in basal ganglia.
Indications/dosage/route: Oral only.
• Parkinson's disease
  – Adults: 25–100 mg combination (1 tablet) t.i.d. Dose may be increased to 1 tablet q.i.d. Maintenance: 2–8 tablets in divided doses. Maximum levodopa: 1000 mg/d.

Adjustment of dosage
• Kidney disease: May need lower dose.
• Liver disease: None.
• Elderly: Lower doses may be necessary due to enhanced sensitivity to L-dopa.
• Pediatric: Safety and efficacy have not been established in children <18 years of age.

Food: Best if taken between meals. The food content should be low in protein because this seems to interfere with absorption of the drug. Patient should be advised that taking food 15 minutes before ingestion can minimize GI upset.
Pregnancy: Category C.
Lactation: No data available. Best to avoid.
Contraindications: Narrow-angle glaucoma, history of melanoma, undiagnosed skin lesions, concurrent therapy with nonselective MAO inhibitors within 14 days of levodopa/carbidopa administration.

Warnings/precautions

- Use with caution in patients with severe renal and hepatic disease, history of MI, arrhythmias, glaucoma, psychiatric illness, psychosis, bronchial asthma, emphysema, active peptic ulcer.
- Stop administration of levodopa at least 12 hours before giving the carbidopa/levodopa combination. If it is necessary to adjust the dosage of a sustained-release product, allow a minimum of 3 days between dosage adjustments.

Advice to patient: Change position slowly, in particular from recumbent to upright to minimize orthostatic hypotension. Sit at the edge of the bed for several minutes before standing, and lie down if feeling faint or dizzy. Avoid hot showers or baths and standing for long periods. Male patients with orthostatic hypotension may be safer urinating while seated on the toilet rather than standing.

Adverse reactions

- Common: dizziness, headache, nausea, vomiting, anorexia, blepharospasm, dysuria, discolored urine and sweating.
- Serious: orthostatic hypotension, arrhythmias, extrapyramidal syndrome (dystonia, dyskinesias), confusion, seizures, hemolytic anemia, agranulocytosis, suicidal tendencies.

Clinically important drug interactions

- Drugs that increase effects/toxicity of levodopa: general anesthetics, MAO inhibitors, sympathomimetic drugs, tricyclic antidepressants.
- Drugs that decrease effects/toxicity of levodopa: anticonvulsants, haloperidol, benzodiazepines, phenothiazines, antacids. Pyridoxine (vitamin B_6) increases peripheral conversion of levodopa.
- Levodopa increases effects/toxicity of antihypertensive drugs.

Parameters to monitor

- Vital signs when changing the drug dosage.
- Signs and symptoms of drug-induced extrapyramidal syndrome (pseudoparkinsonism): akinesia, tremors at rest, pill rolling, shuffling gait, mask-like facies, drooling. If these occur while taking this medication drug discontinuation may

be required. Alternatively, administration of antagonists to this effect such as diphenhydramine and benztropine may be indicated.
• Signs and symptoms of depression.

Editorial comments

• Patient should be advised that a therapeutic response may not be observed for up to 6 months. If the dose is to be increased, this should be done under close supervision by a physician.
• It should be emphasized that if an MAO inhibitor has been used, it should be discontinued for 2–4 weeks before L-dopa treatment is begun.
• There is a possibility that if carbidopa/levodopa treatment is stopped abruptly, a syndrome similar to NMS may develop. Accordingly, it is necessary to monitor such a patient very carefully in such circumstances. Sudden discontinuation of levodopa may also worsen symptoms of Parkinson's disease.
• It may be advisable to institute periodic drug holidays to reestablish the effectiveness of these drugs.
• The properties of the levodopa/carbidopa combination are very similar to those of levodopa alone.

Levofloxacin

Brand name: Levaquin.
Class of drug: Broad-spectrum quinolone antibiotic.
Mechanism of action: Inhibits DNA gyrase, thereby blocking bacterial DNA replication.
Susceptible organisms *in vivo*: *Citrobacter* sp, *Enterobacter* sp, *Escherichia coli, Hemophilus ducreyi, Hemophilus influenzae, Klebsiella pneumoniae, Neisseria gonorrhoeae, Proteus mirabilis, Pseudomonas aeruginosa, Staphylococcus aureus.*
Indications/dosage/route: Oral, IV (same dose for both routes).

- Acute maxillary sinusitis
  - 500 mg once daily for 10–14 days.
- Acute bacterial exacerbation of chronic bronchitis
  - 500 mg once daily for 7 days.
- Community-acquired pneumonia
  - 500 mg once daily for 7–14 days.
- Uncomplicated skin and skin structure infections
  - 500 mg once daily for 7–10 days.
- Complicated UTIs
  - 250 mg once daily for 10 days.
- Acute pyelonephritis
  - 250 mg once daily for 10 days.

Adjustment of dosage
- Kidney disease: Creatinine clearance 50–80 mL/min: no adjustment needed; creatinine clearance 20–49 mL/min: 250 mg q24h, initial dose 500 mg; creatinine clearance 10–19 mL/min: 250 mg q48h, initial dose 500 mg. Complicated UTI/acute pyelonephritis: creatinine clearance >20 mL/min: no adjustment needed; creatinine clearance 10–19 mL/min: 250 mg q48h, initial dose 250 mg.
- Liver disease: None.
- Elderly: None.
- Pediatric: Safety and efficacy have not been established in children <18 years.

Food: Take 1 hour before or 2 hours after meals with a glass of water.

Pregnancy: Category C.

Lactation: Appears in breast milk. Potentially toxic to infant. Avoid breastfeeding.

Contraindications: Hypersensitivity to fluoroquinolone antibiotics or quinolone antibiotics, eg, cinoxacin, nalidixic acid.

Editorial comments
- Levofloxacin is one of the quinolones with improved gram-negative efficiency which allows it to be used in community- acquired pneumonia, acute and chronic sinusitis, as well as otitis media.
- It is less effective than ciprofloxacin for some gram-negative organisms such as *Pseudomonas aeruginosa, Burkholderia*

cepacia, and *Stenotrophomonas maltophilia.* Because of this, ciprofloxacin is the preferred choice for nosocomial infections when *Pseudomonas aeruginosa* is a potential pathogen.
• For additional information, see *norfloxacin,* p. 675.

Levomethadyl

Brand name: Orlaam.
Class of drug: Narcotic analgesic, agonist.
Mechanism of action: Binds to opiate receptors and blocks ascending pain pathways. Reduces patient's perception of pain without altering cause of the pain.
Indications/dosage/route: Oral only.
• Treatment of opioid dependence
– Adults: Initial: 20–40 mg. Subsequent doses at 48- to 72-hour intervals. Adjust by increments of 5–10 mg until steady state is reached (1–2 weeks). Maintenance: Usual dose 60–90 mg, 3 times per week. Maximum: 140 mg every other day.
Adjustment of dosage
• Kidney disease: Use with caution.
• Liver disease: Use with caution.
• Elderly: None.
• Pediatric: Not recommended for use in children <18 years.
Food: May be taken with food to lessen GI upset.
Pregnancy: Category C. Category D if prolonged use or if given in high doses at term.
Lactation: No data available. Potentially toxic to infant. Avoid breastfeeding.
Contraindications: Hypersensitivity to levomethadyl, use other than for treatment of narcotic dependence.
Warnings/precautions
• Use with caution in patients with head injury with increased intracranial pressure, serious alcoholism, prostatic hypertrophy, chronic pulmonary disease, severe liver or kidney disease,

postoperative patients with pulmonary disease, disorders of biliary tract.

- Administer drug before patient experiences severe pain for fullest efficacy.

- Have the following available when treating patient with this drug: naloxone (Narcan) or other antagonist, means of administering oxygen, and support of respiration.

- Nausea, vomiting, and orthostatic hypotension occur most prominently in ambulatory patients. If nausea and vomiting persist, it may be necessary to administer an antiemetic, eg, droperidol or prochlorperazine.

- This drug can cause severe hypotension in a patient who is volume depleted or if given along with a phenothiazine or general anesthetic.

- Careful diagnosis must be made of acute abdominal condition before this drug is administered.

Editorial comments

- This drug is used only for treatment of narcotic addiction and can be dispensed only by treatment programs approved by FDA, DEA, and designated state authorities. The drug is dispensed only in oral form and according to treatment requirements stated in federal regulations.

- This drug should not be used on a daily basis.

- Patient should be warned that use or abuse of CNS depressant drugs including alcohol could be fatal if taken during initiation of treatment or after treatment is ended.

- For additional information, see *morphine*, p. 633.

Levonorgestrel

Brand names: Norplant, Norgestrel II.
Class of drug: Progestational hormone, contraceptive.
Mechanism of action: Inhibits secretion of pituitary gonadotropins (FSH, LH) by positive feedback.

Indications/dosage/route: Subdermal implant.
• Contraception
   – 6 Silastic capsules or 2 rods implanted subdermally in mid-portion of upper arm. Distribute in a fanlike pattern.
Adjustment of dosage
• Kidney disease: None.
• Liver disease: Contraindicated.
• Elderly: None.
• Pediatric: Safety and efficacy have not been determined.
Food: No restrictions.
Pregnancy: Category D.
Lactation: Another drug from this class (medroxyprogesterone) is considered compatible by American Academy of Pediatrics.
Contraindications: Hypersensitivity to progestins, history of thrombophlebitis, active thromboembolic disease, cerebral hemorrhage, liver disease, missed abortion, diagnostic for pregnancy, known or suspected pregnancy (first 4 months), undiagnosed vaginal bleeding, carcinoma of the breast, known or suspected genital malignancy.
Warnings/precautions
• Use with caution in patients with respiratory infection, history of depression, epilepsy, migraine, cardiac disease, renal disease, diabetes.
• Cigarette smoking significantly increases risk of cardiac complications and thrombotic events. At highest risk are women >35 years of age, smoking ≥15 cigarettes per day.
Advice to patient
• Weigh yourself twice a week and report to treating physician if there are any unusual changes in weight.
• If you observe a yellowing of skin or eyes, report to treating physician.
• If you experience changes in mental status suggestive of depression, report to treating physician.
• Discontinue medication if you experience sudden headaches or attack of migraine.

- Discontinue drug and notify physician if you miss a period or experience unusual bleeding.
- If you miss a dose, take the missed dose as soon as possible; do not double the next dose.
- If the drug is used as contraceptive and you miss a dose, stop taking and use an alternative method of contraception until period returns.
- Use good hygiene—flossing, gum massages, regular cleaning by dentist—to avoid gum problems.
- Keep an extra month supply of the drug on hand.
- Do not give this medication to anyone else.

Adverse reactions
- Common: irregular or unpredictable menstrual bleeding (spotting), amenorrhea, breakthrough bleeding, infertility for up to 18 months.
- Serious: thromboembolic events, depression, cholestatic jaundice.

Clinically important drug interactions: Drugs that decrease effects/toxicity of progestins: aminoglutethimide, phenytoin, rifampin, carbamazepine.

Parameters to monitor
- Liver enzymes, cholesterol (total, LDL, HDL), triglycerides.
- Diabetic patient: Monitor blood glucose closely and adjust antidiabetic medication if necessary.
- Signs and symptoms of thromboembolic or thrombotic disorders: pains in leg, sudden chest pain, shortness of breath, migraine, sudden severe headache, vomiting. Discontinue drug.

Editorial comments
- Patient receiving a progesterone for contraceptive purposes should have a complete physical examination performed with special attention to breasts and pelvic organs as well as a Pap test before treatment and annually thereafter. If a patient experiences persistent or abnormal vaginal bleeding while on this drug, perform diagnostic tests including endometrial sampling, to determine cause.

Levorphanol

Brand name: Levo-Dromoran.

Class of drug: Narcotic analgesic, agonist.

Mechanism of action: Binds to opiate receptors and blocks ascending pain pathways. Reduces patient's perception of pain without altering cause of the pain.

Indications/dosage/route: Oral, IM, SC.

• Pain, acute
  – Adults: IM, SC 1–2 mg; repeat in 6–8 hours if needed. PO 2–3 mg; repeat in 6–8 hours if needed.
• Pain, chronic
  – Adults: PO $\frac{1}{15}$ th $-\frac{1}{12}$ th total daily dose of oral morphine previously required.

Adjustment of dosage

• Kidney disease: None.
• Liver disease: None.
• Elderly: None.
• Pediatric: Safety and efficacy have not been established in children <18.

	Onset of Action	Peak Effect	Duration
Oral	30–90 min	0.5–1 h	6–8 h

Food: May be taken with food to lessen GI upset.

Pregnancy: Category B. Category D if prolonged use or if given in high doses at term.

Lactation: Appears in breast milk. Potentially toxic to infant. Avoid breastfeeding.

Contraindications: Hypersensitivity to levorphanol or narcotics of the same chemical class.

Warnings/precautions

• Use with caution in patients with head injury with increased intracranial pressure, serious alcoholism, prostatic hypertrophy, chronic pulmonary disease, severe liver or kidney disease, postoperative patients with pulmonary disease, disorders of biliary tract.

- Administer drug before patient experiences severe pain for fullest efficacy.
- Have the following available when treating patient with this drug: naloxone (Narcan) or other antagonist, means of administering oxygen, and support of respiration.
- Nausea, vomiting, and orthostatic hypotension occur most prominently in ambulatory patients. If nausea and vomiting persist, it may be necessary to administer an antiemetic, eg, droperidol or prochlorperazine.
- This drug can cause severe hypotension in a patient who is volume depleted or if given along with a phenothiazine or general anesthesia.
- Careful diagnosis must be made of acute abdominal condition before this drug is administered.
- For additional information, see *morphine,* p. 633.

Levothyroxine (T$_4$ or L-Thyroxine)

Brand names: Synthroid, Levothyroid.
Class of drug: Thyroid hormone.
Mechanism of action: Levothyroxine stimulates protein synthesis and increases utilization of carbohydrate. Increases cellular metabolic rate.
Indications/dosage/route: Oral, IV.
- Infantile and childhood hypothyroidism
  – For children who cannot swallow intact tablet, crush tablet in small quantity of water or formula. Sprinkle crushed tablet on small amount of food, eg, apple sauce.
- Thyroid hormone replacement
  – Adults, healthy: Initial: PO 1.6 μg/kg/d. Increase dose by 12.5–25 μg/d until serum TSH is normalized.

- Elderly, younger adults with history of cardiovascular disease: Initial: PO 12.5–50 µg/d. Dose is increased by 12.5–25 µg/d every 3–6 weeks until desired response is reached.
- Myxedema or hypothyroid with angina
  - Adults: PO 12.5–25 µg/d. Increase by 25–50 µg/d at 2 to 4-week intervals until desired response is reached.
- Myxedema coma
  - Adults: IV 300–500 µg. Additional 100–300 µg IV if no response in 24 hours. Maintenance: 75–200 µg/d. Begin oral therapy when clinical condition stable.
- Congenital hypothyroidism

Age of Child	Initial Dose/day (µg/kg), PO
0–6 mo	8–15
6–12 mo	6–8
1–5 y	5–6
6–12 y	4–5
>12 y	2–3

Adjustment of dosage
- Kidney disease: None.
- Liver disease: May require decreased dose.
- Elderly: Initial: 12.5–25 µg/d. Increase by 12.5–25 µg every 2–4 weeks. After age 60, initial dose should be 25% lower than usual recommended adult dose.
- Pediatric: See above.

	Onset of Action	Peak Effect	Duration
Oral	3–5 d	3–4 wk	7–10 d

Food: Levothyroxine should be taken as a single dose before breakfast.

Pregnancy: Category A.

Lactation: Appears in breast milk. Potentially beneficial for neonatal hypothyroidism. Probably safe to breastfeed.

Contraindications: Acute MI, untreated thyrotoxicosis, uncorrected adrenal insufficiency, hypersensitivity to thyroid hormones.

Warnings/precautions

- Use with caution in patients with hypertension, angina coronary artery disease, elderly, diabetes.
- Advise parents of children that there may be partial hair loss during levothyroxine therapy. This is generally a self-limited toxic effect.
- Capsules contain tartrazine dye and this may cause hypersensitivity reactions in some patients.
- Superphysiologic doses of levothyroxine should not be prescribed as treatment for obesity. These may predispose to life-threatening toxicity.
- Perform ECG analysis of elderly patients to determine if they have incipient or undetected cardiac problems. This should be done before initiating therapy.

Advice to patients

- Continue to take usual daily dose if a dose is missed. Do not take double doses to make up for missed doses.
- Use only the same product as prescribed; do not switch to other brands.
- Do not discontinue levothyroxine without notifying the physician.
- Avoid iodine-rich foods.
- Report to your physician if you experience any of the following signs of toxicity: irregular or increased heart rate (>100 beats/min), chest pain, persistent headache, weight loss in excess of 5 lb/wk, excessive sweating, heart intolerance.
- Inform your dentist or doctor that you are taking this drug before surgery.
- Notify your physician if you become pregnant.
- If you are diabetic, monitor your blood glucose carefully when you are started on levothyroxine as the dose of hypoglycemic drug may have to be altered.

Adverse reactions
• Common: None.
• Serious: arrythmias, tachycardia.

Clinically important drug interactions
• Drugs that decrease effectiveness of levothyroxine: cholestyramine, phenytoin, estrogens.
• Levothyroxine increases effects/toxicity of oral anticoagulants, sympathomimetics, tricyclic antidepressants.
• Levothyroxine decreases effects/toxicity of theophylline, digoxin, insulin, oral hypoglycemic agents.

Parameters to monitor
• Blood levels of T_3, TSH, T_4, free thyroxine index q6–8wk of therapy. After stabilization, monitor these parameters q6–12mo.
• Symptoms of possible exacerbation of concurrent diseases such as diabetes, adrenal insufficiency, myxedema. These patients may require smaller doses for adequate replacement.
• Signs or symptoms of overdose and toxicity including: nervousness, excessive sweating, chest pain, palpitations, diarrhea.
• Signs and symptoms of hypothyroidism to determine whether treatment is effective.
• Height, weight, and psychomotor development of children.
• Pulse rate. Rates greater than 100/min may require reduction in dose.

Editorial comments
• When switching patients from liothyronine to levothyroxine, the following principles should be noted: (1) The daily dosage of levothyroxine is determined by multiplying the daily dose of liothyronine by 2.5. (2) Liothyronine can be discontinued when levothyroxine administration is instituted. (3) Levothyroxine should be started at a dosage that is lower than the estimated daily dosage and titrated upward as needed.
• Levothyroxine is the drug of choice for thyroid replacement because of its purity, long half-life, and close simulation to normal physiologic hormone.
• Thyroid hormones are ineffective for weight reduction, obesity, or premenstrual tension when used at physiologic doses in euthyroid patients. If used at higher doses, levothyroxine may

produce serious or even life-threatening toxic effects particularly when used with some anorectic drugs. They are therefore contraindicated for these purposes.

• When switching patients from desiccated thyroid to levothyroxine, the daily dosage of levothyroxine in micrograms is approximately the same as the daily dosage of desiccated thyroid in milligrams.

Lidocaine (as Antiarrhythmic)

Brand name: Xylocaine.

Class of drug: Class Ib antiarrhythmic agent.

Mechanism of action: Lidocaine suppresses myocardial conduction automaticity, shortens effective refractory period and action potential duration of His-Purkinje fibers, and inhibits reentry phenomenon.

Indications/dosage/route: IV, IM, topical.

• Ventricular arrthymias, from MI, cardiac glycosides, or long QT: initial drug of choice
  – Adults: IV bolus 50–100 mg, rate 25–50 mg/min. Repeat q3–5min until symptoms are reversed. Maximum: 200–300 mg/h.
  – Adults: IV infusion 20–50 mg/kg, rate 1–4 mg/min. Maximum: 200–300 mg/h.
  – Adults: IM 4.5 mg/kg. Repeat after 60–90 min.
  – Pediatric loading dose: IV 1 mg/kg q5–10min. Maximum: 5 mg/kg.

Adjustment of dosage

• Kidney disease: None.

• Liver disease: In acute hepatitis and uncompensated cirrhosis: decrease dose by 50%.

• Elderly: Use with caution. Initial dose should be reduced by 50% and then increased slowly as needed.

• Pediatric: Safety and efficacy of parenteral preparations have not been established in children <2 years.

	Onset of action	Peak effect	Duration
IV	Immediate	—	10–20 min
IM	5–15 min	—	60–90 min

Pregnancy: Category B.
Lactation: No data available. Best to avoid.
Contraindications: Hypersensitivity to amide local anesthetics, second- or third-degree heart block (when no pacemaker is present), Wolff–Parkinson–White syndrome, Stokes–Adams syndrome, sulfite sensitivity (in epinephrine-containing preparations).
Warnings/precautions

• Use with caution in patients with severe kidney and liver disease, CHF, patients <110 lb, atrial fibrillation, hypovolemia, shock, severe hypoxia, respiratory depression.
• Know all signs of toxicity such as convulsions, confusion, paresthesias. These call for prompt reduction in dosage or cessation of drug administration. Prolonged infusion of the drug could result in seizures and coma. It is necessary to have oxygen and CPR equipment available when lidocaine is administered by IV route. The IV route is preferred for lidocaine. If necessary, and benefits outweigh risks, IM injections should be used. Such injections should be made only into the deltoid muscle and care must be taken to avoid IV injection.
Adverse reactions

• Common: headache, shivering.
• Serious: hypotension, seizures, hallucinations, respiratory arrest, heart block, arrthymias, anaphylaxis, status asthmaticus, coma.
Clinically important drug interactions

• Drugs that increase effects/toxicity of lidocaine: cimetidine, β blockers, other antiarrthymic agents.

- Drugs that decrease effects/toxicity of lidocaine: phenytoin.
- Lidocaine increases effects/toxicity of succinylcholine.

Parameters to monitor

- BP, respiratory status, and ECG continuously during intravenous administration. Monitor continuously until arrhythmia is controlled. If arrhythmia returns, serum level should be measured and dosage increased to the proper range, 2–6 mg/L.
- Serum lidocaine levels periodically throughout prolonged or high-dose therapy. The therapeutic level ranges from 1.5 to 5 µg/mL. If lidocaine blood level increases to 6 mg/mL. The drug should be discontinued immediately.
- Signs of toxicity: paresthesias and somnolence (first signs), severe sinus bradycardia, respiratory depression, convulsions, tinnitus, blurred vision, hypotension, cardiovascular collapse. Treat as follows. Circulatory depression: A vasopressor should be administered as should IV fluids if necessary. Seizures: Respiratory support including endotracheal intubation should be instituted. If seizures continue, diazepam should be administered in 2.5-mg increments. Alternatively, an ultrashort barbiturate such as pentobarbital or thiopental in 50- to 100-mg increments
- Serum electrolytes, creatinine, BUN.
- Signs of excessive blockade of normal cardiac conductivity, eg, sinus node dysfunction.

Editorial comments

- An infusion pump should be used when intravenous lidocaine is given to meter the amount administered precisely. Infusion rate should never exceed 4 mg/min.
- First-pass pharmacokinetics makes dosing of lidocaine complex. This is the reason for subsequent boluses q3–5min after the initial dose. As maintenance therapy is instituted (usually at 2 mg/min), lidocaine active levels rise linearly and accumulate. Thus, after 8 hours, reducing the maintenance dose in half will avoid toxicity while ensuring efficacy with a steady state.

• Lidocaine is an antiarrhythmic drug with no atrial pharmacologic effects and therefore is largely ineffective for the treatment of atrial arrhythmias. The American Heart Association and American College of Cardiology recommend that lidocaine be administered prophylactically for 12–24 hours for patients with a suspected acute MI who experience frequent ventricular premature beats (>6/min). Lidocaine should be used only for asymptomatic arrhythmias occurring in association with acute MI.

Lidocaine (as Anesthetic)

Brand name: Xylocaine (with or without epinephrine for local anesthesia).
Class of drug: Local and regional anesthetic.
Mechanism of action: Reversibly inhibits initiation and conduction of nerve impulses near site of injection.
Indications/dosage/route: Local injection, topical.
• Infiltration anesthesia
  – Percutaneous: Adults: total dose 0.5 or 1% solution: 5–300 mg.
  – IV regional: Adults: total dose 0.5% solution: 50–300 mg (10–60 mL).
• Peripheral nerve blocks:
  – Brachial: Adults: Total dose, 1.5% solution: 225–300 mg (15–20 mL).
  – Paravertebral: Adults: Total dose, 1% solution: 30–50 mg (3–5 mL).
• Paracervical
  – Obstetric-analgesia: Adults: Total dose, 1% solution: 100 mg (10 mL).
• Sympathetic nerve block
  – Lumbar: Adults: Total dose, 1% solution: 50–100 mg (5–10 mL).
• Epidural block
  – Thoracic lumbar: Adults: Total dose, 1% solution: 200–300 mg (20–30 mL).

- Caudal block:
  – Obstetric analgesia: Adults: Total dose, 1% solution: 200–300 mg (20–30 mL).
- Pediatric, all uses:
  – Maximum dose depends on age and weight: 1.5–2 mg/lb.
- Topical anesthesia of skin, mucous membranes for pain from dental extractions.
  – Adults/children: 2–5% solution or ointment 15 mL Xylocaine Viscous q3–4h to oral mucosa.
- Local anesthesia (injected)
  – Dosage based on individual requirements, dependent on tissue, blood flow, procedure duration, etc. Maximum: 4.5 mg/kg.

Adjustment of dosage

- Kidney disease: None.
- Liver disease: Use with extreme caution in severe liver disease.
- Elderly: None.
- Pediatric: See above.

Food: Not applicable.

Pregnancy: Category C.

Lactation: Appears in breast milk. Considered compatible by American Academy of Pediatrics.

Contraindications: Hypersensitivity for amide-type local anesthetic (eg, mepivacaine), sensitivity to sodium metabisulfate (in preparations containing epinephrine).

Warnings/precautions

- Use local anethetics plus vasoconstrictor (eg, epinephrine, norepinephrine) with caution in patients with peripheral vascular disease and hypertension and those receiving general anesthetics.
- Use local anesthetics with or without vasoconstrictor with caution in patients with severe liver disease. Use with extreme caution for lumbar and caudal epidural anesthesia in patients with spinal deformities, existing neurologic disease, severe uncontrolled hypotension, septicemia.
- Epidural anesthesia: A test dose of the local anesthetic should first be given before the full dose is administered to ensure that the catheter is not within a blood vessel. The test dose should include 10–15 µg epinephrine. Any increase in heart rate and

systolic pressure within 45 seconds (the epinephrine response) would indicate that the injection is intravascular.

- Local anesthetics can trigger malignant hyperthermia. Symptoms of this condition include tachycardia, labile BP, tachypnea, muscle rigidity. The necessary means must be available to manage this condition (dantrolene, oxygen, supportive measures).
- A local anesthetic containing a vasoconstrictor should be injected with great caution into areas of the body supplied by end-organ arteries (nose, ears, penis, digits).

Editorial comments: For additional information, see *bupivacaine*, p. 113.

Lindane

Brand names: Kwell, Kwildane, Scabene.
Class of drug: Ectoparasiticide, treatment for scabies (*Sarcoptes scabei*).
Mechanism of action: Directly absorbed by parasites and ova. Mechanism of toxicity unknown.
Indications/dosage/route: Topical only.
- Scabies
  – Adults/children: Apply thin layer to all skin surfaces after bathing with soap and water. Remove drug after 8–12 hours by bathing. Repeat treatment after 1 week if needed.
- Pediculosis
  – Adults/children: Apply shampoo to dry area, wait 4 minutes, add small amount of water, wait 4–5 minutes, and rinse thoroughly. Repeat treatment after 1 week if needed.

Adjustment of dosage
- Kidney disease: None.
- Liver disease: Probably should reduce dose.
- Elderly: Reduce dose, may have increased skin absorption.
- Pediatric: Contraindicated in premature neonates.

Onset of Action	Duration
Rapid	>24 h

Food: No restrictions.

Pregnancy: Category B. Patient should be treated no more than twice during pregnancy.

Lactation: Probably appears in breast milk. Avoid nursing for at least 4 days after treatment.

Contraindications: Premature neonates, known seizure disorders, hypersensitivity to lindane, Norwegian (crusted) scabies.

Warnings/precautions

- Lindane is normally absorbed to a limited extent through human skin. Systemic lindane is toxic to the CNS and may cause seizures and death from overexposure.
- Provide patient with instructions for use along with drug.

Advice to patient

- Use only on cool, dry skin.
- If drug comes in contact with eyes, face, mucous membranes, or urethral meatus, flush immediately with water and call physician for further information.
- Do not inhale vapor.
- Do not use other oils or ointments along with lindane.
- Do not use lindane if there are open wounds, cuts, or sores on groin or scalp. If necessary to use, consult the physician.
- Do not use hair preparations simultaneously as this may promote the absorption of lindane and possible systemic toxicity.
- If lindane is ingested, gastric lavage and general supportive measures should be instituted. Diazepam at a dose of 0.01 mg/kg can be used to control seizures if they occur.
- Examine family members and individuals with close contact with patient for infestation with scabies. Family members and others in close contact with the patient should be treated concurrently.
- Sexual partners should be treated concurrently for scabies.

- Wear gloves when applying lindane.
- Clothing recently worn as well as bed linens and towels should be washed in very hot water or dry cleaned to prevent reinfestation or spreading of the organisms.
- Parents should monitor young children closely during and immediately after treatment for signs of CNS toxicity. Keep medication away from children. Most cases of lindane toxicity occur from oral ingestion.
- Do not re-treat without consulting treating physician.

Adverse reactions
- Common: pruritis.
- Serious: CNS toxicity (dizziness, seizures, death).

Clinically important drug interactions: None reported.

Parameters to monitor: Presence of living lice in hair. If present 7 days after treatment, re-treatment may be necessary.

Editorial comments: Centers for Disease Control and Prevention and FDA do not recommend lindane for children <10 years. Other scabicides such as permethrin and crotamiton should be used rather than lindane.

Lisinopril

Brand names: Prinuvil, Zestril.

Class of drug: ACE inhibitor.

Mechanism of action: Inhibits ACE, thereby preventing conversion of angiotensin I to angiotensin II, resulting in decreased peripheral arterial resistance.

Indications/dosage/route: Oral only.
- Hypertension
  - Initial: 10 mg/d. Can be increased to 20–40 mg/d (initiate therapy at 5 mg/d in patients receiving diuretics).
- CHF
  - Initial: PO 2.5–5 mg/d. Can be increased up to 50 mg/d. Improved survival after MI: 5 mg/d for 2 days, then 10 mg/d for 6 weeks.

Adjustment of dosage
- Kidney disease: Creatinine clearance 10–30 ml/min: 5 mg/d; creatinine clearance <10 ml/min: 2 mg/d.
- Liver disease: None.
- Elderly: Use with caution.
- Pediatric: Safety and efficacy have not been established.

Onset of Action	Peak Effect	Duration
Within 1 h	6 h	24 h

Food: Administer without regard to meals.

Pregnancy: Category C for first trimester. Category D for second and third trimesters.

Lactation: No information available. Likely to be present in breast milk. Other similar agents considered safe.

Contraindications: Hypersensitivity to ACE inhibitors, hereditary or idiopathic angioedema, second and third trimestesrs of pregnancy.

Warnings/precautions
- Use with caution in patients with kidney disease, especially renal artery stenosis, hypovolemia, hyponatremia, cardiac or cerebral insufficiency, collagen vascular disease, lupus erythematosus, scleroderma in patients undergoing dialysis and patients taking drugs that cause bone marrow depression.
- ACE inhibitors have been associated with anaphylaxis and angioedema.
- Use extreme caution in combination with potassium-sparing diuretics (high risk of hyperkalemia).
- Sodium- or volume-depleted patients may experience severe hypotension. Lower initial doses are advised.
- During surgery/anesthesia, the drug may increase hypotension. Volume expansion may be required.
- There may be a profound drop in BP after the first dose is taken. Close medical supervision is necessary once therapy is begun.

Advice to patient
- Do not use salt substitutes containing potassium.

- Use two forms of birth control including hormonal and barrier methods.
- Avoid NSAIDs; may be present in OTC preparations.
- Take BP periodically and report to treating physician if significant changes occur. Stop drug if prolonged vomiting or diarrhea occurs. These symptoms may indicate plasma volume reduction.
- Discontinue drug immediately if signs of angioedema (swelling of face, lips, extremities, breathing or swallowing difficulty) become prominent, and notify physician immediately.
- If chronic cough develops, notify treating physician.

Adverse reactions
- Common: none.
- Serious: bone marrow depression (neutropenia, agranulocytosis), hypotension, angioedema, hyperkalemia, oliguria, chest pain, angina, tachycardia, autoimmune symptom complex (see Editorial Comments), hepatitis, liver failure, pancreatitis, gout, arrhythmia, MI.

Clinically important drug interactions
- Lisinopril increases toxicity of lithium, azothioprine, allopurinol, potassium-sparing diuretics, digoxin.
- Drugs that increase toxicity of lisinopril: potassium-sparing drugs, phenothiazines (eg, chlorpromazine).
- Drugs that decrease effectiveness of lisinopril: NSAIDs, antacids, cyclosporine.

Parameters to monitor
- Electrolytes, CBC with differential and platelets, BUN and creatinine.
- Signs and symptoms of angioedema: swelling of face, lips, tongue, extremities, glottis, larynx. Observe in particular for obstruction of airway, difficulty in breathing. If symptoms are not relieved by an antihistamine, discontinue drug.
- BP closely, particularly at beginning of therapy. Observe for evidence of severe hypotension. Patients who are hypovolemic as a result of GI fluid loss or diuretics may exhibit severe hypotension. Also monitor for orthostatic changes.
- Signs of persistent, nonproductive cough. This may be drug-induced.

- Changes in weight in patients with CHF. Gain of more than 2 kg/wk may indicate edema development.
- Signs and symptoms of infection.
- Possible antinuclear antibody development.
- WBC count monthly for first 3–6 months and at frequent intervals thereafter for patients with collagen vascular disease or renal insufficiency. Discontinue therapy if neutrophil count drops below 1000.
- Signs and symptoms of bone marrow depression.
- Intake of fluids and urinary and other fluid output to minimize renal toxicity. Increase fluid intake if inadequate. Closely monitor electrolyte levels.
- Signs and symptoms of renal toxicity.

Editorial comments
- Unlabeled uses of ACE inhibitors include hypertensive crisis, diagnosis of renal artery stenosis, hyperaldosteronism, Raynaud's phenomenon, angina, diabetic nephropathy.
- ACE inhibitors have been associated with an autoimmune-type symptom complex including fever, positive antinuclear antibody, myositis, vasculitis, and arthritis.
- ACE inhibitors have been a highly efficacious and well-tolerated class of drugs. Nearly every large randomized clinical trial examining their use has been favorable. First, the Consensus trial proved that enalapril decreased mortality and increased quality of life in class II–III CHF patients. Then the SOLVE trial and others proved their benefits in remodeling myocardium post-MI. The DCCT trial of diabetic patients demonstrated the ability of ACE inhibitors to decrease the small vessel damage to retina and glomeruli. Clinical trials looking into primary prevention of cardiac effects are ongoing. Treatment with this class of drugs is the gold standard in patients with left ventricular systolic dysfunction. The two most common adverse effects of ACE inhibitors are cough and angioedema. Transient and persistent rises in antinuclear antibody have been noted. As drugs in this class are vasodilators, orthostasis is another potential problem.

Lithium

Brand names: Eskalith, Lithium carbonate, Lithonate.

Class of drug: Antimanic agent, antidepressant.

Mechanism of action: Alters the reuptake of norepinephrine and/or serotonin in the CNS; alters sodium transport in nerve and muscle cells.

Indications/dosage/route: Oral only. Toxic level: >2.0 mEq/L.

– Adults: Usual: 600 mg t.i.d.

• Acute mania

– Adults: 1800 mg t.i.d. Maintenance: 900–1200 mg/d.

– Children >12 years: 15–60 mg/kg/d, 3–4 divided doses. Maximum: 300–600 mg 3–4 times/d.

– Elderly: Initial: 300 mg b.i.d. or q.i.d. Increase by 300 mg/d in weekly increments. Maintenance: 900–1200 mg/d. Lower doses are indicated, as is more frequent monitoring of blood levels for toxicity.

Adjustment of dosage

– Kidney disease: Creatinine clearance 10–50 mL/min: 50–75% of normal dose; creatinine clearance ≤10 mL/min: 25–50% of normal dose.

– Liver disease: None.

– Elderly: See above.

– Pediatric: See above. Safety and efficacy have not been determined in children <12 years.

Food: Lithium should be taken with food or milk.

Pregnancy: Category D. Lithium should be avoided in pregnancy, especially in the first trimester.

Lactation: Appears in breast milk. Considered contraindicated by American Academy of Pediatrics.

Contraindications: Pregnancy, severe cardiovascular or renal disease, severe debilitation or sodium depletion.

Warnings/precautions

• Use with caution in patients with thyroid disease, kidney or cardiovascular disease, seizure disorders and in patients receiving neuroleptics, diuretics, NSAIDs, or neuromuscular blocking agents.

- If electroconvulsive therapy is contemplated, discontinue lithium.
- Lithium's therapeutic effect may require 1–3 weeks. It may be necessary to administer more rapidly acting drugs during this interim period.
- Lithium tablets contain tartrazine; this dye may precipitate an allergic reaction in susceptible individuals.
- Drugs containing large amounts of sodium (eg, Fleet's phosphosoda) may increase the excretion of lithium and thereby reduce its efficacy.

Advice to patient

- Use two forms of birth control including hormonal and barrier methods.
- Do not drink caffeinated coffee or other beverages containing large amounts of xanthines [theophylline (tea), theobromine (cocoa)].
- Do not stop drug abruptly without consulting physician.
- Maintain adequate salt and fluid intake, particularly during hot weather.
- Avoid driving and other activities requiring mental alertness or that are potentially dangerous until response to drug is known.
- Weigh yourself on the same scale at approximately the same time each day wearing the same amount of clothing.
- Use OTC medications only with approval from treating physician.
- Carry an identification card as well as instructions for treatment overdose.
- Asthmatics who are sensitive to aspirin are particularly susceptible to the development of hypersensitivity reactions to tartrazine.
- Use caution carrying out activities that cause excessive sodium loss such as exercise in hot weather, sauna.
- Inform treating physician if you experience severe persistent diarrhea.

- Do not change brands of lithium without consulting treating physician.

Adverse reactions
- Common: polydipsia, nausea, taste disturbance, diarrhea, fatigue, muscle weakness, tremor.
- Serious: hypothyroidism, diabetes insipidus, renal disease, movement disorder, ECG changes.

Clinically important drug interactions
- Drugs that increase effects/toxicity of lithium: thiazide diuretics, loop diuretics, fluoxetine, phenothiazines, probenecid, NSAIDs, tetracyclines, phenytoin, carbamazepine, methyldopa, caffeine, haloperidol.
- Drugs that decrease effects/toxicity of lithium: acetazolamide, mannitol, theophylline, verapamil.
- Lithium increases effects/toxicity of succinylcholine, pancuronium, atracurium.
- Lithium decreases effects/toxicity of sympathomimetics.

Parameters to monitor
- Renal, hepatic, thyroid, and cardiovascular functions, serum electrolytes, CBC with differential, urinalysis. TSH should be checked prior to therapy, every 6 months for 1 year, and then annually.
- Serum levels of lithium twice weekly until the proper dosage is established for stabilizing the patient. Thereafter monitor the level weekly until patient is on maintenance dose. At that time lithium level may be determined every 2–3 months, particularly as symptoms subside because patient's tolerance for lithium decreases with improvement of depression. Therapeutic level 1.0–1.5 mEq/L.
- Urinalysis on a regular basis.
- Symptoms of lithium toxicity: diarrhea, vomiting, decreased coordination, confusion, visual disturbance, seizures, coma.
- Thyroid enlargement while on lithium treatment.
- Dietary sodium intake. Make sure that intake of sodium is constant because a change in sodium intake may have a deleterious effect on lithium's activity.
- Signs of edema or sudden weight gain.

- Blood glucose levels should be monitored closely in diabetic patients.
- Intake of fluids and urinary and other fluid output to minimize renal toxicity. Closely monitor electrolyte levels.
- Polyuria. In such circumstances the dosage should be reduced by 25%. If this is not successful in reversing polyuria, lithium should be discontinued.

Editorial comments

- It is essential to have facilities for determining lithium serum levels when therapy is instituted; access to close monitoring of lithium levels is necessary. Individualize dosage according to serum levels and clinical response (see Indications/Dosage/Route for therapeutic and toxic levels).
- Divalproex is the treatment of choice for bipolar patients who do not respond to or cannot tolerate lithium.
- Candidates with depression for possible treatment with lithium include (1) patients with a previous good response to electroconvulsive therapy, (2) patients for whom antidepressant drugs are contraindicated or who have suicidal or homicidal tendencies, and (3) patients who have failed previous trials using other pharmacotherapies.
- Lithium is the drug of choice for treating acute mania in bipolar manic–depressive disorder.
- Educate the patient's family concerning the toxic effects of lithium.

Lomefloxacin

Brand name: Maxaquin.
Class of drug: Broad-spectrum quinolone antibiotic.
Mechanism of action: Inhibits DNA gyrase, thereby blocking bacterial DNA replication.
Susceptible organisms *in vivo*: *Citrobacter, Enterobacter, Escherichia coli, Hemophilus ducreyi, Hemophilus influenzae, Klebsiella pneumoniae, Neisseria gonorrhoeae, Proteus mirabilis,*

Pseudomonas aeruginosa, Staphylococcus aureus. Limited activity against *Streptococcus pneumoniae, Streptococcus pyogenes.*

Indications/dosage/route: Oral only.
- Acute bacterial exacerbation of chronic bronchitis
  – 400 mg q.d., 10 days.
- Uncomplicated cystitis cause by *E. coli*
  – Adults (females): 400 mg q.d., 3 days.
- Uncomplicated cystitis caused by *K. pneumoniae, P. mirabilis,* or *Staphylococcus saprophyticus*
  – Adults: 400 mg q.d., 10 days.
- Complicated UTI
  – Adults: 400 mg q.d., 14 days.

Adjustment of dosage
- Kidney disease: Creatinine clearance 10–40 mL/min: 200 mg q.d. Initial loading dose: 400 mg.
- Liver disease: None.
- Elderly: None.
- Pediatric: Safety and efficacy have not been established in children <18 years.

Food: Take 1 hour before or 2 hours after meals with a glass of water.

Pregnancy: Category C.

Contraindications: Hypersensitivity to fluoroquinolone antibiotics or quinolone antibiotics, eg, cinoxacin, nalidixic acid.

Editorial comments
- Lomefloxacin is used for the same indications as ofloxacin but is more likely to produce phototoxicity.
- For additional information, see *norfloxacin*, p. 675.

Lomustine

Brand names: CeeNU, CCNU.
Class of drug: Antineoplastic alkylating agent.

Mechanism of action: Inhibits DNA and RNA synthesis; carbamylates DNA polymerase; causes alkylation of RNA, alteration of tumor proteins.

Indications/dosage/route: Oral only.

- Primary and metastatic brain tumors, Hodgkin's disease, non-Hodgkin's lymphoma, melanoma, renal cell carcinoma, colon cancer, lung cancer
  - Adults: 100–130 mg/m^2.
  - Children: 75–150 mg/m^2.

Adjustment of dosage

- Bone marrow depression: WBC count 2000–2900/mm^3: give 75% of previous dose; WBC count 2000–2900/mm^3: give 50% of previous dose.
- Kidney disease: Creatinine clearance 10–50 mL/min: reduce dose by 25%; creatinine clearance <10 mL/min: reduce dose by 50%.
- Liver disease: None
- Elderly: None
- Pediatric: See above

Food: Lomustine should be administered on an empty stomach at bedtime. No food or drink for 2 hours after taking drug.

Pregnancy: Category D.

Lactation: No data available. Potentially toxic to infant. Avoid breastfeeding.

Contraindications: Hypersensitivity to lomustine, pregnancy.

Warnings/precautions

- Use with caution in patients with reduced bone marrow activity and liver disease and in patients receiving other drugs that cause bone marrow suppression.
- Do not administer more frequently than every 6 weeks, as lomustine-induced bone marrow depression may last this long.
- Advise patient that anorexia may persist 2–3 days after a dose is given. Consider giving an antiemetic drug prophylactically.
- Do not administer to patients with active infections.

Advice to patients
- Use two forms of birth control including hormonal and barrier methods.
- Avoid alcohol.
- Receive vaccinations (particularly live attenuated viruses) only with permission from treating physician.
- Avoid crowds as well as persons who may have a contagious disease.

Adverse reactions
- Common: nausea and vomiting.
- Serious: **bone marrow suppression**, neurotoxicity, disorientation, hepatotoxicity, pulmonary fibrosis, renal failure.

Clinically important drug interactions
- The following drug increases effects/toxicity of lomustine: cimetidine.
- The following drugs decrease effects/toxicity of lomustine: phenobarbital.

Parameters to monitor
- CBC with differential and platelets, serum BUN and creatinine, liver enzymes.
- Signs of hypersensitivity reactions: Urticaria, rash, wheezing, pruritus, hypotension.
- Signs and symptoms of bone marrow depression.
- Discontinue this medication if platelet count falls below $100,000/mm^3$.
- Signs and symptoms of infection.
- Signs and symptoms of pulmonary toxicity: basilar rales, tachypnea, cough, fever, exertional dyspnea.
- Signs and symptoms of thrombocytopenia: excessive bleeding and easy bruising.
- Intake of fluids and urinary and other fluid output to minimize renal toxicity. Increase fluid intake if inadequate. Closely monitor electrolyte levels.
- Signs and symptoms of hepatotoxicity.
- Signs of hyperuricemia.
- Signs and symptoms of renal toxicity:

- Signs and symptoms of stomatitis: mouth sores, painful swallowing, dry mouth, white patchy areas in oral mucosa. Treat with peroxide, tea, topical anesthetics such as benzocaine and lidocaine or anti-fungal drug.
- Pulmonary fibrosis, particularly when cumulative doses are 600–1200 mg.

Editorial comments
- Cumulative bone marrow toxicity manifested by thrombocytopenia is a major concern with lomustine.
- Careful monitoring of platelet counts with discontinuation when platelets fall below $100,000/mm^3$ is strongly advised.

Loracarbef

Brand name: Lorabid.
Class of drug: Cephalosporin, second generation.
Mechanism of action: Binds to penicillin-binding proteins and disrupts or inhibits bacterial cell wall synthesis.
Susceptible organisms *in vivo*: Comparable to cefuroxime axetil, but less effective against *Hemophilus influenzae* and *Moraxella catarrhalis*.
Indications/dosage/route: Oral only.
- Secondary bacterial infection of acute bronchitis (cefuroxime axetil preferred)
  – Adults, children >13 years: 200–400 mg q12h for 7 days.
- Acute bacterial exacerbation of chronic bronchitis
  – Adults, children >13 years: 400 mg q12h for 7 days.
- Pharyngitis, tonsillitis
  – Adults, children >13 years: 200 mg q12h for 10 days (longer for *Streptococcus pyogenes* infection).
  Infants, children 6 months–12 years: 15 mg/kg/d in divided doses q12h for 10 days (longer for *S. pyogenes* infections).
- Sinusitis (cefuroxime axetil preferred)
  – Adults, children >13 years: 400 mg q12h for 10 days.

- Acute otitis media, acute maxillary sinusitis
  - Infants, children 6 months–12 years: 30 mg/kg/d in divided doses q12h for 10 days.
- Skin and skin structure infections (impetigo)
  - Adults: 200 mg q12h for 7 days.
  - Infants, children 6 months–12 years: 15 mg/kg/d in divided doses q12h for 7 days.
- Uncomplicated cystitis
  - Adults, children >13 years: 200 mg q24h for 7 days.

Adjustment of dosage
- Kidney disease: Creatinine clearance 10–49 mL/min: one-half recommended dose at usual dose interval; creatinine clearance <10 mL/min: recommended dose q3–5h.
- Liver disease: None.
- Elderly: None.
- Pediatric: See above.

Food: Take with yogurt or buttermilk (4 oz/d) to maintain bacterial flora and reduce the possibility of severe GI effects.

Pregnancy: Category B for all.

Lactation: No data available. American Academy of Pediatrics considers cephalosporins to be compatible with breastfeeding.

Contraindications: Hypersensitivity to other cephalosporins or related antibiotics, eg, penicillin.

Editorial comments: For additional information, see *cefuroxime*, p. 182.

Loratadine

Brand name: Claritin.
Class of drug: Long-acting H_1 receptor blocker, nonsedating.
Mechanism of action: Antagonizes histamine effects on GI tract, respiratory tract, blood vessels.
Indications/dosage/route: Oral only.
- Allergic rhinitis, chronic urticaria:

- Adults, children >12 years: 10 mg/d.
- Children 6–11 years: 10 mg/d.

Adjustment of dosage
- Kidney disease: Creatinine clearance <10 mL/min: 10 mg every other day.
- Liver disease: Lower initial dose to 10 mg every day.
- Elderly: None.

Pediatric: See above. Safety and efficacy have not been established for children <6 years.

Onset of Action	Peak Effect	Duration
1–3 h	8–12 h	24 h

Food: Take on empty stomach.
Pregnancy: Category B.
Lactation: Appears in breast milk. Should be safe to breastfeed.
Contraindications: Hypersensitivity to loratadine.
Warnings/precautions: Do not use in neonates or premature infants. Infants and young children at risk for overdosage.

Advice to patient
- Avoid driving and other activities requiring mental alertness or that are potentially dangerous until response to drug is known.
- Use caution if used along with alcohol and other CNS depressants such as narcotic analgesics and sedatives (eg, diazepam).
- Drink large quantities of water to minimize drying of secretions.
- If you are experiencing dry mouth, rinse with warm water frequently, chew sugarless gum, suck on an ice cube, or use artificial saliva. Carry out meticulous oral hygiene (floss teeth daily).
- Discontinue drug at least 4 days before skin testing (for allergies) to avoid the possibility of false-negative results.

Adverse reactions
- Common: none.
- Serious: arrhythmias, hypotension, confusion, bronchospasm, hepatitis, depression.

Clinically important drug interactions: None.

Parameters to monitor: Signs of dry mouth, eg, thickened secretions. Increase fluid intake to decrease viscosity of secretion.

Editorial comments: Loratadine has an excellent safety profile. It does not cause the prolongation of the QT interval observed with some nonsedating antihistamines. Interactions with erythromycin, cimetidine, and ketoconazole do not appear to be clinically significant.

Lorazepam

Brand name: Ativan.

Class of drug: Antianxiety agent, hypnotic, benzodiazepine.

Mechanism of action: Potentiates effects of GABA in limbic system and reticular formation.

Indications/dosage/route: Oral, IV, IM.

- Status epilepticus
  - Adults: IV 4 mg (slowly 2 mg/min). Repeat if seizures recur after 10–15 minutes.
- Anxiety disorder
  - Adults: PO 1–3 mg b.i.d. to t.i.d.
- Hypnotic
  - Adults: PO 2–4 mg h.s.
  - Elderly, debilitated patients: Initial: PO 0.5–2 mg/d in divided doses.
- Preoperative sedation
  - Adults: IM 0.05 mg/kg. Maximum: 4 mg 2 hours before surgery.
  - Adults: Initial: IV 0.044 mg/kg or 2 mg 2 hours before surgery.
- Antiemetic in cancer chemotherapy
  - Initial: IV 2 mg 30 minutes before chemotherapy, then 2 mg q4h as needed.

Adjustment of dosage

- Kidney disease: Use caution, especially with repeated doses.

- Liver disease: None.
- Elderly: See above.
- Pediatric: Only limited safety and efficacy data are available for use in children.

Food: No restrictions.

Pregnancy: Category D.

Lactation: Appears in breast milk. Potentially toxic to infant. American Academy of Pediatrics expresses concern about breast-feeding while taking benzodiazepines. Avoid breastfeeding.

Contraindications: Hypersensitivity to benzodiazepines, pregnancy, sleep apnea, respiratory compromise, intra-arterial injection.

Warnings/precautions

- Use with caution in patients with the following conditions: history of drug abuse, severe renal and hepatic impairment, elderly, neonates, infants.
- Benzodiazepines may cause psychologic and physical dependence.
- These drugs may cause paradoxical rage.
- It is best not to prescribe this drug for more than 6 months. If there is a need for long-term therapy, evaluate patient frequently.
- Use only for patients who have significant anxiety without medication, do not respond to other treatment, and are not drug abusers.

Advice to patient

- Avoid driving and other activities requiring mental alertness or that are potentially dangerous until response to drug is known.
- Avoid alcohol and other CNS depressants such as narcotic analgesics, alcohol, antidepressants, antihistamines, barbiturates, when taking this drug.
- Avoid use of OTC medications without first informing the treating physician.
- Cigarette smoking will decrease drug effect. Do not smoke when taking this drug.
- Do not stop drug abruptly if taken longer than 1 month. If suddenly withdrawn, there may be recurrence of the original anxiety or insomnia. A full-blown withdrawal syndrome may

occur consisting of vomiting, insomnia, tremor, sweating, muscle spasms. After chronic use, decrease drug dosage slowly, ie, over a period of several weeks at the rate of 25% per week.

- Avoid excessive use of xanthine-containing beverages (regular coffee, tea, cocoa) as these may counteract the action of the drug.

Adverse reactions

- Common: drowsiness.
- Serious: respiratory depression, depression, bone marrow depression, hypotension, drug dependence, hostile behavior, memory impairment.

Clinically important drug interactions

- Drugs that increase effects/toxicity of benzodiazepines: CNS depressants (alcohol, antihistamines, narcotic analgesics, tricyclic antidepressants, SSRIs, MAO inhibitors), cimetidine, disulfiram.
- Drugs that decrease effects/toxicity of benzodiazepines: flumazenil (antidote for overdose), carbamazepine.

Parameters to monitor

- Signs of chronic toxicity: ataxia, vertigo, slurred speech.
- Dosing to make sure amount taken is as prescribed, particularly if patient has suicidal tendencies.
- Efficacy of treatment: reduced symptoms of anxiety and tension, improved sleep.
- Signs of physical/psychologic dependence, particularly if patient is addiction-prone and requests frequent renewal of prescription or is experiencing a diminished response to the drug.
- Neurologic status including memory (anterograde amnesia), disturbing thoughts, unusual behavior.
- Possibility of blood dyscrasias: fever, sore throat, upper respiratory infection. Perform total and differential WBC counts.

Editorial comments

- Lorazepam is eliminated by the renal route and is not metabolized by cytochrome P450 enzymes. It is therefore safe to use in patients with liver disease. Overall, the side effect profile of lorazepam appears better than those of some other benzodiazepines.

• Seizures may occur if flumazenil is given after long-term use of benzodiazepines.

Losartan

Brand name: Cozaar.
Class of drug: Angiotensin II receptor antagonist, antihypertensive.
Mechanism of action: Blocks binding of angiotensin II to vascular smooth muscle receptors. This results in inhibition of vasoconstriction. Also diminishes aldosterone activity.
Indications/dosage/route: Oral only.
• Hypertension
  – Adults: 25–50 mg/d. Maintenance: PO 25–100 mg daily or b.i.d.

Adjustment of dosage
• Kidney disease: None.
• Liver disease: Initial dose should be 25 mg, maximum daily dose 100 mg.
• Elderly: None.
• Pediatric: Safety and efficacy have not been established in children <18 years of age.

Onset of Action	Peak Effect
1 wk	3–6 wk

Food: Advise patients to limit foods containing large amounts of potassium: sodium substitutes, orange juice, bananas.
Pregnancy: Category C. Category D in second and third trimesters. Discontinue losartan as soon as possible when pregnancy is detected.
Lactation: No data available. Potentially toxic to infant. Avoid breastfeeding.
Contraindications: Hypersensitivity to losartan.

Warnings/precautions

- Use with caution in patients with decreased renal function due to CHF or aldosterone-dependent kidney function, progressive liver disease.
- Losartan is less effective in African-American patients. Losartan's effects may be greater in females than males as plasma levels are higher in females.
- There is an increased risk of hypotension if losartan is given along with concurrent diuretic drug therapy. Under such circumstances, the initial dose should not exceed 25 mg/d.

Advice to patient

- Use two forms of birth control including hormonal and barrier methods.
- Do not discontinue drug abruptly.
- Avoid conditions of extreme heat as this may lead to dehydration and excessive lowering of BP.
- Change position slowly, in particular from recumbent to upright, to minimize orthostatic hypotension. Sit at the edge of the bed for several minutes before standing and lie down if feeling faint or dizzy. Avoid hot showers or baths and standing for long periods. Male patients with orthostatic hypotension may be safer urinating while seated on the toilet rather than standing.
- Notify dentist or treating physician prior to surgery if taking this medication.

Adverse reactions

- Common: none.
- Serious: hypotension, arrhythmia, angina, depression, hypersensitivity.

Clinically important drug interactions

- Drugs that increase effects/toxicity of losartan: cimetidine, ketoconazole, potassium sparing diuretics.
- Drugs that decrease effects/toxicity of losartan: phenobarbital, sulfaphenazole.

Parameters to monitor

- Evaluate patient for orthostasis with BP measurements in the sitting, lying, and standing positions repeatedly before and after initiating therapy.

- Efficacy of antihypertensive action. If daily losartan is not satisfactory at trough, it may be necessary to institute a twice daily regimen at the same dose or else increase the dose until a satisfactory response is obtained.

Editorial comments

- Losartan is not recommended for those patients who cannot tolerate ACE inhibitors.
- Losartan should not be used or should be used at much lower dosages in patients whose intravascular volume is depleted.

Lovastatin

Brand name: Mevacor.

Class of drug: Antilipidemic agent.

Mechanism of action: Inhibits HMG-CoA reductase. Reduces total LDL cholesterol, serum triglyceride levels. There is little if any effect on serum HDL levels.

Indications/dosage/route: Oral only.

- Hypercholesterolemia (types IIA and IIB)
  - Adults, adolescents: Initial: 20 mg with evening meal. Maintenance: 10–80 mg/d in single or two divided doses.

Adjustment of dosage

- Kidney disease: None.
- Liver disease: None.
- Elderly: None.
- Pediatric: Safety and efficacy have not been established in children.

Food: Take with meals.

Pregnancy: Category X. Contraindicated.

Lactation: Appears in breast milk. Contraindicated.

Contraindications: Hypersensitivity to statins, active liver disease or unexplained persistent elevations of serum transaminase, pregnancy, lactation.

Warnings/precautions

- Use with caution in patients with renal insufficiency, history of liver disease, alcohol abusers.

- Discontinue if drug-induced myopathy develops. This is characterized by myalgia, creatinine kinase levels >10 times normal.
- May cause acute renal failure from rhabdomyolysis. May occur more frequently when drug is combined with gemfibrozil or niacin.
- Discontinue drug if patient experiences severe trauma, surgery, or serious illness.

Advice to patient

- Avoid alcohol.
- Use OTC medications only after first informing the treating physician.
- Exercise regularly, reduce fat and alcohol intake, and stop smoking.

Adverse reactions

- Common: None.
- Serious: myopathy, rhabdomyolysis, neuropathy, cranial nerve abnormalities, hypersensitivity reactions, pancreatitis, hepatic injury including hepatic necrosis and cirrhosis, lens opacities.

Clinically important drug interactions

- Drugs that increase effects/toxicity of HMG-CoA reductase inhibitors: gemfibrozil, clofibrate, erthyromycin, cyclosporine, niacin, clarithromycin, itraconazole, protease inhibitors.
- HMG-CoA reductase inhibitors increase effects/toxicity of oral anticoagulants.

Parameters to monitor

- Total cholesterol, LDL and HDL cholesterol, triglycerides. These should be obtained prior to and periodically after treatment begins to ascertain drug efficacy.
- Serum BUN and creatinine.
- Liver enzymes before beginning therapy, at 3, 6, and 12 months thereafter, and semiannually afterward.
- Signs and symptoms of myopathy: unexplained skeletal muscle pain, muscle tenderness or weakness particularly when accompanied by fever or fatigue. Check creatinine kinase levels. If these are markedly elevated or patient is symptomatic, discontinue drug.

- Discontinue drug if transaminase levels exceed 3 times normal values. It may be advisable to take a liver biopsy if transaminase elevation persists after drug is discontinued.
- Ophthalmic status should be evaluated once a year following treatment. If lens opacity occurs, consider discontinuing drug.

Editorial comments: Current literature suggests that the most effective reduction of total and LDL cholesterol occurs with a combination of exercise, weight reduction, low-fat diet, and lipid-lowering agents.

Loxapine

Brand name: Loxitane.
Class of drug: Antipsychotic.
Mechanism of action: Blockade of dopamine receptors in the CNS.
Indications/dosage/route: Oral, IM.
- Psychotic disorders
  – Adults: PO 20–100 mg/d, divided as b.i.d. or q.i.d. Starting dose: 10 mg b.i.d.
  – Adults: IM 12.5–50 mg q4–6h. Maximum: 250 mg/d.

Adjustment of dosage
- Kidney disease: None.
- Liver desease: None.
- Elderly: Lower initial dosage should be given.
- Pediatric: Safety and efficacy have not been established in children <6 years.

Food: Mix oral concentrate in grapefruit or orange juice.
Pregnancy: Category C.
Lactation: No data available. Appears in breast milk in laboratory animals. Avoid breastfeeding.
Contraindications: Severe CNS depression, drug-induced depressed states, coma, hypersensitivity to dibenzoxepines.
Warnings/precautions
- Use with caution in patients with the following conditions: seizures, glaucoma, history of urinary retention, cardiovascular disorders.

- Advise patient that drowsiness and dizziness are transient and will subside after the first weeks of treatment.

Advice to patient

- Avoid alcohol and other CNS depressants such as opiate analgesics and sedatives (eg, diazepam) when taking this drug.
- To minimize possible photosensitivity reaction, apply adequate sunscreen and use proper covering when exposed to strong sunlight.
- Avoid driving and other activities requiring mental alertness or that are potentially dangerous until response to drug is known.
- Do not stop taking medication without consulting the physician.
- If experiencing constipation, increase intake of fluids and consumption of high-fiber foods (bran, whole-grain bread, raw vegetables and fruits).
- Change position slowly, in particular from recumbent to upright, to minimize orthostatic hypotension. Sit at the edge of the bed for several minutes before standing, and lie down if feeling faint or dizzy. Avoid hot showers or baths and standing for long periods. Male patients with orthostatic hypotension may be safer urinating while seated on the toilet rather than standing.
- Symptomatic relief of xerostomia: Rinse mouth with warm water frequently, chew sugarless gum, suck on ice cube, use artificial saliva if necessary, carry out meticulous oral hygiene (floss teeth daily).
- Notify dentist or treating physician prior to surgery if taking this medication.

Adverse reactions

- Common: extrapyramidal reactions, drowsiness, constipation, dry mouth.
- Serious: **orthostatic hypotension**, seizures, bone marrow suppression, NMS, hepatitis, hypotension, urinary retention.

Clinically important drug interactions

- Drugs that increase effects/toxicity of loxapine: β blockers, antacids (aluminum and magnesium types), antidiarrheals.
- Loxapine decreases effects/toxicity of sympathomimetics, appetite suppressants, clonidine, guanabenz, methyldopa, reserpine, bromocriptine, dopamine, levodopa.

• Loxapine increases effects/toxicity of CNS depressants, antiarrhythmics (guanethidine, procainamide), atropine, antidepressants, phenothiazines, antihistamines, lithium.

Parameters to monitor

• CBC with differential and platelets, liver enzymes.
• Orthostasis with BP measurements in the sitting, lying, and standing positions repeatedly before and after initiating therapy.
• Signs and symptoms of NMS: fever, tachycardia, convulsions, respiratory distress, irregular BP, severe muscle spasms. Use supportive measures and administer dantrolene.
• Signs and symptoms of drug-induced extrapyramidal syndrome (pseudoparkinsonism): akinesia, tremors at rest, pill rolling), shuffling gait, mask-like facies, drooling. If these occur while taking this medication drug discontinuation may be required. Alternatively, administration of diphenhydramine and benztropine may be indicated.

Editorial comments

• Tardive dyskinesia, a neuroleptic-induced movement disorder, if it occurs will become apparent after several months or years after treatment. This condition may disappear after drug withdrawal or be present for life. Prevention of the condition is not currently possible.
• Do not give by IV route.
• Do not eat candy or other foods that contain large amounts of sugar because these can result in fungal infections of the mouth or can increase caries.

Mannitol

Brand names: Osmitrol, Resectisol.
Class of drug: Osmotic diuretic.
Mechanism of action: Inhibits tubular resorption of water and electrolytes, increasing urine output.
Indications/dosage/route: IV only.
• Diuresis in drug intoxication, treatment of oliguria, prevention of oliguria or acute renal failure
   – Adults, children >12 years: 50–100 g injected over 90 minutes to several hours.
   – Children <12 years: 2 g/kg.
• Treatment of edema and ascites
   – Adults, children >12 years: 100 g injected over 2–6 hours.
• Increased intracranial pressure (preoperative), reduction of intraocular pressure.
   – 1.5–2 g/kg 1–1.5 hours before surgery.
• Cerebral edema
   – 1.5–2 g/kg over ≥30 minutes. Give as 15–20% solution. Maintain serum osmolality of 310–320 mOsm/kg.
Adjustment of dosage
• Kidney disease: See above.
• Liver disease: None.
• Elderly: May require lower dosage.
• Pediatric: Safety and efficacy have not been established in children <12 years.
• To decrease intracranial pressure: Onset 15 minutes, peak 60–90 minutes, duration 3–8 hours after infusion is stopped.

	Onset of Action	Peak Effect	Duration
Lowering intracranial pressure	15 min	30–60 min	3–8 h
Lowering intraocular pressure	30 min	No data	No data

Food: Not applicable.
Pregnancy: Category C.

Lactation: No data available. Best to avoid.

Contraindications: Severe renal disease, dehydration, pulmonary edema, hypersensitivity to mannitol or its components.

Warnings/precautions

- Use with caution in patients with severe heart failure, severe pulmonary congestion, active intracranial bleeding.
- Do not administer if crystals are present after warming solution.
- Cardiac status should be established before administration.
- Do not mix with blood products.

Adverse reactions

- Common: headache, nausea, vomiting, dizziness, blurred vision, urinary frequency.
- Serious: pulmonary edema, water intoxication, CHF, seizures, hypovolemia, electrolyte imbalance, tissue necrosis.

Clinically important drug interactions

- Mannitol decreases effects/toxicity of lithium.
- Mannitol increases effects/toxicity of cardiac glycosides, other diuretics.

Parameters to monitor

- Vital signs hourly as well as fluid input and output, serum BUN and creatinine, serum and urinary sodium and potassium levels and other electrolytes. Check daily or several times a day.
- Symptoms of CHF.
- Signs of fluid or electrolyte depletion: dry mouth, thirst, weakness, muscle pains or cramps, oliguria, tachycardia, dry mucous membranes.
- Signs of fluid overload: dyspnea, rales/crackles, edema, increased central venous pressure.
- Signs of electrolyte imbalance: muscle weakness, tingling, paresthesia, confusion.

Editorial comments

- Overdose with mannitol is manifested as hypotension and cardiovascular collapse. In such circumstances, infusion should be discontinued, supportive measures used, and, if necessary, hemodialysis initiated. When mannitol is administered for oliguria, the rate at which it is given should be titrated to produce a urine output of 30–50 mL/h.

- Evaluate the following when mannitol is used to reduce intracranial pressure and brain mass: fluid and electrolyte balance, circulatory and renal reserve, total input and output. Such determination should be made before and after the drug is administered.
- This drug is not listed in the *Physician's Desk Reference,* 54th edition, 2000.

Mebendazole

Brand name: Vermox.
Class of drug: Anthelmintic.
Mechanism of action: Inhibits uptake of glucose and other nutrients by parasitic helminths.
Indication/dosage/route: Oral only.
- Pinworms
  - Adults, children >12 years: 100 mg as single dose. Repeat in 2 weeks if infection persists. Treat other family members.
- Roundworms, hookworms, whipworms
  - 100 mg b.i.d. for 3 days. Repeat dose in 3–4 weeks.
- Capillariasis
  - Pediatric: 200 mg b.i.d. for 20 days. Its use in children <2 years is considered a relative contraindication.

Adjustment of dosage: None.
Food: Take with food.
Pregnancy: Category C.
Lactation: Probably present in minute amounts in breast milk. May continue breastfeeding.
Contraindications: Hypersensitivity to mebendazole.
Warnings/precautions: Use with caution in patients with liver disease, ulcerative colitis, Crohn's ileitis.
Advice to patient
- Avoid driving and other activities requiring mental alertness or that are potentially dangerous until response to drug is known.
- Patient and family members should shower frequently if possible.

- Keep hands away from mouth.
- Keep fingernails short and clean.
- Do not shake bedding as this could result in airborne spread of ova.
- Counsel patient's family members to check for worm infestation and treat accordingly.
- Disinfect toilet daily; wash all fruits and vegetables; cook all meats and vegetables thoroughly.
- Wear gloves when preparing food.

Adverse reactions
- Common: diarrhea, abdominal pain, nausea, vomiting.
- Serious: bone marrow suppression, hepatitis, hypersensitivity reactions.

Clinically important drug interactions: Drugs that decrease effects/toxicity of mebendazole: phenytoin, carbamazepine, cimetidine.

Parameters to monitor
- Feces for ongoing pinworm infection. Have patient swab perianal area each morning using transparent tape and bring to your office. Criteria for discontinuity: no additional eggs for 7 consecutive days.
- Appearance of adult worms in perianal area. Cellophane tape swabs should be taken prior to and starting 1 week after treatment to detect ova in the perianal area.

Editorial comments
- Patient and family members should be taught how to avoid reinfestation with these worms. The following measures should be undertaken to avoid reinfection: (1) perianal area should be washed thoroughly; (2) hands and fingernails should be cleaned before meals and after defecation; (3) undergarments and bedclothes should be changed daily.
- Mebendazole is the drug of choice for whipworm; it can produce up to 70% cure with a single treatment. The cure rate for roundworms, pinworms, and hookworms is 90–100%. The criterion for cure is negative perianal swabs for 7 days.
- For those treated for hookworm and whipworm: it may be necessary to take an iron supplement every day and for 6 months following treatment if anemia is present.

Meclizine

Brand names: Antivert, Bonine.
Class of drug: Antihistamine (H_1 blocker), antiemetic.
Mechanism of action: Inhibits impulses from vestibular system to the chemoreceptor trigger zone. Decreases the excitability of the labyrinth in the middle ear. Central anticholinergic.
Indications/dosage/route: Oral only.
- Vertigo, Meniere's disease, labyrinthitis
  – Adults, children ≥12 years: 25–100 mg/d, divided doses.
- Motion sickness
  – Adults, children ≥12 years: 25–50 mg 1 hour before travel. Drug regimen may be repeated throughout period of travel.

Adjustment of dosage
- Liver disease: None.
- Kidney disease: None.
- Elderly: Dosage should be reduced; increased risk for anticholinergic side effects (constipation, drowsiness, confusion).
- Pediatric: Safety and efficacy have not been established in children <12 years.

Onset of Action	Duration
1 h	8–24 h

Food: Take with food, water, or milk.
Pregnancy: Category B.
Lactation: Probably appears in breast milk. Effects on infant unknown. Newborns and premature infants may have increased sensitivity to drug.
Contraindications: Hypersensitivity to meclizine.
Warnings/precautions: Use with caution in patients with closed-angle glaucoma, asthma, BPH, GI obstruction, bladder neck obstruction.

Advice to patients

- Avoid driving and other activities requiring mental alertness or that are potentially dangerous until response to drug is known.
- Avoid alcohol and other CNS depressants such as opiate analgesics and sedatives (eg, diazepam) when taking this drug.
- Symptomatic relief of xerostomia: Rinse mouth with warm water frequently, chew sugarless gum, suck on ice cube, use artificial saliva if necessary, carry out meticulous oral hygiene (floss teeth daily).
- Take meclizine approximately 1 hour before anticipated exposure to conditions causing motion sickness.

Adverse reactions

- Common: drowsiness, dry mouth.
- Serious: urinary retention.

Clinically important drug interactions: Drugs that increase effects/toxicity of meclizine: CNS depressants, alcohol, drugs that cause ototoxicity (aminoglycosides, vancomycin, loop diuretics, cisplatin).

Parameters to monitor

- Patients with motion sickness: nausea and vomiting prior to and 60 minutes after drug is taken.
- Patients with vertigo: monitor periodically.

Editorial comments: Discontinue meclizine if the vertigo does not respond in 1–2 weeks.

Medroxyprogesterone

Brand names: Provera, Depo-provera, Cycrin, Amen.
Class of drug: Progestational hormone, contraceptive.
Mechanism of action: Inhibits secretion of pituitary gonadotropins (FSH, LH) by positive feedback.
Indications/dosage/route: Oral, IM.

- Secondary amenorrhea
  - Adults: PO 5–10 mg/d for 5–10 days. Begin any time during menstrual cycle. If previously estrogen primed, the dose is 10 mg/d for 10 days

- Abnormal uterine bleeding with no pathology
  - Adults: PO 5–10 mg/d for 5–10 days. Begin on day 16 or 21 of menstrual cycle. If previously estrogen primed, the dose is 10 mg/d for 10 days, beginning on day 16 of menstrual cycle.
- Long-acting contraceptive (Depo-provera):
  - Adults: 150 mg of depot form q3mo.
- Endometrial or renal cell carcinoma (unlabeled)
  - Adults: Initial: IM 400–1000 mg/wk.

Adjustment of dosage
- Kidney disease: None.
- Liver disease: Contraindicated.
- Elderly: None.
- Pediatric: Safety and efficacy have not been determined.

Food: No restrictions.

Pregnancy: Category D.

Lactation: Considered compatible by American Academy of Pediatrics.

Contraindications: Hypersensitivity to progestins, history of thrombophlebitis, active thromboembolic disease, cerebral hemorrhage, liver disease, missed abortion, use as diagnostic for pregnancy, known or suspected pregnancy (first 4 months), undiagnosed vaginal bleeding, carcinoma of the breast, known or suspected genital malignancy.

Warnings/precautions
- Use with caution in patients with respiratory infection, history of depression, epilepsy, migraine, cardiac disease, renal disease, diabetes.
- Cigarette smoking significantly increases risk of cardiac complications and thrombotic events. At highest risk are women >35 years of age, smoking ≥15 cigarettes per day.

Advice to patient
- Weigh yourself twice a week and report to treating physician if there are any unusual changes in weight.
- If you observe a yellowing of skin or eyes, report to treating physician.
- If you experience changes in mental status suggestive of depression, report to treating physician.

- Discontinue medication if you experience sudden headaches or attack of migraine.
- Discontinue drug and notify physician if you miss a period or experience unusual bleeding.
- If you miss a dose, take the missed dose as soon as possible; do not double the next dose.
- If the drug is used as a contraceptive and you miss a dose, stop taking and use an alternative method of contraception until period returns.
- Use good hygiene—flossing, gum massages, regular cleaning by dentist—to avoid gum problems.
- Keep an extra month supply of the drug on hand.
- Do not give this medication to anyone else.

Adverse reactions

- Common: irregular or unpredictable menstrual bleeding (spotting), amenorrhea, breakthrough bleeding, infertility for up to 18 months.
- Serious: thromboembolic events, depression, cholestatic jaundice.

Clinically important drug interactions: Drugs that decrease effects/toxicity of progestins: aminoglutethimide, phenytoin, rifampin.

Parameters to monitor

- Liver enzymes, cholesterol (total, LDL, HDL), triglycerides.
- Diabetic patient: Monitor blood glucose closely and adjust antidiabetic medication if necessary.
- Signs and symptoms of thromboembolic or thrombotic disorders: pains in leg, sudden chest pain, shortness of breath, migraine, sudden severe headache, vomiting. Discontinue drug.

Editorial comments

- Prior to initiation of treatment with progestins, female patients should undergo pelvic examination, PAP smear, and breast examinations.
- If a patient experiences persistent or abnormal vaginal bleeding while on this drug, perform diagnostic tests including endometrial sampling, to determine cause.

Mefenamic Acid

Brand name: Ponstel.
Class of drug: NSAID.
Mechanism of action: Inhibits cyclooxygenase, resulting in inhibition of synthesis of prostaglandins and other inflammatory mediators.
Indications/dosage/route: Oral.
• Analgesia, primary dysmenorrhea
  – Adults, children >14 years: Initial: 500 mg. Maintenance: 250 mg q6h.
Adjustment of dosage
• Kidney disease: Do not use.
• Liver disease: None.
• Elderly: May be necessary to reduce dose for patients >65 years.
• Pediatric: Safety and efficacy have not been established in children <14 years.
Food: Take with food or large quantities of water or milk.
Pregnancy: Category C. Category D in third trimester or near delivery.
Lactation: Appears in breast milk. Considered compatible with breastfeeding by American Academy of Pediatrics.
Contraindications: Hypersensitivity to mefenamic acid, active gastric ulcer, renal disease and cross-sensitivity with other NSAIDs and aspirin.
Editorial comments: For additional information, see *ibuprofen*, p. 445.

Megestrol Acetate

Brand name: Megace.

Class of drug: Progestational hormone.

Mechanism of action: Inhibits secretion of pituitary gonadotropins (FSH, LH) by positive feedback.

Indications/dosage/route: Oral only.

- Appetite stimulant for AIDS patients
  - Adults: Initial: 800 mg/d. Maintenance: 400 mg/d after 1 month.
- Breast cancer
  - 40 mg q.i.d.
- Endometrial cancer
  - 40–320 mg/d in divided doses for at least 2 months.

Adjustment of dosage

- Kidney disease: None.
- Liver disease: None.
- Elderly: None.
- Pediatric: Safety and efficacy have not been determined in children.

Food: No restrictions.

Pregnancy: Category D

Lactation: Another drug from this class (medroxyprogesterone) is considered compatible by American Academy of Pediatrics.

Contraindications: Hypersensitivity to progestins, history of thrombophlebitis, active thromboembolic disease, cerebral hemorrhage, liver disease, missed abortion, use as diagnostic for pregnancy, known or suspected pregnancy (first 4 months), undiagnosed vaginal bleeding, carcinoma of the breast, known or suspected genital malignancy.

Warnings/precautions

- Use with caution in patients with respiratory infection, history of depression, epilepsy, migraine, cardiac disease, renal disease, diabetes.
- Cigarette smoking significantly increases risk of cardiac complications and thrombotic events. At highest risk are women > 35 years of age, smoking ≥15 cigarettes per day.

Advice to patient

- Weigh yourself twice a week and report to treating physician if there are any unusual changes in weight.

- If you observe a yellowing of skin or eyes, report to treating physician.
- If you experience changes in mental status suggestive of depression, report to treating physician.
- Discontinue medication if you experience sudden headaches or attack of migraine.
- Discontinue drug and notify physician if you miss a period or experience unusual bleeding.
- If you miss a dose, take the missed dose as soon as possible; do not double the next dose.
- Use good hygiene—flossing, gum massages, regular cleaning by dentist—to avoid gum problems.

Adverse reactions
- Common: irregular or unpredictable menstrual bleeding (spotting), amenorrhea, breakthrough bleeding, infertility for up to 18 months.
- Serious: thromboembolic events, depression, cholestatic jaundice.

Clinically important drug interactions: Drugs that decrease effects/toxicity of progestins: aminoglutethimide, phenytoin, rifampin.

Parameters to monitor
- Response of tumor to therapy increased appetite and weight gain.
- Liver enzymes, cholesterol (total, LDL, HDL), triglycerides.
- Diabetic patient: Monitor blood glucose closely and adjust antidiabetic medication if necessary.
- Signs and symptoms of thromboembolic or thrombotic disorder: pains in leg, sudden chest pain, shortness of breath, migraine, sudden severe headache, vomiting. Discontinue drug.

Editorial comments: Megesterol treatment has been shown to result in increased appetite and weight gain in cachectic patients with advanced HIV infection and carcinoma patients. Addition of weight occurs primarily in the fat compartment.

Melphalan

Brand name: Alkeran.
Class of drug: Alkylating anticancer drug.
Mechanism of action: Forms covalent bond with elements in DNA, preventing separation of strands of DNA during cell division.
Indications/dosage/route: Oral only.
• Multiple myeloma
  – Adults: Initial: 6 mg; dose adjusted on basis of blood counts done at approximately weekly intervals. After 2–3 weeks, discontinue drug for up to 4 weeks during which WBC and platelet counts should be followed. When the WBC and platelet counts rise, maintenance of 2 mg daily may be instituted.
• Epithelial ovarian cancer
  – Adults: Initial: 0.2 mg/kg/d for 5 days depending on response. Course is repeated every 4–5 weeks depending on hematologic tolerance.
Pregnancy: Category D.
Lactation: No data available. Potentially toxic to infant. Contraindicated.
Contraindications: Failure to respond to previously administered drug, hypersensitivity to melphalan and related drugs.
Editorial comments: For additional information, see *busulfan,* p. 120.

Meperidine

Brand name: Demerol.
Class of drug: Narcotic analgesic, agonist.

Mechanism of action: Binds to opiate receptors and blocks ascending pain pathways. Reduces patient's perception of pain without altering cause of the pain.

Indications/dosage/route: Oral, IV, IM.

• Analgesia
  – Adults: IV, IM, PO 50–150 mg q3–4h as needed.
  – Children: 1.0–1.5 mg/kg q3–4h as needed.
• Preoperatively
  – Adults: IM 50–100 mg 30–90 min before anesthesia.
  – Children: IM 1–2 mg/kg 30–90 min before anesthesia.
• Obstetrics
  – Adults: IM 50–100 mg q1–3h.
• Adjunct to anesthesia
  – IV infusion 1–10 mg/mL as needed

Adjustment of dosage

• Kidney disease: Creatinine clearance 10–50 mL/min: give 75% of normal dose; creatinine clearance <10 mL/min: give 50% of normal dose.
• Liver disease: Reduce dose in patients with cirrhosis.
• Elderly: None.
• Pediatric: See above.

Onset of Action	Peak Effect	Duration
10–45 min	0.5–1 h	2–4 h

Food: May be taken with food to lessen GI upset.

Pregnancy: Category B. Category D if prolonged use or if given in high doses at term.

Lactation: Appears in breast milk. Potentially toxic to infant. Considered compatible with breastfeeding by American Academy of Pediatrics.

Contraindications: Hypersensitivity to narcotics of the same chemical class, MAO inhibitors within 14 days.

Warnings/precautions

• Use with caution in patients with head injury with increased intracranial pressure, serious alcoholism, prostatic hypertrophy, chronic pulmonary disease, severe liver or kidney disease, disorders of biliary tract, supraventricular tachycardia, history of convulsive disorder and in postoperative patients with pulmonary disease.

- Administer drug before patient experiences severe pain for fullest efficacy of the drug.
- Have the following available when treating patient with this drug: naloxone (Narcan) or other antagonist, means of administering oxygen, and support of respiration.
- Nausea, vomiting, and orthostatic hypotension occur most prominently in ambulatory patients. If nausea and vomiting persist, it may be necessary to administer an antiemetic, eg, droperidol or prochlorperazine.
- This drug can cause severe hypotension in a patient who is volume depleted or if given along with a phenothiazine or general anesthetic.
- Careful diagnosis must be made of acute abdominal condition before this drug is administered.

Advice to patient

- Avoid alcohol and other CNS depressants such as sedatives (eg, diazepam) when taking this drug.
- Avoid driving and other activities requiring mental alertness or that are potentially dangerous until response to drug is known.
- Change position slowly, in particular from recumbent to upright, to minimize orthostatic hypotension. Sit at the edge of the bed for several minutes before standing, and lie down if feeling faint or dizzy. Avoid hot showers or baths and standing for long periods. Male patients should sit on the toilet while urinating rather than standing.
- Do not increase dose if you are not experiencing sufficient pain relief without approval from treating physician.
- Do not stop medication abruptly when you have been taking this drug for 2 or more weeks. If so, a withdrawal reaction may occur within 24–48 hours. The following are typical symptoms: iritability, perspiration, rhinorrhea, lacrimation, dilated pupils, piloerection ("goose flesh"), bone and muscle aches,

restless sleep ("yen"), increased systolic pressure, hyperpyrexia, diarrhea, hyperglycemia, spontaneous orgasm.

- Take OTC drugs only with approval by treating physician. Some of these may potentiate the CNS depressant effects of the drug.
- If dizziness persists longer than 3 days, decrease dose gradually (over 1–2 days).
- Attempt to void every 4 hours.

Adverse reactions

- Common: constipation, lightheadedness, dizziness, sedation, nausea, vomiting, sweating, dyspnea.
- Serious: **hypotension, bradycardia**, apnea, circulatory depression, respiratory arrest, convulsions (high doses, IV), shock, increased intracranial depression, paralytic ileus, physical and psychologic dependence and addiction.

Clinically important drug interactions: Drugs that increase effects/toxicity of narcotic analgesics: alcohol, benzodiazepines, antihistamines, phenothiazines, butyrophenones, triyclic antidepressants, MAO inhibitors.

Parameters to monitor

- Signs and symptoms of pain: restlessness, anorexia, elevated pulse, increased respiratory rate. Differentiate restlessness associated with pain and that caused by CNS stimulation caused by meperidine. This paradoxical reaction is seen mainly in women and elderly patients.
- Respiratory status prior to and following drug administration. Note rate, depth, and rhythm of respirations. If rate falls below 12/min, withhold drug unless patient is receiving ventilatory support. Consider administering an antagonist, eg, naloxone, 0.1–0.5 mg IV every 2–3 minutes. Be aware that respiratory depression may occur even at small doses. Restlessness may also be a symptom of hypoxia.
- Character of cough reflex. Encourage postoperative patient to change position frequently (at least every 2 hours), breathe deeply, and cough at regular intervals, unless coughing is contraindicated. These steps will help prevent atelectasis.

- Signs and symptoms of urinary retention, particularly in patients with prostatic hypertrophy or urethral stricture. Monitor output/intake and check for oliguria or urinary retention.
- Signs of tolerance or dependence. Determine whether patient is attempting to obtain more drug than prescribed as this may indicate onset of tolerance and possibility of dependence. If tolerance develops to one opiate, there is generally cross-tolerance to all drugs in this class. Physical dependence is generally not a problem if the drug is given <2 weeks.
- BP. If systolic pressure falls below 90 mm Hg, do not administer the drug unless there is ventilatory support. Be aware that the elderly and those receiving drugs with hypotensive properties are most susceptible to sharp fall in BP.
- Heart rate. Withhold drug if adult pulse rate is below 60 beats/min. Alternatively, administer atropine.
- Respiratory status of newborn baby and possible withdrawal reaction. If the mother has received an opiate just prior to delivery, the neonate may experience severe respiratory depression. Resuscitation may be necessary as may a narcotic antgonist, eg, naloxone. Alternatively, the neonate may experience severe withdrawal symptoms 1–4 days after birth. In such circumstances, administer tincture of opium or paregoric.
- Signs and symptoms of constipation. If patient is on drug longer than 2–3 days, administer a bulk or fiber laxative, eg, psyllium, 1 teaspoon in 240 mL liquid/d. Encourage patient to drink large amounts of fluid, 2.5 to 3 L/d.

Editorial comments

- The following considerations should be noted by the clinician. Breakthrough pain: use a sustained-release morphine preparation along with one that provides rapid release. Transdermal therapy may be beneficial.
- Cancer patients who are experiencing severe, unrelieved pain: Administer the drug IV or IM and switch to oral therapy once pain is controlled. Transdermal therapy may be beneficial.

Mephobarbital

Brand name: Mebaral.
Class of drug: Sedative, antiepileptic.
Mechanism of action: Facilitates action of GABA at its receptor. Depresses sensory cortex, cerebellum, decreases motor activity.
Indications/dosage/route: Oral only.

- Epilepsy
  - Adults: 400–600 mg/d.
  - Children <5 years: 16–32 mg t.i.d. or q.i.d.
- Sedation
  - Adults: 32–100 mg t.i.d. or q.i.d.
  - Children: 16–32 mg t.i.d. or q.i.d.

Adjustment of dosage

- Kidney disease: Reduce dose.
- Liver disease: Reduce dose.
- Elderly: Reduce dose.
- Pediatric: See above.

Onset of Action	Duration
10–15 min	3–4 h

Food: Best taken at bedtime. No food restriction.
Pregnancy: Category D. Causes fetal abnormalities. Infants with chronic *in utero* barbiturate exposure are at risk for withdrawal. Administration during labor may cause infant respiratory depression.
Lactation: Appears in breast milk. Classified by American Academy of Pediatrics as potentially causing major adverse effects on infant when breastfeeding. Avoid breastfeeding.
Contraindications: Hypersensitivity to barbiturates, porphyria, preexisting CNS depression, hepatic encephalopathy, severe respiratory disease, compromised respiration, previous addiction to a barbiturate or other sedative–hypnotic (eg, benzodiazepines), pregnancy.

Editorial comments: For additional information, see *phenobarbital*, p. 728.

Mepivacaine

Brand name: Carbocaine.
Class of drug: Local and regional anesthetic.
Mechanism of action: Reversibly inhibits initiation and conduction of nerve impulses near site of injection.
Indications/dosage/route: Local injection only.
• Cervical, brachial, intercostal nerve block
  – Adults: Total dose 1% solution: 50–400 mg (5–40 mL).
• Paracervical block
  – Obstetric analgesia: Adults: Total dose 1% solution: 200 mg (20 mL).
• Caudal and epidural block
  – Adults: Total dose 1% solution: 400 mg (40 mL). Use solution that does not contain preservative.
• Infiltration analgesia
  – Adults: Total dose 1% solution: 400 mg (40 mL).
  – Pediatric, all uses: Children <30 lb: 5–6 mg/kg; maximum: 400 mg. Children <3 years: 0.5–1.5% solutions only should be used.
Adjustment of dosage
• Kidney disease: Use with caution.
• Liver disease: Use with extreme caution in severe liver disease.
• Elderly: Use with caution.
• Pediatric: See above.
Food: Not applicable
Pregnancy: Category C
Lactation: No data available. Use with caution.
Contraindications: Hypersensitivity to amide-type local anesthetic (eg, lidocaine), sensitivity to sodium metabisulfate (in preparations containing epinephrine).

Warnings/precautions
- Use local anesthetics plus vasoconstrictor (eg, epinephrine, norepinephrine) with caution in patients with peripheral vascular disease and hypertension and those receiving general anesthetics. Use local anesthetics with or without vasoconstrictor with caution in patients with severe liver disease. Use with extreme caution for lumbar and caudal epidural anesthesia in patients with spinal deformities, existing neurologic disease, severe uncontrolled hypotension, septicemia.
- Epidural anesthesia: A test dose of the local anesthetic should first be given before the full dose is administered to ensure that the catheter is not within a blood vessel. The test dose should include 10–15 µg epinephrine. Any increase in heart rate and systolic pressure within 45 seconds (the epinephrine response) would indicate that the injection is intravascular.
- Local anesthetics can trigger familial malignant hyperthermia. Symptoms of this condition include tachycardia, labile BP, tachypnea, muscle rigidity. The necessary means must be available to manage this condition (dantrolene, oxygen, supportive measures).
- A local anesthetic containing a vasoconstrictor should be injected with great caution into areas of the body supplied by end-organ arteries (nose, ears, penis, digits).

Editorial comments
- This drug is not intended for use in spinal anesthesia or in dentistry.
- This drug is listed without details in the *Physician's Desk Reference*, 54th edition, 2000.
- For additional information, see *bupivacaine*, p. 113.

Meprobamate

Brand names: Equanil, Miltown.
Class of drug: Antianxiety, sedative.
Mechanism of action: Nonselective CNS depressant similar to

barbiturates. Depresses multiple regions in the CNS including thalamus, hypothalamus, limbic system, and spinal cord.

Indications/dosage/route: Oral only.

• Anxiety and tension; sedative for managing anxiety disorders
  – Adults: 1.2–1.6 g/d, 3 or 4 equal doses. Maximum: 2.4 g/d.
  – Children 6–12 years: 100–200 mg b.i.d. or t.i.d.

Adjustment of dosage

• Kidney disease: Creatinine clearance 10–50 mL/min: administer every 9–12 hours; creatinine clearance <10 mL/min: administer every 12–18 hours.
• Liver disease: Use with caution.
• Elderly: Lowest dose possible should be used.
• Pediatric: Safety and efficacy have not been established in children <6 years.

Onset of Action	Peak Effect	Duration
< 1 h	1–3 h	6–12 h

Food: Take with meals.

Pregnancy: Category D. Increased risk of congenital malformations during the first trimester of pregnancy.

Lactation: Appears in breast milk. Potentially toxic to infant. Avoid breastfeeding.

Contraindications: Hypersensitivity to meprobamate, carisoprodol, mebutamate, tybutamate, or carbromal; history of prophyria.

Warnings/precautions

• Use with caution in elderly and debilitated patients and patients with kidney or liver disease, seizure disorders, suicidal tendencies.
• Drug dependence, abuse, and withdrawal reactions have been documented to occur with meprobamate. Symptoms of withdrawal, which occur generally within 12–48 hours of abrupt discontinuation of meprobamate include: muscle twitching, ataxia, convulsions, hallucinations.
• If there is a history of dermatologic conditions, an allergic reaction may occur. This usually happens by the fourth dose.

• Avoid prolonged use of meprobamate particularly in those who are addiction-prone individuals and alcoholics. The dose prescribed should be carefully supervised and the least amount of drug feasible should be dispensed at any one time. If it is necessary to withdraw the drug, the dose should be reduced gradually over a period of 1–2 weeks, particularly when the drug has been used at high dose for many weeks or months.

Advice to patient

• Use two forms of birth control including hormonal and barrier methods.
• Avoid driving and other activities requiring mental alertness or that are potentially dangerous until response to drug is known.
• Avoid alcohol and other CNS depressants such as opiate analgesics or sedatives (eg, diazepam) when taking this drug.
• Change position slowly, in particular from recumbent to upright, to minimize orthostatic hypotension. Sit at the edge of the bed for several minutes before standing, and lie down if feeling faint or dizzy. Avoid hot showers or baths and standing for long periods. Male patients with orthostatic hypotension may be safer urinating while seated on the toilet rather than standing.

Clinically important drug interactions: Meprobamate increases effects/toxicity of barbiturates, narcotic analgesics, antihistamines, other CNS depressants, alcohol, MAO inhibitors.

Adverse reactions

• Common: drowsiness, dizziness, weakness, overstimulation, nausea, palpitations.
• Serious: seizures, bone marrow depression, severe allergic reactions, arrhythmias, severe hypotension, exacerbation of porphyria.

Parameters to monitor

• Levels of consciousness and vital signs. Such determinations should be made frequently.
• Hematologic status, particularly during long-term therapy.

Editorial comments: This medication is indicated for short-term use. No studies on chronic ingestion (>4 months) have been performed.

Mercaptopurine

Brand name: Purinethol.
Class of drug: Antineoplastic, immunosuppressant.
Mechanism of action: Inhibition of DNA and RNA synthesis by cytotoxic metabolite of mercaptopurine.
Indications/dosage/route: Oral only.
- Acute lymphoblastic leukemia, chronic myelocytic leukemia
  – Adults: PO 2.5 mg/kg/d. Maximum: 5 mg/kg/d. Maintenance: 1.5–2.5 mg/kg/d as single dose.
  – Children ≥5 years: PO 2.5 mg/kg/d. Maximum: 75 mg/m^2/d.
- Off-label indications: autoimmune disorders (eg, rheumatoid arthritis), inflammatory bowel disease

Adjustment of dosage
- Kidney disease: Dose should be reduced to avoid accumulation; specific guidelines are not available.
- Liver disease: Dose should be reduced to avoid accumulation; specific guidelines are not available.
- Elderly: None.
- Pediatric: See above.

Food: Should be taken with meals.
Pregnancy: Category D. It is recommended that contraception be used by females and males taking this drug.
Lactation: No data available. Best to avoid.
Contraindications: Patients with illnesses that have proved resistant to mercaptopurine on previous use, severe liver disease, severe bone marrow depression
Warnings/precautions: Use with caution in patients who have received chemotherapy or radiation therapy and patients with reduced neutrophil or platelet counts or renal or hepatic disease

Advice to patient
- Use two forms of birth control including hormonal and barrier methods.
- Take sufficient fluids, 2000–3000 mL/d.

- Avoid alcohol.
- Avoid crowds as well as patients who may have a contagious disease.
- Inform physician if you experience the following signs of toxicity: fever, sore throat, jaundice, nausea, vomiting, bleeding.
- Do not receive any vaccinations (particularly live attenuated viruses) without permission from treating physician.

Adverse reactions
- Common: nausea, vomiting, diarrhea, oral ulcers, ulcers of the GI tract.
- Serious: **bone marrow depression, intrahepatic cholestasis and centrilobular necrosis,** renal toxicity, pancreatitis, drug fever.

Clinically important drug interactions
- Drugs that increase effects/toxicity of mercaptopurine: allopurinol, other potentially hepatotoxic agents, trimethoprim–sulfamethoxazole, doxorubicin.
- Mercaptopurine decreases effects/toxicity of warfarin, live virus vaccines.

Parameters to monitor
- Signs and symptoms of bone marrow depression, hepatotoxicity, thrombocytopenia, anemia, renal toxicity, infection.
- Signs of hypersensitivity reactions: urticaria, rash, wheezing, pruritis, hypotension.
- Intake of fluids and urinary and other fluid output to minimize renal toxicity. Increase fluid intake if inadequate. Closely monitor electrolyte levels.
- Signs and symptoms of anemia: shortness of breath, dizziness, angina, pale conjunctiva, skin, and nailbeds.

Editorial comments: Randomized, double-blind placebo-controlled trials have demonstrated efficacy of 6-mercaptopurine in active or quiescent Crohn's disease. Patients in these trials were generally able to taper prednisone doses to 5 mg/d or less. Doses for 6-mercpatopurine were generally 1.5 mg/kg/d and were 2.5 mg/kg/d for azathioprine.

Mesalamine

Brand names: Asacol, Pentasa, Rowasa.

Class of drug: GI antiinflammatory.

Mechanism of action: Modulation of GI inflammation via alteration of prostaglandins and leukotrienes.

Indications/dosage/route: Oral, rectal.

- Acute treatment of Crohn's disease, ulcerative colitis, or other inflammatory bowel diseases; maintenance therapy for above

- *Tablet* (pH-sensitive coating, delayed release)
  - Adults: 800 mg t.i.d.
  - Children: 50 mg/kg/d, dose two to three times per day.

- *Capsule* (microspheres in semipermeable membrane, released at pH >6)
  - Adults: 1000 mg q.i.d.

- *Retention enema*
  - Adults: 60 mL (4 g) q.h.s. Retained through the night (approximately 8 hours).

- *Suppository*
  - Adults: 1 suppository (500 mg) b.i.d. or q.h.s.

Adjustment of dosage

- Kidney disease: None.
- Liver disease: None.
- Elderly: None.
- Pediatric: See above.

Pregnancy: Category B.

Lactation: No data available. Use with caution. Some systemic absorption anticipated.

Contraindications: Hypersensitivity to mesalamine or salicylates.

Warnings/precautions

- Use with caution in patients with GI obstruction. Do not use in the setting of toxic megacolon.
- Usage of these agents may be associated with rare but serious complications including pericarditis, pancreatitis, and renal insufficiency.

Advice to patients

- Keep well hydrated while taking this drug.
- Report worsening symptoms of colitis such as increasing abdominal pain, diarrhea, or rectal bleeding to your physician.
- Do not break tablets, capsules, or suppositories. Attempt to retain enemas at least 8 hours. Be sure to unwrap suppository prior to insertion. Avoid excessive handling of suppository or enema preparations.

Adverse reactions

- Common: none.
- Serious: pancreatitis, renal insufficiency, hypersensitivity reactions, severe abdominal pain and bloody diarrhea (acute intolerance syndrome), pericarditis.

Clinically important drug interactions: Mesalamine decreases effects/toxicity of digoxin.

Parameters to monitor

- Serum BUN and creatinine.
- Symptoms of colitis. Gradual improvement in diarrhea, abdominal pain, and rectal bleeding is anticipated with treatment.
- Symptoms of pericarditis including shortness of breath and chest pain.
- Symptoms of hypersensitivity reactions.

Editorial comments

- Newer forms of mesalamine that do not contain sulfapyridine are generally better tolerated than the older 5-ASA agent, sulfasalazine. It does, however, appear that these are somewhat less potent agents. As a general rule, patients with acute severe colitis are not immediately administered 5-ASA agents. Instead, corticosteroids are administered and followed by 5-ASA agents when the severity of the acute flare of colitis has diminished. New studies are investigating the usage of 5-ASA agents as preventive therapy for relapse following surgical resection for refractory Crohn's disease.

Mesna

Brand name: Mesnex.

Class of drug: Bladder mucosa protectant.

Mechanism of action: Mesna is converted in the kidney to a sulfhydryl metabolite which combines with and detoxifies ifosfamide and cyclophosphamide.

Indications/dosage/route: Oral, IV.

- Prevention of ifosfamide-induced and cyclophosphamide-induced hemorrhagic cystitis
  - Adults: 20% (w/w) ifosfamide or cyclophosphamide: IV bolus, 15 minutes before treatment and 4–8 hours after treatment. Maximum daily dose is 60–100% of ifosfamide. May use up to 150% of ifosfamide dose.
  - Oral: 40% of ifosfamide or cyclophosphamide dose. Three doses at 4-hour intervals.
  - Alternative: 20 mg/kg/dose q4h; total of 3 doses.

Adjustment of dosage

- Kidney disease: None.
- Liver disease: None.
- Elderly: Guidelines are not available.
- Pediatric: Safety has not been established.

	Onset of Action	Duration
Oral	Rapid	4 h

Food: Mesna should be diluted in carbonated beverages, juices, or whole milk. Solution stable for 24 hours.

Pregnancy: Category B.

Lactation: No data available. Best to avoid.

Contraindications: Hypersensitivity to mesna or compounds containing the thiol group.

Warnings/precautions
- Examine patient's urine for appearance of blood before ifosfamide or cyclophosphamide is administered.
- If hematuria is present, reduce dose of ifosfamide or discontinue drug.
- Use with caution in patients who may be sensitive to benzyl alcohol.

Adverse reactions
- Common: fatigue, headache, nausea, vomiting, diarrhea, limb pain.
- Serious: hypotension.

Clinically important drug interactions
- Mesna increases effects of aziocillin versus *Pseudomonas aeruginosa*
- Mesna decreases effectiveness of coumadin.

Parameters to monitor: Signs of hematuria before and after mesna administration.

Editorial comments: Reduction or discontinuation of ifosfamide or cyclophosphamide may be required if nausea, vomiting, or diarrhea occurs. If these persist or are severe it may be necessary to reduce the dose or discontinue mesna as well.

Mesoridazine

Brand name: Serentil.
Class of drug: Phenothiazine antipsychotic (neuroleptic).
Mechanism of action: Antagonizes dopamine at dopaminergic receptors in CNS neurons.
Indications/dosage/route: Oral only.
- Psychotic disorders
  - Adults, adolescents: Initial: PO 50 mg t.i.d. Maintenance: 100–400 mg/d.
- Alcoholism
  - Adults: Initial: PO 25 mg b.i.d. Maintenance: 50–200 mg/d.
- Pyschoneurotic disorders

– Adults, adolescents: PO 10 mg t.i.d. Maintenance: 30–150 mg/d.
– Adults, adolescents: Initial: IM 25 mg. Repeat: q30–60min as needed. Maintenance: 25–200 mg/d.

Adjustment of dosage
• Kidney disease: Use with caution. Guidelines not available.
• Liver disease: Use with caution. Guidelines not available.
• Elderly: Use lower doses; increase dosage more gradually.
• Pediatric: Safety and efficacy have not been determined in children <12 years.

Food: No restriction.

Pregnancy: Category C.

Lactation: No data available. Considered to be an agent of concern by American Academy of Pediatrics. Avoid breastfeeding.

Contraindications: Hypersensitivity to phenothiazines, concurrent use of high-dose CNS depressants (alcohol, barbituates, benzodiazepines, narcotics), CNS depression, comatose state.

Editorial comments: For additional information, see *chlorpromazine*, p. 206.

Metaprotenol

Brand name: Alupent.

Class of drug: β-Adrenergic agonist, bronchodilator.

Mechanism of action: Relaxes smooth muscles of the bronchioles by stimulating β_2-adrenergic receptors.

Indications/dosage/route: Oral inhalant.
• Bronchodilation
  – Adults, children >27.2 kg or 9 years: 20 mg t.i.d. to q.i.d.
  – Children <27.2 kg or 6–9 years: 10 mg t.i.d. to q.i.d.
  – Children <6 years: 1.3–2.6 mg/kg/d.
• Bronchodilation: hand nebulizer
  – 5–15 inhalations
• Bronchodilation: IPPB
  – 0.3 mL of 5% solution diluted to 2.5 mL saline or other diluent.

- Bronchodilation: MDI
  - 2–3 inhalations q3–4h. Maximum: 12 inhalations.

Adjustment of dosage
- Kidney disease: None.
- Liver disease: None.
- Elderly: Lower doses may be required.
- Pediatric: See above.

	Onset of Action	Peak Effect	Duration
PO	≈ 30 min	—	4 h
Inhalation	5–30 min	—	2–6 h

Food: Not applicable.

Pregnancy: Category C.

Lactation: No data available. Potentially toxic to infant. Best to avoid.

Contraindications: Hypersensitivity to adrenergic compounds, tachycardia (idiopathic or from digitalis).

Warnings/precautions
- Use with caution in patients with hyperthyroidism, diabetes, coronary insufficiency, ischemic heart disease, cardiac arrhythmias, history of stroke, CHF, hypertension.
- Some preparations contain bisulfite, which may cause an allergic reaction in sensitive individuals.
- Instruct patient in proper technique for using nebulizer and/or inhaler.
- Overuse as bronchodilator is potentially toxic. May cause systemic adrenergic effects including tachycardia.
- This drug can produce paradoxical bronchospasm.

Advice to patient
- Use OTC products only with approval by treating physician.
- Do not use solutions that contain a precipitate or are discolored.
- Wait at least 1 minute after 1 or 2 inhalations before taking a third dose.

- Keep inhalant away from eyes.
- Maintain adequate fluid intake (2000–3000 mL/d) to facilitate clearing of secretions.
- Rinse mouth with water after each inhalation to minimize dry mouth and throat irritation.
- Administer inhalant when arising in the morning and before meals.
- Notify treating physician if more than 3 aerosol inhalations are required to achieve relief within a 24-hour period. Do not increase dose in an attempt to obtain relief.

Adverse reactions

- Common: nervousness (20%), tremor (17%), tachycardia (17%), GI upset, insomnia, hyperactivity.
- Serious: bronchospasm.

Clinically important drug interactions

- Drugs that increase effects/toxicity of β agonists: ipratropium, MAO inhibitors, tricyclic antidepressants.
- Drugs that decrease activity of β agonists: sympathomimetic drugs (nasal decongestants, weight loss drugs, eg, phenyl-propanolamine), anticholinergic drugs, phenothiazines.

Parameters to monitor

- Heart rate, BP.
- Possible development of tolerance with prolonged use. Discontinue drug temporarily and effectiveness will be restored.
- Signs of paradoxical bronchospasm.
- Pulmonary function on initiation and during bronchodilator therapy. Assess respiratory rate, sputum character (color, quantity), peak airway flow, O_2 saturation, and blood gases.
- Efficacy of treatment: improved breathing, prevention of bronchospasm, reduction of asthmatic attacks, prevention of exercise-induced asthma. If no relief is obtained from 3–5 aerosol inhalations within 6–12 hours, reevaluate effectiveness of treatment.
- FEV_1 rate to determine effectiveness of the drug in reversing bronchostriction. Efficacy is indicated by an increase in FEV_1 of 10–20%. In addition such patients, as well as those who

have chronic disease, should be given a peak flow gauge and told to determine peak expiratory flow rate at least twice daily.
• Arterial blood gases if applicable.

Editorial comments: For patients with acute asthma or acute exacerbation of COPD, reduce dose to minimum necessary to control condition after initial relief is achieved. For chronic conditions, the patient should be reassessed every 1–6 months following control of symptoms.

Methadone

Brand name: Dolophine.
Class of drug: Narcotic analgesic, agonist.
Mechanism of action: Binds to opiate receptors and blocks ascending pain pathways. Reduces patient's perception of pain without altering cause of the pain.
Indications/dosage/route: Oral only.
• Analgesia
  – Adults: 2.5–10 mg q3–4h.
• Detoxification treatment of narcotic addiction
  – Adults: Initial: 15–20 mg/d.
• Maintenance treatment of narcotic addiction
  – Adults: Initial: 20–40 mg q4–8h after heroin is stopped. Then increase to maximum 120 mg/d as needed.
  – Children 16–18 years: Admitted to maintenance program under limited conditions only.

Adjustment of dosage
• Kidney disease: Reduce dose.
• Liver disease: Reduce dose.
• Elderly: Reduce dose.
• Pediatric: Safety and efficacy have not been established in children <16 years.

Onset of Action	Peak Effect	Duration
30–60 min	0.5–1 h	4–6 h

Food: May be taken with food to lessen GI upset.

Pregnancy: Category B. Category D if prolonged use or if given in high doses at term.

Lactation: Appears in breast milk. Potentially toxic to infant. Avoid breastfeeding.

Contraindications: Hypersensitivity to methadone or other narcotics of the same chemical class.

Warnings/precautions

• Use with caution in patients with head injury with increased intracranial pressure, serious alcoholism, prostatic hypertrophy, chronic pulmonary disease, severe liver or kidney disease, disorders of the biliary tract, postoperative patients with pulmonary disease.

• Administer drug before patient experiences severe pain for fullest efficacy of the drug.

• Have the following available when treating patient with this drug: naloxone (Narcan) or other antagonist, means of administering oxygen, and support of respiration.

• Nausea, vomiting, and orthostatic hypotension occur most prominently in ambulatory patients. If nausea and vomiting persist, it may be necessary to administer an antiemetic, eg, droperidol or prochlorperazine.

• This drug can cause severe hypotension in a patient who is volume depleted or if given along with a phenothiazine or general anesthesia.

• Careful diagnosis must be made of acute abdominal condition before this drug is administered.

Editorial comments

• When this drug is used for treatment of narcotic addiction it is dispensed only by treatment programs approved by FDA, DEA, and designated state authority. The drug is dispensed only in oral form and according to treatment requirements stated in federal regulations.

- Methadone can produce dependence of the morphine type. It should be prescribed with the same degree of caution as for morphine. A patient who is dependent on methadone will experience a withdrawal reaction if given a narcotic antagonist, the severity of which will depend on the degree of dependence and dose of antagonist.
- Methadone oral concentrate is for oral administration only. As it is in highly concentrated form, this product must not be injected.
- Patients who are on methadone maintenance may experience opioid withdral symptoms if given pentazocine. Symptoms of opioid withdrawal include lacrimation, rhinorrhea, yawning, anxiety, dilated pupils, abdominal cramping, diarrhea, and weight loss. During induction with methadone, these symptoms may occur. Excessive dosing of methadone may produce severe opiate toxicity including respiratory depression and cardiovascular collapse.
- For additional information, see *morphine*, p. 633.

Methicillin

Brand name: Staphcillin.
Class of drug: Antibiotic, penicillin family.
Mechanism of action: Inhibits bacterial cell wall synthesis.
Susceptible organisms *in vivo*: MSSA, streptococci.
Indications/dosage/route: IV, IM.
- Systemic infections caused by susceptible organisms
  - Adults: 4–12 g/d in divided doses q4–6h.
  - Children: 100–300 mg/kg in divided doses q4–6h.
  - Infants >7 days, weight >2000 g: 100 mg/kg in divided doses q6h.
- Meningitis
  - Infants >7 days, weight >2000 g: 200 mg/kg/d.
  - Infants >7 days, weight <2000 g: 150 mg/kg/d.
  - Infants <7 days, weight <2000 g: 100 mg/kg/d.

Adjustment of dosage
- Kidney disease: Would not use because of the risk of acute

interstitial nephritis. Creatinine clearance less than 10 mL/min (adults): 1 g q8–12h.
- Liver disease: None.
- Elderly: None.
- Pediatric: None.

Food: Not applicable.
Pregnancy: Category B.
Lactation: No data available. Best to avoid.
Contraindications: Hypersensitivity to penicillin or cephalos-porins.
Editorial comments: Methicillin is used only for the treatment of penicillin G-resistant *Staphylococcus aureus.* It frequently causes more interstitial nephritis, so nafcillin is the preferred agent. The microbiology lab reports susceptibility to methicillin (which appropriately predicts susceptibility to nafcillin).

This drug is not listed in the *Physician's Desk Reference,* 54th edition, 2000.

For additional information, see *penicillin G*, p. 708.

Methimazole

Brand name: Tapazole.
Mechanism of action: Inhibits synthesis of thyroid hormone.
Indications/dosage/route: Oral only.
- Mild hyperthyroidism
  – Adults: Initial: 15 mg/d.
- Moderately severe hyperthyroidism
  – Adults: Initial: 30–40 mg/d.
- Severe hyperthyroidism
  – Adults: Initial: 60 mg/d. Maintenance: 5–15 mg/d. Maximum: 30 mg/d.
  – Children: 0.4–0.5 mg/kg/d, once daily or divided in two doses. Maintenance: 0.2 mg/kg/d q8h. Maximum: 30 mg/d.
- Thyrotoxic crisis
  – Adults: 15–20 mg/d q4h along with other supportive treatments, eg, β-blocker.

Adjustment of dosage
- Dosage should be adjusted to achieve and maintain serum T_3, T_4, and TSH in normal range.
- Kidney disease: None.
- Liver disease: None.
- Elderly: Use with caution as they are particularly at risk for toxicity from methimazole.
- Pediatric: See above.

Onset of Action	Duration
30–40 min	2–4 h

Food: Patient should take methimazole with meals if GI upset occurs.
Pregnancy: Category D.
Lactation: Appears in breast milk. Potentially toxic to infant. Considered compatible by American Academy of Pediatrics.
Contraindications: Hypersensitivity to methimazole.

Warnings/precautions
- Use with caution in patients receiving drugs known to cause bone marrow suppression, particularly agranulocytosis, or in patients with decreased bone marrow reserve.
- Avoid doses >40 mg/d.
- Use with caution in patients >40 years.

Advice to patient
- Use two forms of birth control including hormonal and barrier methods.
- Avoid driving and other activities requiring mental alertness or that are potentially dangerous until response to drug is known.
- Carry identification card at all times describing disease, treatment regimen, name, address, and telephone number of treating physician.
- Report to treating physician if you experience any of the following: chills, unexplain bleeding, fever, sore throat.
- Limit intake of iodine in foods: shell fish, iodized salt, cabbage, turnips.
- Check weight on the same scale 2–7 times per month. Notify physician if there is a significant change in body weight.

Adverse reactions
- Common: fever, skin rash.
- Serious: **leukopenia,** bone marrow suppression, agranulocytosis, thrombocytopenia, lupus-like syndrome, urticaria, cholestasis, nephrotic syndrome.

Clinically important drug interactions
- Drugs that increase effects/toxicity of methimazole: drugs causing bone marrow depression, lithium, potassium iodide, glycerol.
- Methimazole increases effects/toxicity of oral anticoagulants.

Parameters to monitor
- Signs and symptoms of bone marrow depression.
- Signs and symptoms of hepatotoxicity.
- Symptoms of hyperthyroidism or thyrotoxicosis: palpations, tachycardia, insomnia, sweating, weight loss.
- Symptoms of hypothyroidism: constipation, dry skin, intolerance to cold, weakness, fatigue. Adjust dosage as required.
- Signs and symptoms of hypersensitivity.
- Thyroid function prior to and weekly during first month of therapy, then monthly for 3 months, and then q2–3 mo.
- In children, appropriate growth and development every 6 months.

Editorial comments
- Methimazole and other antithyroid thioamides have been replaced by radioactive iodine as treatment for hyperthyroidism.
- This drug is listed without details in the *Physician's Desk Reference*, 54th edition, 2000.

Methotrexate

Brand names: Folex, Mexate, Rheumatrex, MTX, Amethopterin.
Class of drug: Antineoplastic antimetabolite.
Mechanism of action: Inhibits DNA, RNA, and protein synthesis.

Indications/dosage/route: Oral, IV, IM.

• Acute lymphoblastic leukemia, meningeal leukemia, head and neck cancers, rheumatoid arthritis, psoriasis, ectopic pregnancy, trophoblastic tumors, inflammatory bowel disease.

Note: Physician is advised to check the current literature for updated recommended protocols. A variety of protocols are available for many tumor types. Dosage individualization is expected.

• Trophoblastic tumors
  – Adults: PO, IM 15–30 mg/d for 5 days. Repeat after 1 or more weeks depending on response or toxicity. Three to five courses commonly used.

• Acute lymphocytic leukemia
  – Adults, children: Loading dose: 100 mg/m^2/d infused for 35 hours.

• Meningeal leukemia
  – Adults, children >3 years: Intrathecal 10–15 mg/m^2. Maximum: 15mg q2–5d until CSF counts are normal, and then weekly for 2 weeks. Monthly treatments follow.
  – Children <3 years: 3–12 mg.

• Burkitt's lymphoma
  – Adults: PO 10–25 mg/d, 4–8 days.

• Psoriasis
  – Adults: IM 10–25 mg once a week or 2.5–5.0 mg q12h, 3 doses/wk.

• Rhematoid arthritis (refractory to other drug treatments)
  – Adults: PO 7.5–15 mg/wk, single or divided doses. Maximum: 20 mg/wk.
  – Elderly: PO 2.5–7.5 mg/wk as tolerated. Maximum: 20 mg/ wk.

Adjustment of dosage

• Kidney disease: Creatinine clearance 50–80 mL/min: 70–75% standard dose; creatinine clearance 10–50 mL/min: 30–50% standard dose; creatinine clearance <10 mL/min: contraindicated.

• Liver disease: Bilirubin 3.1–5.0 mg/dL or AST >180 units: 75% of standard dose; bilirubin >5 mg/dL: contraindicated. Avoid if evidence of severe hepatic dysfunction.

• Elderly: Monitor carefully because of increased risk of toxicity.

• Pediatric: See above.

Pregnancy: Category D.

Lactation: Appears in breast milk. Considered contraindicated by American Academy of Pediatrics.

Contraindications: Pregnancy, lactation, severe renal or hepatic impairment, severe bone marrow depression in patients with psoriasis, rheumatoid arthritis, AIDS.

Warnings/precautions

• Use with caution in patients with liver or kidney disease, bone marrow suppression, anemia, peptic ulcer, ulcerative colitis, folic acid deficiency, infections.

• Avoid in women of childbearing age unless benefits outweigh risk of pregnancy. Remind female patients with childbearing potential to practice two forms of birth control.

• Hydrate patient prior to high-dose therapy with 1–2 L of IV fluid.

• Urine should be alkalinized to prevent precipitation of methotrexate. Administer dose of bicarbonate to keep urine pH >7 for 24 hours or longer after high dose.

Advice to patient

• Use two forms of birth control including hormonal and barrier methods.

• Avoid alcohol.

• Avoid aspirin-containing products and all NSAIDs when taking this drug.

• Receive vaccinations (particularly live attenuated viruses) only with permission from treating physician.

• Use good mouth care to prevent infections of the oral cavity.

• Maintain adequate fluid intake.

Adverse reactions

Chemotherapy

• Common: rash, hyperpigmentation, photosensitivity, hyperuricemia, decreased oogenesis and spermatogenesis, stomatitis, glossitis, nausea, diarrhea, anorexia, mucositis, alopecia.

• Serious: **vasculitis, bone marrow depression, renal failure, arachnoiditis (intrathecal only), subacute CNS toxicity (intrathecal only—motor paralysis, cranial nerve palsy,**

seizure, coma), seizures, renal failure, pulmonary toxicity, nephropathy, diabetes, hepatitis, hepatic fibrosis, cirrhosis, necrotizing demyelinating leukoencephalopathy, intestinal perforation, pneumonitis, anaphylaxis, secondary infections.

Rheumatoid arthritis

- Common: elevated liver enzymes, nausea.
- Serious: thrombocytopenia, leukopenia, pancytopenia, arachnoiditis with subacute cerebral toxicity (with intrathecal administration).

Note: Toxicity is generally related to dose and frequency of administration.

Clinically important drug interactions

- Drugs that increase effects/toxicity of methotrexate: vincristine, salicylates, NSAIDs, sulfonamides, probenecid, penicillins, cyclosporine.
- Drugs that decrease effects/toxicity of methtrexate: folic acid, chloramphenicol, tetracyclines, broad-spectrum antibiotics, corticosteroids.
- Methotrexate decreases effects/toxicity of phenytoin.
- Methotrexate increases effects/toxicity of live virus vaccines, cytarabine, cyclosporine.

Parameters to monitor

- Chronic use: CBC with differential and platelets, serum BUN and creatinine, liver enzymes every 3 months. Consider liver biopsy after cumulative oral dose of 1.5 g.
- High-dose treatment: Monitor patient's temperature daily and note whether patient is coughing and has dyspnea, cyanosis, or symptoms of pneumonitis.
- Urinary output, BUN and serum creatinine. Drug should be stopped if BUN is >30 mg/dL or serum creatinine is >2 mg/dL. Give IV fluids, bicarbonate.
- GI symptoms: oral ulcerations, abdominal pain, stomatitis, vomiting; consider peptic ulcer perforation. Therapy may have to be discontinued if these persist.
- Signs of infection: fever, sore throat, cough, low back pain, difficulty in urination.
- Signs of hypersensitivity reactions.

- Hepatic function: AST, ALT, bilirubin, LDH, prior to and throughout course of therapy.

Editorial comments

- In the event hemapoietic toxicity develops, the treatment is highly specific. Patient should be administered calcium leucovorin within 24 hours of administration of high dose of methotrexate. The dosage of leucovorin should be such as to produce serum concentrations that are higher than those of methotrexate. (See *leucovorin*, p. 497).
- Chemotherapy with methotrexate requires the signature of attending physician before the drug is dispensed by a pharmacy.
- Intramuscular methotrexate has been shown to be effective for the treatment of Crohn's disease at doses up to 25 mg/wk. Long-term efficacy has not been fully established.

Methoxsalen

Brand names: Oxsoralen, 8-MOP.
Class of drug: Photoactive agent, psoralen compound.
Mechanism of action: After photoactivation, forms conjugates and covalent bonds with DNA. Inhibits DNA synthesis and decreases cell proliferation.
Indications/dosage/route: Oral only.

- Severe, disabling psoriasis that is not responsive to other therapy; palliation in cutaneous T-cell lymphoma
  - Adults: Dosage depends on weight. 30–50 kg: 20 mg; 51–65 kg: 30 mg; 66–80 kg: 40 mg. Doses are given 1.5–2 hours before exposure to high-intensity UVA light, 3 times/wk. Treatments are given 48 hours apart.
- Idiopathic vitiligo
  - Adults, children >12 years: 20 mg 2–4 hours before exposure to UVA light or sunlight.

Adjustment of dosage: Pediatric: Safety and efficacy have not been established in children <12 years.

Food: Patient should be advised to take methoxalen with food and milk. However, the following foods may increase the toxicity of methoxalen: carrots, figs, celery, mustard, parsley. These foods should be avoided.

Pregnancy: Category C.

Lactation: No data available. Best to avoid.

Contraindications: Light-sensitive diseases including porphyria cutanea tarda, xeroderma pigmentosa, systemic lupus erythematosus, melanoma, variegate aphakia (absence of the lens of the eye), squamous cell carcinoma of the skin, cataract, invasive squamous cell cancer.

Warnings/precautions: Use with caution in patients with basal cell carcinoma of the skin, prior radiation therapy, arsenic exposure, liver disease, cardiac disease.

Advice to patients

• Wear UVA-protective glasses for several hours following treatment.

• Protect the skin and avoid direct or indirect sunlight for at least 24 hours after oral therapy and 48 hours after topical therapy. Wraparound sunglasses should be worn for 24 hours after UVA treatment.

Clinically important drug interactions: Drugs that increase effects/toxicity of methoxalen: tetracyclines, thiazide diuretics, griseofulvin, coal tars, phenothiazines, halogenated salicylamides, organic dyes (methylene blue).

Adverse reactions

• Common: nausea.

• Serious: depression.

When combined with UVA

• Common: nausea, pruritis, erythema, headache, malaise, leg cramps.

• Serious: squamous cell carcinoma (skin), cataracts if proper eye wear is not used.

Parameters to monitor

• Serum level of antinuclear antibody, CBC, liver enzymes, BUN, creatinine. Check these prior to therapy and every 6 months thereafter.

- Baseline ophthalmologic status should be established. Periodic eye examinations at regular intervals during extended therapy.
- Signs and symptoms of burning or blistering. Discontinue methoxsalen treatment temporarily if this occurs.
- Effectiveness of therapy including frequent examinations of the skin.

Editorial comments: Methoxsalen lotion should be applied only under the direct supervision of the treating physician and should not otherwise be dispensed to the patient.

Methyclothiazide

Brand names: Aquatensen, Enduron.
Class of drug: Thiazide diuretic.
Mechanism of action: Inhibits sodium resorption in distal tubule, resulting in increased urinary excretion of sodium, potassium, and water.
Indications/dosage/route: Oral only.
- Diuretic
  - Adults: 2.5–10 mg/d. Maximum: 10 mg/d.
  - Children: 20–200 µg/kg/d.
- Hypertension
  - Adults: 2.5–5 mg/d.
  - Children: 50–200 µg/d.

Adjustment of dosage
- Kidney disease: Use with caution. Ineffective in severe renal failure.
- Liver disease: Use with caution. May cause electrolyte imbalance.
- Elderly: Use with caution because of age-related impairment of kidney function.
- Pediatric: See above.

Onset of Action	Peak Effect	Duration
2 h	4–6 h	24 h

Food: Should be taken with food.
Pregnancy: Category D.
Lactation: Thiazides are excreted in breast milk. Hydrochlorothiazide (another thiazide diuretic) is considered compatible by American Academy of Pediatrics. Thiazide diuretics may suppress lactation.
Contraindications: Anuria, hypersensitivity to thiazides or sulfonamide-derived drugs.
Editorial comments: For additional information, see *hydrochlorothiazide*, p. 426.

Methyldopa

Brand name: Aldomet.
Class of drug: Centrally acting hypertensive.
Mechanism of action: Activates central inhibitory α-adrenergic receptors.
Indications/dosage/route: Oral, IV.
• Moderate to severe hypertension
  – Adults: Initial: PO 250 mg b.i.d. or t.i.d. Increase or decrease prn q2d. Maintenance: 500 mg to 3 g/d in 2–4 divided doses; Maximum: 3 g/d. IV: 250–500 mg q6h. Maximum; 1 g q6h (crisis).
  – Children: 10 mg/kg/d. Increase dose q2d until desired response is obtained. Maximum: 65 mg/kg/d.
Adjustment of dosage
• Kidney disease: Creatinine clearance >50 mL/min: dose q8h; creatinine clearance 10–50 mL/min: dose q8–12h.
• Liver disease: None.
• Elderly: Reduce dosage. Initiate at 125 mg q.d. or b.i.d. Increase dose by 125 mg q2–3d.
• Pediatric: Safety and efficacy have not been established.

Onset of Action	Peak Effect	Duration
12–24 h	4–6 h	24–48 h

Food: Take before meals.

Pregnancy: Category D.

Lactation: Appears in breast milk. Considered compatible by American Academy of Pediatrics.

Contraindications: Hypersensitivity to methyldopa, active liver disease, pheochromocytoma, MAO inhibitor therapy.

Warnings/precautions

- Use with caution in patents with history of liver disease, kidney disease, elderly.
- Methyldopa has been associated with hemolytic anemia.
- Do not administer methyldopa by the IM or SC route; IV administration is acceptable for emergency purposes.
- Twenty to forty-three percent of patients taking methyldopa develop positive Coombs tests.
- Advise patient to take methyldopa at bedtime to avoid daytime sedation.
- Increase in dosage should be made with the evening dose.

Advice to patient

- Use two forms of birth control including hormonal and barrier methods.
- Avoid driving and other activities requiring mental alertness or that are potentially dangerous until response to drug is known.
- Avoid alcohol and other CNS depressants such as opiate analgesics and sedatives (eg, diazepam) when taking this drug.
- May discolor urine
- Change position slowly, in particular from recumbent to upright, to minimize orthostatic hypotension. Sit at the edge of the bed for several minutes before standing, and lie down if feeling faint or dizzy. Avoid hot showers or baths and standing for long periods. Male patients should sit on the toilet while urinating rather than standing.

Adverse reactions

- Common: headache, dizziness, sedation, dry mouth, edema, drug fever, anxiety, nightmares.
- Serious: bone marrow suppression, hemolytic anemia, hepatitis, cholestasis, cirrhosis, hepatic necrosis, angina, myocarditis,

hemolytic anemia, depression, anxiety, orthostatic hypotension, lupus-like syndrome.

Clinically important drug interactions

- Drugs that increase effects/toxicity of methyldopa: diuretics, levodopa, verapamil, MAO inhibitors.
- Drugs that decrease effects/toxicity of methyldopa: iron salts, NSAIDs, phenothiazines, tricyclic antidepressants.
- Methyldopa increases the effects/toxicity of other antihypertensive agents, lithium, phenylpropanolamine, haloperidol, phenoxybenzamine.

Parameters to monitor

- Hematocrit, hemoglobin, RBC count, liver enzymes periodically.
- Signs of hepatotoxicity. These may be observed 2–4 weeks after methyldopa administration.
- Signs of drug-induced depression.
- Intake of fluids and urinary and other fluid output to minimize renal toxicity. Closely monitor electrolyte levels.
- Perform Coombs test between 6th and 10th months of drug administration. Discontinue methyldopa if positive.
- Body temperature during therapy to assess whether drug fever is occurring. Drug fever from methyldopa has the following characteristics: eosinophilia, liver enzyme abnormalities. It is recommended to examine liver enzymes and prothrombin time if unexplained fever occurs.
- Signs and symptoms of bone marrow depression.

Editorial comments

- The parenteral form of methyldopa should no longer be used for emergency purposes because of its slow onset of action.
- Tolerance to the antihypertensive effects of methyldopa may occur between 2 and 3 months of administration. This may be averted by adding a diuretic or by increasing the dose of methyldopa.
- Some of the methyldopa products contain alcohol or bisulfites; accordingly, these products should not be administered to patients who have a known sensitivity to these substances.

• Methyldopa is no longer considered to be a first-line drug for the treatment of hypertension because of its side effect profile.
• Elderly are at high risk for CNS toxicity.

Methylphenidate

Brand name: Ritalin.

Class of drug: Therapeutic agent for ADHD, narcolepsy, antidepressant.

Mechanism of action: Stimulant, blocks reuptake of norepinephrine at nerve terminals.

Indication/dosage/route: Oral only.

• ADHD
  – Children >6 years: 2.5–5 mg (or 0.3 mg/kg) before breakfast and lunch. Increase by 5- to 10-mg increments (or 0.1 mg/kg) per week prn. Maximum: 2 mg/kg or 60 mg/d.
• Narcolepsy
  – Adults: 10 mg b.i.d. to t.i.d. 30–45 minutes before meals. Maintenance: 40–50 mg/d.
• Depression (unlabeled use).
  – Adults: 2.5 mg every morning. Increase by 2.5–5 mg q2–3d. Maximum: 20 mg/d. Last dose prior to noon.

Adjustment of dosage: Pediatric: Safety and efficacy have not been established in children under 6 years of age.

Onset of Action	Duration
2 h	4–6 h

Food: Take before meals.

Pregnancy: Category C.

Lactation: Probably appears in breast milk. Potentially toxic to infant. Avoid breastfeeding.

Contraindications: Hypersensitivity to methylphenidate, suicidal or homicidal tendencies, marked anxiety, agitation, glaucoma, motor tics, hyperthyroidism, family history or diagnosis of Tourette's syndrome.

Warnings/precautions: Use with caution in patient's with hypertension, diabetes, seizure disorders, history of drug abuse, EEG abnormalities, dementia.

Advice to patient
- Take the last dose with lunch to reduce the possibility of insomnia.
- Avoid the use of OTC medications without first informing the treating physician.
- Do not drink caffeinated beverages including coffee and colas.

Adverse reactions
- Common: insomnia, anorexia.
- Serious: **tachycardia,** hypertension, seizures, thrombocytopenia, arrhythmias, dermatitis, erythema multiforma, worsening of Tourette's syndrome, psychosis, growth retardation.

Clinically important drug interactions
- The following drugs increase effects/toxicity of methylphenidate: sympathomimetics (decongestants, vasoconstrictors), MAO inhibitors.
- Methylphenidate increases effects/toxicity of tricyclic antidepressants, anticonvulsants, warfarin, caffeine.
- Methylphenidate decreases effects/toxicity of guanethidine, bretylium.

Parameters to monitor
- BP, pulse rate, respiratory function before administering methylphenidate and periodically thereafter.
- Height and weight of children on long-term therapy.
- Effectiveness of methylphenidate because tolerance occurs rapidly. Dose should not be increased as this may result in dependence. Determine if the symptoms are sufficiently controlled to warrant continuation.
- Signs of Tourette's syndrome.
- Hematologic status when drug is administered long-term.

Editorial comments
- Methylphenidate is the drug of choice for ADHD. Its use should be reassessed at puberty and generally discontinued at that time.
- It may be advisable to institute periodic holidays from the drug to determine its efficacy as well as to decrease the possibility of tolerance and dependence.
- It is most important that the psychologic evaluation of the child before instituting therapy does not show evidence of a psychotic condition.

Methylprednisolone

Brand name: Solu-Medrol.
Class of drug: Corticosteroid, systemic.
Mechanism of action: Inhibits migration of polymorphonuclear leukocytes, stabilizes lysosomal membranes, inhibits production of products of arachidonic acid cascade.
Indications/dosage/route: Oral, IM.
- Rheumatoid arthritis
  - Adults: PO 6–16 mg/d. Decrease dose gradually as condition improves.
  - Children: PO 6–10 mg/d.
- Acute rheumatic fever
  - Adults: PO 1 mg/kg in 4 equally divided doses after meals and h.s.
- Rheumatoid arthritis
  - Adults: IM 40 mg q2wk.
- Dermatitis, dermatologic diseases
  - Adults: IM 40–100 mg/wk, 1–4 weeks.
- Allergic states
  - Adults: IM 80–120 mg.
Adjustment of dosage
- Kidney disease: None.
- Liver disease: None.

- Elderly: None.
- Pediatric: Children on long-term therapy must be monitored carefully for growth and development.

Food: Administer with food to minimize GI upset.

Pregnancy: Category B.

Lactation: Steroids appear in breast milk. American Academy of Pediatrics considers prednisone to be compatible with breast-feeding.

Contraindications: Systemic fungal, viral, or bacterial infections, severe cardiovascular disease.

Editorial comments

For additional information, see *prednisone*, p. 760.

   This drug is listed without details in the *Physician's Desk Reference,* 54th edition, 2000.

Methyltestosterone

Brand names: Android, Estratest, Testred.

Class of drug: Androgenic hormone.

Mechanism of action: Stimulates receptors in androgen-responsive organs, thereby promoting growth and development of male sex organs. Maintains secondary male characteristics in deficit states.

Indications/dosage/route: Oral only.

Males

- Hypogonadism, impotence
  - PO 10–40 mg/d.
- Androgen deficiency
  - PO 10–50 mg/d.
- Postpubertal cryptorchidism
  - PO 30 mg/d.

Females

- Postpartum breast pain and engorgement
  - PO 80 mg/d for 3–5 days.

- Breast cancer
  - PO 50–200 mg/d (25–100 mg buccal).
- Inoperable breast carcinoma
  - 10–40 mg daily in divided doses.
- Prevention of postpartum breast pain and engorgement
  - 2.5 mg shortly after delivery, then 5–10 mg daily in divided doses for 4–5 days.

Adjustment of dosage

- Kidney disease: None.
- Liver disease: None.
- Elderly: Use with caution because of possibility of developing prostatic hypertrophy and prostatic carcinoma.
- Pediatric: Use with great caution. Drug should be administered only by a physician who is aware of possible adverse effects of drug on bone maturation. Hand and wrist should be examined radiologically every 6 months.

Food: Information not available.

Pregnancy: Category X. Contraindicated.

Lactation: No data available. Best to avoid.

Contraindications: Hypersensitivity to testosterones, males with carcinoma of the breast, known or suspected carcinoma of the prostate, serious cardiac, renal, or hepatic decompensation; women who are or may become pregnant.

Warnings/precautions: Prolonged use of androgens has been associated with peliosis hepatitis, cholestatic jaundice, hepatic neoplasms.

Advice to patient

- Notify physician for persistent erections in males, excessive facial hair, menstrual irregularities in women.

Adverse reactions

- Common: pruritis, edema, acne, gynecomastia, priapism, breast tenderness.
- Serious: cerebrovascular accident, CHF, hyperlipidemia, hyponatremia, peliosis, hepatic carcinoma, anaphylaxis (rare).

Clinically important drug reactions

- Drugs that increase effects/toxicity of testosterones: ACTH,

corticosteroids, oral hypoglycemic drugs, hepatotoxic drugs.
• Testosterones increase effects/toxicity of oral anticoagulants, oxyphenbutazone.
• Testosterones decrease effects/toxicity of propranolol.

Parameters to monitor
• Intake of fluids and urinary and other fluid output to minimize renal toxicity. Increase fluid intake if inadequate. Closely monitor electrolyte levels.
• Male patients for breast enlargement, priapism, increased urinary urgency, difficulty in urination (elderly men). Reduce dose if these occur.
• Women for virilism: unusual hair growth, acne, menstrual irregularity, enlargement of clitoris. Discontinue to avoid irreversible clitoral enlargement or deepening of voice.
• Patients treated for metastatic cancer: serum and urine calcium levels and serum alkaline phosphatase to avoid hypercalcemia (nausea, vomiting, weakness).
• Signs and symptoms of hepatitis.
• Elderly patients for possible development of symptomatic prostatic hyperplasia or carcinoma. If these occur, drug must be discontinued.
• Bone age during treatment of prepubertal males by performing periodic x-ray examinations (q6mo).

Editorial comments: Physicians who prescribe androgens including progesterone for nonapproved indications may be subject to criminal prosecution.

Methysergide

Brand name: Sansert.
Class of drug: Ergot alkaloid, vasoconstrictor, 5-HT inhibitor.
Indications/dosage/route: Oral only.

- Prevention of vascular headaches, eg, migraine and cluster headaches
  - Adults: 4–8 mg/d.

Editorial comments

- Methysergide is seldom used.
- Serious toxic effects of methysergide include inflammatory fibrosis (retroperitoneal, endocardial, pleuropulmonary).
- This drug is not listed in the *Physician's Desk Reference*, 54th edition, 2000.

Metoclopramide

Brand name: Reglan.
Class of drug: GI stimulant, antiemetic.
Mechanism of action: GI-stimulating effect: Sensitizes GI smooth muscles to acetylcholine; increases esopahgeal sphincter tone; increases amplitude of gastric contractions. Antiemetic: Raises threshold stimulation of chemoreceptor trigger zone in medulla.
Indications/dosage/route: Oral, IV.

- Emesis from chemotherapy
  - Adults: PO, IV 1–2 mg/kg, 30–60 minutes before chemotherapy, q2–4h afterward.
- Postoperative emesis
  - Adults: IM 10 or 20 mg 30 minutes before and during surgery.
- Gastroesophageal reflux
  - Adults: PO 10–15 mg q.i.d. 30 minutes before meals and h.s.
- Delayed gastric emptying secondary to diabetic gastroparesis
  - Adults: PO 30 minutes before meals and h.s. for 2–8 weeks.
- Small bowel intubation (aid to radiologic examination)
  - Adults: IV 10 mg over 1–2 minutes.
  - Children 6–14 years: IV 2.5–5 mg.
  - Children <6 years: IV 0.1 mg/kg.

Adjustment of dosage
- Kidney disease: Creatinine clearance <40 mL/min: administer 50% of dose.
- Liver disease: None.
- Elderly: Reduce dose. At higher risk for toxicity.
- Pediatric: See above. Only use in children is for facilitation of intubation.

	Onset of Action	Duration
IV	1–3 min	1–2 h
IM	10–15 min	1–2 h
PO	30–60 min	1–2 h

Food: Should be taken 30 minutes before meals.

Pregnancy: Category B.

Lactation: Appears in breast milk. Potentially toxic to infant. Considered a drug of concern during lactation by American Academy of Pediatrics.

Contraindications: GI hemorrhage, obstruction or perforation, pheochromocytoma, epilepsy, drugs causing extrapyramidal symtoms (eg, phenothiazines).

Warnings/precautions
- Use with caution in patients with hypertension, kidney disease.
- Administer IV drug slowly or else it my cause feelings of restlessness or anxiety.
- To prevent extrapyramidal reactions, pretreat with diphenhydramine 50 mg PO or IV or benztropine 1–2 mg IV or PO q4–6h before chemotherapy. Young adults and elderly are more likely to develop extrapyramidal reactions. Lower doses are recommended for these populations of patients.

Advice to patient
- Do not drive or operate machinery for several hours after taking this drug.
- If you experience twitching or involuntary movements, report to treating physician.

• Avoid alcohol and other CNS depressants (phenothiazines, barbiturates, narcotic analgesics).

Adverse reactions

• Common: restlessness, drowsiness, fatigue, dizziness, diarrhea.
• Serious: depression, extrapyramidal reactions, tardive dyskinesia, hypotension, galactorrhea.

Clinically important drug interactions

• Drugs that increase effects/toxicity of metoclopramide: narcotic analgesics, phenothiazines, haloperidol.
• Drugs that decrease effects/toxicity of metoclopramide: anticholinergic drugs.

Parameters to monitor

• BP, pulse.
• Signs of tremor, restlessness, tardive dyskinesia.
• Development of depression.

Editorial comments: In the majority of patients >65 years, treatment with metoclopramide should generally be avoided. In general, its use as chronic treatment should be limited.

Metolazone

Brand names: Mykrox (rapid-release tablet), Zaroxolyn (slow-release tablet).

Class of drug: Thiazide-like diuretic.

Mechanism of action: Inhibits sodium reabsorption at critical dilution site of renal tubule.

Indications/dosage/route: Oral only.

• Mild to moderate hypertension
  – Mykrox: Adults: Initial: 0.5 mg once daily in a.m. Increase to maximum of 1 mg once daily if needed.
  – Zaroxolyn: Adults: 2.5–5 mg once daily.
• Edema of cardiac failure, renal disease
  – Zaroxolyn: Adults: 5–20 mg once daily.

Adjustment of dosage
- Kidney disease: None.
- Liver disease: None.
- Elderly: None.
- Pediatric: Not recommended.

Food: No restriction.

Pregnancy: Category B.

Lactation: Appears in breast milk. Other thiazide diuretics are considered compatible by American Academy of Pediatrics. Thiazide diuretics suppress lactation.

Contraindications: Anuria, hepatic coma or precoma, hypersensitivity to metolazone.

Editorial comments
- Zaroxolyn must not be interchanged with other metolazone formulations as these differ greatly in bioavailability and thus are not bioequivalent.
- For additional information, see *hydrochlorothiazide*, p. 426.

Metoprolol

Brand names: Lopressor, Troprol XL.

Class of drug: β-Adrenergic receptor blocker.

Mechanism of action: Competitive blocker of β-adrenergic receptors in heart and blood vessels.

Indications/dosage/route: Oral, IV.
- Angina pectoris
  - Initial: PO 100 mg/d in a single dose. Increase at weekly intervals until optimum effect is reached. Maximum: 400 mg/d.
- Hypertension
  - Initial: PO 50–100 mg/d in a single dose with or without a diuretic. Increase weekly until maximum effect is achieved. Maximum: 400 mg/d.
- Prophylaxis of migraine
  - PO 50–100 mg b.i.d.

- Ventricular arrhythmias
  - PO 200 mg/d.
- Early treatment of MI
  - 3 IV bolus injections of 5 mg each at approximately 2-minute intervals. Then, PO 50 mg q6h beginning 15 minutes after the last IV dose; continue for 48 hours.
- Late treatment of MI
  - PO 100 mg b.i.d. Continue for 1–3 months.

Adjustment of dosage
- Kidney disease: None.
- Liver disease: None.
- Elderly: None.
- Pediatric: Safety and efficacy have not been established.

Food: No restriction.

Pregnancy: Category C.

Lactation: Appears in breast milk. Potentially toxic to infant. Wait at least 3–4 hours after dose before breastfeeding. Considered compatible by American Academy of Pediatrics. Observe infant for bradycardia, hypotension.

Contraindications: Cardiogenic shock, asthma, CHF unless it is secondary to tachyarrhythmia treatable with a β blocker, sinus bradycardia and AV block greater than first degree, severe COPD.

Warnings/precautions
- Use with caution in patients with diabetes, kidney disease, liver disease, COPD, peripheral vascular disease.
- Do not stop drug abruptly as this may precipitate arrhythmias, angina, MI or cause rebound hypertension. If necessary to discontinue, taper as follows: Reduce dose and reassess after 1–2 weeks. If status is unchanged, reduce by another 50% and reassess after 1–2 weeks.
- Drug may mask symptoms of hyperthyroidism, mainly tachycardia.
- Drug may exacerbate symptoms of arterial insufficiency in patients with peripheral or mesenteric vascular disease.

Advice to patient
- Avoid driving and other activities requiring mental alertness or that are potentially dangerous until response to drug is known.

- Dress warmly in winter and avoid prolonged exposure to cold as drug may cause increased sensitivity to cold.
- Avoid drinks that contain xanthines (caffeine, theophylline, theobromine) including colas, tea, and chocolate because they may counteract the effect of drug.
- Restrict dietary sodium to avoid volume expansion.
- Drug may blunt response to usual rise in BP and chest pain under stressful conditions such as vigorous exercise and fever.

Adverse reactions
- Common: fatigue, dizziness.
- Serious: symptomatic bradycardia, CHF, worsened AV block, hypotension, depression, bone marrow, depression, lupus-like condition, bronchospasm, Peyronie's disease, hepatitis.

Clinically important drug interactions
- Drugs that increase effects/toxicity of β blockers: reserpine, bretylium, calcium channel blockers.
- Drugs that decrease effects/toxicity of β blockers: aluminum salts, calcium salts, cholestyramine, barbiturates, NSAIDs, rifampin.

Parameters to monitor
- Liver enzymes, serum BUN and creatinine, CBC with differential and platelets.
- Pulse rate near end of dosing interval or before the next dose is taken. A reasonable target is 60–80 beats/min for resting apical ventricular rate. If severe bradycardia develops, consider treatment with glucagon, isoproterenol, IV atropine (1–3 mg in divided doses). If hypotension occurs despite correction of bradycardia, administer vasopressor (norephinephrine, dopamine or dobutamine).
- Symptoms of CHF. Digitalize patient and administer a diuretic or glucagon.
- Efficacy of treatment: decreased BP, decreased number and severity of anginal attacks, improvement in exercise tolerance. Confirm control of arrhythmias by ECG, apical pulse, BP, circulation in extremities and respiration. Monitor closely when changing dose.
- CNS effects. If patient experiences mental depression reduce dosage by 50%. The elderly are particularly sensitive to adverse CNS effects.

- Signs of bronchospasm. Stop therapy and administer large doses of β-adrenergic bronchodilator, eg, albuterol, terbutaline, or aminophylline.
- Signs of cold extremities. If severe, stop drug. Consider β blocker with sympathomimetic properties.

Editorial comments

- Stopping a β blocker before surgery is controversial. Some advocate discontinuing the drug 48 hours before surgery; others recommend withdrawal for a considerably longer time. Notify anesthesiologist that patient has been on β blocker.
- β blockers are first-line treatments for hypertension, particularly in patients with the following conditions: previous MI, ischemic heart disease, aneurysm, atrioventricular arrhythmias, migraine. These are drugs of first choice for chronic stable angina, used in conjunction with nitroglycerin.
- Many studies indicate benefit from administration of a β blocker following an MI.
- β Blockers are considered to be first-line drugs for prophylaxis of migraine headache in patients who have two or more attacks per month.

Metronidazole

Brand name: Flagyl.
Class of drug: Antibacterial, antiprotozoan, amebicide.
Mechanism of action: Inhibits nucleic acid synthesis and disrupts DNA structure. Causes loss of helical DNA structure and breakage of DNA strands.
Susceptible organisms *in vivo*: Anaerobes: *Bacteroides fragilis* and DOT group. *Fusobacterium, Clostridium* species including *C. difficile; Proprionibacterium acne* and *Actinomyces* are not susceptible. Also, *Treponema pallidum,* oral spirochetes, *Campylobacter fetus, Gardnerella vaginalis, Helicobacter pylori.* Parasites: *Trichomonas vaginalis, Giardia lamblia, Entamoeba histolytica.*

Indications/dosage/route: Oral, IV.
• Intestinal amebiasis
– Adults: PO 750 mg t.i.d., 5–10 days.
Note: It is recommended that iodoquinol be added at a dosage of 650 mg PO t.i.d. for 20 days for infection or abscess or both.
• Amoebic hepatic abscess
– Adults: PO 500–750 mg t.i.d., 5–10 days.
– Children: PO 35–50 mg/kg/d (divided in 3 doses), 10 days.
• *Trichomonas* infections
– Adults: PO 350 mg b.i.d. for 7 days or PO 2g b.i.d.
• Infections caused by anaerobic microorganisms
– Adults: IV, Oral 500 mg q6–8h. Maximum: 4 g/d.
– Children: IV 7.5 mg/kg q6h. Maximum: 4 g/d.
• Prophylaxis of postoperative infection
– Adults: IV 15 mg/kg, infused 30–60 minutes, completed 1 hour before surgery; then 7.5 mg/kg infused 30–60 minutes, 6–12 hours after initial dose.
• *Clostridium difficile*
– Adults: PO 750–2000 mg/d, 3–4 divided doses, 7–14 days.
• *Helicobacter pylori*: associated with peptic ulcer
– Adults: PO 250–500 mg t.i.d. in combination with bismuth subsalicylate 525 mg and tetracycline 500 mg q.i.d. Other combinations anticipated.
– Children: PO 15–20 mg/kg/d, divided in 2 doses, 4 weeks, combine with bismuth subsalicylate and amoxicillin. Other combinations anticipated.

Adjustment of dosage
• Kidney disease: Creatinine clearance <10 mL/min: reduce dose by 50%. Administer after dialysis.
• Liver disease: Mild: no change in dose. Severe: reduce dose.
• Elderly: Prone to intolerance, use lower doses.
• Pediatric: Neonates require lower doses than infants and children. Safety and efficacy in children have not been established except in treatment of amebiasis.

Food: Take drug with food or milk.

Pregnancy: Category B. Considered contraindicated in the first trimester of pregnancy when used for trichomoniasis.

Lactation: Appears in breast milk. Potentially mutagenic. American Academy of Pediatrics recommends caution with use. Patient should discontinue breastfeeding for 12–24 hours after single 2-g dose.

Contraindications: Hypersensitivity to metronidazole.

Warnings/precautions: Use with caution in patients with alcoholism, kidney disease, severe hepatic disease, CHF, blood dyscrasias, CNS infections, retinal visual field problems, seizures or neurologic problems, predisposition to edema (IV preparation).

Advice to patient

- Avoid driving and other activities requiring mental alertness or that are potentially dangerous until response to drug is known.
- Use OTC medications only if approved by the treating physician.
- If treated for trichomioniasis, abstain from intercourse or use barrier protection to prevent reinfection.
- Do not use alcohol for 72 hours after discontinuing therapy.

Adverse reactions

- Common: headache, abdominal pain, anorexia, dizziness, vomiting.
- Serious: seizures, peripheral neuropathy, pancreatitis, leukopenia, ataxia.

Clinically important drug interactions

- Drugs that decrease effects/toxicity of metronidazole: barbiturates, phenytoin.
- Metronidazole increases effects/toxicity of oral anticoagulants, hydantoins, cimetidine, astemizole, lithium, phenytoin, and alcohol (disulfiram-like reaction).
- Drug that increases effects/toxicity of metronidazole: cimetidine.

Parameters to monitor

- Signs and symptoms of neuropathy.
- Use of yogurt (4 oz/d) may be helpful in prevention of superinfection.
- Differential leukocyte counts before and after therapy.

Editorial comments
- Off-label use of metronidazole includes treatment of Crohn's disease, especially with fistulization. Doses of 20 mg/kg/d for 3 months have been shown to prevent recurrence of Crohn's disease following ileal resection.
- Peripheral neuropathy developing with long-term use may be irreversible.

Mexiletine

Brand name: Mexitil.
Class of drug: Class 1b antiarrhythmic agent.
Mechanism of action: Suppresses automaticity and shortens effective refractory period in His-Purkinje conducting system. Increases effective refractory period/action potential duration ratio. Reduces premature ventricular beats.
Indications/dosage/route: Oral.
- Life threatening ventricular arrhythmias
  – Adults: PO 200 mg q8h. Increase or decrease dose based on efficacy and/or side effects. Maximum daily dose: 1200 mg.
Adjustment of dosage
- Kidney disease: None.
- Liver disease: Reduce dose; specific guidelines not available.
- Elderly: Reduce dosage.
- Pediatric: Safety and efficacy have not been established.

Onset of Arrhythmic Action	Peak Effect	Duration
30 min–2 h	2–3 h	8–12 h

Food: Take with food or antacid.
Pregnancy: Category C.
Lactation: Appears in breast milk. Should avoid.

Contraindications: Second- or third-degree AV block in absence of pacemaker, cardiogenic shock.

Warnings/precautions

- Use with caution in patients with hypotension, CHF, cardiogenic shock, acute MI, first-degree heart block, history of seizure disorders, liver disease, impaired AV node function.
- Mexiletine may worsen hypotension as well as CHF. Use with caution if these are present.
- Has been associated with severe liver disease including hepatic necrosis. Patients with underlying CHF at highest risk.
- May cause bone marrow depression, particularly when combined with procainamide.

Advice to patient

- Avoid driving and other activities requiring mental alertness or that are potentially dangerous until response to drug is known.
- Carry identification card at all times describing disease, treatment regimen, name, address, and telephone number of treating physician.

Adverse reactions

- Common: blurred vision, dizziness, tremor, nervousness, headache, GI upset (nausea, vomiting, heartburn, diarrhea, dry mouth).
- Serious: arrhythmias, hepatic necrosis.

Clinically important drug interactions

- Drugs that increase effects/toxicity of mexiletine: cimetidine, other antiarrhythmic drugs, metoclopramide.
- Drugs that decrease effects/toxicity of mexiletine: opioids, atropine, phenytoin, rifampin, phenobarbital.
- Mexiletine increases effects/toxicity of theophylline.

Parameters to monitor

- Cardiovascular parameters, including ECG, pulse, BP, continuous Holter monitoring is suggested when initiating mexiletine. If pulse rate falls to less than 50 beats/min or becomes irregular reduce or discontinue mexiletine.
- Signs and symptoms of bone marrow depression.
- Signs and symptoms of hepatotoxicity.

Editorial comments

• Mexiletine currently is not a mainstay antiarrhythmic drug. Frequently debilitating GI side effects limit its usefulness. Still, in cases of ventricular arrhythmias refractory to class III antiarrhythmics, mexiletine may be added synergistically at doses of 100–150 mg b.i.d. to t.i.d. for effect. These patients usually have an ICD and are receiving therapy frequently with the device despite high doses of amiodarone or sotalol.

• Mexiletine,because of its class 1b sodium channel blockade and shortening of the His-Purkinje action potential (similar to lidocaine), can be useful in selected cases of the long QT syndrome. This condition should be managed by a cardiac electrophysiologist.

Mezlocillin

Brand name: Mezlin.
Class of drug: Antibiotic, penicillin family plus β-lactamase inhibitor.
Mechanism of action: Inhibits bacterial cell wall synthesis.
Susceptible organisms *in vivo*: *Streptococcus pneumoniae,* beta-hemolytic streptococci, *Enterococcus faecalis, Escherichia coli, Hemophilus influenzae, Klebsiella* sp, *Neisseria gonorrhoeae, Proteus mirabilis, Salmonella* sp, *Shigella* sp, *Morganella morganii, Proteus vulgaris, Providencia rettgeri, Providencia stuartii, Enterobacter* sp, *Citrobacter* sp, *Pseudomonas aeruginosa, Serratia* sp, *Acinetobacter* sp, *Clostridium* sp, *Peptococcus* sp, *Peptostreptococcus* sp, *Bacteroides* sp, *Fusobacterium* sp, *Eubacterium* sp, *Veillonella* sp.
Indications/dosage/route: IV, IM.
• Serious infections
  – Adults: 3 g q4h or 4 g q6h.
  – Infants, children 1 month–12 years: 50 mg/kg q4h over 30 minutes.

- Infants >2 kg and <1 week or <2 kg and <1 week: 75 mg/kg q12h.
- Infants <2 kg and >1 week: 75 mg/kg q8h.
- Infants >2 kg and >1 week: 75 mg/kg q6h.
• Life-threatening infections
  – Adults: 350 mg/kg/d. Maximum: 24 g/d.
• Uncomplicated UTIs
  – IV, IM 1.5–2 g q6h.
• Complicated UTIs
  – IV 3 g q6h.
• Lower respiratory tract infection, intraabdominal infection, gynecologic infection, skin and skin structure infections, septicemia
  – Adults: IV 4 g q6h or 3 g q4h.
• Gonococcal urethritis
  – Adults: 1–2 g with probenecid.
• Prophylaxis of postoperative infection
  – Adults: 4 g 30–90 minutes prior to surgery, then IV 4 g 6 and 12 hours later.
• Prophylaxis of infection in patients undergoing cesarean section
  – IV 4 g when cord is clamped, second and third doses, IV 4 g, 4 and 8 hours after the first dose.

Adjustment of dosage
• Kidney disease.

Creatinine Clearance	Uncomplicated UTI	Complicated UTI	Serious Systemic Infection
>30 mL/min	Usual dose	Usual dose	Usual dose
10–30 mL/min	1.5 g q8h	1.5 g q6h	3 g q8h
<10 mL/min	1.5 g q8h	1.5 g q8h	2 g q8h

• Liver disease: None.
• Elderly: None.
• Pediatric: Children >1 month up to age 12: IV, IM 50 mg/kg q4h, slow infusion.
Food: Not applicable.
Pregnancy: Category B.

Lactation: No data available. Best to avoid.

Contraindications: Hypersensitivity to penicillin or cephalosporins.

Editorial comments

- Mezlocillin is used to treat aerobic gram-negative infections. It covers *Pseudomonas aeruginosa*. It can be used in noscomial pneumonia and neutropenic fever (in combination with an aminoglycoside), bacteremia, complicated UTI, and surgical infections of the abdomen.
- Mezlocillin is not as effective as piperacillin against *P. aeruginosa*.
- Like piperacillin, mezlocillin also covers *Enterococcus faecalis*.
- This drug causes a smaller increase in bleeding time than carbenicillin.
- For additional information, see *penicillin G*, p. 708.

Miconazole

Brand name: Monistat.

Class of drug: Antifungal agent.

Mechanism of action: Thickens cell wall, thereby altering permeability of fungal cell membrane.

Susceptible organisms *in vitro*: *Coccidioides immitis, Candida albicans, Cryptococcus neoformans, Histoplasma, Paracoccidioides, Brasiliensis*.

Indications/dosage/route: IV, topical.

- Severe systemic fungal infections caused by susceptible organisms resistant to other azoles
  - Adults: IV 300–600 mg daily.
  - Children >1 year: IV 20–40 mg/kg daily. Maximum dose per infusion: 15 mg/kg.
  - Children <1 year: 15–30 mg/kg daily in 3 or 4 divided doses.
- Cutaneous or mucocutaneous fungal infections caused by susceptible organisms
  - Adults: Topical: Cover affected areas b.i.d., 2–4 weeks.
  - Adults: Vaginal use: 200-mg suppository, h.s., 3 days.

Adjustment of dosage
- Kidney disease: None.
- Liver disease: None.
- Elderly: None.
- Pediatric: Safety and efficacy in children <1 year have not been established.

Food: No restrictions.

Pregnancy: Category C (IV form).

Lactation: No data available. Potentially toxic to infant. Avoid breastfeeding.

Contraindications: Hypersensitivity to miconazole.

Warnings/precautions
- Use with caution in patients with hepatic insufficiency.
- Inject IV form very slowly (over 30–60 minutes) to avoid arrhythmias. IV administration is carried out in hospital under strictly monitored conditions.
- Use only to treat severe systemic fungal disease.
- Before IV administration, ascertain whether patient is hypersensitive to the drug.
- Premedicate with an antiemetic to lessen or avoid nausea and vomiting.
- Advise patient about the symptoms of fungal infections.
- If a pruritic rash develops, it may persist long after drug is stopped. Diphenhydramine may be useful in counteracting this condition.

Advice to patient: Continue topical application for at least 1 month. If no improvement, consult treating physician.

Adverse reactions
- Common: nausea, vomiting, diarrhea, rash.
- Serious: anaphylactoid reaction, phlebitis at injection site, arrhythmias, cardiorespiratory arrest.

Clinically important drug interactions
- Miconazole increases effects/toxicity of oral anticoagulants, sulfonylureas, phenytoin.
- Drugs that increase effects/toxicity of miconazole: ketoconazole, cyclosporine.
- Drugs that decrease effects/toxicity of ketoconazole: rifampin.

Parameters to monitor: Cardiorespiratory arrest and anaphylaxis.

Editorial comments
- Used mainly as topical drug for yeast infections.
- IV (for infectious disease specialist only) for unusual mold infections such as *Pseudallescheria boydii* and highly resistant strains of fungi.
- IV form of this drug is not listed in *Physician's Desk Reference,* 54th edition, 2000.

Midazolam

Brand name: Versed.
Class of drug: Benzodiazepine.
Mechanism of action: Potentiates effects of GABA in limbic system and reticular formation.
Indications/dosage/route: IV only.
- Preoperative sedation
  - Adults: 0.07–0.08 mg/kg 1 hour before surgery.
  - Children: 0.08–0.2 mg/kg 1 hour before surgery.
- Conscious sedation for endoscopic or cardiovascular procedures
  - Adults <60 years: Initial: 0.5–2.5 mg given over 2 minutes. If needed, administer small increments q2min. Maximum: 5 mg.
  - Adults >60, debilitated patients: Initial: 0.5–1.5 mg given over 2 minutes. If needed, administer 1-mg increments over 2 minutes q2min. Maximum: 3.5 mg.
  - Children: Individualize.
- Induction of general anesthesia before general anesthetic
  - Adults ≤55 years: Initial: 0.2–0.35 mg/kg over 5–30 seconds. If needed, administer up to 0.6 mg/kg in small increments.
  - Adults >55 years: Initial: 0.15–0.3 mg/kg over 20–30 seconds.
  - Debilitated adults >55 years: Initial: 0.15–0.25 mg/kg.
- Maintenance of balanced anesthesia (short procedures)
  - Adults, children: 25% of dose used for induction as needed for maintaining surgical anethesia.

Adjustment of dosage
- Kidney disease: Use with caution.
- Liver disease: Use with caution.
- Elderly: See above.
- Pediatric: See above.

Food: Not applicable.

Pregnancy: Category D.

Lactation: Appears in breast milk. Potentially toxic to infant. American Academy of Pediatrics expresses concern about breast-feeding while taking benzodiazepines. Avoid breastfeeding.

Contraindications: Hypersensitivity to benzodiazepines, pregnancy, narrow-angle glaucoma.

Editorial comments: For additional information, see *diazepam,* p. 273.

Milrinone

Brand name: Primacor.

Class of drug: Inotropic agent, vasodilator.

Mechanism of action: Milrinone inhibits phosphodiesterase, increases cyclic AMP, and increases level of intracellular ionized calcium. These effects result in increased force of cardiac muscle contraction and vasodilation.

Indications/dosage/route: IV.
- CHF
  – Adults: Loading dose: IV 50 µg/kg over 10-minute period, followed by continuous IV infusion of maintenance dose 0.375–0.75 µg/kg/min. Maintenance dose titrated to clinical effect.

Adjustment of dosage
- Kidney disease: Creatinine clearance <50 mL/min: reduce infusion rate of milrinone; creatinine clearance 50 mL/min per 1.73 m^2: 0.43 µg/kg/min; creatinine clearance 40 mL/min per 1.73 m^2: 0.38 µg/kg/min; creatinine clearance 30 mL/min per 1.73 m^2: 0.33 µg/kg/min; creatinine clearance 20

mL/min per 1.73 m^2: 0.28 µg/kg/min; creatinine clearance 10 mL/min per 1.73 m^2: 0.20 µg/kg/min.

- Liver disease: None.
- Elderly: None
- Pediatric: Safety and efficacy have not been established.
- Food: Not applicable.

Pregnancy: Category C.

Lactation: No data available. Potentially toxic to infant. Avoid breastfeeding.

Contraindications: Severe aortic valvular disease, acute MI, pheochromocytoma, hypertrophic subaortic stenosis, hypersensitivity to milrinone.

Warnings/precautions: Use with caution in patients with ventricular arrhythmias, atrial fibrillation or flutter, obstructive disorders of the aortic or pulmonic valve, renal impairment, electrolyte abnormalities.

Adverse reactions

- Common: **ventricular arrhythmias**.
- Serious: **ventricular arrhythmias**, sustained ventricular tachycardia, ventricular fibrillation, supraventricular tachycardia, thrombocytopenia, hypokalemia.

Clinically important drug interactions: None reported.

Parameters to monitor

- Renal function, fluid and electrolytes, especially potassium carefully during therapy. Correct hypokalemia before or during use of this drug.
- ECG continuously during milrinone infusion. Be aware of arrhythmias, which are common and may be life-threatening.
- Platelet count.
- Efficacy of treatment: improvement of signs and symptoms of CHF.

Editorial comments: Milrinone is a useful intravenous inotropic cardiac drug in patients with advanced CHF caused by systolic dysfunction. Its largely sympathomimetic effects also makes it a proarrhythmic drug. The proarrhythmic effects can be seen even after infusion has ceased. Hence, care should be taken to monitor patients carefully during and shortly after infusion.

Minocycline

Brand names: Dynacin, Minocin.
Class of drug: Antibiotic, tetracycline.
Mechanism of action: Inhibits bacterial protein synthesis after specific ribosomal binding.
Susceptible organisms *in vivo*: *Borrelia burgdorferi, Borrelia recurrentis, Brucella* sp, *Calymmatobacterium granulomatis, Chlamydia pneumoniae, Chlamydia psittaci, Chlamydia trachomatis, Ehrlichia* sp, *Helicobacter pylori,* Q fever, *Rickettsia* sp, *Vibrio* sp.
Indications/dosage/route: Oral, IV.
  – Adults: PO, IV 200 mg, then 100 mg q12h. Maximum: 400 mg/d.
  – Children >8 years: PO, IV 4 mg/kg, then 2 mg/kg 1–3 times/d.
Adjustment of dosage
• Kidney disease: None.
• Liver disease: None.
• Elderly: None.
• Pediatric: Not to be used in children <8 years unless all other drugs are either ineffective or contraindicated.
Food: Take 1 hour before or 2 hours after meals. Dairy products interfere with tetracycline absorption.
Pregnancy: Category D.
Lactation: Appears in breast milk. Considered compatible by American Academy of Pediatrics.
Contraindications: Hypersensitivity to any tetracycline, patients with esophageal obstruction, children <8 years.
Editorial comments: For more information, see *tetracycline*, p. 885.

Minoxidil

Brand names: Loniten, Rogaine, Minoxidil.
Class of drug: Antihypertensive, vasodilator, hair growth stimulator.

Mechanism of action: Causes arteriolar smooth muscle relaxation, resulting in decreased BP, increased peripheral resistance. Stimulates hair follicles by increasing blood flow to skin.

Indications/dosage/route: Oral, topical.

• Hypertension (combination, usually with diuretic and β blocker)
  – Adults, children >12 years: Initial: PO 5 mg/d. Slowly increase dose q3d to optimum BP response. Maintenance: 10–40 mg/d. Maximum: 100 mg/d.
  – Children <12 years: 0.1–0.2 mg/kg/d as single dose (maximum: 5 mg). Gradually increase q3d to 0.25–1 mg/kg/d in single or divided doses (maximum 50 mg/d).

• Topical male and female pattern boldness
  – 1 ml (2 or 5% solution) bid to area with loss of hair.

Adjustment of dosage

• Kidney disease: Reduce dose by one-third usual in renal failure.
• Liver disease: None.
• Elderly: Initial dose reduced to 2.5 mg daily. Slow dosage increases.
• Pediatric: See above.

Onset of Action	Peak Effect	Duration
30 min	2–3 h	2–5 d

Food: May be taken with or without food.

Pregnancy: Category C.

Lactation: Appears in breast milk. Potentially toxic to infant. Avoid breastfeeding.

Contraindications: Hypersensitivity to minoxidil, pheochromocytoma, MI (within 1 month), dissecting aortic aneurysm.

Warnings/precautions

• Use with caution in patients with coronary artery disease, renal disease (severe), pulmonary hypertension, CHF.
• Prior to discontinuation, consult treating physician.
• To minimize possible photosensitivity reaction, apply adequate sunscreen and use proper covering when exposed to strong sunlight.

Advice to patient: Do not take magnesium-containing antacids.

Adverse reactions

- Common: edema, tachycardia, breast tenderness, weight gain, hypertrichosis.
- Serious: **predisposition to CHF**, pericardial effusion, Stevens–Johnson syndrome, fluid and electrolyte disturbance, angina, bone marrow suppression.

Clinically important drug interactions

- Drugs that increase effects/toxicity of minoxidil: guanethidine, diuretics, other antihypertensives.
- Drugs that decrease effects/toxicity of minoxidil: NSAIDs.

Parameters to monitor

- BP and pulse for orthostasis, checking supine, seated, and standing BPs. Significant changes, eg, heart rate increase >20 beats/min, probably require reduction of dosage.
- Intake of fluids and urinary and other fluid output to minimize renal toxicity. Closely monitor electrolyte levels.
- Signs of CHF.
- Signs and symptoms of Stevens–Johnson syndrome.

Editorial comments

- Minoxidil should be given along with a diuretic unless the patient is on hemodialysis.
- Use should be limited to those patients who do not respond to maximum doses of diuretics and to other antihypertensive agents.
- Minoxidil should be administered under close supervision by the treating physician.
- A β blocker is generally given concomitantly to prevent tachycardia.
- Oral and topical forms of minoxidil have been used to treat male pattern baldness. Minoxidil stimulates resting hair follicles and increases cutaneous blood flow via its vasodilatory properties.
- This drug is listed without details in the *Physician's Desk Reference*, 54th edition, 2000.

Misoprostol

Brand name: Cytotec.

Class of drug: Prostoglandin analogue, gastric mucosal protectant.

Mechanism of action: Enhances gastric mucosal blood flow. Increases mucus and bicarbonate production. Decreases basal and stimulated gastric acid secretion.

Indications/dosage/route: Oral only.

- Prevention of NSAID-induced gastric and duodenal ulcer
  - Adults: 200 µg q.i.d. Reduce to 100 µg q.i.d. if intolerance to side effects develops.

Adjustment of dosage

- Kidney disease: Adjust dosage according to side effects only.
- Liver disease: Adjust dosage according to side effects only.
- Pediatric: Safety has not been established in children <18 years.

Onset of Action	Duration
30 min	3–6 h

Food: Misoprostol should be administered with meals and at bedtime.

Pregnancy: Category X.

Lactation: No data available. Potentially toxic to infant. Avoid breastfeeding.

Contraindications: Pregnancy, hypersensitivity to misoprostol.

Warnings/precautions

- Misoprostol should not be prescribed for a female patient who is potentially capable of childbearing unless patient understands effect of misoprostol in causing abortion, is capable of complying with recommended contraception, and has a negative pregnancy test within 2 weeks of initiating therapy.
- To initiate misoprostol use in women of childbearing age, ideally begin on the second or third day of the next menstrual period following a negative pregnancy test in the prior 2 weeks.

Advice to patient: Use two forms of birth control including hormonal and barrier methods.

Adverse reactions
- Common: diarrhea, nausea, abdominal pain, headache, body aches, anxiety, arthralgia.
- Serious: miscarriage, anaphylaxis.

Clinically important drug interactions: None.

Parameters to monitor: Signs of diarrhea. This tends to be self-limited and can be minimized by giving the drug with meals.

Editorial comments
- Usage of misoprostol to prevent NSAID-induced ulcers will probably decline with development of the COX-2 inhibitors, a new class of antiinflammatory agents (see *celecoxib, rofecoxib*).
- Off-label use includes treatment of refractory constipation.
- Misoprostol is also available on the market in a combination preparation with diclofenac (Arthrotec).

Mitomycin

Brand name: Mutamycin.

Class of drug: Antineoplastic antibiotic.

Mechanism of action: Crosslinks strands of DNA, thereby inhibiting DNA synthesis. Inhibits RNA and protein synthesis.

Indications/dosage/route: IV only.
- Disseminated gastric and pancreatic adenocarcinoma (used in conjunction with other chemotherapeutic agents)
  - Single agent: Adults, children: 10–20 mg/m^2 as a single daily dose. Repeat q6–8wk.
- Combination chemotherapy
  - 10 mg/m^2 q6–8wk.
- Single dose of 40–50 mg/m^2 may be used in bone marrow transplant patients.

Adjustment of dosage
- Kidney disease: Creatinine clearance <10 mL/min: administer 75% of usual dose.

- Liver disease: None.
- Elderly: None.
- Pediatric: See above.

Pregnancy: Category C.

Lactation: No data available. Potentially toxic to infant. Avoid breastfeeding.

Contraindications: Hypersensitivity to mitomycin, coagulation disorders, platelet count <75,000/mm^3, WBC count <3000/ mm^3, serum creatinine >1.7 mg/dL.

Warnings/precautions

- Use with caution in patients with active infection, kidney or liver disease, respiratory disorders, decreased bone marrow reserve.
- This drug has been noted to cause hemolytic uremic syndrome (HUS). Patients with this syndrome develop irreversible kidney failure, microangiopathic hemolytic anemia with low platelet counts.
- This agent is severely toxic to bone marrow.

Advice to patient

- Receive vaccinations (particularly live attenuated viruses) only with permission from treating physician.
- Avoid alcohol.

Adverse reactions

- Common: nausea, vomiting (occurs in most patients), stomatitis, diarrhea.
- Serious: **bone marrow suppression**, interstitial pneumonitis, renal toxicity, pulmonary fibrosis (7% of patients), septicemia, hemolytic anemia, hemolytic uremic syndrome, renal failure, hypertension, hepatitis, CHF.

Clinically important drug interactions: Drugs that increase effects/toxicity of mitomycin: vinca alkaloids (respiratory toxicity), doxorubicin (cardiac toxicity).

Parameters to monitor

- CBC, differential. If initial nadir of WBC count is 2000–3000 and/or platelet count is 25,000–75,000, reduce next dose by 30%. If initial nadir of WBC count is <2000 and/or platelet count is <25,000, reduce next dose by 50%.
- Signs and symptoms of infection: fever, sore throat, backache.

- Symptoms of internal bleeding: bleeding gums, easy bruising, blood in stools, urine, emesis.
- Symptoms of hemolytic uremic syndrome which may be fatal: thrombocytopenia, renal failure, hypertension.
- Urine output, BUN and creatinine.
- Symptoms of interstitial pneumonitis or pulmonary fibrosis: dry cough, progressive dyspnea. Check periodic chest radiographs. If toxicity is suspected, discontinue mitomychin and administer corticosteroids.

Editorial comments

- Use latex gloves and safety glasses when handling cytotoxic drugs. Avoid contact with skin and inhalation. If possible, prepare in biologic hood.
- Mitomycin is not to be used for primary therapy or to replace surgery or radiotherapy.
- Reevaluate patient after each course of therapy because of the possibility of cumulative bone marrow suppression, especially of platelets.
- This drug is also used to treat non-small cell lung cancer and advanced breast cancer.
- This drug is a vesicant: severe pain and tissue necrosis may occur if drug extravasates from vein during injection. It should ideally be injected through a central line.

Mitotane

Brand name: Lysodren.
Class of drug: Antineoplastic.
Mechanism of action: Inhibits adrenal organ function; does not cause adrenal organ destruction.
Indications/dosage/route: Oral only.

- Inoperable adrenocortical cancer
  – Adults: Initial: 2–6 g/d, divided t.i.d. or q.i.d. Maintenance: 8–10 g/d.

Adjustment of dosage
• Kidney disease: None.
• Liver disease: None.
• Elderly: None.
• Pediatric: Safety and efficacy have not been established.

Food: May be administered with or without food. Advise patient to avoid fatty meals.

Pregnancy: Category C.

Lactation: No data available. Potentially toxic to infant. Avoid breastfeeding.

Contraindications: Contraindicated in patients with hypersensitivity to mitotane; should be discontinued in patients following shock or trauma.

Warnings/precautions
• Use with caution in patients with liver disease, obesity.
• Tumor tissue should be removed surgically before mitotane is given, as tumor infarction and hemorrhage may occur following drug administration.

Advice to patient
• Avoid alcohol.
• Avoid taking NSAIDs.
• Avoid driving and other activities requiring mental alertness or that are potentially dangerous until response to drug is known.
• Carry identification card at all times describing disease, treatment regimen, name, address, and telephone number of treating physician.
• Use method of birth control other than oral contraceptives.

Adverse reactions
• Common: anorexia, vertigo, nausea, vomiting, diarrhea, lethargy, depression, transient rash.
• Serious: depression, optic injury (lens opacification, retinopathy), hemorrhagic cystitis, orthostatic hypotension.

Clinically important drug interactions
• Drugs that increase effects/toxicity of mitotane: alcohol, antihistamines, opioids, sedative–hypnotics, antidepressants.
• Mitotane decreases effects/toxicity of warfarin, phenytoin.

• Drugs that decrease effects/toxicity of mitotane: spironolactone.

Parameters to monitor

• Signs of GI or skin reactions. If these are severe, reduce dosage.

• Symptoms of adrenal insufficiency: nausea or vomiting, diarrhea, fatigue, hypotension, darkening of skin.

• Signs of infection. Supplemental steroids should be prescribed or it may be necessary to discontinue mitotane.

• Signs of neurotoxicity when used on a prolonged basis ($\geq$2 years). Patients require periodic neurologic and behavioral testing. May cause permanent brain damage with prolonged use.

• Periodic ophthalmologic examinations.

Editorial comment

• Because mitotane distributes mainly in body fat, it may be necessary to prescribe higher doses than standard for obese patients. Such patients may experience a much longer duration of adverse reactions.

• Patients receiving mitotane frequently develop adrenal insufficiency. Some have advocated coadministration of adrenocorticosteroids with mitotane; others have suggested treatment when documented adrenal insufficiency develops. Steroids should be given to patients receiving mitotane who develop shock or have experienced trauma because of increased steroid requirements.

Mitoxantrone

Brand name: Novantrone.

Class of drug: Antibiotic antineoplastic.

Mechanism of action: Inhibits DNA and RNA synthesis by binding to nucleic acids and causing template abnormalities. Also binds to DNA topoisomerase II, decreasing replication of tumor cells.

Indications/dosage/route: IV only.

• Treatment of acute nonlymphocytic leukemia in combination with other approved drugs; other leukemias, breast cancer, lymphoma, pediatric sarcomas (Varies according to individual protocols.)

– Children, adults: 12 mg/m^2/d for 3 days. Acute relapse: 8–12 mg/m^2/d for 4–5 days.

- Solid tumors
  – Children: 18–20 mg/m^2 q3–4wk or 5–8 mg/m^2 weekly.
  – Adults: 12–14 mg/m^2 q3–4wk or 2–4 mg/m^2/d × 5 days.
  – Maximum lifetime dose: 80–120 mg/m^2 for patients at risk for cardiotoxicity (see Warnings and Precautions); otherwise, 160 mg/m^2.

Adjustment of dosage

- Kidney disease: None.
- Liver disease: Dosage adjustment is recommended. A suggested algorithm is 50% dose reduction for bilirubin 1.5–3.0 mg/dL and a 75% dose reduction for more severe bilirubin elevation or other evidence of severe disorder.
- Pediatric: See above. Some protocols have included mitoxantrone for children <2 years.

Pregnancy: Category D.

Lactation: Appears in breast milk. A similar agent (doxorubicin) is considered contraindicated by American Academy of Pediatrics.

Contraindications: Hypersensitivity to mitoxantrone.

Warnings/precautions: Use with caution in patients at risk for cardiotoxicity from mitoxantrone, in patients previously exposed to anthracyclines or other cardiotoxic drugs, in patients who have had mediastinal radiation, and in patients with cardiovascular disease, active infections, radiation therapy, ongoing depressed bone marrow, other forms of anemia, liver disease.

Advice to patient

- Use two forms of birth control including hormonal and barrier methods.
- Drink large quantities of fluid, 1.5–2 L/d.
- Avoid alcohol.
- Be aware that mitoxantrone may cause urine and sclera to turn blue-green.

• Receive vaccinations (particularly live attenuated viruses) only with permission from treating physician.

Adverse reactions
• Common: abdominal pain, headache, alopecia, nausea, vomiting, diarrhea, dyspnea, petechiae, urine discoloration, liver enzyme elevation, cough, fever.
• Serious: **GI bleeding, sepsis**, seizures, CHF, arrhythmias, renal failure, shortness of breath, bone marrow suppression.

Clinically import ant drug interactions: Drugs that increase effects/toxicity of mitoxantrone: daunorubicin, idarubicin, doxorubicin.

Parameters to monitor
• CBC with differential and platelets, serum uric acid, liver enzymes.
• Serial echocardiography or radionuclide evalution of ejection fraction (MUGA scan).
• Signs and symptoms of bone marrow depression.
• Symptoms of gout: increased uric acid levels, joint pain, swelling. Treat accordingly if symptoms develop.
• Symptoms of CHF.

Editorial comments: Cardiac toxicity occurs less frequently with mitoxantrone than doxorubicin. It is important to identify patients at risk for cardiac toxicity (see Warnings/Precautions).

Mivacurium

Brand name: Mivacron.
Class of drug: Nondepolarizing neuromuscular blocker.
Mechanism of action: Blocks nicotinic acetylcholine receptors at neuromuscular junction resulting in skeletal muscle relaxation and paralysis.
Indications/dosage/route: IV only.
• Facilitation of tracheal intubation
   – Adults: 0.15 mg/kg over 5–15 seconds. Maintenance: 0.1 mg/kg.

– Children 2–12 years: Initial: 0.2 mg/kg over 5–15 seconds.
• Facilitation of tracheal intubation using continuous IV infusion
  – Adults: Initial: 6–10 µg/kg/min.
  – Children: 5–31 µg/kg/min.
• Use with reduced cholinesterase activity
  – Initial dose: 0.3 mg/kg.
• Use with isoflurane or enflurane anesthesia
  – Initial: 0.15 mg/kg.
• Use in burn patients
  – 0.015–0.02 mg/kg.

Adjustment of dosage

• Kidney disease: Slower recovery anticipated.
• Liver disease: Decrease infusion rate required (by as much as 50%).
• Elderly: None.
• Pediatric: Safety and efficacy have not been determined for children <2 years.

	Onset of Action	Peak Effect	Duration
Children	—	15–20 min	25–30 min
Adults	—	6–15 min	—

Food: Not applicable.
Pregnancy: Category C.
Lactation: No data available. Best to avoid.
Contraindications: Hypersensitivity to mivacurium and chemically related drugs.
Editorial comments: For additional information see *rocuronium*, p. 824.

Moexipril

Brand name: Univasc.
Class of drug: ACE inhibitor.

Mechanism of action: Inhibits ACE, thereby preventing conversion of angiotensin I to angiotensin II resulting in decreased peripheral arterial resistance.

Indications/dosage/route: Oral.

- Adults: Initial: 7.5 mg/d. May be increased as needed. Usual range is 7.5–30 mg/day b.i.d. Initiate therapy at 3.75 mg in patients receiving diuretics.

Adjustment of dosage

- Kidney disease: Creatinine clearance <40 mL/min: initial, 3.75 mg/d; maximum, 15 mg/d.
- Liver disease: Reduce dose.
- Elderly: None
- Pediatric: Safety and efficacy have not been established.

Onset of Action	Peak Effect	Duration
1 h	3–6 h	24 h

Food: Administer without regard to meals.

Pregnancy: Category C for first trimester. Category D for second and third trimesters.

Lactation: No information available. Likely to be present in breast milk. Other similar agents considered safe.

Contraindications: Hypersensitivity to ACE inhibitors, hereditary or idiopathic angioedema, second and third trimesters of pregnancy.

Editorial comments: For additional information, see *Enalapril*, p. 317.

Molindone

Brand name: Moban.
Class of drug: Antipsychotic, neuroleptic.
Indications/dosage/route: Oral only.

- Psychotic disorders
  - Adults: 50–75 mg/d. Maximum: 225 mg/d. Maintenance: 5–15 mg t.i.d. or q.i.d.; severe disease, 225 mg/d.

Editorial comments: This drug is seldom used. For information about other neuroleptic agents, see *haloperidol*, p. 415.

Montelukast

Brand name: Singulair.
Class of drug: Antiasthmatic.
Mechanism of action: Competitive antagonist of leukotriene (LTD_4).
Indications/dosage/route: Oral only.
- Oral prophylaxis and chronic treatment of asthma
  - Adults, children >15 year: 10 mg/d, in the evening.
  - Children 6–14 years: 5 mg/d, in the evening.

Adjustment of dosage
- Kidney disease: None.
- Liver disease: None.
- Elderly: None.
- Pediatric: Safety and efficacy have not been determined in children <6 years.

Food: No restrictions.
Pregnancy: Category B.
Lactation: No data available. Best to avoid.
Contraindications: Use as terminating agent during acute asthma attack or status asthmatics, hypersensitivity to montelukast.

Editorial comments
- A short-acting inhalation β-adrenergic agonist should be used to treat acute attacks of asthma.
- Montelukast also has been shown to have fewer drug interactions than zafirlukast or zileuton. It does not inhibit the cytochrome P450 enzymes. At this time, no data are available on interactions with highly potent cytochrome P450 enzyme

inducers such as rifampin or potent cytochrome P3A4 inhibitors such as ketoconazole.
- Montelukast has been shown to be less effective than inhaled corticosteroids in terms of antiasthmatic activity but it is more convenient to take.
- This drug has a distinct advantage over zafirlukast and zileuton in that its use has not been associated with hepatotoxicity. Montelukast and zafirlukast have rarely caused eosinophilia and vasculitis (Chung–Strauss syndrome).
- For additional information, see *zafirlukast*, p. 948.

Moricizine

Brand name: Ethmozine.
Class of drug: Class Ic antiarrhythmic.
Mechanism of action: Reduces the fast inward current carried by sodium ions; local anesthetic action stabilizes myocardial membrane.
Indications/dosage/route: Oral.
- Treatment of life-threatening documented ventricular arrthymias, sustained ventricular tachycardia
  – 600–900 mg/d q8h in equally divided doses.

Adjustment of dosage
- Kidney disease: Use caution when administering. Start with lower doses, eg, ≤600 mg/d.
- Liver disease: Drug is cleared by the liver. Dosage reduction suggested. Start with ≤600 mg/d.
- Pediatric: Safety has not been established.

Onset of Action	Peak Effect	Duration
—	0.5–2 h	8–12 h

Food: May be administered with or without food.
Pregnancy: Category B.

Lactation: No data available. Best to avoid.

Contraindications: Hypersensitivity to moricizine, second- or third-degree AV block, right bundle branch block with left hemiblock (bifascicular block) unless artificial pacemaker is present, cardiogenic shock.

Warnings/precautions

- Use with caution in patients with kidney or liver disease, coronary artery disease, sick sinus syndrome.
- Withdraw previous antiarrhythmic therapy prior to starting moricizine.
- If it is necessary to adjust dosage do so at least 3 days apart.
- Correct preexisting hypokalemia, hyperkalemia, hypomagnesemia before starting therapy.

Advice to patient

- Carry identification card at all times describing disease, treatment regimen, name, address, and telephone number of treating physician.

Adverse reactions

- Common: dizziness, nausea.
- Serious: ventricular arrthymias, supraventricular tachycardia, sudden death, heart failure, hypotension, bradycardia, pulmonary embolism, MI, seizure, depression, coma, apnea, urticaria.

Clinically important drug interactions

- Drugs that increase effects/toxicity of moricizine: digoxin, cimetidine.
- Moricizine decreases effects of theophylline.

Parameters to monitor

- Cardiac function by ECG or Holter before and periodically throughout therapy. Check for new arrythmia or worsening of present arrhythmia.
- Signs of orthostasis: Measure BP in the sitting, lying, and standing positions repeatedly before and after initiating therapy.
- Intake of fluids and urinary and other fluid output to minimize renal toxicity. Increase fluid intake if inadequate. Closely monitor electrolyte levels.

- Symptoms of CHF.
- Signs and symptoms of renal toxicity.
- Signs and symptoms of hepatotoxicity.
- Electrocardiographic response 1 week after beginning therapy. If QRS interval is prolonged more than 25% as compared with baseline values, moricizine dosage should be reduced by 50 mg q8h.

Editorial comments

- Moricizine should be administered, its dosage adjusted, or discontinued only after consulting a cardiologist or cardiac electrophysiologist.
- Used for treating life-threatening ventricular tachycardia only in patients for whom the following conditions apply: no history of MI or ischemic heart disease; failure to respond to antiarrhythmic drugs in class IA (quinidine or procanamide) or class IB drugs (mexiletine) or a combination of class IA and 1B drugs.
- The National Heart Lung and Blood Institute's Cardiac Arrhythmia Suppression Trial (CAST II) revealed that patients with asymptomatic, non-life-threatening arrhythmias (with an MI between 4 and 90 days prior to study entry and a left ventricular ejection fraction <10%) had no evidence of improved survival when treated with moricizine compared with placebo. Additionally a trend toward higher mortality (due to proarrhythmia) in the drug arm of the trial has effectively stopped the utilization of class I antiarrhythmics prophylactically and has certainly curtailed their overall use in a highly symptomatic patient population unless an ICD is already implanted.

Morphine

Brand names: Astramorh, Duramorph, Infumorph, Oramorph, Roxanol.
Class of drug: Narcotic analgesic, agonist.

Mechanism of action: Binds to opiate receptors and blocks ascending pain pathways. Reduces patient's perception of pain without altering cause of the pain.

Indications/dosage/route: Oral, IV, IM.

• Analgesia
  – Adults: PO 30–50 mg q4h.
  – Sustained-release tablets: Adults: 30–100 mg q8–12h.
  – Adults: IV, IM 5–20 mg/70 kg q4h.
  – Children: IV, IM 100–200 µg/kg. Maximum: 15 mg
  – Adults: IV 2–10 mg/70 kg body wt.

Adjustment of dosage

• Kidney disease: None.
• Liver disease: None.
• Elderly: Use with caution.
• Pediatric: See above.

	Onset of Action	Peak Effect	Duration
IV	15–60 min	0.5–1 h	3–7 h

Food: May be taken with food to lessen GI upset.

Pregnancy: Category B. Category D if prolonged use or if given in high doses at term.

Lactation: Appears in breast milk. Potentially toxic to infant. Avoid breastfeeding.

Contraindications: Hypersensitivity to narcotics of the same chemical class, respiratory depression in the absence of resuscitation equipment, premature infant, labor prior to delivery of premature infant.

Warnings/precautions

• Use with caution in patients with head injury with increased intracranial pressure, serious alcoholism, prostatic hypertrophy, chronic pulmonary disease, severe liver or kidney disease, disorders of biliary tract and postoperative patients with pulmonary disease.

• Administer drug before patient experiences severe pain for fullest efficacy of the drug.

- Have the following available when treating patient with this drug: naloxone (Narcan) or other antagonist, means of administering oxygen, and support of respiration.
- Nausea, vomiting, and orthostatic hypotension occur most prominently in ambulatory patients. If nausea and vomiting persist, it may be necessary to administer an antiemetic, eg, droperidol or prochlorperazine.
- This drug can cause severe hypotension in a patient who is volume depleted or if given along with a phenothiazine or general anesthesia.
- Careful diagnosis must be made of acute abdominal condition before this drug is administered.

Advice to patient
- Avoid alcohol and other CNS depressants such as sedatives (eg, diazepam) when taking this drug.
- Avoid driving and other activities requiring mental alertness or that are potentially dangerous until response to drug is known.
- Change position slowly, in particular from recumbent to up-right, to minimize orthostatic hypotension. Sit at the edge of the bed for several minutes before standing, and lie down if feeling faint or dizzy. Avoid hot showers or baths and standing for long period. Male patients should sit on the toilet while urinating rather than standing.
- Do not increase dose if you are not experiencing sufficient pain relief without approval from treating physician.
- Do not stop medication abruptly when you have been taking it for ≥2 weeks. If so, a withdrawal reaction may occur within 24–48 hours. The following are typical symptoms: irritability, perspiration, rhinorrhea, lacrimation, dilated pupil, piloerection ("goose flesh"), bone and muscle aches, restless sleep ("yen"), increased systolic pressure, hyperpyrexia, diarrhea, hyperglycemia, spontaneous orgasm.
- Do not take OTC drugs without approval by treating physician. Some of these may potentiate the CNS depressant effects of the drug.

- If dizziness persists more than 3 days, decrease dose gradually (over 1–2 days).
- Attempt to void every 4 hours.

Adverse reactions
- Common: constipation, lightheadedness, dizziness, sedation, nausea, vomiting, sweating, dysplasia, emphoma.
- Serious: **hypotension, bradycardia**, apnea, circulatory depression, respiratory arrest, convulsions (high doses, IV), shock, increased intracranial depression, paralytic ileus, physical and psychologic dependence and addiction.

Clinically important drug interactions: Drugs that increase effects/toxocity of narcotic analgesis: alcohol, benzodiazepines, antihistamines, phenothiazines, butyrophenones, triyclic antidepressants, MAO inhibitors.

Parameters to monitor
- Signs and symptoms of pain: restlessness, anorexia, elevated pulse, increased respiratory rate. Differentiate restlessness associated with pain from that caused by CNS stimulation caused by morphine. This paradoxical reaction is seen mainly in women and elderly patients.
- Respiratory status prior to and following drug administration. Note rate, depth, and rhythm of respirations. If rate falls below 12/min, withhold drug unless patient is receiving ventilatory support. Consider administering an antagonist, eg, naloxone 0.1–0.5 mg IV every 2–3 minutes. Be aware that respiratory depression may occur even at small doses. Restlessness may also be a symptom of hypoxia.
- Character of cough reflex. Encourage postoperative patient to change position frequently (at least every 2 hours), breathe deeply, and cough at regular intervals, unless coughing is contraindicated. These steps will help prevent atelectasis.
- Signs and symptoms of urinary retention, particularly in patients with prostatic hypertrophy or urethral stricture. Monitor output/intake and check for oliguria or urinary retention.
- Signs of tolerance or dependence. Determine whether patient is attempting to obtain more drug than prescribed as this may

indicate onset of tolerance and possibility of dependence. If tolerance develops to one opiate, there is generally cross-tolerance to all drugs in this class. Physical dependence is generally not a problem if the drug is given <2 weeks.

- BP. If systolic pressure falls below 90 mm Hg, do not administer the drug unless there is ventilatory support. Be aware that the elderly and those receiving drugs with hypotensive properties are most susceptible to sharp fall in BP.
- Heart rate. Withhold drug if adult pulse rate is below 60 beats/min. Alternatively, administer atropine.
- Respiratory status of newborn baby and possible withdrawal reaction. If the mother has received an opiate just prior to delivery, the neonate may experience severe respiratory depression. Resuscitation may be necessary as may a narcotic antgonist, eg, Narcan. Alternatively, the neonate may experience severe withdrawal symptoms 1–4 days after birth. In such circumstances, administer tincture of opium or paregoric.
- Signs and symptoms of constipation. If patient is on drug longer than 2–3 days, administer a laxative.
- For patients on long-term therapy, administer a bulk or fiber laxative, eg, psyllium, 1 teaspoon in 240 mL liquid/d. Encourage patient to drink large amounts of fluid, 2.5 to 3 L/d.

Editorial comments
- Morphine is the drug of choice for the following conditions: treatment of severe pain, pain of terminal cancer when treatment with other drugs is not effective, noncancer pain when treatment with other drugs is not effective, postoperative pain, postmyocardial pain, pulmonary edema.
- The following considerations should be made in the event of pain or in unusual circumstances, eg, breakthrough pain: use a sustained release morphine preparation along with one that provides rapid release. Transdermal therapy may be beneficial.
- Cancer patients who are experiencing severe, unrelieved pain: Administer the drug IV or IM and switch to oral therapy once pain is controlled. Transdermal therapy may be beneficial.

Mycophenolate Mofetil

Brand name: CellCept.
Class of drug: Immunosuppressant, used for prevention and treatment of posttransplant organ rejection.
Mechanism of action: Inhibits lymphocyte proliferation; decreases lymphocyte purine synthesis.
Indications/dosage/route: Oral.
- Prophylaxis for organ rejection in patients receiving renal or heart transplant.
  - Adults: Initial: 1 g b.i.d. within 72 hours of transplant.
- Mycophenolate is used in combination with corticosteroids and cyclosporine.
  - Children: Studies recommend 15–27 mg/kg b.i.d.

Adjustment of dosage
- Kidney disease: Do not exceed dose of 2 g/d.
- Liver disease: None.
- Elderly: Guidelines are not available.
- Pediatric: See above. Limited data available.

Food: Take on empty stomach, 1 hour before or 2 hours after meals.
Pregnancy: Category C.
Lactation: Probably appears in breast milk. Potentially toxic to infant. Avoid breastfeeding.
Contraindications: Hypersensitivity to mycophenolate mofetil, mycophenolic acid.
Warnings/precautions: Use with caution in patients with kidney disease, serious GI diseases.

Advice to patients
- Use two forms of birth control including hormonal and barrier methods. Contraception should be initiated before, during, and for at least 6 weeks after discontinuing therapy.
- Avoid contact with individuals with contagious infections.
- Do not take OTC medication (such as antacids) along with mycophenolate unless approved by the treating physician.

Adverse reactions

- Common: headache, fever, edema, diarrhea, constipation, nausea, hypercholesterolemia, dyspnea, fever, back pain, oral candidiasis, dizziness, hyperglycemia, tremor.
- Serious: **bone marrow depression, urinary tract infection, hematuria, respiratory infection**, sepsis, hypophosphatemia, hypokalemia, hyperkalemia, pneumonia, dyspnea.

Clinically important drug interactions

- Drugs that increase effects/toxicity of mycophenolate: acyclovir, gancyclovir, probenecid, salicylates (all potentially increase drug level).
- Drugs that decrease effects/toxicity of mycophenolate: cholestyramine, antacids.
- Mycophenolate increases effects/toxicity of oral contraceptives.

Parameter to monitor

- Liver enzymes, CBC with differential and platelets, serum creatinine.
- Signs of organ rejection: laboratory abnormalities, fever, fatigue, jaundice, heart failure, kidney failure.
- Signs and symptoms of infections.

Editorial comments

- The initial dose of mycophenolate should be given within 72 hours of transplant.
- Unapproved uses of mycophenolate include resistant psoriasis and other inflammatory conditions.
- This drug is teratogenic. Accordingly, capsules should not be opened or crushed and patient should be warned not to inhale or come in direct contact with the drug on skin or mucous membranes. If such contact occurs, skin should be washed with soap and water, and eyes rinsed with plain water.

Nabumetone

Brand name: Relafen.
Class of drug: NSAID.
Mechanism of action: Inhibits cyclooxygenase, resulting in inhibition of synthesis of prostaglandins and other inflammatory mediators.
Indications/dosage/route: Oral only.
• Osteoarthritis, rheumatoid arthritis
  – Adults: 1000–2000 mg/d in 1 or 2 doses. Maximum: 2000 mg/d.
Adjustment of dosage
• Kidney disease: None.
• Liver disease: None.
• Elderly: May be necessary to reduce dose for patients >50 years.
• Pediatric: Safety and efficacy have not been established.
Food: Take with food or large quantities of water or milk.
Pregnancy: Category C. Category D in third trimester or near delivery.
Lactation: May appear in breast milk. Best to avoid.
Contraindications: Hypersensitivity to nabumetone and cross-sensitivity with other NSAIDs and aspirin.
Editorial comments: For additional information, see *ibuprofen*, p. 445.

Nadolol

Brand name: Corgard.
Class of drug: β-Adrenergic receptor blocker.
Mechanism of action: Competitive blocker of β-adrenergic receptors in heart and blood vessels.

Indications/dosage/route: Oral only.
• Hypertension
– Initial: 40 mg/d. Increase in 40- to 80-mg increments until optimum response is obtained. Maintenance: 40–320 mg/d.
• Angina pectoris
– Initial: 40 mg/d. Maintenance: 40–240 mg/d.
Adjustment of dosage
• Kidney disease: Creatinine clearance >50 mL/min: dose q24h; creatinine clearance 31–50 mL/min: dose q24–36h; creatinine clearance 10–30 mL/min: dose q24–48h; creatinine clearance <10 mL/min: dose q40–60h.
• Liver disease: None.
• Elderly: None.
• Pediatric: Safety and efficacy have not been established.
Food: No restriction.
Pregnancy: Category C.
Lactation: Appears in breast milk. Potentially toxic to infant. Considered compatible by American Academy of Pediatrics. Observe infant for hypotension, bradycardia, etc.
Contraindications: Cardiogenic shock, asthma, CHF unless it is secondary to tachyarrhythmia treated with a β blocker, sinus bradycardia and AV block greater than first degree, severe COPD.
Editorial comments: For additional information, see *propranolol*, p. 790.

Nafcillin

Brand names: Unipen, Nallpen.
Class of drug: Antibiotic, penicillin family.
Mechanism of action: Inhibits bacterial cell wall synthesis.
Susceptible organisms *in vivo*: *Staphylococcus aureus* (not MRSA), other staphylococci, viridans streptococci, *Streptococcus pneumoniae*, beta-hemolytic streptococci.

Indications/dosage/route: PO, IV, IM.
- Systemic infections caused by susceptible organisms
  - Adults: IV 0.5–1 g q4h.
  - Adults: IM 0.5 g q4–6h.
  - Children, infants <40 kg: IM 25 mg/kg b.i.d.
  - Neonates >2000 g and <7 days: IM 100 mg/kg/d in 2 divided doses.
  - Neonates >7 days: IM 100 mg/kg/d in 3 divided doses.
  - Neonates <2000 g: IM 20 mg/kg q8h.
- Mild to moderate infections
  - Adults: PO 50–500 mg q4–6h.
- Severe infections
  - Adults: PO up to 1 g q4–6h.
- Pneumonia/scarlet fever
  - Children: PO 25 mg/kg/d in 4 divided doses.
- Staphylococcal infections
  - Children: PO 50 mg/kg/d in 4 divided doses.
  - Neonates: PO 10 mg/kg t.i.d. to q.i.d.
- Streptococcal pharyngitis
  - Children: PO 250 mg t.i.d. for 10 days.

Adjustment of dosage: None.
Food: Not applicable.
Pregnancy: Category B.
Lactation: No data available. Best to avoid.
Contraindications: Hypersensitivity to penicillin or cephalosporins.
Editorial comments
- Nafcillin is the drug of choice for severe *St. aureus* infections, such as bacteremia, endocarditis, spinal osteomyelitis, and epidural abscess. Although it is not effective against MRSA, it is more effective than vancomycin against MSSA and is the drug of choice for MSSA endocarditis. In right-sided endocarditis caused by MSSA, nafcillin in combination with gentamicin is effective as a short course of therapy (2 weeks). In intravenous catheter infection, a minimum of 2 weeks of intravenous nafcillin is recommended when the blood cultures are positive for MSSA.

- Nafcillin is also very effective against *S. aureus* (MSSA) epidural abscess.
- For most other indications, nafcillin can be changed to oral dicloxacillin.
- This drug is not listed in the *Physicians' Desk Reference*, 54th edition, 2000.
- For additional information, see *penicillin G*, p. 708.

Nalbuphine

Brand name: Nubain.
Class of drug: Narcotic analgesic, agonist.
Mechanism of action: Binds to opiate receptors and blocks ascending pain pathways. Reduces patient's perception of pain without altering cause of the pain.
Indications/dosage/route: IV, IM, SC.
- Analgesia
  – Adults: IV, IM, SC 10 mg/70 kg q3–6h as needed.
  – Nontolerant adults: Maximum single dose: 20 mg. Maximum daily dose: 160 mg.
Adjustment of dosage
- Kidney disease: Use with caution.
- Liver disease: Use with caution.
- Elderly: Use with caution.
- Pediatric: Safety and efficacy have not been established in children <18 years.

	Onset of Action	Peak Effect	Duration
IM, SC	<15 min	60 min	3–6 h
IV	2–3 min	30 min	3–6 h

Food: May be taken with food to lessen GI upset.
Pregnancy: Category B. Category D if prolonged use or if given in high doses at term.

Lactation: No data available. Potentially toxic to infant. Avoid breastfeeding.

Contraindications: Hypersensitivity to narcotics of the same chemical class.

Warnings/precautions

- Use with caution in patients with head injury with increased intracranial pressure, serious alcoholism, prostatic hypertrophy, chronic preliminary disease, severe liver or kidney disease, disorders of biliary tract, and in postoperative patients with pulmonary disease.
- Administer drug before patient experiences severe pain for fullest efficacy of the drug. Have the following available when treating patient with this drug: naloxone (Narcan) or other antagonist, means of administering oxygen, and support of respiration.
- Nausea, vomiting, and orthostatic hypotension occur most prominently in ambulatory patients. If nausea and vomiting persist, it may be necessary to administer an antiemetic, eg, droperidol or prochlorperazine.
- This drug can cause severe hypotension in a patient who is volume depleted or if given along with a phenothiazine or general anesthesia.
- Careful diagnosis must be made of acute abdominal condition before this drug is administered.

Editorial comments

- Administration of nalbuphine in narcotic-dependent individuals may result in withdrawal reaction.
- When used during pregnancy, administer atropine proportionally to reduce incidence of bradycardia.
- For additional information, see *morphine*, p. 633.

Naloxone

Brand name: Narcan.
Class of drug: Narcotic (opioid) antagonist.

Mechanism of action: Competitive antagonist of narcotic analgesics (opioids) at one or more receptor sites in the CNS. Reverses CNS and respiratory depression in suspected or known opioid overdose.

Indications/dosage/route: IM, IV.

• Postoperative respiratory depression
  – Adults: IV 0.4–2 mg q2–3min until response is obtained. Repeat dose q20–60min as needed. Discontinue if no response after 10 mg total dose.
  – Children: IV 5–10 µg. Repeat 2–3 minutes until response is obtained. May repeat q1–2h if needed.

• Postanesthetic opioid reversal of respiratory depression
  – Opioid overdose: IV 0.4 mg q2–3min. Maximum: 10 mg. If ineffective, respiratory depression is probably caused by nonopioid source.

• Opioid overdose
  – Infants, children: 0.01 mg/kg; repeat 2 or 3 times as needed.
  – Neonates (asphyxia, neonatorum): IV 0.01 mg/kg into umbilical vein; repeat q2–3min. Maximum: 3 doses.
  – Adults: IV 0.4–2 mg q2–3min as needed. Repeat dose q20–60min. If no response is observed after 10 mg, the diagnosis of opioid overdose is questionable.
  – Children: IV 0.5–2 µg/kg.

• Naloxone challenge for diagnosing opioid dependence
  – Adults: IM 0.16 mg. Signs of withdrawal should be observed after 20–30 minutes. If this does not occur, give another dose of 0.24 mg IV.

Adjustment of dosage: None.

Food: Not applicable.

Pregnancy: Category B.

Lactation: Present in breast milk. Best to avoid.

Contraindications: Hypersensitivity to naloxone.

Warnings/precautions

• Use with caution in patients with opioid addiction, cardiac irregularities. May precipitate full-blown opioid withdrawal at high doses in patients receiving an opioid longer than 1 week.

- Failure of naloxone to produce a significant reversal of symptoms of opioid overdose, in particular respiratory depression, may indicate that symptoms are nonopioid effects (eg, CNS disease, overdose of other drugs).
- Naloxone's duration of action is much shorter than those of the opioids. Accordingly, vigilance is required and repeated doses are usually necessary to manage acute narcotic overdose.
- The occurrence of narcotic usage must be determined in the mother giving birth to a baby with respiratory depression. Naloxone must be used with great caution in such patients to avoid precipitating withdrawal symptoms in the neonate.
- Naloxone should be used with caution postoperatively when opioids are used in surgery to avoid reversal of anesthesia and rapid increases in BP and pain.

Advice to patient: None.

Adverse reactions
- Common: none.
- Serious: ventricular tachycardia and fibrillation, cardiac arrest, seizures, pulmonary edema. (These are seen in postoperative patients with cardiovascular disorders or after abrupt withdrawal in patients with narcotic addiction.)

Clinically important drug interactions
- Naloxone may precipitate severe withdrawal reaction in patients.
- Naloxine increases the toxicity of cardiotoxic drugs.

Parameters to monitor
- Monitor all vital signs and level of consciousness frequently for 3–4 hours after peak blood concentrations of naloxone. Peak activity occurs 45 minutes after administration.
- Level of pain when used to treat postoperative respiratory depression.
- Signs and symptoms of opioid withdrawal: diarrhea, abdominal cramps, restlessness, increased BP.

Editorial comments
- When treating drug overdose, adjuvant therapy using the following may be necessary: mechanical ventilation, oxygen, vasopressors, nasogastric lavage.

- Naloxone is a safe drug to administer in patients with respiratory depression of unknown cause.
- Higher concentrations of naloxone (ie, 0.4 mg/mL preparations) may be required in neonates to avoid fluid accumulation.
- Naloxone is the drug of choice for intentional or unintentional opioid overdose.

Naltrexone

Brand name: Revia.
Class of drug: Narcotic (opioid) antagonist, long-acting.
Mechanism of action: Competitive binding at opioid receptor sites reduces euphoria and drug craving without supporting the addiction.
Indications/dosage/route: Oral only.
- Management of opioid dependence
  - Adults: Initial: PO 25 mg. Maintenance: 50 mg q24h, single dose.
- Alcoholism
  - Adults: 50 mg/d.
Adjustment of dosage
- Kidney disease: None.
- Liver disease: None.
- Elderly: None.
- Pediatric: Use in children <18 years has not been established.

Onset of Action	Duration
5 min–1 h	24 h

Food: May be taken with food.
Pregnancy: Category C.
Lactation: No data available. Best to avoid breastfeeding.
Contraindications: Naltrexone is contraindicated in patients with ongoing opioid use, dependence on opioids, opioid withdrawal,

positive toxicology screen for opioids, acute hepatitis or hepatic failure, failure of naloxone challenge (see *naloxone*, p. 644).

Warnings/precautions

• Use with caution in patients with history of liver disease.

• Test patient for dependence by administering a naloxone challenge (see Naloxone). If patient shows signs of withdrawal, naltrexone should not be used.

Advice to patient

• Carry an identification card indicating you are undergoing naltrexone therapy.

Adverse reactions

• Common: nausea.

• Serious: liver toxicity, depression, suicide attempt or ideation, idiopathic thrombocytopenic purpura.

Clinically important drug interactions

• Drugs that increase effects/toxicity of naltrexone: Thioridazine.

• Naltrexone decreases effects/toxicity of opioids used as antidiarrheals, analgesics or antitussives.

Parameters to monitor

• Evidence of suicidal tendency (higher risk in opiate abusers).

• Signs of withdrawal: muscle cramps, perspiration, rhinorrhea, nausea, diarrhea, abdominal cramps, restlessness, increased BP.

Editorial comments: It is necessary to determine when the patient last received an opioid. Such patients should be free of opioids for a minimum of 7–10 days before starting naloxone. This opioid-free status should be confirmed by means of the naloxone challenge.

Naproxen

Brand names: Aleve, Naprosyn, Anaprox (Naproxen sodium).
Class of drug: NSAID.

Mechanism of action: Inhibits cyclooxygenase, resulting in inhibition of synthesis of prostaglandins and other inflammatory mediators.

Indications/dosage/route: Oral only.

• Rheumatoid arthritis, osteoarthritis, ankylosing spondylitis, dysmenorrhea, tendinitis, bursitis
  – Adults: 250–500 mg b.i.d.
  – Delayed-release tablets: 375–500 mg b.i.d.
  – Naproxen sodium: 275–550 mg b.i.d.
  – Controlled-release tablets: Adults: 750 or 1000 mg/d.

• Acute gout
  – Adults: Initial: 750 mg. Maintenance: 250 mg q8h.
  – Controlled-release tablets: Adults: 1000–1500 mg once daily.
  – Naproxen sodium: Adults: Initial: 825 mg. Maintenance: 275 mg q8h.

• Juvenile rheumatoid arthritis
  – 10 mg/kg/d.

Adjustment of Dosage

• Kidney disease: None.
• Liver disease: None.
• Elderly: May be necessary to reduce dose for patients >65 years.
• Pediatric: Safety and efficacy have not been established in children <2 years.

Food: Take with food or large quantities of water or milk.

Pregnancy: Category B. Category D in third trimester or near delivery.

Lactation: No data available. Best to avoid.

Contraindications: Hypersensitivity and cross-sensitivity with other NSAIDs and aspirin.

Warnings/precautions

• Use with caution in patients with history of GI bleeding, decreased renal function, rhinitis, urticaria, hay fever, nasal polyps, asthma.
• Administer this drug with caution in patients with infections or other diseases as the drug may mask symptoms of the disease, eg, fever, inflammation.

- NSAIDs may cause severe allergic reactions including urticaria and vasomotor collapse. Cross-reactivity may occur in patients allergic to aspirin.

Advice to patient

- Avoid use of alcohol.
- Notify physician if your stool turns dark, if you develop abdominal pain, or if you vomit blood or dark material.
- Notify dentist or treating physician prior to surgery if taking this medication.
- Avoid taking OTC products that contain aspirin or other NSAIDs, eg, Alka-Seltzer.
- Take drug with full glass of water and sit up for 15–30 minutes to avoid lodging of tablet in esophagus.
- If pain occurs with physical activity, take drug 30 minutes before physical therapy or other planned exercise.

Adverse reactions

- Common: nausea, indigestion, dizziness, fatigue.
- Serious: GI bleeding (peptic ulcer, diverticular NSAID colitis), acute renal failure, bronchospasm, Stevens–Johnson syndrome, renal or hepatic toxicity, GI perforation.

Clinically important drug interactions

- Drugs that increase effects/toxicity of NSAIDs: alcohol, insulin, cimetidine.
- Drugs that decrease effects/toxicity of NSAIDs: barbiturates, corticosteroids, antacids.
- NSAIDs increase effects/toxicity of oral anticoagulants, cyclosporine, lithium, methotrexate, sulfonamides, streptokinase, valproic acid, oral hypoglycemics.
- NSAIDs decrease effects/toxicity of β blockers, calcium channel blockers, loop diuretics, probenecid, sulfinpyrazone.

Parameters to monitor

- CBC, liver enzymes, stool hemoccult, serum BUN and creatinine.
- Efficacy of treatment: pain reduction, decreased temperature, improved mobility. Assess pain reduction 1 or 2 hours after taking drug.

- Rhinitis, asthma, urticaria before beginning treatment. Such patients are at increased risk of developing hypersensitivity reaction to NSAID.
- Blood glucose of diabetic patients taking oral hypoglycemic drugs. An NSAID may potentiate the hypoglycemic effect of oral hypoglycemic drugs.
- Signs and symptoms of auditory toxicity, in particular tinnitus in elderly patients. Stop drug to avoid irreversible hearing loss. Restart at 50% of previous dose after reversal occurs.
- Symptoms of iron deficiency anemia, particularly in patients on long-term, high-dose drug. Perform hematocrit and guaiac tests periodically.
- Signs and symptoms of renal toxicity.
- Signs and symptoms of hepatotoxicity.
- Symptoms of GI toxicity: occult blood loss, hematochezia, melena, abdominal pain.
- Efficacy in treating rheumatoid arthritis. Increase dose if drug is not effective within 7 days. If maximum dose is not effective, change to another NSAID. If a second- or third-line drug is required, the NSAID should not be stopped.

Editorial comments

- Some rheumatologists consider aspirin to be the first-line drug for treatment of rheumatoid arthritis. Patient should be given 14-day trial at dose of 3.2 g/d; if ineffective, another drug should be used.
- It is recommended that misoprostol should be given prophylactically for the following patients requiring long-term treatment with an NSAID: those >60 years of age, those with past history of peptic ulcer disease, those concurrently receiving anticoagulants or corticosteroids. Misoprostol has also been shown to reduce the incidence of NSAID-induced ulcers in younger patients.
- Concomitant acid-blocking agents (H_2 blockers, proton pump inhibitor) may reduce the incidence of duodenal ulcer but not gastric ulcer in patients on chronic NSAID therapy. They may also reduce NSAID-induced GI symptoms.

- Treat *Helicobacter plyori* if present in patients developing active ulcer on NSAID therapy; use proton pump inhibitor plus two additional antibiotics.
- Newer COX-2 inhibitors are potential alternatives for patients requiring chronic NSAID therapy.
- For additional information see *celecoxib,* p. 186, and *rofecoxib,* p. 827.

Neostigmine

Brand name: Prostigmin.
Class of drug: Cholinesterase inhibitor.
Mechanism of action: Inhibits acetylcholinesterase, thereby increasing acetylcholine at cholinergic receptor sites.
Indications/dosage/route: Oral, IV, IM, SC.
- Symptomatic control of myasthenia gravis
  – Adults: Initial: IM, SC 0.5 mg. Subsequent doses are based on response.
  – Adults: Initial: PO 15 mg. Subsequent doses are based on response.
- Prevention of postoperative distension and urinary retention
  – Adults: Initial: IM, SC 0.25 mg as soon after operation as possible. Repeat q4–6h, 2–3 days.
- Urinary retention
  – Adults: Initial: IM, SC 0.5 mg. Catheterize patient if no response within 1 hour. After voiding continue with 0.5-mg injection q3–5h.
- Reversal of nondepolarizing blocking agent (curare-type drug) postanesthesia
  – Adults: Slow IV injection: Initial: 0.5–2 mg. Repeat as required. Maximum: 5 mg. Administer simultaneously IV 0.6–1.2 mg atropine via separate syringe.
Adjustment of dosage
- Kidney disease: None.
- Liver disease: None.
- Elderly: None.

• Pediatric: Safety and efficacy have not been established.

Food: Oral form should be taken with food or milk to lesson GI side effects.

Pregnancy: Category C.

Lactation: It is not known if this drug is excreted in milk. Avoid breastfeeding.

Contraindications: Hypersensitivity to neostigmine or bromides, peritonitis, mechanical obstruction of intestinal or urinary tract.

Warnings/precautions

• Use with caution in patients with the following conditions: epilepsy, bronchial asthma, bradycardia, recent coronary occlusion, hyperthyroidism, cardiac arrhythmias, peptic ulcer.

• If large doses of neostigmine are needed, inject atropine IV prior to or simultaneously with the drug.

• Atropine as well as means of treating anaphylaxis should be available before neostigmine administration.

• It is essential to distinguish between myasthenic and cholinergic crises before administering a cholinesterase inhibitor.

• Identify all drugs patient is taking to avoid unfavorable drug–drug interactions.

• Determine whether patient is allergic to bromide if neostigmine bromide is to be used.

• When the drug is to be used as an antidote for excessive drug-induced neuromuscular blockade, use assisted ventilation and maintain a patent airway.

• Provide patient with a printed list of most serious adverse reactions to the drug. Indicate which of these should be reported immediately.

• Avoid use of a cholinesterase inhibitor if succinylcholine is used during surgery.

• Stop all other cholinergic drugs during therapy with cholinesterase inhibitor.

Advice to patient

• Keep record of periods of muscle strength and weakness. This will enable the physician to evaluate the dosage and, if necessary, make adjustments. Take your doses exactly as prescribed to avoid myasthenic or cholinergic crisis.

- Report any signs of muscle weakness immediately to treating physician.
- Carry identification card indicating your condition, medication, name and address of treating physician.

Adverse reactions
- Common: bowel cramps, salivation, diarrhea, fasciculations, muscle cramps.
- Serious: cardiac arrest, AV block, bradycardia, hypotension, bronchospasm, respiratory arrest, anaphylaxis, seizures, laryngospasm.

Clinically important drug interactions
- Drugs that increase effects/toxicity of cholinesterase inhibitors: aminoglycosides (neomycin, streptomycin, kanamycin), local anesthetics, general anesthetics, magnesium salts.
- Drugs that increase effects/toxicity of cholinesterase inhibitors: atopine and other anticholinergics, antihistamines, phenothiazines, quinidine, disopyramide, procainamide.
- Cholinesterase inhibitors increase effects/toxicity of succinylcholine, decamethonium, organophosphate pesticides.

Parameters to monitor
- Status of muscle strength to differentiate between myasthenic and cholinergic crises. Onset of weakness 1 hour after taking the drug indicates drug overdose (cholinergic crisis). Onset of weakness 3 hours or more after taking drug indicates drug underdosage (myasthenic crisis).
- Vital signs during the beginning of therapy. If pulse rate falls below 80, stop drug administration. If patient becomes hypotensive, maintain in recumbent position until BP stabilizes.

Editorial comments: Unapproved use of neostigmine includes treatment of intestinal pseudo-obstruction (Ogilve's syndrome).

Netilmicin

Brand name: Netromycin.
Class of drug: Antibiotic, aminoglycoside.

Mechanism of action: Binds to ribosomal units in bacteria, inhibits protein synthesis.

Susceptible organisms *in vivo*: Staphylococci (penicillinase and nonpenicillinase), *Acinetobacter* sp, *Citrobacter* sp, *Enterobacter* sp, *Escherichia coli*, *Klebsiella* sp, *Neisseria* sp, *Proteus* sp, *Pseudomonas* sp, *Salmonella* sp, *Serratia* sp, *Shigella* sp.

Indications/dosage/route: IV, IM.

• Complicated UTIs
  – Adults: 1.5–2.0 mg/kg q12h.
• Serious systemic infections
  – Adults: 2.0–3.25 mg/kg q12h.
• For all infections
  – Neonates <6 weeks: 2.0–3.25 mg/kg q12h.
  – Infants, children 6 weeks–12 years: 2.7–4.0 mg/kg q12h.

Adjustment of dosage

• Kidney disease: Creatinine clearance 40–50 mL/min: administer 50% of usual dose q8h; creatinine clearance 30–40 mL/min: administer 35% of usual dose q8h; creatinine clearance 20–30 mL/min: administer 25% of usual dose q8h.
• Liver disease: None.
• Elderly: None.
• Pediatric: See above.

Contraindications: Hypersensitivity to netilmicin.

Editorial comments: For additional information, see *amikacin*, p. 33.

Nicardipine

Brand name: Cardene IV.

Class of drug: Calcium channel blocker.

Mechanism of action: Inhibits calcium movement across cell membranes.

Indications/dosage/route: IV, PO.

• Hypertension
  – IV 5 mg/h. Increase to 15 mg/h. Maintenance: 3 mg/h.
  – PO 30 mg b.i.d.

• Angina
  – PO 20–40 mg b.i.d.

Adjustment of dosage
• Kidney disease: Reduce dose.
• Liver disease: Reduce dose in severe liver disease.
• Elderly: None.
• Pediatric: Safety and efficacy in children <18 years have not been established.

Onset of Action	Peak Effect	Duration
30 min	1–2 h	8 h

Food: No restriction.
Pregnancy: Category C.
Lactation: No data available. Potentially toxic to infant. Avoid breastfeeding.
Contraindications: Hypersensitivity to calcium blockers, advanced aortic stenosis.

Editorial comments
• Cardene IV is indicated only for short-term use when oral therapy is not feasible.
• Oral medication should be administered as soon as clinical condition permits.
• For additional information, see *nifedipine*, p. 656.

Nifedipine

Brand name: Procardia.
Class of drug: Calcium channel blocker.
Mechanism of action: Inhibits calcium movement across cell membranes.
Indications/dosage/route: Oral only.
• Hypertension
  – Adults, individualized: 30–60 mg/d. Maximum: 180 mg/d.

- Angina
  - Adults: 30–120 mg/day.
  - Elderly: 30–120 mg/day.

Adjustment of dosage

- Kidney disease: None.
- Liver disease: Use with caution. Monitor carefully.
- Elderly: Use with caution.
- Pediatric: Safety and efficacy have not been established.

Onset of Action	Peak Effect	Duration
0.5–1 h	2 h	8 h

Food: No restriction.

Pregnancy: Category C.

Lactation: Probably appears in breast milk. Potentially toxic to infant. Avoid breastfeeding.

Contraindications: Hypersensitivity to calcium blockers.

Warnings/precautions

- Use with caution in patients with CHF, severe left ventricular dysfunction and in those concomitantly receiving β blockers or digoxin, liver disease.
- Do not withdraw drug abruptly, as this may result in increased frequency and intensity of angina.
- For the diabetic patient, the drug may interfere with insulin release and therefore produce hyperglycemia.
- Patient should be tapered off β blockers before beginning calcium channel blockers to avoid exacerbation of angina from abrupt withdrawal of the β blocker.

Advice to patient

- Use two forms of birth control including hormonal and barrier methods.
- Change position slowly, in particular from recumbent to upright, to minimize orthostatic hypotension. Sit at the edge of the bed for several minutes before standing, and lie down if feeling faint or dizzy. Avoid hot showers or baths and standing for long periods.

Male patients should sit on the toilet while urinating rather than standing.

- Avoid driving and other activities requiring mental alertness or that are potentially dangerous until response to drug is known.
- Use OTC medications only with approval from treating physician.
- Determine BP and heart rate aproximately at the same time each day and at least twice a week, particularly at the beginning of therapy.
- Be aware of the fact that this drug may also block or reduce anginal pain, thereby giving a false sense of security on severe exertion.
- Include high-fiber foods to minimize constipation.
- Limit consumption of xanthine-containing drinks: regular coffee (fewer than 5 cups/d), tea, cocoa.

Adverse reactions
- Common: headache, edema.
- Serious: CHF, arrhythmias, hypotension, depression.

Clinically important drug interactions
- Drugs that increase effects/toxicity of calcium blockers: cimetidine, β blockers, cyclosporine.
- Drugs that decrease effects of calcium blockers: barbiturates.

Parameters to monitor
- BP during initial administration and frequently thereafter. Ideally, check BP close to the end of dosage interval or before next administration.
- Status of liver and kidney function. Impaired renal function prolongs duration of action and increases tendency for toxicity.
- Intake of fluids and urinary and other fluid output to minimize renal toxicity. Increase fluid intake if inadequate. Closely monitor electrolyte levels.
- Efficacy of treatment for angina: decrease in frequency of angina attacks, need for nitroglycerin, episodes of PST segment deviation, anginal pain.
- If anginal pain is not reduced at rest or during effort reassess patient as to medication.

- GI side effects: Use alternative.
- ECG for development of heart block.
- Symptoms of CHF.

Nimodipine

Brand name: Nimotop.
Class of drug: Calcium channel blocker.
Mechanism of action: Inhibits calcium movement across cell membranes.
Indications/dosage/route: Oral only.
- Subarachnoid hemorrhage from ruptured congenital aneurysm
  – Adults: 60 mg q4h beginning within 96 h of subarachnoid hemorrhage and continue for 21 consecutive days.

Adjustment of dosage
- Kidney disease: None.
- Liver disease: Reduce dose to 30 mg q4h.
- Elderly: Reduce dose.
- Pediatric: Safety and efficacy have not been established.

Onset of Action	Peak Effect	Duration
Rapid	1 h	4 h

Food: No restriction.
Pregnancy: Category C.
Lactation: Probably appears in breast milk. Potentially toxic to infant. Avoid breastfeeding.
Contraindications: None.
Editorial comments
- Use with caution in cerebral edema or if intracranial pressure is severely raised. Condition may worsen.
- For additional information, see *nifedipine*, p. 656.

Nitrofurantoin

Brand names: Furadantin, Macrobid, Macrodantin, Nephrondx.
Class of drug: Urinary tract germicide.
Mechanisms of action: Inhibits acetyl coenzyme A and bacterial cell wall synthesis.
Indications/dosage/route: Oral only.
• UTI
  – Adults: 50–100 mg q.i.d. Maximum: 600 mg/d.
  – Children ≥1 month: 5–7 mg/kg/d, 4 equal doses.
• UTI prophylaxis
  – Adults: 50–100 mg h.s.
  – Children ≥1 month: 1 mg/kg/d h.s. or 2 divided doses.
Adjustment of dosage
• Kidney disease: None.
• Liver disease: None.
• Elderly: None.
• Pediatric: See above.
Food: Take with food or milk. Oral suspension may be prepared with water, fruit juice, or milk.
Pregnancy: Category B. Contraindicated in women near term.
Lactation: Appears in breast milk. Considered compatible by American Academy of Pediatrics.
Contraindications: Pregnancy at term, imminent labor, during labor and delivery, anuria, anemia.
Warnings/precautions
• Use with caution in patients with G6PD deficiency, anemia, B vitamin deficiency, diabetes mellitus, electrolyte abnormalities.
• Prolonged therapy may result in pulmonary damage.
• Administer capsules instead of suspension if GI upset occurs.
Advice to patient: Report following to treating physican: flu-like symptoms, numbness in extremities, difficulty breathing, jaundice.

Adverse reactions
- Common: chest pain, fever, nausea, diarrhea, cough, fatigue, dizziness, discolored urine.
- Serious: peripheral neuropathy, hemolysis, anemia in patients with G6PD deficiency, bone marrow suppression, hepatic toxicity, asthmatic attacks (patients with history of asthma), exfoliative dermatitis, anaphylactic shock.

Clinically important drug interactions
- Drugs that increase effects/toxicity of nitrofurantoin: sulfinpyrazone, anticholinergic drugs, probenecid.
- Drugs that decrease effects/toxicity of nitrofurantoin: antacids containing magnesium trisilicate.

Parameters to monitor
- Signs and symptoms of UTI: burning sensation on urination, fever, cloudy or foul-smelling urine. Such assessment should be made before and throughout course of treatment.
- Intake of fluids and urinary and other fluid output to minimize renal toxicity. Closely monitor electrolyte levels.
- Signs and symptoms of bone marrow depression.
- Signs and symptoms of hepatic toxicity.
- Signs of hypersensitivity reactions.
- Signs and symptoms of antibiotic-induced bacterial or fungal superinfection. Use of yogurt (4 oz/d) may be helpful in prevention of superinfection.
- Signs and symptoms of pulmonary toxicity: basilar rales, tachypnea, cough, fever, exertional dyspnea.

Editorial comments
- It is recommended that therapy be continued for at least 3 days after urine specimens are shown to be sterile.

Nitrofurazone

Brand name: Furacin.
Class of drug: Topical antibacterial agent.

Mechanism of action: Inhibits bacterial carbohydrate metabolism.
Indications/dosage/route: Topical only.
• Major burns particularly those resistant to other antibacterial drugs; prevention of skin graft infection
  – Adults, children: Apply ointment, topical solution, or cream once daily or every few days.
Pregnancy: Category C.
Lactation: No data available. Best to avoid.
Contraindications: Hypersensitivity to nitrofurazone.
Warnings/precautions
• Use with caution in patients with renal disease, G6PD deficiency, serious liver dysfunction.
• Advise patient to store medication so as to avoid exposure to excessive heat, fluorescent lighting, or direct sunlight.
Adverse reactions
• Common: pruritis, erythema, contact dermatitis.
• Serious: none.
Parameters to monitor: Possible overgrowth of fungi or other organisms that are not susceptible to nitrofurazone action.
Editorial Comments
• This drug is not listed in the *Physician's Desk Reference*, 54th edition, 2000.

Nitroglycerin IV

Brand names: Tridil, Nitro-Bid, IV.
Class of drug: Antianginal, vasodilator, IV nitrate.
Mechanism of action: Reduces peripheral resistance (arterial and venous) by vasodilation; decreases left ventricular pressure.
Indications/dosage/route: IV only.
• Hypertension associated with surgery, CHF after acute MI, intractable angina
  – Adults: Initial: 5 µg/min by infusion pump. Increase dose until response is noted.

Adjustment of dosage
- Kidney disease: None.
- Liver disease: None.
- Elderly: None.
- Pediatric: Safety and efficacy have not been established in children.

Onset of Action	Peak Effect	Duration
1–2 min	—	3–5 min

Food: Not applicable.
Pregnancy: Category B.
Lactation: No data available. Best to avoid.
Contraindications: Hypersensitivity to nitrates or nitrites, hypotension or uncorrected hypovolemia, increased intracranial pressure, inadequate cerebral circulation, constrictive pericarditis and pericardial tamponade.

Warnings/precautions
- Use with caution in patients with severe liver or kidney disease, depleted blood volume, increased intraocular pressure, severe obliterative vascular disease, low systolic BP (below 90 mmg Hg), coronary artery disease, heart rate <50 beats/min.
- Nitroglycerin for IV injection is highly concentrated. It must be diluted in dextrose 5% or 0.9% sodium chloride before administration.

Editorial comments
- This drug is not listed in *Physician's Desk Reference*, 54th edition, 2000.
- For additional information, see *isosorbide dinitrate*, p. 473.

Nitroglycerin (Sublingual)

Brand name: Nitrostat.
Class of drug: Antianginal, vasodilator, oral nitrate.

Mechanism of action: Reduces peripheral resistance (arterial and venous) by vasodilation; decreases left ventricular pressure.
Indications/dosage/route: Sublingual only.
• Acute angina
  – 150–600 μg under the tongue, at first sign of attack. Repeat in 5 min. if necessary. Maximum: 3 tablets within 15 min.
• Angina prophylaxis
  – Take 5–10 min before activities that may provoke an attack.
Adjustment of dosage
• Kidney disease: None.
• Liver disease: None.
• Elderly: Lower doses may be required.
• Pediatric: Safety and efficacy have not been established.

Onset of Action	Duration
1–3 min	30–60 min

Food: Not applicable.
Pregnancy: Category B.
Lactation: No data available. Best to avoid.
Contraindications: Hypersensitivity to nitrates or nitrites, very low BP, shock, acute MI with low ventricular filling pressure.
Editorial comments: For additional information, see *isosorbide dinitrate*, p. 473.

Nitroglycerin (Sustained Release)

Brand names: Nitrong, Nitroglyn.
Class of drug: Antianginal, vasodilator, oral nitrate.
Mechanism of action: Reduces peripheral resistance (arterial and venous) by vasodilation; decreases left ventricular pressure.
Indications/dosage/route: Oral only.
• Prophylaxis or treatment of anginal attacks
  – Capsules: 2.5–9 mg q8–12h.
  – Tablets: 1.3–6.5 mg q8–12h.

Adjustment of dosage
- Kidney disease: None.
- Liver disease: None.
- Elderly: Lower doses may be required.
- Pediatric: Safety and efficacy have not been established.

Onset of Action	Duration
20–45 min	3–8 h

Food: Take 1 hour before or 2 hours after meals with full glass of water.

Pregnancy: Category B.

Lactation: No data available. Best to avoid.

Contraindications: Hypersensitivity to nitrates or nitrites, very low BP, shock, acute MI with low ventricular filling pressure.

Advice to patient
- Be aware of disulfiram reaction after drinking alcohol. Symptoms include: headache, facial flush, abdominal cramps, tachycardia. These symptoms generally occur within 2–3 minutes of alcohol ingestion and may last 1–4 hours. Contact treating physician.
- Change position slowly, in particular from recumbent to upright, to minimize orthostatic hypotension. Sit at the edge of the bed for several minutes before standing, and lie down if feeling faint or dizzy. Avoid hot showers or baths and standing for long periods. Male patients should sit on the toilet while urinating rather than standing.
- Avoid alcohol.
- Carry identification card at all times describing disease, treatment regimen, name, address, and telephone number of treating physician.
- Sit when taking a nitrate drug to avoid injury from dizziness or syncope.
- Headache may frequently accompany use of the drug. Use acetaminophen or aspirin to treat. Notify physician if headache is persistent or severe.

- Do not stop taking the drug abruptly as this may precipitate angina.
- Use OTC medications only with approval by treating physician.
- Avoid abrupt withdrawal as this may precipitate angina.

Adverse reactions
- Common: none.
- Serious: hypotension, methemoglobinemia, anaphylactic reactions.

Clinically important drug interactions
- Drugs that increase effects/toxicity of nitrates: alcohol, antihypertensive drugs, aspirin, β blockers, calcium channel blockers, vasodilators.
- Drugs that decrease effects/toxicity of nitrates: sympathomimetics.

Parameters to monitor
- Symptoms of angina, CHF.
- Frequency and severity of anginal attacks. Monitor for development of tolerance as shown by worsening coronary disease.
- Signs and symptoms of hypotension. BP should be monitored every 5 minutes when the drug is used for an acute angina attack and every 20–30 minutes thereafter. Maximal drug effect is achieved when systolic BP decreases by 15 mm Hg, diastolic BP decreases by 10 mm Hg, or pulse increases by 10 beats/min.
- Signs and symptoms of methemoglobinemia: blood becomes dark colored, mucosa and nails turn bluish, dyspnea, headache, vertigo. This condition requires immediate attention.
- Changes in intraocular pressure. Patient should be monitored periodically if long-term use is required.
- When changing dosage, monitor BP and pulse rate.

Editorial comments
- Nitrates, including nitroglycerin, are the drugs of choice for chronic stable angina. This includes patients with the following preexisting conditions: COPD, asthma, CHF, diabetes.
- This drug is "possibly effective" for the prophylaxis and treatment of angina attacks.

• This drug is not listed in *Physician's Desk Reference*, 54th edition, 2000.
• For additional information see *isosorbide dinitrate*, p. 473.

Nitroglycerin (Transdermal)

Brand names: Nitro-Derm, Transderm-Nitro, Minitran.
Class of drug: Antianginal, vasodilator, transdermal nitrate.
Mechanism of action: Reduces peripheral resistance (arterial and venous) by vasodilation; decreases left ventricular pressure.
Indications/dosage/route: Transdermal only.
• Prophylaxis of angina
  – Adults: One patch on for 12–24 hours; off 10–12 hours (eg, at night). Start with patch delivering 0.2–0.4 mg/h.

Adjustment of dosage
• Kidney disease: None.
• Liver disease: None.
• Elderly: None.
• Pediatric: Safety and efficacy have not been established.

Onset of Action	Peak Effect	Duration
30–60 min	—	8–24 h

Food: No restriction.
Pregnancy: Category B.
Lactation: No data available. Best to avoid.
Contraindications: Hypersensitivity to nitrates or nitrites or to adhesive in patch.
Editorial comments
• This product will not abort an acute attack of angina.
• The patch must be removed before defibrillation as it may explode.

- Advise patient not to stop patch application without consulting treating physician.
- For additional information, see *isosorbide dinitrate*, p. 473.

Nitroglycerin (Topical)

Brand name: Nitrol.
Class of drug: Antianginal, vasodilator, topical nitrate.
Mechanism of action: Reduces peripheral resistance (arterial and venous) by vasodilation; decreases left ventricular pressure.
Indications/dosage/route: Topical.
- Prophylaxis or treatment of anginal attacks
  – Topical ointment (2%): Apply 1–2 inches q8h. Maximum: 4–5 inches q4h.
Adjustment of dosage
- Kidney disease: None.
- Liver disease: None.
- Elderly: Lower doses may be required.
- Pediatric: Safety and efficacy have not been established.

Onset of Action	Duration
30–60 min	2–12 hr

Food: No restrictions.
Pregnancy: Category B.
Lactation: No data available. Best to avoid.
Contraindications: Hypersensitivity to nitrates or nitrites, very low BP, shock, acute MI with low ventricular filling pressure.
Editorial comments
- Determine optimum dose as follows: Begin with 0.5 inch every 8 hours; increase by 0.5 inch until appearance of headache. Reduce dose to that amount that does not cause headache. Rotate sites of application to avoid irritation.

- When drug is terminated, reduce amount applied as well as frequency of application over a period of 4–6 weeks to prevent withdrawal reaction.
- This drug is not listed in the *Physician's Desk Reference*, 54th edition, 2000.
- For additional information, see *isosorbide dinitrate*, p. 473.

Nitroprusside

Brand names: Nipride, Nitropress.
Class of drug: Vasodilator, antihypertensive drug.
Mechanism of action: Direct effect on vascular smooth muscle to produce vasodilation.
Indications/dosage/route: IV.
- Hypertensive emergency
  – Adults, children: Initial: 0.3–0.5 µg/kg/min. Incremental increases based on hemodynamics.
  – Standard dose: 3–10 µg/kg/min. Maximum infusion rate: 10 mg/kg/min, 10 minutes. Patients receiving >4 µg/kg/min are at risk for development of cyanide poisoning. Also seen when total of 500 µg/kg nitroprusside accumulates when rate is >2 µg/kg.

Adjustment of dosage
- Elderly: These patients are more sesitive to the effects of nitroprusside.
- Kidney disease: Use with caution.
- Liver disease: Use with caution.
- Pediatric: No information available.

Onset of Action	Peak Effect	Duration
Immediate	Rapid	1–20 min

Pregnancy: Category C.
Lactation: No data available, best to avoid.

Contraindications: Congenital optic atrophy, tobacco amblyopia, inadequate cerebral circulation, coarctation of the aorta, arteriovenous shunt, hypersensitivity to nitroprusside.

Warnings/precautions

• Use with caution in patients with severe kidney or hepatic disease, hypothyroidism, increased intracranial pressure, low serum vitamin B_{12}, hyponatremia.

• Patients taking other antihypertensive drugs may have increased sensitivity to the effects of nitroprusside.

• Solutions of nitroprusside are highly sensitive to light; if exposed to light a highly colored solution may result. A blue color indicates almost complete degradation of nitroprusside to cyanide and such solutions should not be used.

• Sudden discontinuation of nitroprusside administration may result in hypertensive crises.

Adverse reactions

• Common: headache, dizziness, nausea, abdominal pain, tinnitus, chest pain.

• Serious: increased intracranial pressure, methemoglobinemia, cyanide toxicity, thiocyanate toxicity, psychosis, hypoxia.

Clinically important drug interactions

• Nitroprusside increases effects/toxicity of other antihypertensive drugs, general anesthetics.

• Drugs that increase effects/toxicity of nitroprusside: ganglionic blockers.

Parameters to monitor

• Cardiovascular function continuously including Swan–Ganz catheter.

• BP should be evaluated every 5 minutes at the start of infusion and every 15 minutes thereafter.

• Signs of rebound hypertension after discontinuing nitroprusside.

• Signs and symptoms of thiocyanate toxicity: psychosis, tinnitus, confusion, seizures, coma.

• Acid–base status: metabolic acidosis may be the earliest sign of cyanide toxicity.

• Signs of frank cyanide toxicity: lactic acidosis, tachycardia, seizures, odor of almonds on breath. Give 4–6 mg/kg sodium nitrite over 2–4 minutes, followed by an infusion of sodium thiosulfate 150–200 µg/kg. Repeat in 2 hours at approximately 50% of initial dose.

Editorial comments

• Sodium nitroprusside is a potent vasodilator and cardiac afterload reducer. Its rapid effectiveness and short half-life make it ideal for critical care use in hypertensive emergencies or acute cardiac compromise (ie, aortic insufficiency, mitral regurgitation) requiring rapid afterload reduction to promote forward flow. Simultaneous addition of another vasodilator drug regimen either oral or IV should be considered because of the cumulative toxicity of nitroprusside.

• An antidote to nitroprusside toxicity is sodium thiosulfate, which effectively binds the thiocyanate and cyanide by-products, allowing use in renally impaired patients and those patients requiring longer infusion time.

• Infusion >4 days or doses >4 µg/kg/min: monitor thiocyanate and cyanide levels in the plasma. Serum thiocynate 35–100 µg/mL = toxicity, >200 µg/mL = fatal. Cyanide >2 µg/mL = toxicity, >3 µg/mL = possibly fatal.

• This drug is not listed in the *Physician's Desk Reference*, 54th edition, 2000.

Nizatidine

Brand name: Axid.
Class of drug: H_2 receptor blocker.
Mechanism of action: Competitively blocks H_2 receptors on parietal cells, thereby blocking gastric acid secretion.
Indications/dosage/route: Oral only.

• Active duodenal ulcer
 – Adults: 300 mg once daily h.s. or 150 mg b.i.d.
• Prophylaxis
 – Adults: 150 mg/day h.s.
• Benign gastric ulcer

– Adults: 150 mg b.i.d. or 300 mg h.s.
• Erosive and ulcerative esophagitis
– Adults: 150 mg b.i.d.

Adjustment of dosage

• Kidney disease: creatinine clearance 20–50 mL/min: 150 mg/d. Maintenance: 150 mg every other day; creatinine clearance <20 mL/min: 150 mg every other day. Maintenance: 150 mg every third day.
• Liver disease: None.
• Elderly: Adjust dosage accordingly to creatinine clearance.
• Pediatric: Safety and effectiveness have not been determined.

Onset of Action	Peak Effect	Duration
30 min	0.5–3 h	8–12 h

Food: Take with food.
Pregnancy: Category B.
Lactation: Appears in breast milk. Cimetidine (another H_2 blocker) is considered compatible by American Academy of Pediatrics.
Contraindications: Hypersensitivity to H_2 blockers.

Editorial comments

• Primarily because of renal clearance, dosage adjustments of nizatidine are probably not required in patients with chronic liver diseases, making it the drug of choice in this patient group.
• For additional information see *ranitidine*, p. 810.

Norethindrone

Brand name: Aygestin.
Class of drug: Progestational hormone.
Mechanism of action: Inhibits secretion of pituitary gonadotropins (FSH, LH) by positive feedback.
Indications/dosage/route: Oral only.

• Secondary amenorrhea; abnormal uterine bleeding caused by hormone imbalance with no pathology
  – Adults: 2.5–10 mg starting day 5 of menstrual cycle, ending on 25th day
• Endometriosis
  – Adults: Initial: 5 mg/d for 2 weeks. Increase by 2.5 mg/d q2wk until 15 mg/d is reached.

Adjustment of dosage
• Kidney disease: None.
• Liver disease: Contraindicated.
• Elderly: None.
• Pediatric: Safety and efficacy have not been determined.

Food: No restrictions.

Pregnancy: Category X.

Lactation: Another drug from this class (medroxyprogesterone) is considered compatible by American Academy of Pediatrics.

Contraindications: Hypersensitivity to progestins, history of thrombophlebitis, active thromboembolic disease, cerebral hemorrhage, liver disease, missed abortion, use as diagnostic for pregnancy, known or suspected pregnancy (first 4 months), undiagnosed vaginal bleeding, carcinoma of the breast, known or suspected genital malignancy.

Warnings/precautions
• Use with caution in patients with respiratory infection, history of depression, epilepsy, migraine, cardiac disease, renal disease, diabetes.
• Cigarette smoking significantly increases risk of cardiac complications and thrombotic events. At highest risk are women >35 years of age, smoking ≥15 cigarettes per day.

Advice to patient
• Weigh yourself twice a week and report to treating physician if there are any unusual changes in weight.
• If you observe a yellowing of skin or eyes, report to treating physician.
• If you experience changes in mental status suggestive of depression, report to treating physician.

- Discontinue medication if you experience sudden headaches or attack of migraine.
- Discontinue drug and notify physician if you miss a period or experience unusual bleeding.
- If you miss a dose, take the missed dose as soon as possible; do not double the next dose.
- If the drug is used as contraceptive and you miss a dose, stop taking and use an alternative method of contraception until period returns.
- Use good hygiene—flossing, gum massages, regular cleaning by dentist—to avoid gum problems.
- Keep an extra month supply of the drug on hand.
- Do not give this medication to anyone else.

Adverse reactions
- Common: irregular or unpredictable menstrual bleeding (spotting), amenorrhea, breakthrough bleeding, infertility for up to 18 months.
- Serious: thromboembolic events, depression, cholestatic jaundice.

Clinically important drug interactions: Drugs that decrease effects/toxicity of progestins: aminoglutethimide, phenytoin, rifampin.

Parameters to monitor
- Liver enzymes, cholesterol (total, LDL, HDL), triglycerides.
- Diabetic patient: Monitor blood glucose closely and adjust antidiabetic medication if necessary.
- Signs and symptoms of thromboembolic or thrombotic disorder: pains in leg, sudden chest pain, shortness of breath, migraine, sudden severe headache, vomiting. Discontinue drug.

Editorial comments
- Patient receiving a progesterone for contraceptive purposes should have a complete physical examination performed with special attention to breasts and pelvic organs as well as a Pap test before treatment and annually thereafter. If a patient experiences persistent or abnormal vaginal bleeding while on this drug, perform diagnostic tests, including endometrial sampling, to determine cause.

Norfloxacin

Brand name: Noroxin.

Class of drug: Broad-spectrum quinolone antibiotic.

Mechanism of action: Inhibits DNA gyrase, thereby blocking bacterial DNA replication.

Susceptible organisms *in vivo*: *Citrobacter* sp, *Enterobacter* sp, *Escherichia coli, Klebsiella pneumoniae, Neisseria gonorrhoeae, Proteus mirabilis, Proteus vulgaris, Pseudomonas aeruginosa* (variable), *Serratia marcescens, Staphylococcus aureus* (less than ciprofloxacin), *Staph.* epidermidis, *Staph.* hemolyticus, *Staph.* saprophyticus, *staph.* agalactiae, *Streptococcus faecalis*.

Indications/dosage/route: Oral only.

- Uncomplicated UTIs (*E. coli, K. pneumoniae, P. mirabilis*)
  – Adults: 400 mg q12h, 3 days.
- Uncomplicated UTIs caused by other indicated organisms
  – Adults: 400 mg q12h, 7–10 days.
- Uncomplicated UTIs
  – Adults: 400 mg q12h, 10–21 days.
- Uncomplicated gonorrhea
  – Adults: 800 mg, single dose.
- Prostatis, acute or chronic
  – Adults: 400 mg q12h, 28 days.

Adjustment of dosage

- Kidney disease: Creatinine clearance <30 mL/min: 400 mg q day, 4–7 days.
- Liver disease: None.
- Elderly: None.
- Pediatric: Safety and efficacy have not been established in children <18 years.

Food: Take 1 hour before or 2 hours after meals with a glass of water.

Pregnancy: Category C.

Lactation: Likely to appear in breast milk. Potentially toxic to infant. Avoid breastfeeding.

Contraindications: Hypersensitivity to fluoroquinolone or quinolone antibiotics.

Warnings/precautions

- Use with caution in patients with CNS disorders (epilepsy), kidney disease.
- Therapy should be continued for 2–4 days after symptoms have disappeared.
- Achilles and other tendon rupture have occurred in patients taking fluoroquinolones.
- Serious and fatal hypersensitivity reactions have occurred with these drugs, even after the first dose.
- Reserve use of this drug for infections that are difficult to treat by other means.

Advice to patient

- Limit intake of caffeinated products including coffee and colas.
- Drink a great deal of fluids during therapy with this drug.
- Do not undertake strenuous exercise while taking this drug.
- To minimize possible photosensitivity reaction, apply adequate sunscreen and use proper covering when exposed to strong sunlight.

Adverse reactions

- Common: None.
- Serious: hypersensitivity reaction (anaphylaxis), seizures, pseudomembranous colitis, cholestatic jaundice, renal failure, pulmonary edema, pulmonary embolism, cardiovascular collapse, pharyngeal edema.

Clinically important drug interactions

- Drugs that increase effects/toxicity of fluoroquinolones: cyclosporine, probenecid.
- Drugs that decrease effects/toxicity of fluoroquinolones: antacids, antineoplastic agents, didanosine, sucralfate, iron salts, zinc salts, caffeine.
- Fluoroquinolones increase effects/toxicity of oral anticoagulants, theophylline, caffeine.

Parameters to monitor

• Renal, hepatic, and hemopoietic systems should be monitored periodically during prolonged therapy.

• Intake of fluids and urinary and other fluid output to minimize renal toxicity. Increase fluid intake if inadequate. Closely monitor electrolyte levels.

• Signs of hypersensitivity reactions.

• Signs and symptoms of antibiotic-induced bacterial or fungal superinfection: Use of yogurt (4 oz/d) may be helpful in prevention of superinfection.

• Signs and symptoms of tendon pain. These may be an indication of tendon rupture.

• Monitor patients for evidence of development of microbial resistance with loss of effectiveness.

Editorial comments

• Use of norfloxacin is limited to treatment of UTI, prostatitis, and uncomplicated gonorrhea.

• This drug is recommended as an alternative to aminoglycosides when clinically relevant.

Nortriptyline

Brand name: Pamelor.

Class of drug: Tricyclic antidepressant.

Mechanism of action: Inhibits reuptake of CNS neurotransmitters, primarily serotonin and norepinephrine.

Indications/dosage/route: Oral only.

• Depression

– Adults: 25 mg t.i.d. to q.i.d. Increase as needed. Doses above 150 mg/d are not recommended.

– Elderly, adolescents: 30–50 mg/d as single or divided doses.

Adjustment of dosage

• Kidney disease: None.

• Liver disease: Lower dose; titrate slowly.

• Elderly: See above.
• Pediatric: Not recommended for children <12 years.
Food: No restrictions.
Pregnancy: Category D.
Lactation: Appears in breast milk. American Academy of Pediatrics expresses concern over use when breastfeeding.
Contraindications: Hypersensitivity to tricyclic antidepressants, acute recovery from MI, concurrent MAO inhibitor.
Editorial comments
• Therapeutic level: 50–150 mg/mL; toxic level: >500 mg/mL.
• This drug is listed without details in the *Physician's Desk Reference*, 54th edition, 2000.
• For additional information, see *amitriptyline*, p. 39.

Nystatin

Brand names: Mycostatin, Mytrex, Nilstat, Nystex.
Class of drug: Antifungal.
Mechanism of action: Disrupts fungal cell membrane, causing leakage of cellular components.
Indications/dosage/route: Oral, vaginal tablet, topical.
• GI Infections
  – Oral tablets: Adults: 500,000–1,000,000 units t.i.d.
• Vaginal and intestinal infections caused by susceptible organisms
  – Oral suspension: Adults: 500,000–1,00,000 units t.i.d.
  – Oral suspension: Children, infants >3 months: 250,000–500,000 units q.i.d.
  – Oral suspension: Newborn, premature infants: 100,000 units q.i.d.
• Cutaneous candidal infections
  – Topical: Apply to affected area 2–3 times/d.
  – Vaginal tablet: 100,000 units b.i.d., 14 days.
  – PO: Adults, children: 400,000–600,000 units q.i.d.

– PO: Infants: 200,000 units q.i.d.
– PO: Infants, premature low-birth-weight infants: 100,000 units q.i.d.

Adjustment of dosage: None.

Food: Not affected by food.

Pregnancy: Category B.

Lactation: Poorly absorbed, not likely to appear in breast milk. May breastfeed.

Contraindications: Hypersensitivity to nystatin. Some nystatin products contain ethyl alcohol or benzyl alcohol. Such preparations should be avoided in patients who may have hypersensitivity to these additives.

Advice to patient

• Notify treating physician if you experience vaginal irritation, redness, or swelling.
• Use a barrier method of contraception when taking this drug.
• Keep vaginal inserts in the refrigerator and protected from extreme temperatures, moisture, and light.
• Let troches dissolve in mouth; do not chew or swallow.
• When troche form is used in children or the elderly, ensure that entire dose is dissolved with each use.

Adverse reactions

• Common: none.
• Serious: urticaria, Stevens–Johnson syndrome.

Clinical important drug interactions: None.

Parameters to monitor: Mucous membranes (oral, esophageal) frequently throughout therapy. It may be necessary to discontinue nystatin if there is increased irritation of membranes.

Ofloxacin

Brand name: Floxin.
Class of drug: Broad-spectrum quinolone antibiotic.
Mechanism of action: Inhibits DNA gyrase, thereby blocking bacterial DNA replication.
Susceptible organisms *in vivo*: *Citrobacter* sp, *Enterobacter* sp, *Escherichia coli, Hemophilus ducreyi, Hemophilus influenzae, Klebsiella pneumoniae, Neisseria gonorrhoeae, Proteus mirabilis, Pseudomonas aeruginosa, Staphylococcus aureus.* Limited activity against *Streptococcus pneumoniae* and *Streptococcus pyogenes.*
Indications/dosage/route: Oral, IV (same doses by both routes), topical (ophthalmic).
- Acute bacterial exacerbation of chronic bronchitis, community-acquired pneumonia, uncomplicated skin and skin structure infections
  – Adults: 400 mg q12h, 10 days.
- Acute uncomplicated urethral and cervical gonorrhea
  – Adults: 400 mg, single dose, 1 day.
- Nongonococcal cervicitis/urethritis, mixed infection of urethra and cervix
  – Adults: 300 mg q12h, 7 days.
- Acute pelvic inflammatory disease, uncomplicated cystitis (*E. coli, K. pneumoniae*, other approved pathogens), complicated UTIs
  – 200 mg q12h, 3–10 days.
- Prostatitis (*E. coli*)
  – 300 mg q12h, 6 weeks.
- Conjunctivitis
  – Ophthalmic solution (0.3%): Initial: 1–2 drops in affected eye(s) q2–4h, first 2 days. Then 1–2 drops q.i.d. for 5 additional days.

Adjustment of dosage
- Kidney disease: Creatinine clearance 10–50 mL/min: dosage interval: 24 hours; creatinine clearance <10 mL/min: one-half dosage q24h.

- Liver disease: None.
- Elderly: None.
- Pediatric: Safety and efficacy have not been established in children <18 years.

Food: Take 1 hour before or 2 hours after meals with a glass of water.

Pregnancy: Category C.

Lactation: Appears in breast milk. Potentially toxic to infant. Avoid breastfeeding.

Contraindications: Hypersensitivity to fluoroquinolone antibiotics or quinolone antibiotics, eg, cinoxacin, nalidixic acid.

Editorial comments

- Ofloxacin offers no advantages over ciprofloxacin, but is less active against *Pseudomonas aeruginosa*.
- Levofloxacin (an L-isomer of ofloxacin) is much more effective against gram-positive organisms.
- For additional information, see *norfloxacin*, p. 675.

Omeprazole

Brand name: Prilosec.

Class of drug: Gastric proton pump inhibitor.

Mechanism of action: Irreversibly blocks H^+K^+-ATPase. This enzyme promotes transport of hydrogen ions across the parietel cell membrane into the gastric lumen.

Indications/dosage/route: Oral only.

- GERD
  - Adults: 20 mg q.d. or b.i.d. (4–8 weeks). Doses to 80 mg/d used. Maintenance: same (long term) as for peptic ulcer disease.
- Peptic ulcer disease
  - Adults: 20 mg q.d. or b.i.d. (6–12 weeks), may be combined with antibiotics for *Helicobacter pylori* toxicity.
- Hypersecretory conditions
  - Adults: up to 120 mg t.i.d.

- Prophylaxis for NSAID-induced GI injury
  - Adults: 20 mg q.d. or b.i.d. (unapproved use). May be administered via nasogastric tubes in acid medium, eg, in orange juice.
- Combination therapy for *H. pylori* (various antibiotics)
  - Adults: 20 mg b.i.d., 7–14 days. Maintenance: 20 mg/d for 14 days more.

Onset of Action	Peak Effect	Duration
1 h	2 h	50% maximum effect remains at 24 h

Food: Should be taken 30 minutes before meal. Some theoretical advantage with consumption 60 minutes after morning meal in patients with GERD.

Pregnancy: Category C. *Note:* Avoid combined omeprazole–clarithromycin.

Lactation: Probably appears in breast milk. Potentially toxic to infant. Avoid breastfeeding.

Contraindications: Prior hypersensitivity reaction to omeprazole, maintenance therapy for duodenal ulcer.

Warnings/precautions: Relief of symptoms by omeprazole does not preclude a gastric malignancy.

Advice to patient

- Avoid alcohol because it predisposes to ulcer formation.
- Avoid NSAIDs because they predispose to ulcer formation.
- Avoid caffeine as it may promote GERD.

Adverse reactions

- Common: headache.
- Serious: bone marrow depression, jaundice, elevated liver enzymes.

Clinically important drug interactions

- Omeprazole increases effects/toxicity of warfarin, phenytoin, benzodiazepines, cyclosporine, carbamazepine, digoxin.
- Omeprazole decreases effects/toxicity of ketoconazole, itraconazole, iron.

Parameters to monitor: Efficacy of treatment: relief of symptoms of GERD and peptic ulcer.

Editorial comments

- Long-term use in individuals infected with *H. pylori* may possibly predispose to the development of gastric intestinal metaplasia and vitamin B_{12} malabsorption. Otherwise, long-term use of proton pump inhibitors appears to be safe.
- Be aware of potential interactions of this drug due to inhibition of cytochrome P450.
- Omeprazole may prolong elimination of diazepam, warfarin, phenytoin, and cyclosporine.
- Previous concerns regarding the development of enterochromaffin cell-like tumors in rats are clinically irrelevant.
- Approved treatment protocols for *H. pylori* infection include combination of omeprazole with clarithromycin and other agents. This combination should be avoided in pregnant women (clarithromycin is category D).

Ondansetron

Brand name: Zofran.

Class of drug: Serotonin receptor antagonist, antiemetic.

Mechanism of action: Selective serotonin 5-HT_3 receptor antagonist at the chemoreceptor trigger zone and peripheral vagal nerve terminals.

Indications/dosage/route: Oral, IV.

- Antiemetic for cancer chemotherapy and postoperative nausea and vomiting
  - Adults, children 4–18 years: IV 0.15 mg/kg infused over 15 minutes. Start 30 minutes before chemotherapy and 4–8 hours after first dose. Alternative: 32-mg dose.
  - Adults, children >12: PO 8 mg b.i.d. Start 30 minutes before chemotherapy, and administer next dose 8 hours later. Then 8 mg q12h 1–2 days after chemotherapy.

– Children 4–12: PO 4 mg t.i.d. Dosing regimen same as for adults.
- Prevention of postoperative nausea and vomiting
  – Adults: PO 15 mg 1 hour before anesthesia.

Adjustment of dosage
- Kidney disease: None.
- Liver disease: Severe hepatic impairment: single IV dose of 8 mg recommended.
- Elderly: None.
- Pediatric: There is limited information for use in children <3 years.

Onset of Action	Peak Effect	Duration
Rapid	15–30 min	4 h

Food: Take without regard to meals.
Pregnancy: Category B.
Lactation: Appears in breast milk. Best to avoid.
Contraindications: Hypersensitivity to ondansetron.

Warnings/precautions
- Use with caution in patients with liver disease.
- Use only in the first 24–48 hours following chemotherapy.
- Do not use in delayed nausea and vomiting.
- Use on a regular schedule, not on prn basis.

Advice to patients: Avoid alcohol and other CNS depressant drugs.

Adverse reactions
- Common: headache, diarrhea, fatigue, dizziness, constipation, musculoskeletal pain.
- Serious: hypersensitivity reactions, arrhythmias, liver toxicity, prolonged QT interval, extrapyramidal syndrome, seizures.

Clinically important drug interactions
- Drugs that increase effects/toxicity of ondansetron: cimetidine, allopurinol, disulfiram.
- Drugs that decrease effects/toxicity of ondansetron: barbiturates, carbamazepine, rifampin, phenytoin.

Parameters to monitor

- Signs and symptoms of drug-induced extrapyramidal syndrome (pseudoparkinsonism): akinesia, tremors resting, pill rolling), shuffling gait, masklike facies, drooling. If these occur while taking this medication drug discontinuation may be required. Alternatively, administration of diphenhydramine and benztropine may be indicated.
- Monitor potassium serum level for possible hypokalemia.

Editorial comments

- Ondansetron is useful as an alternative to metoclopramide in patients likely to develop extrapyramidal reactions from metoclopramide. It has proven very useful in patients receiving highly emetogenic chemotherapy.
- When ondansetron is used for the prophylaxis or treatment of post-operative nausea and vomiting, the drug is generally administered by an anesthesiologist.
- Efficacy of ondansetron for patients receiving chemotherapeutic agents with low emetogenic potential (bleomycin, busulfan, low-dose cyclophosphamide, 5-fluorouracil, vinblastine, vincristine) has not been established.
- Evaluate patient for etiology of emesis and be aware that this drug may mask signs of overdose with other drugs or underlying pathology.

Orlistat

Brand name: Xenical.
Class of drug: Anti-obesity agent.
Mechanism of action: Reduces absorption of fat from GI tract by inhibiting pancreatic lipase.
Indications/dosage/route: Oral only.

- Obesity in patients with body mass index ≥ 30 kg/m^2 in association with hypertension, diabetes, dyslipidemias

– 120 mg t.i.d.

Adjustment of dosage: No data available.

Food: Should be taken with meals.

Pregnancy: No data.

Lactation: No data.

Contraindications: Chronic malabsorption syndrome, cholestasis.

Warnings/precautions: None.

Advice to patient: Take fat-soluble vitamin supplements (vitamins A, D, E, and K) at least 2 hours before or after taking orlistat.

Adverse reactions
• Common: flatulence, fecal urgency.

Serious: none.

Clinically important drug interactions: Orlistat reduces absorption of fat-soluble vitamins.

Parameters to monitor: Weight of patient to determine whether drug is losing effectiveness.

Editorial comments
• The benign side effect profile of this drug makes it a safe antiobesity agent.
• At present, it is not known what effect long-term chronic steatorrhea has on neoplastic potential or in patients with inflammatory bowel disease. There are no data concerning the safety or efficacy of combining this drug with other anti-obesity drugs such as phentermine.

Oxacillin

Brand names: Bactocill, Prostaphlin.

Class of drug: Antibiotic, penicillin family.

Mechanism of action: Inhibits bacterial cell wall synthesis.

Susceptible organisms *in vivo*: MSSA, streptococci.

Indications/dosage/route: IV, IM.
• Mild to moderate infections of upper respiratory tract, skin, soft tissue

- Adults, children >20 kg: PO 500 mg q4–6h at least 5 days.
- Children <20 kg: PO 50 mg/kg/d in equally divided doses q6h.
• Mild to moderate infections
  - Adults, children >40 kg: IM, IV 250–500 mg q4–6h.
  - Children <40 kg: IM, IV 50 mg/kg/d in equally divided doses q6h.
• Severe infections of lower respiratory tract or disseminated infections
  - Adults, children >40 kg: IM, IV 1 g q4–6h.
  - Children <40 kg: IM, IV 100 mg/kg/d in equally divided doses q4–6h.
  - Neonates, premature infants <2000 g: IM, IV 50 mg/kg/d divided q12h if <7 days of age.
  - Neonates, premature infants >2000 g: IM, IV 75 mg/kg/d divided q8h if <7 days of age.
  - Maximum daily dose: Adults: 12 g; children: 100–300 mg/kg.

Adjustment of dosage: None.
Food: Take on empty stomach 1 hour before or 2 hours after eating.
Pregnancy: Category B.
Lactation: Appears in breast milk. Use with caution.
Contraindications: Hypersensitivity to penicillin or cephalosporins.
Editorial comments
• This drug is not listed in the *Physicians' Desk Reference*, 54th edition, 2000.
• For additional information, see *dicloxacillin*, p. 279.

Oxaprozin

Brand name: Daypro.
Class of drug: NSAID.
Mechanism of action: Inhibits cyclooxygenase, resulting in inhibition of synthesis of prostaglandins and other inflammatory mediators.
Indications/dosage/route: Oral only.

• Rheumatoid arthritis, osteoarthritis
  – 1200 mg once a day. Maximum: 1800 mg/d in divided doses.

Adjustment of dosage
• Kidney disease: None.
• Liver disease: None.
• Elderly: May be necessary to reduce dose for patients >65 years.
• Pediatric: Safety and efficacy have not been established.

Food: Take with food or large quantities of water or milk.

Pregnancy: Category C. Category D in third trimester or near delivery.

Lactation: No data available. Best to avoid.

Contraindications: Hypersensitivity to oxaprozin and cross-sensitivity with other NSAIDs and aspirin.

Editorial comments: For additional information, see *ibuprofen*, p. 445.

Oxazepam

Brand name: Serax.

Class of drug: Antianxiety agent, hypnotic.

Mechanism of action: Potentiates effects of GABA in limbic system and reticular formation.

Indications/dosage/route: Oral only.
• Anxiety disorders, mild to moderate
  – Adults: 10–15 mg t.i.d. to q.i.d.
• Anxiety disorders, severe
  – Adults: 15–30 mg t.i.d. to q.i.d.
  – Elderly and debilitated patients: Initial: 10 mg t.i.d. Increase to 15 mg t.i.d. to q.i.d. as needed.
• Alcohol withdrawal
  – Adults: 15–30 mg t.i.d. to q.i.d.

Adjustment of dosage
• Kidney disease: Use caution.

- Liver disease: Use caution.
- Elderly: See above.
- Pediatric: Safety and efficacy have not been established in children <6 years. Pediatric doses in other age groups have not been established.

Food: No restrictions.

Pregnancy: Category D.

Lactation: Appears in breast milk. Potentially toxic to infant. American Academy of Pediatrics expresses concern about breast-feeding while taking benzodiazepines. Avoid breastfeeding.

Contraindications: Hypersensitivity to benzodiazepines, pregnancy.

Editorial comments

- This drug is listed without details in the *Physician's Desk Reference*, 54th edition, 2000.
- For additional information, see *diazepam*, p. 273.

Oxybutinin

Brand name: Ditropan.

Class of drug: Anticholinergic.

Mechanism of action: Blocks acetylcholine effects at muscarinic receptors throughout the body.

Indications/dosage/route: Oral only.

- Neurogenic bladder (relief of symptoms)
  - Adults: Initial: 5 mg once per day. Increase to maximum of 30 mg/d as needed.

Adjustment of dosage:

- Kidney disease: None.
- Liver disease: None.
- Elderly: None.
- Pediatric: Safety and efficacy have not been established.

Pregnancy: Category C.

Lactation: No data available. Potentially toxic to infant. Avoid breastfeeding.

Contraindications: Myasthenia gravis, narrow-angle glaucoma, GI obstruction, megacolon, active ulcerative colitis, obstructive uropathy, hypersensitivity to atropine-type compounds (belladonna alkaloids).

Editorial comments: For additional information, see *atropine*, p. 67.

Oxycodone

Brand names: Roxicodone, Oxycentin.

Class of drug: Narcotic analgesic, agonist.

Mechanism of action: Binds to opiate receptors and blocks ascending pain pathways. Reduces patient's perception of pain without altering cause of the pain.

Indications/dosage/route: Oral only.

• Analgesia
  – Adults, opioid naive: 10-30 mg q4h.
  – Adults, opioid naive, extended-release tablets: 10 mg q12h.
  – For patients using regular opioid doses, start at 10–20 mg q12h. Those receiving larger doses may require up to 40 mg q12h.
• Breakthrough pain
  – Adults: 5–60 mg, immediate-release oxycodone.
• Analgesia, severe
  – Adults: 30 mg q4h or additional as needed.

Adjustment of dosage

• Kidney disease: None.
• Liver disease: None.
• Elderly: Use with caution.
• Pediatric: Should not be used in children.

Onset of Action	Peak Effect	Duration
15–30 min	1 h	4–6 h

Food: May be taken with food to lessen GI upset.

Pregnancy: Category B. Category D if prolonged use or if given in high doses at term.

Lactation: Appears in breast milk. Potentially toxic to infant. Avoid breastfeeding.

Contraindications: Hypersensitivity to oxycodone or other narcotics of the same chemical class, respiratory depression, severe bronchial asthma, paralytic ileus.

Warnings/precautions

- Use with caution in patients with: head injury with increased intracranial pressure, serious alcoholism, prostatic hypertrophy, chronic pulmonary disease, severe liver or kidney disease, disorders of biliary tract, supraventricular tachycardia, history of convulsion disorder, postoperative patients with pulmonary disease.
- Administer drug before patient experiences severe pain for fullest efficacy of the drug.
- Have the following available when treating patient with this drug: naloxone (Narcan) or other antagonist, means of administering oxygen, and support of respiration.
- Nausea, vomiting, and orthostatic hypotension occur most prominently in ambulatory patients. If nausea and vomiting persist, it may be necessary to administer an antiemetic, eg, droperidol or prochlorperazine.
- This drug can cause severe hypotension in a patient who is volume depleted or if given along with a phenothiazine or general anesthesia.
- Careful diagnosis must be made of acute abdominal condition before this drug is administered.

Editorial comments

- Oxycodone is metabolized by cytochrome P450 CYP2D6. Inhibitors of CYP2D6 including some cardiac drugs and antidepressants; these may raise levels of this drug.
- Patient should not break, chew, or crush sustained-release tablets. These must be swallowed whole.
- For additional information, see *morphine*, p. 633.

Oxymorphone

Brand name: Numorphan.
Class of drug: Narcotic analgesic, agonist.
Mechanism of action: Binds to opiate receptors and blocks ascending pain pathways. Reduces patient's perception of pain without altering cause of the pain.
Indications/dosage/route: IV, IM, SC, suppository.
• Analgesia
  – Adults, Initial: IM, SC 1–1.5 mg q4–6h.
  – Adults: Suppository: 5 mg q4–6h.
• Analgesia during labor
  – Adults: IM 0.5–1.0 mg.
Adjustment of dosage
• Kidney disease: None.
• Liver disease: Use lower doses.
• Elderly: Use with caution. Lower doses or longer intervals may be necessary.
• Pediatric: Safety and efficacy have not been established in children <18 years.

Onset of Action	Peak Effect	Duration
5–10 min	0.5–1 h	No data

Food: May be taken with food to lessen GI upset.
Pregnancy: Category B. Category D if prolonged use or if given in high doses at term.
Lactation: Appears in breast milk. Potentially toxic to infant. Avoid breastfeeding.
Contraindications: Hypersensitivity to narcotics of the same chemical class, paralytic ileus, acute asthmatic attack, severe respiratory depression, upper urinary tract obstruction, pulmonary edema secondary to chemical respiratory irritant.

Warnings/precautions

- Use with caution in patients with head injury with increased intracranial pressure, serious alcoholism, prostatic hypertrophy, chronic pulmonary disease, severe liver or kidney disease, disorders of biliary tract, and in postoperative patients with pulmonary disease.
- Administer drug before patient experiences severe pain for fullest efficacy of the drug.
- Have the following available when treating patient with this drug: naloxone (Narcan) or other antagonist, means of administering oxygen, and support of respiration.
- Nausea, vomiting, and orthostatic hypotension occur most prominently in ambulatory patients. If nausea and vomiting persist, it may be necessary to administer an antiemetic, eg, droperidol or prochlorperazine.
- This drug can cause severe hypotension in a patient who is volume depleted or if given along with a phenothiazine or general anesthesia.
- Careful diagnosis must be made of acute abdominal condition before this drug is administered.

Editorial comments: For additional information, see *morphine*, p. 633.

Oxytocin

Brand names: Pitocin, Syntocinon.
Class of drug: Oxytocic, lactation stimulant.
Mechanism of action: Oxytocic action: stimulates contractions of uterine smooth muscle. Lactation stimulation: contracts epithelial cells around breast alveoli.
Indications/dosage/route: IV, IM.

- Induction of labor
  - Adults: IV infusion; 1–2 milliunits/min. Increase by 1–2 milliunits q15–30min until contraction pattern is occurring. Maximum: 20 milliunits/min.

- Reduction of postpartum bleeding
  - Adults: IV 10–40 milliunits/L. Infuse at rate to control uterine action.
  - Alternate: IM 10 units.
- Abortion.
  - Adults: IV 10 units.
- Promote lactation
  - Adults: 1 spray or 1 drop of nasal solution 2–3 minutes before breastfeeding.

Adjustment of dosage
- Kidney disease: None.
- Liver disease: None.
- Elderly: Not applicable.
- Pediatric: Not applicable.

	Onset of Action	Peak Effect	Duration
IV	Immediate	40 min	20 min after stopping infusion
IM	3–5 min	40 min	2–3 h

Food: Not applicable.
Pregnancy: Category X (contraindicated).
Lactation: Used in postpartum period. Promotes lactation.
Contraindications: Hypersensitivity to oxytocin, fetal distress, severe toxemia, total placenta previa, anticipated nonvaginal delivery (invasive cervical cancer), prolapse, active herpes genitalis, unfavorable fetal position, hyperactive uterus, contraindicated vaginal delivery, women with four or more previous deliveries.
Warnings/precautions
- Use systemic form with caution in patients in the first and second stages of labor and patients with history of cervical or uterine surgery, overdistended uterus, cervical cancer, nausea, vomiting, PVCs, other arrhythmias, pelvic hematoma.
- May potentially cause uterine rupture.

• Prolonged infusion (>24 hours) may cause water intoxication associated with seizures, coma, and death.

Adverse reactions

• Common: none.
• Serious: Maternal: seizures, coma, arrhythmias, hypotension, anaphylactic reactions, postpartum hemorrhage, fatal afibrinogenemia, pelvic hematoma, death. Fetal: arrhythmias, intracranial hemorrhage, hypoxia, death.

Clinically important drug interactions: Drugs that increase effects/toxicity of oxytocin: sympathomimetics, vasoconstrictors, cyclopropane, thiopental.

Parameters to monitor

• Fetal maturity, presentation, adequacy of pelvis before administration of oxytocin for labor induction.
• Frequency, character, duration of uterine contractions, fetal heart rate.
• Signs and symptoms of fetal anoxia.
• Fetal cardiovascular status throughout.
• Signs of water intoxication: drowsiness, confusion, headache, anuria.
• Maternal electrolytes.

Editorial comments

• Oxytocin is not indicated for elective induction of labor.
• Physicians prescribing oxytocin should be aware of all important toxic effects of this agent.
• This drug is not listed in the *Physician's Desk Reference*, 54th edition, 2000.

Paclitaxel

Brand name: Taxol.

Class of drug: Antineoplastic.

Mechanism of action: Inhibits normal reorganization of micro-tubules required for mitosis, thus inhibiting tumor cell division.

Indications/dosage/route: IV only.

• Ovarian cancer, metastatic breast cancer, after failure of combination therapy or rapid relapse, AIDS-associated Kaposi's sarcoma.

  – Adults: IV 135 mg/m^2 or IV 175 mg/m^2 over 3 hours q3wk. Maximum: 250 mg/m^2.

Note: This course of treatment should not be repeated unless the neutrophil count is at least 1500 mm^3 or platelet count is 100,000/mm^3.

Adjustment of dosage

• Kidney disease: None.

• Liver disease: Increased toxicity; use extreme caution. May need to decrease dose.

• Elderly: Use with caution.

• Pediatric: Safety and effectiveness have not been established.

Onset of Action	Peak Effect	Duration
No data	11 days	3 wk

Food: Not applicable.

Pregnancy: Category D.

Lactation: Probably appears in breast milk. Potentially toxic to infant. Avoid breastfeeding.

Contraindications: Contraindicated in patients with hypersensitivity to paclitaxel or polyoxyethylated castor oil (excipient), neutrophil count <1500 mm^3, pregnancy.

Warnings/precautions

• Use with caution in patients with radiation therapy, decreased bone marrow reserve, chronic debilitating illness, active infections, liver disease.

- Paclitaxel has been associated with severe allergic reactions requiring discontinuation in 2% of patients in clinical studies. Pretreatment of patients with corticosteroids and H_1 and H_2 blockers is advised.

Advice to patient: Use two forms of birth control including hormonal and barrier methods.

Adverse reactions

- Common: nausea, vomiting, diarrhea, alopecia, myalgia, phlebitis, erythema at site of injection.
- Serious: **bone marrow depression, hypersensitivity reactions, hypotension, ECG abnormalities, peripheral neuropathy, infections**, anaphylaxis, bradycardia, hypertension, skin exfoliation and necrosis at injection site, severe cardiovascular events, paralytic ileus.

Clinically important drug interactions

- Cisplatin increases the effects/toxicity of paclitaxel.
- Inhibitors of cytochrome P450 subgroups C4P2C8 and C4P3A4 could increase toxicity: these include ketoconazole, verapamil, diazepam, quinidine, dexamethasone, cyclosporine, etoposide, vincristine, protease inhibitors.
- Paclitaxel increases drug level of doxorubicin.

Parameters to monitor

- Monitor vital signs frequently, particularly during the 24 hours of infusion.
- Hypersensitivity reactions during infusion. It is recommended that all patients should receive one of the following prior to administration of paclitaxel: diphenhydramine, an H_2 blocker, dexamethasone. Infusion should be stopped if patient manifests dyspnea, chest pain, hypotension. Institute measures to counteract anaphylactic reaction.
- Signs of infection.
- Signs of platelet reduction.
- Signs and symptoms of anemia.
- Intake of fluids and urinary and other fluid output to minimize

renal toxicity. Increase fluid intake if inadequate. Closely monitor electrolyte levels.

• Signs and symptoms of neuropathy: burning, tingling, numbness in hands or feet, loss of peripheral sensation, motor weakness, discoordination, ataxia, diminished deep tendon reflexes, foot or wrist drop; paralytic ileus. If medication-induced neuropathy is suspected, discontinue treatment immediately.

• Pain suggesting arthralgia or myalgia. Administer NSAID or opioid if pain is severe.

Editorial comments: This is a major addition to the oncology drug armamentarium. Paclitaxel is active in breast cancer, ovarian cancer, non-small cell lung cancer, and head and neck cancers. In combination with cisplatin or carboplatin, it is the drug of choice for ovarian cancer. It is also approved for adjuvant chemotherapy for lymph node-positive breast cancer. The cumulative toxicity of peripheral neuropathy is common and dose limiting.

Pancuronium

Brand name: Pavulon.
Class of drug: Nondepolarizing neuromuscular blocker.
Mechanism of action: Blocks nicotinic acetylcholine receptors at neuromuscular junction, resulting in skeletal muscle relaxation and paralysis.
Indications/dosage/route: IV only.
• Muscle relaxation during anesthesia
 – Adults, children >1 month of age: Initial: 0.04-0.1 mg/kg. Additional doses of 0.01 mg/kg administered as required
 – Neonates: Administer a test dose of 0.02 mg/kg.
• Tracheal intubation
 – Adults: 0.06–0.1 mg/kg.
Adjustment of dosage: None.

Onset of Action	Peak Effect	Duration
<45 s	3–4.5 min	35–45 min

Food: Not applicable.
Pregnancy: Category C.
Lactation: No data available. Best to avoid.
Contraindications: Hypersensitivity to pancuronium and chemically related drugs.
Editorial comments
• This drug is listed without details in the *Physician's Desk Reference*, 54th edition, 2000.
• For additional information, see *rocuronium*, p. 824.

Para-Aminosalicylic Acid (PAS)

Brand name: PAS Sodium.
Class of drug: Antitubercular drug.
Indications/dosage/route: Oral only.
   – Adults: 14–16 g/d, 2–3 divided doses.
   – Children: 275–420 mg/kg/d, 3–4 divided doses.
Editorial comments
• This drug is seldom used.
• The following drugs are alternatives to PAS for treatment of tuberculosis: ethambutol, isoniazide, pyrazinamide, rifampin, rifabutin, streptomycin.
• This drug is not listed in the *Physician's Desk Reference*, 54th edition, 2000.

Paromomycin

Brand name: Humatin.
Class of drug: Antibacterial aminoglycoside.
Indications/dosage/route: Oral only.
• Amebiasis
   – Adults: 25–35 mg/kg/d in 3 divided doses.
• Hepatic coma

– 4 g/d in divided doses.
• Adjustment of dose: No data available.

Editorial comments
• Alternative drugs for amebiasis include amikacin, gentamicin, kanamycin, neomycin, streptomycin, tobramycin.
• Several studies have suggested efficacy of paromomycin in the treatment of cryptosporidiosis in patients with AIDS.
• This drug is not listed in the *Physicians' Desk Reference*, 54th edition, 2000.

Paroxetine

Brand name: Paxil.
Class of drug: SSRI.
Mechanism of action: Inhibits reuptake of serotonin into CNS neurons.
Indications/dosage/route: Oral only.
• Depression, obsessive–compulsive disorder
  – Adults: 20 mg/d. Increase as needed to maximum 50 mg/d.
• Panic disorders
  – Adults: Initial: 10 mg/d given in the morning. Maintenance: 40 mg/d. Maximum: 60 mg/d.

Adjustment of dosage
• Kidney disease: Initial: 10 mg/d. Maximum: 40 mg/d.
• Liver disease: Initial: 10 mg/d. Maximum: 40 mg/d.
• Elderly: Initial: 10 mg/d. Maximum: 40 mg/d.
• Pediatric: Contraindicated in children <6 years.

Food: May be taken with meals.
Pregnancy: Category B.
Lactation: Appears in breast milk. Best to avoid. American Academy of Pediatrics expresses concern with use during breast-feeding.
Contraindications: MAO inhibitor taken within 14 days, hypersensitivity to paroxetine.

Warnings/precautions
- Use with caution in patients with diabetes mellitus, seizures, liver, kidney disease.
- Advise patient that effectiveness of the drug may not be apparent until 4 weeks of treatment.
- A withdrawal syndrome has been described after abrupt withdrawal of this drug. Symptoms include blurred vision, diaphoresis, agitation, and hypomania.
- Mania or hypomania may be unmasked by SSRIs.

Advice to patient
- Avoid driving and other activities requiring mental alertness or that are potentially dangerous until response to drug is known.
- Avoid alcohol and other CNS depressants such as opiate analgesics and sedatives (eg, diazepam) when taking this drug.
- Take this drug in the morning as it may cause insomnia.

Adverse reactions
- Common: drowsiness, nausea, diarrhea, constipation, dry mouth, male sexual dysfunction, tremor.
- Serious: hypertension, tachycardia, arrhythmias, hypoglycemia, hyponatremia, suicidal tendency, extrapyramidal reactions, psychosis.

Clinically important drug interactions
- Drugs that increase effects/toxicity of paroxetine: MAO inhibitors (combination contraindicated), clarithromycin, tryptophan.
- Paroxetine increase effects/toxicity of tricyclic antidepressants, diazepam, dextromethorphan, encainide, haloperidol, perphenazine, propafenone, thioridizine, trazadone, warfarin, carbamazepine, lithium.
- Drug that decreases effects/toxicity of paroxetine: buspirone.

Parameters to monitor
- Progressive weight loss. Recommend dietary management to maintain weight. This may be particularly important in underweight patients.
- Signs of hypersensitivity reactions.
- Signs and symptoms of hypoglycemia.

Editorial comments

- SSRIs are recommended for patients who are at risk for medication overdose because they are safer than tricyclic antidepressants.
- SSRIs may be a better choice than tricyclic antidepressants for the following patients: those who cannot tolerate the anticholinergic effects or excessive daytime sedation of tricyclic antidepressants and those who experience psychomotor retardation or weight gain. These drugs are generally well tolerated.
- If coadministered with a tricyclic antidepressant, dosage of the latter may need to be reduced and blood levels monitored.
- Do not administer for at least 14 days after discontinuing a MAO inhibitor. Do not initiate MAO inhibitor until at least 5 weeks after discontinuing this agent.
- SSRIs have generally replaced other antidepressants (tricyclics, MAO inhibitors) as drugs of choice for depression.

Pemoline

Brand name: Cylert.
Class of drug: CNS stimulant. This is a controlled substance, Schedule IV.
Mechanism of action: Inhibits reuptake of dopamine, thereby increasing dopamine concentrations in the CNS.
Indications/dosage/route: Oral only.
- ADHD
  - Maintenance dose range: 56–75 mg/d. Maximum: 112.5 mg/d.
  - Children ≥6 years: Initial: 37.5 mg, a.m.
Adjustment of dosage
- Kidney disease: Creatinine clearance <50 mL/min: avoid.
- Liver disease: Contraindicated.
- Elderly: Use with caution.
- Pediatric: Safety and efficacy in children under 6 years of age have not been established.
Food: May take with morning meal.

Pregnancy: Category B.

Lactation: No data available. Potentially toxic to fetus. Avoid breastfeeding.

Contraindications: Liver disease, hypersensitivity to pemoline.

Warnings/precautions

• Use with caution in patients with kidney disease.

• This drug can cause severe, life-threatening hepatotoxicity.

Advice to patient

• Take medication in the morning. If a dose is missed, it should be taken as soon as possible. Do not double the dose if it is missed on a particular day.

• Do not discontinue abruptly as this may cause symptoms of withdrawal: mental depression, fatigue.

• Do not take large amounts of caffeine and related xanthines present in coffee, colas, chocolate, tea.

• Avoid driving and other activities requiring mental alertness or that are potentially dangerous until response to drug is known.

• Diabetic patient should monitor blood glucose closely, as pemoline may increase the need for insulin.

• Notify physician immediately if fatigue, yellow skin, and/or dark urine develops.

Adverse reactions

• Common: insomnia, anorexia and weight loss (transient).

• Serious: seizures, aplastic anemia, liver injury, liver failure, precipitation of Tourette's syndrome, growth suppression in children, hypertension, arrythmias.

Clinically important drug interactions

• Drugs that increase effects/toxicity of pemoline: CNS stimulants, sympathomimetics.

• Pemoline decreases effects/toxicity of anticonvulsants.

Parameters to monitor

• Serum SGOT, SGPT, alkaline phosphatase, bilirubin at baseline and every two weeks during therapy.

• Signs and symptoms of Tourette's syndrome.

• Cardiovascular status for signs of overdose.

• Height and weight when on long-term therapy.

- Response to drug: attention span, impulse control, motor or vocal tics.
- Signs of sleep disturbance.
- Neurologic status: tremors, nervousness, restlessness, insomnia, anorexia. If these become severe, adjustment of dosage is necessary.

Editorial comments

- Pemoline is not recommended as first-line therapy in ADHD (a parental consent form has been provided by the manufacturer [Abbott Laboratories] and is available by phoning 847-937-7302).
- There have has been 15 cases of reported liver failure while taking pemoline, including 12 deaths. Avoid administration if baseline liver enzymes are abnormal and discontinue immediately if abnormalities develop during therapy. If therapy is discontinued and then resumed, baseline liver enzymes and continuous monitoring are required.

Penicillamine

Brand names: Cuprimine, Depen.
Class of drug: Heavy metal detoxifying agent, antirheumatologic agent.
Mechanism of action: Wilson's disease: chelates copper into a complex readily excreted by the kidneys, thus decreasing blood and tissue levels; decreases circulating IgM rheumatoid factor and depresses T-cell activity; these result in suppression of active inflammation. Antirheumatic action: enhances lymphocyte function. Cystinurea: forms a soluble complex with cystine, preventing formation of cystine calculi.
Indications/dosage/route: Oral only.

- Wilson's disease

- Adults: 250 mg q.i.d, 30–60 minutes before meals. Maximum: 2 g/d.
- Children: 20 mg/kg/d divided into 4 doses, 30–60 minutes before meals.
- Cystinuria
  - Adults: 250 mg/d divided into 4 doses. Maintenance: 1–4 g/d.
  - Children: 30 mg/kg/d, divided into 4 doses, 30–60 minutes before meals.
- Rheumatoid arthritis
  - Adults: Initial: 125–250 mg/d. Maintenance: 120–250 mg/d. Maximum: 1.5 g/d.
- Heavy metal poisoning (lead, mercury, copper)
  - Children, adults: 23–35 mg/kg/d, 3 or 4 divided doses.

Adjustment of dosage

- Kidney disease: Creatinine clearance <50 mL/min: avoid use.
- Liver disease: None.
- Elderly: Maximum: 750 mg/d.
- Pediatric: Has not been established as treatment for juvenile rheumatoid arthritis.

Onset of Action	Duration
May be delayed for 2–3 mo in treatment for rheumatoid arthritis	No data

Food: Should be taken 1 hour before or 2 hours after meals. Pyridoxine supplementation with doses of 25 mg/d is recommended in patients with Wilson's disease or cystinuria receiving pencillamine. Capsules may be opened and given in 1–2 tablespoons of juice or pureed fruit.

Pregnancy: Category D.

Lactation: No data available. Potentially toxic to infant. Avoid breastfeeding.

Contraindications: Hypersensitivity to penicillamine, history of adverse reaction to penicillamine (aplastic anemia or agranulocytosis) or penicillins, concurrent use of a variety of drugs as listed below (see Clinically Important Drug Interactions); concurrent use of iron, rheumatoid arthritis with renal insufficiency.

Warnings/precautions

- Use with caution in patients with history of aplastic anemia due to penicillin, patients requiring surgery; kidney disease; elderly.
- Patients started on penicillamine should not have an interruption of even a few days as hypersensitivity has been observed following reinstitution of therapy.
- Patient with Wilson's disease should observe dietary restrictions; ie, a low-copper diet may be necessary. Foods rich in copper should be avoided. These include shellfish, liver, chocolate, broccoli, foods enriched with copper (cereals). If drinking water contains >100 µg/L of copper, patient should take only demineralized or distilled water.
- Patients with cystinuria should drink large amounts of water.

Advice to patient

- Use two forms of birth control including hormonal and barrier methods.
- Use electric razor and soft toothbrush to prevent excessive bleeding.
- Drink large amounts of fluids (2–3 L/d).

Adverse reactions

- Common: anorexia, nausea, vomiting, abdominal pain, taste disorders, skin rash.
- Serious: neuropathy, bone marrow depression, severe allergic reactions (urtiaria, exfoliative dermatitis, pemphigus, thyroiditis, hypoglycemia), liver damage, pancreatitis, thrombotic throm-bocytopenic purpura, hemolytic anemia, thrombocytosis, proteinuria, nephrotic syndrome, optic neuritis, Guillain–Barré syndrome, myasthenia gravis, Goodpasture's syndrome, hemorrhagic alveolitis and glomerular nephphritis, pulmonary fibrosis, interstitial alveolitis, leukemia, drug-induced lupus erythematosus.

Clinically important drug interactions

- Drugs that are contraindicated for use with penicillamine: gold

salts, antimalarial drugs, cytotoxic drugs, oxphenybutazone, phenylbutazone. These increase the toxic effects of penicillamine.
- Drugs that decrease effects/toxicity penicillamine: iron salts.
- Penicillamine increases effects/toxicity of digoxin.

Parameters to monitor
- CBC with differential and platelets; liver function every 6 months during the first 1–1.5 years of therapy.
- Intake of fluids and urinary and other fluid output to minimize renal toxicity. Closely monitor electrolyte levels.
- Urinalysis for protein and cells, every 2 weeks during the first 6 months of therapy, monthly afterward.
- Monitor cystinuria patients annually for stone formation.
- Signs of allergic reactions. Approximately 33% of patients may experience such reactions.
- Signs and symptoms of bone marrow depression.
- Response in Wilson's disease: determine urinary copper levels before and soon after initiation of therapy, every 3 months afterward.
- Response in cystinuria: Monitor urinary cystine levels. Urinary excretion of cystine should be maintained at <100 mg/d. Examine annually for stone formation.
- Response in arthritis. It may be necessary to adjust dosage every 2–3 months. If no improvement is seen after several months of therapy (3–4 months) at 1–1.5 mg/d, discontinue penicillamine.
- Signs and symptoms of Stevens–Johnson syndrome: urticaria, edema of mucous membranes including lips and genital organs, headache, high fever, conjunctivitis, rhinitis, stomatitis.

Editorial comments
- This agent has a high potential for severe toxicity. It should be administered only by physicians familiar with all potentially toxic reactions as well as proper monitoring of patients receiving the drug. It is not a first-line treatment for rheumatoid arthritis.
- Penicillamine often causes iron deficiency and may cause zinc deficiency.

• This agent causes delayed wound healing; dose should be diminished or discontinued prior to surgery. Full dosage should be resumed only after completion of wound healing.

Penicillin G

Brand name: Pfizerpen.
Class of drug: Antibiotic, penicillin family, natural penicillin.
Mechanism of action: Inhibits bacterial cell wall synthesis.
Susceptible organisms *in vivo*: Beta-hemolytic streptococci, viridans streptococci, *Streptococcus pneumoniae* (increasing lack of susceptibility), *Enterococcus faecalis*, *Neisseria meningitidis*, *Treponema pallidum* (syphilis), *Listeria monocytogenes*. Unusual infections: *Corynebacterium diphtheriae*, *Bacillus anthracis*, *Clostridium* sp, *Erisipelothrix rhusiopathiae*, *Actinomyces*, *Streptococcus bovis*, *Pasteurella multicoda*, *Streptobacillus moniliformis*, *Spirillum minus*.
Indications/dosage/route: Continuous IV, IM.
• Severe infections caused by susceptible strains of streptococci, staphylococci, pneumococci; bacteremia, pneumonia, endocarditis, empyema, meningitis, gonorrheal meningitis
  – Adults: Minimum: 5×10^6 units/d.
• Meningococcal meningitis
  – Adults: IM $1–2 \times 10^6$ units q2h or $20–30 \times 10^6$ units, continuous IV.
• Actinomycosis, cervicofacial
  – Adults: $1–6 \times 10^6$ units/d.
• Actinomycosis, thoracic, abdominal
  – Adults: $10–20 \times 10^6$ units/day
• Clostridial infections
  – Adults: 20×10^6 units/d.
• Severe infections (fusospirochetal) of oropharynx, lower respiratory tract, genital area

  –Adults: $5–10 \times 10^6$ units/d.
- *Listeria* infections
  – Neonates: 500,000 to 1×10^6 units/d.
- Adults with meningitis
  – $15–20 \times 10^6$ units/d, 2 weeks.
- Adults with endocarditis
  – $15–20 \times 10^6$ units/d, 4 weeks.
- Bacteremia, meningitis (Pasteurella)
  – Adults: $4–6 \times 10^6$ units/d, 2 weeks.
- Endocarditis (erysipeloid)
  – Adults: $2–20 \times 10^6$ units/d, 4–6 weeks.
- Bacteremia (gram-negative baccilli)
  – Adults: $20–80 \times 10^6$ units/d.
- Diphtheric (carrier state)
  – Adults: 300,000–400,000 units/d in divided doses, 10–12 days.
- Anthrax
  – Adults: $\geq 5 \times 10^6$ units/d in divided doses until cure is effected.
- Prophylaxis against bacterial endocarditis (patients with congenital heart disease, rheumatic fever)
  – Adults: IM 1×10^6 units of penicillin G 30 minutes to 1 hour before dental or surgical procedures.
  – Children: IM 600,000 units 30 minutes to 1 hour before dental or surgical procedures.

Adjustment of dosage: None.

Food: Take oral dosage with food.

Pregnancy: Category B.

Lactation: Appears in breast milk. Use with caution.

Contraindications: Hypersensitivity to penicillin or cephalosporins.

Warnings/precautions

- Allergic reactions are more likely to occur in patients with asthma, hay fever, allergy to cephalosporins, history of allergy for penicillin. Consider skin testing with major and minor antigenic components of penicillin in such patients to assess the possibility of a hypersensitivity reaction. If patient is given the drug parenterally, observe for at least 20 minutes for possible anaphylactic reaction.

- Negative history of penicillin hypersensitivity does not preclude a patient from reacting to the drug.
- Administer at least 1 hour before a bacteriostatic agent is given (eg, tetracycline, erythromycin, chloramphenicol).
- IV infusion: Make sure no other drugs are added or mixed into the infusing solution. Do not use solution containing precipitate or foreign matter.

Advice to patient

- If you are receiving an oral contraceptive, use an alternative method of birth control.
- If you are allergic to a penicillin or cephalopsporin, carry an identification card with this information.

Adverse reactions

- Common: None.
- Serious: Stevens–Johnson syndrome, anaphylaxis, angioedema, laryngospasm, pseudomembraneous colitis, myoclonus.

Clinically important drug interactions

- Drug that increases effects/toxicity of penicillins: probenecid.
- Drugs that decrease effects/toxicity of penicillins: antacids, tetracyclines.
- Penicillins increase effects of oral anticoagulants, heparin.
- Penicillins decrease effects of oral contraceptives.

Parameters to monitor

- Signs and symptoms of anaphylactic shock.
- Signs and symptoms of allergic reaction.
- Signs and symptoms of pseudomembranous colitis.
- Intake/output of fluid.
- Renal, hepatic, and hematologic status for patients on high-dose prolonged therapy.

Editorial comments

- Penicillin G no longer is recommended for the empiric treatment of *Staphylococcus aureas* infections (90% produce penicillinase), *Neisseria gonorrhoeae* (frequent penicillinase production), anaerobic infections even above the diaphragm (frequent penicillinase production by oral anaerobes), *Streptococcus pneumoniae* meningitis or endocarditis due to modification of penicillin-binding proteins.

- Penicillin G is the preferred penicillin against gonorrhea. Inject penicillin G benzathine 1.4×10^6 units IM into each buttock. This regimen is not used for penicillinase-producing *Neisseria gonorrhoeae*.
- Penicillin G is also the drug of choice for treatment of syphilis. In neurosyphilis, penicillin is the only recommended drug; therefore, patients with allergy to penicillin are usually tested and desensitized if needed.
- Tonsillitis possibly or proven to be caused by *Streptococcus pyogenes* (group A) should be treated with oral penicillin VK.
- In severe infection of the soft tissues with *Streptococcus pyogenes* (necrotizing fasciitis), clindamycin may be preferred because of its antitoxin effect.
- Penicillin G is the drug of choice against a number of unusual inections, such as diphtheria, rat bite fever, actinomycosis, anthrax, and gas gangrene (caused by *Clostridia* sp).
- Penicillin G is also still a first-choice antibiotic against *Neisseria meningitidis*.

Penicillin G Benzathine

Brand name: Bicillin L-A.
Class of drug: Antibiotic, penicillin family.
Mechanism of action: Inhibits bacterial cell wall synthesis.
Susceptible organisms *in vivo*: See *pencillin G*.
Indications/dosage/route: IM only.
- Upper respiratory tract infection caused by group A streptococcus
  - Adults: 1.2×10^6 units as single dose.
  - Older children: 900,000 units.

  – Children <27 kg: 300,000–600,000 units as single dose.
  – Neonates: 50,000 units/kg as single dose.
- Early syphilis (primary, secondary, or latent of less than 1-year duration)
  – Adults: 2,400,000 units as single dose.
  – Children: 50,000 units/kg, up to adult dose.
- Gummas and cardiovascular syphilis
  – Adults: 2,400,000 units q7d for 3 weeks.
  – Children: 50,000 units/kg up to adult dose.
- Neurosyphilis
  – Adults: Aqueous penicillin G IV 1.8–2.4×10^7 units/d for 10–14 days followed by penicillin G benzathine, IM 2.4×10^6 units every week for 3 weeks.
- Yaws, bejel, pinta
  – Adults: 1.2×10^6 units in single dose.
- Prophylaxis of rheumatic fever
  – Adults: 1.2×10^6 units once a month or 600,000 units q2wk.

Adjustment of dosage: None.

Food: Not applicable.

Pregnancy: Category B.

Lactation: Appears in breast milk. Use with caution.

Contraindications: Hypersensitivity to penicillin or cephalosporins, IV injections.

Editorial Comments
- Penicillin G benzathine is injected IM to reach low levels in the plasma for a long period.
- It is used in latent syphilis (unknown duration or duration >1 year) as a course of 3 injections given weekly.
- Treatment failures do occur and the response is monitored by quantitative syphilis tests (eg, rapid plasma reagin).
- Neurosyphilis is treated with IV penicillin G to reach the high CSF levels needed for eradication of *Treponema pallidum* organisms. Some physicians add IM penicillin G benzathine after a full IV course.
- Penicillin G benzathine is frequently used as single-dose

therapy in upper respiratory infections with group A streptococci.

- For additional information, see *penicillin G*, p. 708.

Penicillin G Procaine

Brand names: Wycillin, Bicillin.
Class of drug: Antibiotic, penicillin family.
Mechanism of action: Inhibits bacterial cell wall synthesis.
Susceptible organisms *in vivo*: See *Penicillin G*.
Indications/dosage/route: IM only.
- Pneumococcal, staphylococcal, streptococcal infections, erysipeloid, rat bite fever, anthrax, fusospirochetosis
  - Adults: Usual: 600,000 to 1×10^6 units/d for 10–14 days.
  - Children <27.2 kg: 300,000 units/d.
- Diphtheria carrier state
  - 300,000 units/day for 10 days.
- Diphtheria, adjunct with antitoxin
  - 300,000–600,000 units/day.
- Anthrax, erysipeloid, rat bite fever
  - 600,000 to 1×10^6 uints/d.
- Fusospirochetosis, Vincent's gingivitis, pharyngitis
  - 600,000 to 1×10^6 units/d.
- Gonococcal infections
  - 4.8×10^6 units plus 1 g PO probenecid 30 minutes before injection.
- Neurosyphilis
  - 2.4×10^6 units/d for 10–14 days with PO probenecid 500 mg q.i.d., then benzathine penicillin G 2.4×10^6 units/wk for 3 weeks (see Editorial Comments).
- Congenital syphilis in infants
  - 50,000 units/kg/d for 10 days.
Adjustment of dosage: None.
Food: Not applicable.

Pregnancy: Category B.
Lactation: Appears in breast milk. Use with caution.
Contraindications: Hypersensitivity to penicillin, cephalosporins or procaine, IV injections.
Editorial comments
• Penicillin G procaine is used as a second choice in neurosyphilis when the patient refuses a 10- to 14-day intravenous course of penicillin G (which requires hospitalization or home IV therapy).
• For additional information, see *penicillin G*, p. 708.

Penicillin V Potassium

Brand name: Pen-Vee K.
Class of drug: Antibiotic, penicillin family plus B-lactamase inhibitor.
Mechanism of action: Inhibits bacterial cell wall synthesis.
Susceptible organisms *in vivo*: Spectrum like that of penicillin G. Used orally to treat infections from susceptible organisms such as group A streptococci, tonsillitis, and skin infections. Used as prophylaxis against recurrences of rheumatic fever, pneumoccocal infections in splenectomized patients, and recurrent streptococcal cellulitis.
Indications/dosage/route: Oral only.
• Systemic infections
  – Children <12 years: 25–50 mg/kg/d in divided doses q6–8h.
  – Adults, children >12 years: 125–500 mg q6–8h.
• Prophylaxis of recurrent rheumatic fever, prophylaxis of pneumoccocal infection
  – Children <5 years: 125 mg b.i.d.
  – Adults, children ≥5 years: 250 mg b.i.d.
Adjustment of dosage: None.
Food: Best to take on empty stomach.

Pregnancy: Category B.

Lactation: Appears in breast milk. Considered compatible by American Academy of Pediatrics.

Contraindications: Hypersensitivity to penicillin or cephalosporins, IV injections.

Editorial comments: For additional information, see *penicillin G*, p. 708.

This drug is listed without details in the *Physician's Desk Reference,* 54th edition, 2000.

Pentamidine

Brand names: NebuPent, Pentam-300.

Class of drug: Antiprotozoal, antiinfective.

Mechanism of action: Inhibits synthesis of DNA, RNA phospholipids, proteins in protozoa.

Indications/dosage/route: IV, IM aerosolized.

- Treatment of *Pneumocystis carinii* pneumonia, trypanosomiasis, visceral leishmaniasis
  - Adults, children: IV 4 mg/kg/d, 10–21 days; in AIDS patients, longer treatment may be required.
- Prophylaxis of *P. carinii* pneumonia
  - Adults, children >5 years: IV or IM 4 mg/kg/mo or q2wk; 300 mg q4wk using Respirgard II.
  - Children <5 years: 4 mg/kg.
  - Infants: (2.27 mg/kg × nebulizer output × wt)/alveolar ventilation.

Adjustment of dosage

- Kidney disease: Half-life prolonged in severe impairment. Reduce dose, prolong interval.
- Liver disease: None.
- Elderly: Consider reduced dose.
- Pediatric: See above.

Food: Not applicable.

Pregnancy: Category C.

Lactation: No data available. Potentially toxic to fetus. Avoid breastfeeding.

Contraindications: Previous anaphylactic reaction to pentamidine.

Warnings/precautions

- Use with caution in patients with hyperglycemia, hypoglycemia hypocalcemia, leukopenia, thrombocytopenia, kidney disease, hypotension, asthma, diabetes, cardiovascular disease, bone marrow depression, previous radiation therapy, pancreatitis, Stevens–Johnson syndrome, anemia.
- Severe hypotension may be produced by a single dose of pentamidine.
- Patient must be adequately hydrated before administering pentamidine.

Advice to patient

- Avoid crowds as well as persons who may have a contagious disease.
- Avoid alcohol.
- Avoid aspirin and aspirin-containing prescriptions.
- Change position slowly, in particular from recumbent to upright, to minimize orthostatic hypotension. Sit at the edge of the bed for several minutes before standing and lie down if feeling faint or dizzy. Avoid hot showers or baths and standing for long periods. Male patients may be safer urinating while seated on the toilet rather than standing.
- Patients on glucose-lowering agents should carry sugar or sugar-containing candy. Patients should wear a bracelet identifying their condition and possibility of developing hypoglycemia.

Adverse reactions

- Common: anxiety, headache, chest pain, dizziness, hypotension, nausea, vomiting, pain at injection site.
- Serious: **hyperkalemia, bronchospasm, hypotension**, arrhythmias, nephrotoxicity, hypoglycemia, hypocalcemia, acute renal failure, pancreatitis, bone marrow depression, pneumothorax,

Jarisch–Herxheimer-like reaction, extrapulmonary pneumo-cystitis infection.

Clinically important drug interactions: Drugs that increase effects/toxicity of pentamidine: aminoglycosides, amphotericin B, vancomycin, antineoplastic drugs, didanosine, foscarnet, erthromycin, NSAIDs, colistin, polymyxin B, methoxyfurane.

Parameters to monitor

- Signs and symptoms of bone marrow depression.
- Respiratory status: lung sounds, rate and character of respiration throughout therapy.
- BP frequently when giving drug IM or IV.
- Signs and symptoms of hypoglycemia: nervousness, involuntary shaking, abnormal sleep pattern, abdominal discomfort, hypotension, coma. If symptoms of hypoglycemia occur at home, advise patient to take a glass of fruit juice, honey (2–3 teaspoons), 1 or 2 sugar tablets, or corn syrup dissolved in water.
- Signs and symptoms of hyperglycemia.
- Pulse rate and ECG periodically.
- Signs and symptoms of renal toxicity.
- Serum calcium and magnesium prior to and every 3 days during therapy.
- Signs and symptoms of infection.
- Monitor patient taking aerosol drug for signs of wheezing or cough. Administer a bronchodilator 5 minutes before pentamidine.
- Signs and symptoms of pancreatitis.

Editorial comments

- Fatalities have been reported from severe hypoglycemia, hypotension, and cardiac arrhythmias when pentamidine is administered IM or IV. Pentamidine should be limited to patients in whom *P. carinii* pneumonia has been fully demonstrated. Pancreatitis may occur with aerosolized as well as parenteral pentamidine administration.
- This drug is not listed in the *Physician's Desk Reference*, 54th edition, 2000.

Pentazocine

Brand name: Talwin.

Class of drug: Narcotic analgesic, agonist/antagonist.

Mechanism of action: Binds to opiate receptors and blocks ascending pain pathways. Reduces patient's perception of pain without altering cause of the pain.

Indications/dosage/route: Oral only.

• Analgesia

  – Adults: 50–100 mg q3–4h. Maximum: 600 mg/d.

Adjustment of dosage

• Kidney disease: None.

• Liver disease: None.

• Elderly: Use with caution.

• Pediatric: Not recommended.

Onset of Action	Peak Effect	Duration
15–30 min	1–3 h	3 h

Food: May be taken with food to lessen GI upset.

Pregnancy: Category C. Category D if prolonged use or if given in high doses at term.

Lactation: Appears in breast milk. Potentially toxic to infant. Avoid breastfeeding.

Contraindications: Hypersensitivity to pentazocine.

Warnings/precautions

• Use with caution in patients with head injury with increased intracranial pressure, serious alcoholism, prostatic hypertrophy, chronic pulmonary disease, severe liver or kidney disease, disorders of biliary tract, and in postoperative patients with pulmonary disease.

• Administer drug before patient experiences severe pain for fullest efficacy of the drug.

- Have the following available when treating patient with this drug: naloxone (Narcan) or other antagonist, means of administering oxygen, and support of respiration.
- Nausea, vomiting, and orthostatic hypotension occur most prominently in ambulatory patients. If nausea and vomiting persist, it may be necessary to administer an antiemetic, eg, droperidol or prochlorperazine.
- This drug can cause severe hypotension in a patient who is volume depleted or if given along with a phenothiazine or general anesthesia.
- Careful diagnosis must be made of acute abdominal condition before this drug is administered.

Advice to patient

- Avoid alcohol and other CNS depressants such as sedatives (eg, diazepam) when taking this drug.
- Avoid driving and other activities requiring mental alertness or that are potentially dangerous until response to drug is known.
- Change position slowly, in particular from recumbent to upright, to minimize orthostatic hypotension. Sit at the edge of the bed for several minutes before standing, and lie down if feeling faint or dizzy. Avoid hot showers or baths and standing for long periods. Male patients should sit on the toilet while urinating rather than standing.
- Do not increase dose if you are not experiencing sufficient pain relief without approval from treating physician.
- Do not stop medication abruptly when you have been taking it for ≥2 weeks. If so, a withdrawal reaction may occur within 24–48 hours. The following are typical symptoms: irritability, perspiration, rhinorrhea, lacrimation, dilated pupil, piloerection ("goose flesh"), bone and muscle aches, restless sleep ("yen"), increased systolic pressure, hyperpyrexia, diarrhea, hyperglycemia, spontaneous orgasm.
- Use OTC drugs only with approval by treating physician. Some of these may potentiate the CNS depressant effects of the drug.

- If dizziness persists more than 3 days, decrease dose gradually (over 1–2 days).
- Attempt to void every 4 hours.

Adverse reactions

- Common: constipation, lightheadedness, dizziness, sedation, nausea, vomiting, sweating, dysplasia, euphoria.
- Serious: **hypotension, bradycardia**, apnea, circulatory depression, respiratory arrest, convulsions (high doses, IV), shock, increased intracranial depression, paralytic ileus, physical and psychologic dependence and addiction.

Clinically important drug interactions: Drugs that increase effects/toxocity of narcotic analgesics: alcohol, benzodiazepines, antihistamines, phenothiazines, butyrophenones, triyclic antidepressants, MAO inhibitors.

Parameters to monitor

- Signs and symptoms of pain: restlessness, anorexia, elevated pulse, increased respiratory rate. Differentiate restlessness associated with pain from that caused by CNS stimulation caused by morphine. This paradoxical reaction is seen mainly in women and elderly patients.
- Respiratory status prior to and following drug administration. Note rate, depth, and rhythm of respirations. If rate falls below 12/min, withhold drug unless patient is receiving ventilatory support. Consider administering an antagonist, eg, naloxone IV 0.1–0.5 mg every 2–3 minutes. Be aware that respiratory depression may occur even at small doses. Restlessness may also be a symptom of hypoxia.
- Character of cough reflex. Encourage postoperative patient to change position frequently (at least every 2 hours), breathe deeply, and cough at regular intervals, unless coughing is contraindicated. These steps will help prevent atelectasis.
- Signs and symptoms of urinary retention, particularly in patients with prostatic hypertrophy or urethral stricture. Monitor output/intake and check for oliguria or urinary retention.
- Signs of tolerance or dependence. Determine whether patient is attempting to obtain more drug than prescribed as this may indicate onset of tolerance and possibility of dependence. If tolerance

develops to one opiate, there is generally cross-tolerance to all drugs in this class. Physical dependence is generally not a problem if the drug is given less than 2 weeks.

- BP. If systolic pressure falls below 90 mm Hg, do not administer the drug unless there is ventilatory support. Be aware that the elderly and those receiving drugs with hypotensive properties are most susceptible to sharp fall in BP.
- Heart rate. Withhold drug if adult pulse rate is below 60 beats/min. Alternatively, administer atropine.
- Respiratory status of newborn baby and possible withdrawal reaction. If the mother has received an opiate just prior to delivery, the neonate may experience severe respiratory depression. Resuscitation may be necessary as may a narcotic antagonist, eg, naloxone. Alternatively, the neonate may experience severe withdrawal symptoms 1–4 days after birth. In such circumstances, administer tincture of opium or paregoric.
- Signs and symptoms of constipation. If patient is on drug more than 2–3 days, administer a laxative.
- For patients on long-term therapy, administer a bulk or fiber laxative, eg, psyllium 1 teaspoon in 240 mL liquid/d. Encourage patient to drink large amounts of fluid, 2.5 to 3 L/d.

Editorial comments

- For cancer patients who are experiencing severe, unrelieved pain, administer the drug IV or IM and switch to oral therapy once pain is controlled. Transdermal therapy may be beneficial.
- This drug is available only in combination with acetaminophen, aspirin or naloxone.

Pentobarbital

Brand name: Nembutal.
Class of drug: Sedative, hypnotic.
Mechanism of action: Facilitates action of GABA at its receptor. Depresses sensory cortex, cerebellum; decreases motor activity.

Indications/dosage/route: Oral, IM, IV.
• Sedation
  – Adults: PO 20 mg t.i.d. to q.i.d.
  – Children: PO 2–5 mg/kg/d.
• Preoperative sedation
  – Adults: PO 100 mg.
  – Children: 2–6 mg/kg/d. Maximum: 100 mg.
• Hypnotic
  – Adults: PO 100 mg h.s.
• Hypnotic/preoperative sedation
  – Adults: IM 150–200 mg.
  – Children: IM 2–5 mg/kg. Maximum: 100 mg.
• Sedative/hypnotic
  – Adults: IV 100 mg. Increase as needed to 200–500 mg. Maximum: 500 mg.

	Onset of Action	Duration
IV	10–15 min	3–4 h

Adjustment of dosage: Reduce dose in severe liver disease.
Pregnancy: Category D. Causes fetal abnormalities. Infants with chronic *in utero* barbiturate exposure are at risk for withdrawal. Administration during labor may cause infant respiratory depression.
Lactation: Appears in breast milk. Potentially toxic to infant. Avoid breastfeeding.
Contraindications: Hypersensitivity to barbiturates, porphyria, hepatic encephalopathy, severe respiratory disease, compromised respiration, previous addiction to a barbiturate or other sedative–hypnotics (eg, benzodiazepines).
Warnings/precautions
• Use with caution in patients with acute or chronic pain, hepatic or renal disease, depression, suicidal tendencies, history of drug abuse.
• When given to a patient with severe pain, this drug may cause excitement or agitation.

- Elderly are particularly sensitive to barbiturates. They develop confusion, depression, or pardoxical excitement.
- Children may exhibit excitement and irritability rather than sedation.
- Limit treatment to 2 weeks. Tolerance and/or psychologic and/or physical dependence may occur when used continuously as treatment for insomnia for more than 2 weeks.

Advice to patient

- Withdrawal symptoms can be very severe or even cause death; abrupt withdrawal should be avoided.
- Avoid driving and other activities requiring mental alertness or that are potentially dangerous until response to drug is known.
- Avoid alcohol and other CNS depressants such as narcotic analgesics and sedatives (eg, diazepam) when taking this drug.
- Use two forms of birth control including hormonal and barrier methods.

Adverse reactions

- Common: lethargy, drowsiness, CNS excitation.
- Serious: hypoventilation, apnea, Stevens–Johnson syndrome, angioedema, hypotension, confusion, psychiatric disturbance, arrhythmias, gangrene from intraarterial injection, laryngospasm, respiratory depression, bone marrow suppression, hypothermia, oliguria.

Clinically important drug interactions

- Barbiturates increase effects/toxicity of antihistamines, other sedative–hypnotics, opioids, alcohol, antidepressants.
- Barbiturates decrease effects/toxicity of oral anticoagulants, corticosteroids, oral contraceptives, theophylline, griseofulvin, phenytoin, doxycycline.
- Drugs that increase effects/toxicity of barbiturates: disulfiram, valproic acid, MAO inhibitors.
- Drug that decreases effects/toxicity of barbiturates: rifampin.

Parameters to monitor

- CBC with differential and platelets, phenobarbital levels.
- Signs and symptoms of dermatologic reactions which may be fatal: fever, severe headache, rhinitis, stomatitis. Discontinue drug.

- Signs and symptoms of allergic reaction: angioedema, Stevens–Johnson syndrome, toxic epidermal necrolysis. Discontinue drug and withdraw slowly.
- Signs and symptoms of acute overdose: respiratory depression, Cheynes–Stokes respiration, peripheral vascular collapse. Maintain adequate airway, institute gastric lavage or gastric aspiration (if drug has been ingested within 4 hours). Do not induce emesis as this may cause aspiration pneumonia.
- If there is evidence of blood dyscrasias (agranulocytosis, megaloblastic anemia, thrombocytopenia), discontinue drug.
- Drug levels: Therapeutic levels: 15–40 µg/mL. Toxic levels: ataxia 35–80 µg/mL; coma >65 µg/mL.

Editorial comments: In general, barbiturates have been replaced by benzodiazepines. Their usage should remain restricted.

Pergolide

Brand name: Permax.
Class of drug: Dopamine agonist, anti-Parkinson agent.
Mechanism of action: Potent dopaminergic agonist. Causes direct stimulation of postsynaptic dopaminergic receptors of the substantia nigra and other portions of the CNS.
Indications/dosage/route: Oral only.

- Parkinsonism
  - Adults: 0.05 mg/d, initial 2 days of therapy. Gradually increase dosage by 0.1 or 0.15 mg/d every third day for 12 days. Then increase dosage by 0.25 mg every third day until optimum response is obtained. Maintenance: 1–3 mg/d. Maximum: 5 mg/d in 3 divided doses.

Adjustment of dosage

- Kidney disease: Metabolized in the kidney. Use cautiously; consider decreased dosage.
- Liver disease: None.
- Elderly: None.
- Pediatric: Safety and efficacy have not been established.

Food: Take with meals.

Pregnancy: Category B.

Lactation: No data available. Inhibits lactation and is therefore not compatible.

Contraindications: Hypersensitivity to pergolide or ergot-type compounds.

Warnings/precautions: Use with caution in patients with arrhythmias, pulmonary fibrosis, pleural effusions, pericarditis, confusional state, hallucinations, kidney disease.

Advice to patient

- Avoid driving and other activities requiring mental alertness or that are potentially dangerous until response to drug is known.
- Change position slowly, in particular from recumbent to upright, to minimize orthostatic hypotension. Sit at the edge of the bed for several minutes before standing, and lie down if feeling faint or dizzy. Avoid hot showers or baths and standing for long periods. Male patients should sit on the toilet while urinating rather than standing.

Adverse reactions

- Common: somnolence, nausea, constipation, rhinitis.
- Serious: **dyskinesia, hallucinations, dystonia, confusion**, orthostatic hypotension, pericarditis, pleural effusions, pulmonary fibrosis, retroperitoneal fibrosis, orthostatic hypotension, anemia.

Clinically important drug interactions

- Drugs that increase effects/toxicity of pergolide: antihypertensives, drugs highly bound to plasma proteins.
- Drugs that decrease effects of pergolide: phenothiazines, haloperidol, metoclopramide, other dopamine antagonists.

Parameters to monitor

- Signs and symptoms of drug-induced extrapyramidal syndrome (pseudoparkinsonism): akinesia, resting tremors, pill rolling), shuffling gait, masklike facies, drooling. If these occur while taking this medication drug discontinuation may be required. Alternatively, administration of diphenhydramine and benztropine may be indicated.

- Signs of confusion or hallucinations.
- Cardiovascular status (ECG, BP) when adjusting dosage as well as periodically during therapy.

Editorial comments
- Pergolide is ordinarily taken along with levodopa/carbidopa for the treatment of Parkinson's disease.
- Following addition of pergolide to levodopa/carbidopa regimen, the dose of the latter can usually be decreased.

Permethrin

Brand names: Actinin Cream, Elimite Cream, Nix Creme.
Class of drug: Pediculicide.
Mechanism of action: Depolarizes nerve cell membranes, causing paralysis and death of ticks, lice, fleas, mites, arthopods.
Indications/dosage/route: Topical only.
- Head lice
  - Adults, children >2 years: Apply 1% lotion to hair for 10 minutes, rinse.
- Scabies
  - Adults, children: Massage 5% cream into skin surfaces for 8–14 hours, wash off.

Adjustment of dosage
- Kidney disease: None.
- Liver disease: None.
- Elderly: None.
- Pediatric: Safety and efficacy in children <2 months have not been established.

Food: Not applicable.
Pregnancy: Category B.
Lactation: No data available. Best to avoid.
Contraindications: Hypersensitivity to permethrin, pyrethrins, isopropyl alcohol (excipient), chrysanthemums.
Warnings/precautions: None.

Advice to patient
- If the cream comes in contact with the eyes, flush eyes thoroughly with water.
- Check family members or others living in the home for lice.
- Use the following methods to prevent reinfestation: Machine wash all clothes, linens, etc, in very hot water and dry in a hot dryer for at least 10 minutes to kill the mites.
- Drug should not come in contact with mucous membranes.

Adverse reactions
- Common: burning, stinging of skin, pruritis.
- Serious: none.

Clinically important drug interactions: None reported.

Parameters to monitor
- Examine scalp for head lice and nits before, and 1 week after, applying permethrin.
- Signs of scabies before and after therapy.
- Examine scalp for itching, redness, rash.

Editorial comments
- Permethrin is at least as effective as lindane in treating head lice and is a far safer agent.
- Ordinarily a single treatment is sufficient for eliminating lice. However, a second application may be necessary if lice reappear 7 days after the initial treatment.

Perphenazine

Brand names: Trilafon, Etrafon.
Class of drug: Phenothiazine antipsychotic (neuroleptic).
Mechanism of action: Antagonizes dopamine at dopaminergic receptors in CNS neurons.
Indications/dosage/route: Oral, IM, IV (seldom used).
- Psychotic disorders
  - Nonhospitalized patients: PO 4–8 mg t.i.d.
  - Hospitalized patients: PO 8–16 mg b.i.d. to q.i.d. Maximum: 64 mg/d.

- Nonhospitalized adults, adolescents: IM 5 mg q6h. Maximum: 15 mg/d.
- Hospitalized patients: Initial: IM 5–10 mg. Maximum: 30 mg.

• Nausea and vomiting
  - Adults: IV 6–18 mg/d in divided doses. Maximum: 24 mg/d.

Adjustment of dosage
• Kidney disease: None.
• Liver disease: None.
• Elderly: None.
• Pediatric: Safety and efficacy have not been established in children <12 years. Children >12 years should be administered lowest adult dose.

Pregnancy: Category C.

Lactation: Appears in breast milk. Considered to be an agent of concern by American Academy of Pediatrics. Avoid breastfeeding.

Contraindications: Hypersensitivity to phenothiazines, concurrent use of high-dose CNS depressants (alcohol, barbituates, benzodiazepines, narcotics), CNS depression, comatose state.

Editorial Comments: For additional information, see *chlorpromazine,* p. 206.

Phenobarbital

Brand names: Solfoton, Luminal.
Class of drug: Sedative, hypnotic, antiepileptic barbiturate.
Mechanism of action: Facilitates action of GABA at its receptor. Depresses sensory cortex, cerebellum; decreases motor activity.
Indications/dosage/route: Oral, IM, IV.
• Sedation
  - Adults: PO 30–120 mg/d in 2 to 3 divided doses.
  - Children: PO 2 mg/kg t.i.d.

- Hypnotic
  - Adults: PO 100–200 mg h.s.
  - Children: dose based on age and weight.
- Anticonvulsant
  - Adults: PO 60–200 mg/d in single or divided doses.
  - Children: PO 3–6 mg/kg/d in single or divided doses.
- Sedation
  - Adults: IM, IV 30–120 mg/d in 2 or 3 divided doses.
- Preoperative sedation
  - Adults: IM 100–200 mg 60–90 minutes before surgery.
  - Children: IM 1–3 mg/kg 60–90 minutes before surgery.
- Hypnotic
  - Adults: IM, IV 100–320 mg.
- Status epilepticus
  - Adults: IV 15–20 mg/kg given over 10–15 minutes. Repeat if needed.
  - Children: IV 15–20 mg/kg given over a 10- to 15-minute period.

Adjustment of dosage

- Kidney disease: Creatinine clearance <10 mL/min, dose q12–16h.
- Liver disease: Use with caution. At higher risk for side effects.
- Elderly: Use with caution.
- Pediatric: See above.

	Onset of Action	Duration
Oral	1 h	10–12 h

Food: Drug levels increase on protein-restricted diets and decrease with vitamin C-containing fruits. Increase vitamin D intake or take supplement.

Pregnancy: Category D. Causes fetal abnormalities. Infants with chronic *in utero* barbiturate exposure are at risk for withdrawal. Administration during labor may cause infant respiratory depression.

Lactation: Appears in breast milk. Classified by American

Academy of Pediatrics as potentially causing major adverse effects on infant when breastfeeding. Avoid breastfeeding.

Contraindications: Hypersensitivity to barbiturates, porphyria, preexisting CNS depression, hepatic encephalopathy, severe respiratory disease, compromised respiration, previous addiction to a barbiturate or other sedative–hypnotic (eg, benzodiazepines), pregnancy.

Warnings/precautions

- Use with caution in patients with acute or chronic pain, hepatic or renal disease, depression, suicidal tendencies, history of drug abuse.
- When given to a patient with severe pain, this drug may cause excitement or agitation.
- Elderly are particularly sensitive to barbiturates. Then develop confusion, depression, or paradoxical excitement.
- Children may exhibit excitement and irritability rather than sedation.
- Limit treatment to 2 weeks. Tolerance and/or psychologic and/or physical dependence may occur when used continuously as treatment for insomnia more than 2 weeks.

Advice to patient

- Withdrawal symptoms can be very severe or even cause death; abrupt withdrawal should be avoided.
- Avoid driving and other activities requiring mental alertness or that are potentially dangerous until response to drug is known.
- Avoid alcohol and other CNS depressants such as narcotic analgesics and sedatives (eg, diazepam) when taking this drug.
- Use two forms of birth control including hormonal and barrier methods.

Adverse reactions

- Common: lethargy, drowsiness, CNS excitation.
- Serious: hypoventilation, apnea, Stevens–Johnson syndrome, angioedema, hypotension, confusion, psychiatric disturbance, arrhythmias, gangrene from intraarterial injection, larygospasm,

respiratory depression, bone marrow suppression, hypothermia, oliguria.

Clinically important drug interactions

- Barbiturates increase effects/toxicity of antihistamines, other sedative–hypnotics, opioids, alcohol, antidepressants.
- Barbiturates decrease effects/toxicity of oral anticoagulants, corticosteroids, oral contraceptives, theophylline, griseofulvin, phenytoin, doxycycline.
- Drugs that increase effects/toxicity of barbiturates: disulfiram, valproic acid, MAO inhibitors.
- Drugs that decrease effects/toxicity of barbiturates: rifampin.

Parameters to monitor

- CBC with differential and platelets, phenobarbital levels.
- Signs and symptoms of dermatologic reactions which may be fatal: fever, severe headache, rhinitis, stomatitis. Discontinue drug.
- Signs and symptoms of allergic reaction: angioedema, Stevens–Johnson syndrome, toxic epidermal necrolysis. Discontinue drug and withdraw slowly.
- Signs and symptoms of acute overdose: respiratory depression, Cheynes–Stokes respiration, peripheral vascular collapse. Maintain adequate airway, institute gastric lavage or gastric aspiration (if drug has been ingested within 4 hours). Do not induce emesis as this may cause aspiration pneumonia.
- Signs and symptoms of blood dyscrasias (agranulocytosis, megaloblastic anemia, thrombocytopenia): discontinue drug.
- Drug levels: Therapeutic levels: 15–40 µg/ml. Toxic levels: ataxia 35–80 µg/ml; coma >65 µg/ml.

Editorial comments

- In general, barbiturates have been replaced by benzodiazepines for their sedative and hyponotic actions. Their usage should remain restricted.
- Phenobarbital is an ingredient of Donnatal (combined with hyoscyamine, atropine, and scopolamine).
- This drug is not listed in the *Physicians' Desk Reference*, 54th edition, 2000.

Phentermine

Brand names: Adipex-P, Fastin, Ionamine.
Class of drug: Anti-obesity agent, anorectic, sympathomimetic.
(Controlled substance, Schedule IV.)
Mechanism of action: Exact mechanism in promoting weight loss is unknown.
Indications/dosage/route: Oral only.
  – Adults: 18.75–37.5 mg/d as single dose or b.i.d.
Adjustment of dosage
• Kidney disease: None.
• Liver disease: None.
• Elderly: Reduced dosage is advisable.
• Pediatric: Safety and efficacy have not been established. Not recommended for children <16 years.
Food: Take before meals or 2 hours after meals.
Pregnancy: Category C. Safe use in pregnancy has not been established.
Lactation: Probably appears in breast milk. Considered contraindicated because of potential toxicity to the infant.
Contraindications: Hyperthyroidism, moderate to severe hypertension, advanced arteriosclerosis, glaucoma, hypersensitivity to sympathomimetic amines, administration within 14 days of taking MAO inhibitor, agitated patients, history of drug abuse.
Warnings/precautions
• Use with caution in patients with mild hypertension and insulin-requiring diabetics.
• Indicated only for short-term therapy.
• Primary pulmonary hypertension and valvular heart disease have to be ruled out before drug is administered.
Advice to patient
• Take last dose at least 6 hours before bedtime.
• Do not take the drug more frequently or at doses higher than those prescribed.

- Avoid driving and other activities requiring mental alertness or that are potentially dangerous until response to drug is known.
- The anorexigenic effects of phentermine persist only a few weeks after stopping the drug.
- Avoid alcohol.
- Diabetic patients should monitor their blood glucose closely as alteration in body weight may require a change in antidiabetic drug.
- Alter eating habits to maintain reduced body weight.

Adverse reactions
- Common: insomnia, palpitations, tachycardia, restlessness.
- Serious: psychosis, primary pulmonary hypertension, regurgitant valvular heart disease, urticaria.

Clinically important drug interactions
- Drugs that increase effects/toxicity of phentermine: MAO inhibitors (contraindicated), caffeine, general anesthetics, antacids, acetazolamide, phenothiazines, haloperidol.
- Phentermine decreases effects/toxicity of guanethidine.

Parameters to monitor
- Weight before and during administration of phentermine. If tolerance develops to the drug's effect, do not increase dose; discontinue.
- Vital signs regularly, in particular for evidence of increased BP and other signs of increased sympathetic activity.
- Signs of pulmonary toxicity.

Editorial comments
- The safety of combining phentermine with SSRIs has not been established.
- Therapy should generally not be continued beyond 6 months. Because of abuse potential, only dispense sufficient supply until next patient visit. Avoid use in patients with potential for drug abuse.
- Pulmonary hypertension and valvular heart disease have been reported in patients receiving phentermine combined with fenfluramine or dexfenfluramine. The latter agents have been removed from the market.

Phentolamine

Brand name: Regitine.
Class of drug: Sympatholytic, antihypertensive.
Mechanism of action: Blocks α-adrenergic receptors; causes vascular dilation.
Indications/dosage/route: IV, IM, intercavernosal.

• Hypertension, immediately before or during surgery for pheochromocytoma
  – Adults: IM or IV 5 mg 1–2 hours before surgery; IV 5 mg during surgery.
  – Children: IM or IV 1 mg, 0.1 mg/kg, or 3 mg/m^2, 1–2 hours before surgery. During surgery repeat indicated dosage.
• Diagnosis of pheochromocytoma
  – Adults: IV or IM 5 mg.
  – Children: IV 1 mg or IM 3 mg or 0.1 mg/kg or 3 mg/m^2.
• Treatment of dermal necrosis from extravasation after IV administration of drugs.
  – Adults, children: 5–10 mg injected into affected area.
• Adjunct therapy of impotence
  – Adults: Intercavernosal 0.5–1 mg along with 30 mg papaverine. Maximum: 3 treatments/wk.
• Hypertensive crisis caused by MAO inhibitor–sympathomimetic amine interaction
  – Adults: IM or IV 5–20 mg.

Adjustment of dosage
• Kidney disease: None.
• Liver disease: None.
• Elderly: Use with extreme caution.
• Pediatric: See above.

Onset of Adrenergic Blockade	Peak effect	Duration
Immediate	2 min	15–30 min

Food: Not applicable.

Pregnancy: Category C.

Lactation: No data available. Best to avoid.

Contraindications: Coronary artery disease with angina or coronary insufficiency, history of MI, cerebrovascular disease.

Warnings/precautions

- Use with caution in patients with active peptic ulcer, tachycardia, elderly.
- May precipitate MI or cerebrovascular occlusion.

Advice to patient: Change position slowly, in particular from recumbent to upright, to minimize orthostatic hypotension. Sit at the edge of the bed for several minutes before standing, and lie down if feeling faint or dizzy. Avoid hot showers or baths and standing for long periods. Male patients should sit on the toilet while urinating rather than standing.

Adverse reactions

- Common: nausea, vomiting, nasal congestion, abdominal pain.
- Serious: **arrythmias, angina, orthostatic hypotension**, cerebral vascular spasm, severe hypotension (may be prolonged), MI, worsening of peptic ulcer.

Clinically important drug interactions

- Phentolamine decreases effects/toxicity of norepinephrine, epinephrine (vasoconstrictor and hypertensive effects), ephedrine, metaraminol, phenylephrine, dopamine.
- Phentolamine increases effects/toxicity of guanethidine, guanadrel.

Parameters to monitor: Cardiovascular function (BP, pulse, ECG) every 2 minutes during IV administration.

Editorial comments

- Phentolamine has been used along with papaverine to treat men with impotence. This method requires special training. There is a risk of priapism.
- When testing for pheochromocytoma, a positive response occurs when the BP decreases by 35 mm Hg systolic, 20–25 mm Hg diastolic.
- All other medication including antihypertensives, analgesics, and sedatives should be withdrawn 48–72 hours before the phentolamine test is instituted. The test may not be administered to normotensive patients.

• If severe hypotension occurs, do not administer epinephrine. Norepinepherine or other vasopressors may be used.
• This drug is not listed in the *Physician's Desk Reference*, 54th edition, 2000.

Phenylephrine

Brand name: Neo-Synephrine.
Class of drug: Sympathomimetic.
Mechanism of action: Phenylephrine constricts blood vessels, resulting in increased total peripheral resistance, increased BP.
Indications/dosage/route: IV, IM, topical (ophthalmic).
• Hypotensive emergencies during spinal anesthesia
  – Adults: Initial: IV 0.1–0.2 mg.
  – Children: 0.5–1 mg/25 lb body wt.
• Mild to moderate hypotension
  – Adults: SC or IM 1–2 mg. Additional doses may be administered in 1–2 hours.
• Severe hypotension or shock
  – Adults: IV infusion 0.1–0.18 µg/min. Maintenance: 0.04–0.06 µg/min. prn.
• Paroxysmal supraventricular tachycardia
  – Adults: Initial: IV 0.5 mg. Dosage may be increased at increments of 0.1–0.2 mg. Maximum: 1 mg.
• Midriasis
  – Adults: 1–2 drops 2.5 or 10% solution before procedure. May be repeated in 10–60 minutes if needed.
• Posterior synechia
  – Adults: 1 drop 10% solution, ≥3 times/d, along with atropine.
• Diagnosis of Horner's or Raeder's syndrome
  – Adults: 1 or 10% solution instilled in both eyes.
• Conjunctival congestion
  – Adults: 1–2 drops 0.08 to 0.25% solution in conjunctivae q3–4h prn.

Adjustment of dosage
- Kidney disease: None.
- Liver disease: None.
- Elderly: Use with caution. Use lower initial dosages.
- Pediatric: 10% ophthalmic solution is contraindicated for use in infants.

Onset of Vasopressor Action	Duration
Immediate	15–20 min

Food: Not applicable.

Pregnancy: Category C.

Lactation: No data available. Potentially toxic to fetus. Avoid breastfeeding.

Contraindications: Severe hypertension, ventricular tachycardia and other ventricular tachyarrthymias, hypersensitivity to phenylephrine or bisulfites (parenteral), camphor, eucalyptol, thimerosal in ophthalmic preparations. Opthalmic preparations contraindicated in patients with angle-closure glaucoma and those who are wearing soft contact lenses.

Warnings/precautions: Use with caution in patients with hyperthyroidism, cardiac disease, diabetes (type I), hypertension, bradycardia, elderly.

Advice to patient
- Ophthalmic preparations may make eyes more sensitive to light. If this occurs, wear dark glasses.
- Correct any hypovolemic state before phenylephrine is administered.
- Phenylephrine solutions exposed to air or strong light may no longer be effective. Store such solutions away from heat, light, and high humidity, ie, not in a bathroom medicine cabinet.
- Do not use solutions that have a brown color or contain a precipitate.

Adverse reactions
- Common: headache, palpitations, burning, brow ache, photophobia.
- Serious: arrthymias, MI, PVCs, asthmatic attack, anaphylaxis.

Clinically important drug interactions

- Drugs that increase effects/toxicity of phenylephrine: MAO inhibitors, ergonovine, general anesthetics, cardiac glycosides, levodopa, tricyclic antidepressants, oxytocics, ergot alkalyoids.
- Drugs that decrease effects of phenylephrine: α-adrenergic blockers, atropine.

Parameters to monitor

- Monitor ECG continuously during IV administration for presence of arrthymias.
- Signs and symptoms of side effects such as headache, dyspnea, pain, dizziness during IV infusion. Discontinue if these become serious.
- Monitor patient receiving ophthalmic preparation for signs of systemic effects: dizziness, chest pain. If this occurs, drug should be discontinued.
- Monitor BP, heart rate, arterial blood gases, and central venous pressure when administering IV.

Editorial comments

- Phenylephrine is a component of a large number of prescription and OTC cold preparations.
- The parenteral form of this drug is listed without details in the *Physician's Desk Reference,* 54th edition, 2000.

Phenytoin

Brand name: Dilantin.
Class of drug: Anticonvulsant, antiarrhythmic.
Mechanism of action: Stabilizes hyperexcitable CNS neurons by inhibiting sodium influx and promoting sodium neuronal efflux. This limits seizure activity.
Indications/dosage/route: Oral, IV.

- Generalized tonic–clonic seizures, status epilepticus, partial complex seizures; prevention and treatment of seizures associated with neurosurgical procedures

– Adults: IV: Loading dose 10–15 mg/kg; maximum 50 mg/min. PO: Loading dose 1 g, divided into 3 doses, 2-hour intervals; Maintenance 300–600 mg/d.

– Children: IV: Loading dose 15–20 mg/kg, maximum 50 mg/min. PO: 15–20 mg/kg q8–12h; maintenance dose 4–8 mg/kg; maximum 300 mg/d.

• Arrhythmias

– Adults: IV 200–400 mg/d, PO 300–600 mg/d.

• Neuritic pain (eg, trigeminal neuralgia, Bell's palsy).

– Adults: PO 200–600 mg/d, in divided doses.

Note: Dosages must be individualized based on response and monitoring of serum phenytoin levels. Therapeutic range for serum levels is 10–20 mg/mL.

Adjustment of dosage

• Kidney disease: None.

• Liver disease: Higher risk for toxicity. Use lower doses and monitor closely.

• Elderly: May require lower doses. At higher risk for toxicity.

• Pediatric: See Indications/Dosage/Route.

	Onset of Arrhythmic Action	Duration
IV	Rapid	≤24 h

Food: Administer phenytoin with food or immediately after meals or with milk. Large doses of vitamin C decrease effectiveness of phenytoin. Therefore, it is best to avoid foods with high vitamin C content. Phenytoin interferes with vitamin D metabolism, necessitating supplementation with vitamin D (4000 units/week). Hypocalcemia may occur in patients on prolonged phenytoin therapy. It may be necessary to supplement the diet with calcium.

Pregnancy: Category D.

Lactation: Appears in breast milk. Considered compatible by American Academy of Pediatrics.

Contraindications: Hypersensitivity to phenytoin or hydantoins, porphyria.

Warnings/precautions

- Use with caution in patients with liver disease, diabetes, respiratory depression, myocardial insufficiency.
- Advise patient to avoid sudden withdrawal as this may precipitate status epilepticus. Withdrawal of phenytoin should occur over several months. The following schedule of withdrawal is suggested: Decrease the dose by 100 mg/d each month until withdrawal is complete.

Advice to patient

- Use two forms of birth control including hormonal and barrier methods.
- Avoid driving and other activities requiring mental alertness or that are potentially dangerous until response to drug is known.
- Avoid alcohol.
- Carry identification card at all times describing disease, treatment regimen, name, address, and telephone number of treating physician.
- Maintain good dental hygiene and see a dentist frequently to prevent gum disorders.
- Do not take phenytoin along with antacids or antidiarrheals. Allow 2–3 hours before taking these drugs.
- Diabetic patient should monitor blood glucose carefully and notify treating physician if there are any significant changes.
- Change brands of phenytoin only after consulting treating physician.
- Practice good skin care as phenytoin may cause acne to develop.
- If you experience weakness, headaches, feelings of faintness, notify your treating physician as these may be signs of folic acid deficiency.

Adverse reactions

- Common: ataxia, nystagmus, diplopia, slurred speech, hypotension, nausea, gingival hyperplasia, rashes.
- Serious: bone marrow depression, dyskinesias, sensory neuropathy, severe dermatitis (Stevens–Johnson syndrome, toxic epidermal necrolysis, exfoliative or bullous dermatitis),

lymphoma, Hodgkin's disease, coarsened facial features, periarteritis nodosa, hepatitis, lupus, immunoglobulin alteration.

Clinically important drug interactions

- Drugs that increase effects/toxicity of phenytoin: acute alcohol, isoniazid, chloramphenicol, benzodiazepines, succinamides, amiodarone, estrogens, cimetidine, halothane, methylphenidate, phenothiazines, salicylates, succinamides, sulfonamides, tolbutamide, trazodone, disulfiram.
- Drugs that decrease effects/toxicity of phenytoin: chronic alcohol, carbamazepine, reserpine, sucralfate, molindone (Moban), calcium-containing antacids.
- Phenytoin decreases effects of digitalis glycosides, oral contraceptives, estrogens, corticosteroids, doxycycline, quinidine, rifampin, furosemide, dicumarol.
- Phenobarbital and valproic acid may either increase or decrease phenytoin levels.

Parameters to monitor

- Serum liver enzymes, CBC with differential and platelets, serum calcium.
- Effectiveness in suppressing seizure activity: Use EEG monitoring.
- Signs of progressive toxicity: nystagmus, confusion, ataxia.
- Signs of skin rash. If rash is purpuric or exfoliative, discontinue treatment.
- Serum glucose levels for hyperglycemia.
- Signs of gingival hyperplasia. Advise patient to practice good oral hygiene, including gum massage, and make regular dental visits.
- Signs of hypertrichosis and coarsening of facial features. Administer vitamin D, calcium, and folic acid to resverse these effects.
- Evaluate patient for orthostasis using BP measurements in the sitting, lying, and standing positions repeatedly before and after initiating therapy.

Editorial comments

- Phenytoin is the drug of choice if the EEG shows partial seizures that generalize in a secondary fashion.

- It is the drug of choice if parenteral administration is required.
- Only the extended-release capsules are approved for single daily dosing. Other forms are given in divided doses q8–12 h.
- Avoid administration by the IM route as it is painful and absorption is erratic by this route.
- Phenytoin is used to prevent seizures after neurosurgery or head trauma. It is also used for ventricular arrhythmia from digoxin toxicity and following pediatric cardiac surgery. Off-label use includes treatment of epidermolysis bullosa. It is not to be used for preventing alcohol withdrawal seizures.

Physostigmine

Brand names: Eserine (physostigmine sulfate), Antilirium (physostigmine salicylate).
Class of drug: Cholinesterase inhibitor.
Mechanism of action: Inhibits acetylcholinesterase thereby increasing acetylcholine at cholinergic receptor sites.
Indications/dosage/route: IV, IM topical (ophthalmic).
- Anticholinergic drug overdose
  - Adults: IV, IM 0.5–2 mg injected at 1 mg/min. Repeat if necessary.
  - Children: IV, IM 0.02 mg/kg (slow IV injection). Repeat at 5–10 minutes if necessary. Maximum: 2 mg.
- Reversal of nondepolarizing blocking agent (curare-type drug) postanesthesia
  - Adults: IV, IM 0.5–1 mg (slow IV injection, <1 mg/min). Repeat at 10- to 30-minute intervals and monitor return of respiratory function.
- Glaucoma
  - Adults, children: Apply 1 cm of 0.25% physostigmine sulfate (ointment) to lower fornix up to t.i.d.
Adjustment of dosage
- Kidney disease: None.
- Liver disease: None.

- Elderly: None.
- Pediatric: Safety and efficacy have not been established.

	Onset of Action	Peak Effect	Duration
ophthalmic	20–30 min	2–6 h	12–36 h

Food: Not applicable.

Pregnancy: Category C.

Lactation: No data available. Potentially toxic to infant. Avoid breastfeeding.

Contraindications

- Parenteral administration: hypersensitivity to physostigmine, peritonitis, mechanical obstruction of intestinal or urinary tract.
- Ophthalmic administration: active uveal inflammation, inflammatory disease of iris or ciliary body, glaucoma associated with iridocyclitis.

Editorial comments

- Use ophthalmic preparation with caution in patients with angle-closure glaucoma, patients with narrow angles.
- Use parenteral preparations with caution in patients with hypersensitivity to sulfites, epilepsy, bronchial asthma, bradycardia, recent coronary occlusion, hyperthyroidism, cardiac arrhythmias, peptic ulcer.
- Be aware that benzyl alcohol in parenteral product may cause "gasping syndrome," which could be fatal in premature infant.
- Systemic administration to children should be reserved for life-threatening situations.
- Advise patient to store ophthalmic ointment in tightly closed container in a cool place.
- Advise patient receiving ophthalmic preparation that night vision may be impaired.
- This drug is not listed in the *Physician's Desk Reference*, 54th edtion, 2000.
- For additional information, see *neostigmine*, p. 652.

Phytonadione

Brand names: AquaMephyton, Mephyton.

Class of drug: Vitamin K substitute. Antidote for oral anticoagulant overdose.

Mechanism of action: Promotes synthesis of clotting factors II, VII, IX, X in the liver.

Indications/dosage/route: Oral, IV, IM, SC.

- Hemorrhagic disease of newborns.
  - Neonates: SC, IM 0.5–1.0 mg within 1 hour of birth; may be repeated in 6–8 hours. Maintenance: 1–2 mg/d.
- Oral anticoagulant overdose
  - Children, adults: PO, IM, SC, IV 2.5–10 mg. Repeat in 6–8 hours if necessary if given by IM, IV, SC route. Repeat 12–48 hours if given by oral route.
- Vitamin K deficiency secondary to malabsorption, antibiotics or drug-induced
  - Infants, children: PO 2.5–5.0 mg/d.
  - Adults: PO 5–25 mg/d. Occasional doses of 50 mg/d used. IM, IV 10 mg/d.

Adjustment of dosage

- Kidney disease: None.
- Liver disease: Repeated dose to correct coagulopathy not advised. Patients may be vitamin K unresponsive.
- Elderly: None.
- Pediatric: See above.

	Onset of Action	Duration
Oral	6–12 h	—
Parenteral	1–2 h	—

Food: Not applicable.

Pregnancy: Category C.

Lactation: Appears in breast milk. Considered compatible by American Academy of Pediatrics.

Contraindications: Hypersensitivity to phytonadione or excipients (benzyl alcohol or polysorbate).

Warnings/precautions
- Not to be used to reverse heparin-induced coagulopathy.
- Use of phytonadione may precipitate thromboses in patients receiving anticoagulants.
- In general IV doses should be avoided unless deemed absolutely necessary. If used, IV, doses should be given at the slow rate of <1 mg/min.
- Patients with bile salt malabsorption will likely have decreased oral phytonadione absorption.
- Do not use large doses of vitamin K in an attempt to correct hypoprothrombinemia associated with severe liver disease (hepatitis or cirrhosis) as this may result in further depression of prothrombin levels.

Advice to patient
- Carry identification card at all times describing disease, treatment regimen, name, address, and telephone number of treating physician.
- Avoid alcohol.
- Notify dentist or treating physician prior to surgery if taking this medication.
- Avoid aspirin and aspirin-containing products and other NSAIDs.
- Use electric razor and soft toothbrush.
- Avoid flossing.

Adverse reactions
- Common: None.
- Serious: Anaphylaxis (following rapid IV administration), hyperbilirubinemia in newborn (high doses), hypotension, cyanosis.

Clincially important drug interactions
- Drugs that increase the requirement for phytonadione: quinidine, quinine, high-dose salicylates, sulfonamides, antibiotics.
- Drugs that decrease effects/toxicity of phytonadione: cholestyramine, colestipol, sucralfate, mineral oil.
- Phytonadine decreases effects of oral anticoagulants.

Parameters to monitor

- PT and PTT prior to and during therapy with phytonadione.
- Liver enzymes.
- Pulse and BP frequently.
- Symptoms of unusual bleeding or bruising, including nosebleeds, black tarry stools, excessive menstrual flow.

Editorial comments

- Because phytonadione has a slow onset of action, it may be necessary to administer whole blood or plasma if there is an emergency need due to severe bleeding.
- Fatalities have occurred during and immediately after IV injection of phytonadione. These resemble anaphylactic reactions. For this reason the IV route is restricted to situations where other routes are not feasible and the possibility of serious risk is justified.
- It is essential to use great caution when counteracting warfarin overdose with phytonadione as the original condition from thrombosis might be restored if excessive amounts of phytonadione are used. The dosage should be kept as low as possible and PT checked regularly to ensure proper anticoagulation.
- Phytonadione is the vitamin K analogue of choice to treat overdose with an oral anticoagulant.

Pindolol

Brand name: Visken.
Class of drug: β-Adrenergic receptor blocker.
Mechanism of action: Competitive blocker of β-adrenergic receptors in heart and blood vessels.
Indications/dosage/route: Oral only.

- Hypertension

– Adults: Initial: 5 mg b.i.d. Increase by 10 mg/d q3–4wk to a maximum of 60 mg/d.

Adjustment of dosage
- Kidney disease: None.
- Liver disease: None.
- Elderly: None.
- Pediatric: Safety and efficacy have not been established.

Food: No restriction.

Pregnancy: Category B.

Lactation: Appears in breast milk. Best to avoid. Observe infant for bradycardia, hypotension.

Contraindications: Cardiogenic shock, asthma, CHF unless it is secondary to tachyarrhythmia treated with a β blocker, sinus bradycardia and AV block greater than first degree, severe COPD.

Editorial comments
- Note that this drug is pregnancy category B; most β blockers are category C.
- For additional information, see *propranolol*, p. 790.
- This drug is listed without details in the *Physician's Desk Reference*, 54th edition, 2000.

Piperacillin

Brand name: Pipracil.

Class of drug: Antibiotic, penicillin family.

Mechanism of action: Inhibits bacterial cell wall synthesis.

Susceptible organisms *in vivo*: Staphylococci, *Staphylococcus aureus, Streptococcus pneumoniae*, beta-hemolytic streptococci, *Escherichia coli, Hemophilus influenzae, Klebsiella* sp, *Neisseria gonorrhoeae, Proteus mirabilis, Enterobacter* sp, *Pseudomonas aeruginosa, Serratia* sp, *Clostridium* sp (*Bacteriodes* sp generally are resistant).

Indications/dosage/route: IV, IM.
- Polymicrobial infections such as noscomial pneumonia, intra-abdominal infections; septicemia; gynecologic, skin, and soft tissue infections.
  – IV 12–14 g/d in divided doses q4–6h.
- Complicated UTIs
  – IV 8–16 g/d in divided doses q6–8h.
- Uncomplicated UTIs and infections and community-acquired pneumonia
  – IM, IV 6–8 g/d in divided doses q6–12h.
- Uncomplicated gonorrhea infections
  – IM 2 g.

Adjustment of dosage
- Kidney disease

Creatinine Clearance	UTI (uncomplicated)	UTI (complicated)	Serious Systemic Infection
>30 mL/min	<No dosage adjustment necessary>		
30–40 mL/min	No dosage adjustment necessary	3 g q8h	4 g q8h
<20 mL/min	3 g q12h	3 g q12h	4 g q12h

Liver disease: None.
Elderly: None.
Pediatric: Dosage in children <12 has not been established.
Food: Not applicable
Pregnancy: Category B.
Lactation: Appears in breast milk. Use with caution.
Contraindications: Hypersensitivity to penicillin or cephalosporins, IV injections.

Editorial comments
- Piperacillin is generally used for noscomial pneumonia, septicemia, endocarditis, and soft tissue infections due to susceptible organisms, especially aerobic gram-negative bacteria or *Enterococcus faecalis*.

- Piperacillin is also combined with tazobactam (Zosyn). Addition of tazobactam inhibits the β–lactamase of *Staphylococcus aureas* (MSSA), *Hemophilus influenzae, Branhamella catarrhalis*, and anaerobes (including *Bacteroides fragilis* and oral anaerobes).
- Piperacillin/tazobatam is used as a very broad-spectrum antibiotic in mixed infections. Good examples of appropriate use would be intraabdominal infections after surgery, ventilator-associated pneumonia, or multiple site infections in ICU patients. Unfortunately, extended-spectrum β-lactamases are produced by more and more aerobic gram-negative bacteria found in noscomial infections. For these, imipenem is a better choice.
- For additional information, see *penicillin G,* p. 708.

Piroxicam

Brand name: Feldene.
Class of drug: NSAID.
Mechanism of action: Inhibits cyclooxygenase, resulting in inhibition of synthesis of prostaglandins and other inflammatory mediators.
Indications/dosage/route: Oral only.
- Osteoarthritis, rheumatoid arthritis, ankylosing spondylitis
  – Adults: 20 mg/d in one or more divided doses.
Adjustment of dosage
- Kidney disease: None.
- Liver disease: None.
- Elderly: May be necessary to reduce dose for patients >65 years.
- Pediatric: Safety and efficacy have not been established in children <14 years.
Food: Take with food or large quantities of water or milk.
Pregnancy: Category B. Category D in third trimester or near delivery.

Lactation: Appears in breast milk. Considered compatible with breastfeeding by American Academy of Pediatrics.

Contraindications: Hypersensitivity to piroxicam, and cross-sensitivity with other NSAIDs and aspirin.

Editorial comments: For additional information, see *ibuprofen*, p. 445.

Potassium Chloride

Brand names: K-Dur, K-Lor, Micro-K, Klor-Con, many others.
Class of drug: Potassium supplement.
Mechanism of action: Replaces potassium lost for various reasons.
Indications/dosage/route: Oral, IV.

• Hypokalemia
  – Adults, children: PO 40–100 mEq divided into 2–4 doses/d. Maximum: 150 mEq/d for adults, 3 mEq/kg for children. Additional dosing is based on serum potassium levels and blood pH.
• Prevention of hypokalemia.
  – Adults, children: PO 16–24 mEq/d in divided doses. Dosage is adjusted based on serum potassium levels. Normal serum potassium level is 3.5–5.0 mEq/L.
• Potassium replacement
  – Adults, children: IV 10–15 mEq/h. Maximum: 400 mEq/d.
• Adults: PO 40–100 mEq/d.

Adjustment of dosage

• Kidney disease: Use with caution. Reduce dose.
• Liver disease: None.
• Elderly: Reduce doses relative to decreased creatinine clearance.
• Pediatric: Safety and effectiveness of oral preparations are not fully established.

Food: Oral doses should be taken with or after meals.

Pregnancy: Category C.

Lactation: Does not appear in breast milk. Safe to use.

Contraindications: Hyperkalemia, severe kidney disease, aneuria, acute dehydration, Addison's disease, hyper- or hypokalemic form of periodic paralysis, use of solid oral form in GI obstruction and/or esophageal obstruction (intrinsic or extrinsic).

Warnings/precautions

- Use with caution in patients with cardiac or renal disease, dysphagia, esophageal compression from left atrial enlargement.
- Do not give immediately after surgery unless urine flow is established.
- Gastric acid intestinal ulceration and bleeding may occur with controlled-release potassium agents.
- It may be difficult for a patient who has esophageal compression from left atrial enlargement to swallow tablets and capsules. Such patients should be prescribed potassium preparations that can be dissolved in liquid or are in liquid form.
- Provide patient with printed information describing symptoms of hypo- and hyperkalemia. Inform patient of foods and other substances that are high in potassium.

Advice to patient

- Do not use potassium-containing salt substitutes without consulting treating physician.
- Do not use potassium-containing salt substances if taking a potassium-sparing diuretic such as spironolactone or triamterene.
- Limit intake of high-potassium foods: Brussels sprouts, spinach, tomato juice, celery, citrus juices, bananas, raisins, nuts.
- Patient should ingest potassium-rich foods once potassium supplementation is discontinued if increased intake is required. Such foods include the following: citrus juices, apricots, bananas, raisins, nuts. It may be necessary to have a dietitian work with the patient to ensure the proper dietary regimen.

Adverse reactions

- Common: nausea, vomiting, abdominal pain, diarrhea.
- Serious: hyperkalemia, arrhythmias, cardiac arrest, respiratory paralysis, GI ulceration, bleeding and perforation.

Clinically important drug interaction: Drugs that increase toxicity of potassium chloride: potassium-sparing diuretics, ACE inhibitors, salt substitute containing potassium, excessive potassium-containing foods, drugs containing potassium.

Parameters to monitor

• Serum potassium level. Maintain between 3.5 and 5.0 mg/L.

• Signs and symptoms of hypokalemia: U wave on ECG, arrhythmias, polyurea.

• Signs and symptoms of hyperkalemia: fatigue, muscle weakness, irregular heartbeat, paresthesias, dyspnea, depressed ST segments, prolonged QT segments, widened QRS complex, loss of P waves. Treatment of overdose (serum potassium >6.5 mEq/L): Discontinue administration of potassium and administer sodium bicarbonate 50–100 mEq IV infusion over 5 minutes. Repeat after 10–15 minutes if ECG abnormalities persist. For patients not on digitalis, administer calcium gluconate or other calcium salt: infuse 0.5–1 g IV over 2-minute period. Also administer glucose and insulin by IV infusion: 3 g glucose with 1 unit regular insulin. Administer sodium polystyrene sulfonate, hemodialysis, or peritoneal dialysis. Institute such procedures to remove potassium from the body.

• Signs and symptoms of toxicity: severe vomiting, abdominal pain, GI distention, bleeding. Drug should be discontinued under such conditions.

• Kidney function periodically: BUN, serum creatinine, serum pH, intake and output of fluids.

• Symptoms of adrenal insufficiency or extensive tissue breakdown.

• Serum magnesium levels. Hypomagnesemia should be corrected prior to administration of potassium for replacement purpose.

Editorial comments

• Oral replacement therapy for hypokalemia is preferable to parenteral. Daily potassium requirement is 2–3 mEq/kg, maximum 80–120 mEq.

• Solutions containing concentrations of 1.5 or 2mEq/mL must not be administered in undiluted form as these can cause fatalities.

Physician should be aware that such concentrated solutions have a black cap on the vial or black stripes around the constriction; such products are labeled with the warning to dilute before administration. The concentration to be administered is limited to 40 mEq/L.

• The following conditions of hypokalemia require use of different potassium salts: If hypokalemia is associated with alkalosis, potassium chloride should be used. If acidosis is present, the following salts of potassium should be used: bicarbonate, acetate, gluconate, citrate.

Potassium Iodide

Brand name: SSKI.
Class of drug: Cation, mineral.
Mechanism of action: Inhibits thyroid secretion, decreases viscosity of mucus.
Indication/dosage/route: Oral only.
• Preoperative for thyroidectomy
  – Adults, children: 50–250 mg q8h, 10–14 days before surgery.
• Thyrotoxicosis.
  – Adults, children: 300–500 mg q8h.
  – Infants <1 year: 150–250 mg q8h.
• Lugol's solution
  – 1 mL in water t.i.d.
• Expectorant
  – Children: 60–250 mg q6–8h. Maximum single dose: 500 mg.
  – Adults: 300–650 mg 2–4 times/d.
Adjustment of dosage
• Kidney disease: Decrease dose.
• Liver disease: None.
• Elderly: None.
• Pediatric: See above.

Onset of Action	Peak Effect	Duration
24–48 h	10–15 d	—

Food: Take with food or milk. Dilute with large quantity of fluids, eg, water, milk, fruit juice. Use at least 8 oz of fluid.

Pregnancy: Category D.

Lactation: Appears in breast milk. Considered compatible by American Academy of Pediatrics.

Contraindications: Hypersensitivity to iodine, hyperkalemia, tuberculosis, active bronchitis, pulmonary edema, GI obstruction, renal failure.

Warnings/precautions
- May contain sulfite. Warn patient if allergic.
- May downregulate thyroid hormone production, leading to hypothyroidism.

Advice to patient: Use two forms of birth control including hormonal and barrier methods.

Adverse reactions
- Common: GI upset, acne.
- Serious: Urticaria, angioedema, hypothyroidism with goiter.

Clinically important drug interaction: Potassium iodide increases effects/toxicity of antithyroid drugs (methimazole, propylthiouracil), potassium-sparing diuretics, ACE inhibitors, potassium supplements.

Parameters to monitor
- Signs and symptoms of iodism: metallic taste, skin lesions, GI upset.
- Symptoms of hypothyroidism: weight gain, lethargy, hair loss, hirsuitism.
- Monitor serum potassium level periodically.

Pralidoxime

Brand name: Protopam chloride.

Class of drug: Antidote for organophosphate cholinesterase poisoning as well as overdose from drugs used to treat myasthenia gravis.

Mechanism of action: Pralidoxime reactivates organophosphate inhibited cholinesterase.

Indications/dosage/route: IV only.

• Organophosphate poisoning
  – Adults: IV 1–2 g over 15–30 minutes. Repeat in 1–2 hours if muscle weakness is not reversed. Repeat in 10–12 hours after first or second dose if needed.
  – Children: IV 20–40 mg/kg over 15–30 minutes. Repeat in 1 hour if muscle weakness is not reversed. Repeat in 10–12 hours after first or second dose if needed.

Adjustment of dosage

• Kidney disease: Reduce dose because of decreased creatinine clearance.
• Liver disease: None.
• Elderly: Give reduced dose because of decreased creatinine clearance.
• Pediatric: See above.

Food: Not applicable.

Pregnancy: Category C.

Lactation: No data available. Best to avoid.

Contraindications: Hypersensitivity to praldoxime (relative contraindication), poisoning with inorganic phosphates, phosphorus, organic phosphates that are not cholinesterase inhibitors.

Warnings/precautions: May precipitate myasthenic crises when used for treatment of overdose of antimyasthenic drugs (neostigmine, ambenonium, pyridostigmine). Use cautiously in this setting.

Adverse reactions

• Common: pain at injection site, visual disturbances, nausea, dizziness, hypertension, tachycardia, muscle weakness.
• Serious: anaphylaxis.

Clinically important drug interactions: Drugs that increase effects/toxicity of pralidoxime: morphine, theophyline, succinylcholine, reserpine, phenothiazines, skeletal muscle relaxants, barbiturates.

Parameters to monitor
• Vital signs during IV administration. Continue monitoring for at least 24 hours after drug administration.
• Serum cholinesterase levels before giving pralidoxime.
• ECG during administration of pralidoxime to assess whether heart block has occurred because of the organophosphate poisoning.

Editorial comments
• When pralidoxime is administered for a suspected organophosphate poisoning, the following principles should be observed:
  1. Treatment should begin immediately.
  2. Measurements of para-nitrophenol in the urine as well as plasma and RBC cholinesterase level are used to guide therapy. RBC cholinesterase <50% of normal is considered diagnostic.
  3. Atropine 2–6 mg should be given IV or IM q5–50min for patients demonstrating overt muscarinic effects, eg, dyspnea, cough, bronchospasm, salivation. Continue until all symptoms subside.
  4. Some degree of anticholinergic action by atropine should be maintained for at least 48 hours.
  5. It may be necessary to administer additional doses of pralidoxime q3–8h for several days.
• It should be recognized that pralidoxime is not very effective against the muscarinic effects of organophosphate poisoning. It is primarily effective against the nicotinic manifestations. Accordingly, it must be administered with atropine to block the muscarinic symptoms directly, particularly within the respiratory and cardiovascular centers in the CNS.
• Pralidoxime may be given IM or SC in patients with pulmonary edema or when IV administration is not feasible, generally in conjunction with atropine. Patients should be observed for 1–3 days after poisoning episode for recurrence of symptoms.

Pravastatin

Brand name: Pravachol.

Class of drug: Antilipidemic agent.

Mechanism of action: Inhibits HMG-CoA reductase enzyme. Reduces total LDL cholesterol, serum triglyceride levels. There is little if any effect on serum HDL levels.

Indications/dosage/route: Oral only.

– Adults: Initial: 10–20 mg h.s. Maintenance: 10–40 mg h.s.

– Elderly: 10 mg h.s. Maintenance: ≤20 mg/d.

Adjustment of dosage

• Kidney disease: 10 mg/d.

• Liver disease: 10 mg/d.

• Elderly: See above.

• Pediatric: Safety and efficacy have not been established.

Pregnancy: Category X. Contraindicated.

Lactation: Appears in breast milk. Contraindicated.

Contraindications: Hypersensitivity to statins, active liver disease or unexplained persistent elevations of serum transaminase, pregnancy, lactation.

Editorial comments

For additional information, see *lovastatin*, p. 543.

Prazosin

Brand name: Minipress.

Class of drug: α-adrenergic blocker antihypertensive agent.

Mechanism of action: Blocks α_1-adrenergic receptors, resulting in decreased BP.

Indications/dosage/route: Oral only.

• Hypertension

– Adults, initial: 1 mg b.i.d. or t.i.d. Maintenance: 6–15 mg/d 2 or 3 divided doses. Maximum: 40 mg/d.

– Children: 0.25–0.5 mg b.i.d. or t.i.d.

– Concomitant therapy with a diuretic or other antihypertensive drug: reduce dose initially and titrate up until desired effect is produced.

Adjustment of dosage
- Kidney disease: None.
- Liver disease: None.
- Elderly: Use with caution.
- Pediatric: See above.

Onset of Action	Peak Effect	Duration
2 h	1–3 h	6–12 h

Food: Take with meals or milk to minimize GI upset.
Pregnancy: Category C.
Lactation: Present in breast milk. Best to avoid.
Contraindications: Hypersensitivity to prazosin and other quinazoline drugs (doxazosin and terazosin).

Warnings/precautions
- Use with caution in patients with pulmonary embolism, aortic and mitral valve stenosis.
- Syncope may occur with first dose because of orthostatic hypotension.
- Use with caution when adding another antihypertensive agent to this drug or adding this drug to another antihypertensive regimen to avoid rapid fall in BP.

Advice to patient
- Avoid driving and other activities requiring mental alertness or that are potentially dangerous until response to drug is known.
- Limit alcohol intake.
- Avoid standing for long periods of time, especially during hot weather.
- Take first dose at bedtime; lie down shortly after first dose.
- Use caution when going from lying down or seated position to standing, especially when dosage is being adjusted.
- Avoid excessive intake of caffeine (regular coffee), theobromine (cocoa, chocolates), and theophylline (regular tea).
- Report significant weight gain or ankle edema to treating physician.
- Notify physician if prolonged penile erection occurs.

Adverse reactions
• Common: dizziness, headache, fatigue.
• Serious: orthostatic hypotension, depression, priapism, angina, arrhythmias, retinopathy, pancreatitis.

Clinically important drug interactions
• Drugs that increase effects/toxicity of α blockers: β blockers, diuretics, verapamil.
• Drugs that decrease effects/toxicity of α blockers: NSAIDs.
• α Blockers decrease effects of clonidine.

Parameters to monitor
• BP for possible first-dose orthostatic hypotension and syncope, particularly when increasing dose.
• Efficacy of treatment for patient with BPH: decreased nocturia, urgency, and frequency of urination.

Prednisolone

Brand names: Hydeltrasol, Pediapred, Prelone, many others.
Class of drug: Corticosteroid, systemic, intra-articular.
Mechanism of action: Inhibits migration of polymorphonuclear leukocytes; stabilizes lysosomal membranes; inhibits production of products of arachidonic acid cascade.
Indications/dosage/route: Oral, IM, IV intra-articular, intralesional.
• Most uses
  – Adults: PO, IM, IV 5–60 mg/d depending on disease.
• Multiple sclerosis
  – Adults: PO Initial: 200 mg/d, 1 week; then 80 mg on alternate days for 1 month.
• Pleurisy of tuberculosis
  – Adults: PO 0.75 mg/kg/d along with antituberculosis therapy.
• Joint diseases
  – Adults, intraarticular, intralesional: 4–100 mg depending on size of joint.

Adjustment of dosage
- Kidney disease: None.
- Liver disease: None.
- Elderly: None.
- Pediatric: Children on long-term therapy must be monitored carefully for growth and development.

Food: Administer with food to minimize GI upset.

Pregnancy: Category B.

Lactation: Steriods appear in breast milk. American Academy of Pediatrics considers prednisone to be compatible with breast-feeding.

Contraindications: Systemic fungal infections.

Editorial comments: For additional information, see *prednisone*, p. 760.

Prednisone

Brand names: Deltasone, Meticorten, Orasone.

Class of drug: Glucocorticoid, antiinflammatory.

Mechanism of action: Inhibits migration of polymorphonuclear leukocytes; stabilizes lysosomal membranes; inhibits production of products of arachidonic acid cascade.

Indications/dosage/route: Oral only. Dosages of corticosteroids are variable. These should be individualized according to the disease being treated and the response of the patient.
- Oral antiinflammatory immunosuppressant
- Acute severe conditions
  - Initial: 5–60 mg/d. Maintenance: 5–10 mg or discontinue altogether until symptoms recur. Larger doses may be required.
- COPD
  - 30–60 mg/d for 1–2 weeks.
- Ophthalmopathy due to Graves' disease
  - 60 mg/d. Maintenance: 20 mg/d.

- Duchenne's muscular dystrophy
  - 0.75–1.5 mg/kg/d.

Adjustment of dosage
- Kidney disease: None.
- Liver disease: None.
- Elderly: None.
- Pediatric: Children on long-term therapy must be monitored carefully for growth and development.

Food: Administer with food to minimize GI upset.

Pregnancy: Category B.

Lactation: Appears in breast milk. Considered compatible by American Academy of Pediatrics.

Contraindications: Systemic fungal, viral, or bacterial infections, Cushing's syndrome.

Warnings/precautions
- Use with caution in patients with diabetes mellitus, cardiovascular disease, hypertension, thrombophlebitis, renal or hepatic insufficiency.
- Skin test patient for tuberculosis before beginning treatment if patient is at high risk.
- For long-term treatment consider alternative-day dosing. However, if the disease flares, may need to return to initial daily dose.
- Observe neonates for signs of adrenal insufficiency if mother has taken steroids during pregnancy.
- Tapering is always required when administration of a steroid is stopped. A variety of procedures for tapering after long-term therapy have been suggested. For example, taper dose by 5 mg/wk until 10 mg/d is reached. Then 2.5 mg/wk until therapy is discontinued or lowest dosage giving relief is reached. Longer tapering periods may be required for some patients. Adrenal insufficiency may persist for up to 1 year.
- Attempt dose reduction periodically to determine if disease can be controlled at a lower dose. When every-other-day therapy is initiated, twice the daily dose should be administered on alternate days in the morning.
- Check whether patient is allergic to tartrazine.

Advice to patient

- It is best to take steroid medication before 9 a.m.
- Adhere to dosing schedule and do not increase dose or time interval between recommended doses without consulting physician.
- Maintain a salt-restricted diet high in potassium. Consume citrus fruits and bananas for extra potassium.
- Pay attention to foot care and report if easy bruising and skin abrasions are experienced.
- Use caution during excessive physical activity if being treated for arthritis. Because the drug may decrease joint pain, you may feel an exaggerated sense of security concerning the effects of too-vigorous exercise. Permanent damage could result.
- Use OTC medications only with approval from the treating physician.
- Increase intake of calcium and vitamin D to minimize bone loss. Intake of 1500 mg/d calcium and 400 IU vitamin D twice a day is recommended.
- Carry identification card at all times describing disease, treatment regimen, name, address, and telephone number of treating physician.
- Receive vaccinations (particularly live attenuated viruses) only with permission from treating physician.

Adverse reactions

- Common: dyspepsia, appetite stimulation, insomnia, anxiety, fluid retension, cushinoid facies.
- Serious: Cushing-like syndrome, adrenocortical insufficiency, muscle wasting, osteoporosis, immunosuppression with increased susceptibility to infection, potassium loss, glaucoma, cataracts (nuclear, posterior, subcapsular), hyperglycemia, hypercorticism, peptic ulcer, psychosis, insomnia, skin atrophy, thrombosis, seizures, angioneuritic edema. Children: growth suppression, pseudotumor cerebri (reversible papilledema, visual loss, nerve paralysis [abducens or oculomotor]), vascular bone necrosis, pancreatitis.

Clinically important drug interactions

- Drugs that increase effects/toxicity of corticosteroids: broad-spectrum antibiotics, anticholinergics, oral contraceptives, cyclosporine, loop diuretics, thiazide diuretics, NSAIDs, tricyclic antidepressants.
- Drugs that decrease effects of corticosteroids: barbiturates, cholestyramine, ketoconazole, phenytoin, rifampin.
- Corticosteroids increase effects/toxicity of digitalis glycosides, neuromuscular blocking drugs.
- Corticosteroids decrease effects of vaccines and toxoids.

Parameters to monitor

- Serum electrolytes, glucose.
- BP: Check at least twice daily during period of dose adjustment.
- Signs and symptoms of hypokalemia: cardiac arrythmias, flaccid paralysis, tetany, polydipsia.
- Signs and symptoms of adrenal insufficiency: weakness, diarrhea, electrolyte disturbances.
- Perform periodic opthalmoscopic examinations. Long-term use may cause cataracts, glaucoma, secondary fundal or viral infections.
- Signs of infection.
- Fluid and electrolyte balance: Check for salt and water retention. Weigh patient on regular basis.
- Symptoms of peptic ulcer.
- Signs and symptoms of Cushing's syndrome: moon face, obesity, hirsuitism, ecchymoses, hypertension, muscle atrophy, diabetes, cataracts, peptic ulcer, fluid and electrolyte imbalance.
- Rheumatoid arthritis patients: Assess patient's symptoms and x-rays each month for the first 2 months, every 3 months for 6 months after the disease is under control, and every 6 months thereafter.
- Signs and symptoms of drug-induced psychologic disturbances: changes in mood (eg, depression), behavior (aggression) or orientation, agitation, hallucinations, suicidal tendencies, sleep disturbances, lethargy.

Editorial comments

- Corticoid treatment remains challenging for clinicians because of commonly occurring short-term and long-term side effects. With chronic use, adrenal suppression may persist for up to 1 year. These drugs produce accelerated bone reabsorption as well as decreased bone formation, resulting in overall bone loss with chronic use. Individuals <40 years on high-dose therapy are at highest risk for bone loss. Ongoing monitoring is suggested and treatment with bisphosphonates or calcitonin is suggested when decreased bone mineral density occurs.

- There is controversy regarding the use of steroids in patients who have tuberculosis or fungal infections of the skin, cutaneous or systemic viral infections, eg, varicella, herpes simplex of the eye. However, if the infection is being treated with appropriate antimicrobials, antifungals, or antiviral agents, steroid may be prescribed by experienced clinicians.

- This drug is listed without details in the *Physician's Desk Reference*, 54th edition, 2000.

Primidone

Brand names: Mysoline, Myidone, Sertan.
Class of drug: Anticonvulsant, barbiturate analog.
Mechanism of action: Acts as nonspecific CNS depressant. Decreases neuronal excitability by unknown mechanism.
Indications/dosage/route: Oral only.

- Tonic–clonic seizures, focal seizures, psychomotor seizures
  – Adults, children >8 years: 100–125 mg, h.s. Increase by 125–250 mg/d every 3–7 days to maintenance dose of 250–500 mg t.i.d. on day 10. Maximum: 2 g/d.
  – Children <8 years: 50–125 mg, h.s. Increase by 50–125 mg/d every 3–7 days to maintenance dose of 125–250 mg t.i.d. or 10–25 mg/kg/d on day 10.
- Benign essential tremor

– Adults: 750 mg/d, in 3 doses.

Adjustment of dosage

- Kidney disease: Creatinine clearance 50–80 mL/min: administer q8h; creatinine clearance 10–50 mL/min: administer q8–12h; creatinine clearance <10 mL/min: administer q12–24h.
- Liver disease: Use with caution.
- Elderly: Close monitoring advised; dose adjusted accordingly.
- Pediatric: See above.

Food: Administer with food.

Pregnancy: Category D.

Lactation: Appears in breast milk. American Academy of Pediatrics advises caution with breastfeeding.

Contraindications: Hypersensitivity to primidone or phenobarbital, porphyria.

Warnings/precautions: Use with caution in patients with kidney or liver disease, pulmonary insufficiency.

Advice to patients

- Use two forms of birth control including hormonal and barrier methods.
- Avoid driving and other activities requiring mental alertness or that are potentially dangerous until response to drug is known.
- Avoid alcohol and other CNS depressants such as opiate analgesics and sedatives (eg, diazepam) when taking this drug.
- Change position slowly, in particular from recumbent to upright, to minimize orthostatic hypotension. Sit at the edge of the bed for several minutes before standing and lie down if feeling faint or dizzy. Avoid hot showers or baths and standing for long periods. Male patients with orthostatic hypotension may be safer urinating while seated on the toilet rather than standing.
- Carry identification card at all times describing disease, treatment regimen, name, address, and telephone number of treating physician.
- Do not discontinue drug without consulting treating physician.

Adverse reactions

- Common: drowsiness, diplopia, nausea, vomiting, ataxia, sedation, headache.

- Serious: leukopenia, lymphoma-like syndrome, red cell hypoplasia, megaloblastic anemia responsive to folate, lupus-like syndrome, impotence.

Clinically important drug interactions

- Drugs that increase effects/toxicity of primidone: alcohol, phenytoin, isoniazid, valproic acid.
- Drugs that decrease effects/toxicity of primidone: succinimides (eg, ethosuximide).
- Primidone decreases effects/toxicity of oral contraceptives, oral anticoagulants, corticosteroids, estrogens, methadone, β blockers, metronidazole, nifedipine, quinidine, theophylline, griseofulvin, carbamazepine.

Parameters to monitor

- Signs of allergic reaction to phenobarbital (a metabolite of primidone).
- Signs and symptoms of folic acid deficiency (fatigue, weakness, mental dysfunction, neuropathy, megaloblastic anemia). Administer folic acid if these symptoms occur.
- Signs and symptoms of bone marrow depression.
- Monitor blood levels closely. Therapeutic level is 5–12 µg/mL in adults, 7–10 µg/mL in children >5 years.
- Signs of hypersensitivity reactions.
- Signs and symptoms of paradoxical excitement.

Editorial comments: Primidone is used alone or in combination with other anticonvulsants.

Probenecid

Brand names: Benemid, Probalan.
Class of drug: Uricosuric agent; adjunct to antibiotic use.
Mechanism of action: Uricosuric action: inhibits active tubular reabsorption of uric acid. Adjunctive to antibiotic therapy: inhibits

tubular secretion of weak organic acids including penicillins, cephalosporins, and fluoroquinolones.

Indications/dosage/route: Oral only.

- Adjunct to antibiotic therapy (penicillins, cephalosporins)
  - Adults, children >14 years: 500 mg q.i.d.
  - Children 2–14 years: 25 mg/kg/d. Maintenance: 40 mg/kg/d, divided q.i.d.
- Hyperuricemia associated with gout; prevention of recurrence of gouty arthritis; hyperuricemia secondary to thiazide therapy.
  - Adults: 250 mg b.i.d. Maintenance: 500 mg b.i.d. Maximum: 2–3 g/d.

Adjustment of dosage

- Kidney disease: Avoid if creatinine clearance <50 mL/min.
- Liver disease: None.
- Elderly: Lower doses suggested.
- Pediatric: Contraindicated in children <2 years.

Onset of Blockade of Penicillin Excretion	Peak Effect	Duration
2 h	—	8 h

Food: Take with food or antacid. Patient should be on a low-urate (low protein) diet.

Pregnancy: Category B.

Lactation: No data available; best to avoid.

Contraindications: Hypersensitivity to probenicid, blood dyscrasias, acute gout, uric acid kidney stones, children <2 years, concomitant administration of salicylates.

Warnings/precautions

- Probenecid may initially cause an exacerbation of gout. If this occurs, colchicine or another appropriate agent should be administered.
- Probenecid may cause a hypersensitivity reaction in individuals who have an allergy to sulfa drugs or other sulfonamides.
- Probenecid should not be used with antibiotics in patients who have severe renal impairment (creatinine clearance <50 mL/min).

- Therapy should not be started with probenecid until an acute attack of gout has subsided.

Advice to patient
- Do not discontinue drug without consulting treating physician.
- Drink large quantities of fluid, 8–10 glasses/d.
- Avoid OTC products containing aspirin or other salicylates.
- Diabetic patient should use glucose oxidase method (KETO-diastix Test Tape) to monitor urinary glucose.
- Avoid regular coffee.
- Avoid alcohol.

Adverse reactions
- Common: headache, nausea, vomiting.
- Severe: hemolytic anemia (especially in G6PD deficiency), aplastic anemia, anaphylaxis, hepatic necrosis, nephrotic syndrome, uric acid stones.

Clinically important drug interactions
- Probenecid increases effects/toxicity of penicillins, cephalosporins, sulfonamides, fluoroquinolones, sufonylureas, dapsone, methotrexate, nitrofurantoin, zidovudine, acyclovir, indomethacin, acetaminophen, lorazepam, rifampin.
- Probenecid decreases effects/toxicity of loop diuretics.
- Drugs that decrease effects of probenecid: pyrazinamide, salicylates.

Parameters to monitor
- Kidney function.
- Uric acid levels. Adjust dose of probenecid to the lowest one that maintains uric acid levels within the normal range (<5 mg/dL).
- Signs and symptoms of uric acid stones. Maintain sufficient hydration and alkalinization of urine.
- Symptoms of probenecid toxicity: headache, nausea, vomiting, anorexia. Decrease dose or discontinue if these signs of toxicity persist.
- Signs of hypersensitivity reactions.

Editorial comments: The following are recommended combinations of probenecid with antibiotics for treatment of selected diseases:

- Gonorrhea: probenecid 1 g immediately before 4.8×10^6 units penicillin G, divided into 2 doses.
- Pelvic inflammatory disease: cefoxitin IM 2 g plus probenecid PO 1 g concomitantly.
- Disseminated gonococcal infection: probenecid 1 g immediately before 10×10^6 units penicillin G/d for 3 days or until symptom resolution. May follow with ampicillin 500 mg q7d.
- Neurosyphilis: aqueous procaine penicillin G IM $2–4 \times 10^6$ units/d plus probenecid 500 mg q.i.d. both given for 10–14 days.

Procainamide

Brand names: Pronestyl, Procanbid, Promine.
Class of drug: Class Ia antiarrhythmic agent.
Mechanism of action: Primarily increases the effective refractory period of atrial and ventricular sodium-dependent tissue.
Indications/dosage/route: Oral, IV, IM.
- Life-threatening ventricular tachycardia—adults
  - IV: 50–200 mg q5min, slow IV push; effective loading dose 500–1000 mg, followed by 1–6 mg/min.
  - IM: 50 mg/kg, divided doses q3–6h during surgery.
  - PO: 50 mg/kg/d, divided doses q3h.
- Prevention of ventricular tachycardia—
  - Adults: Initial PO: 50 mg/kg/d divided doses, q3h. Maximum: 1–1.5 g q4–6h.
- Dosages suggested for children
  - PO: 15–50 mg/kg/d divided doses, q4–6h. Maximum: 4 g/d.
  - IM: Not recommended.
  - IV: Loading dose: 3–6 mg/kg over 5 minutes. Maintenance: 20–80 µg/kg/min. Maximum: 100 mg/dose or 2 g/d.

Adjustment of dosage
- Kidney disease: Creatinine clearance 10–50 mL/min; administer q6–12h; creatinine clearance <10 mL/min: administer q8–24h.

- Liver disease: Reduce dose by 50%.
- Elderly: May require reduced dosage. Serum levels should be monitored as metabolism is variable in elderly patients.
- Pediatric: Dosage guidelines have not been established. For suggested dosage see above.

	Onset of Action	Peak Effect	Duration
IM	10–30 min	15–30 min	≤6 h
Oral	5–10 min	60–90 min	≤12 h
IV	Immediate	Immediate	≤6 h

Food: Oral dose should be taken with full glass of water on empty stomach, ie, 1 hour before or 2 hours after meals.

Pregnancy: Category C.

Lactation: Appears in breast milk. Considered compatible by American Academy of Pediatrics.

Contraindications: Hypersensitivity to procaine and ester-type local anesthetics, complete heart block in absence of pacemaker, first-degree AV block after procainamide, systemic lupus erythematosus, Torsade de pointes, long QT syndrome, sulfite or tartrazine allergy (see Warnings/Precautions).

Warnings/precautions

- Use with caution in patients with heart failure, bundle branch heart block, kidney or liver disease, bone marrow insufficiency, digitalis intoxication, other concurrent antiarrhythmic agents, renal insufficiency, myasthenia gravis.
- Because of procainamide's ability to enhance AV conduction, simultaneous administration of an AV blocking agent is necessary (eg, β blocker, calcium channel blocker, or digitalis).
- Use cardioversion or digitalize a patient having atrial flutter or fibrillation before administering procainamide; this reduces the possibility of a sudden rise in ventricular rate.
- *N*-Acetylprocainamide is an active metabolite and promotes most of the toxicity as it tends to accumulate over time. Its level must be closely monitored.

- Some preparations of procainamide contain tartrazine and/or sulfite. Such preparations should be avoided in patients who have demonstrated previous hypersensitivity reactions to these substances.
- Use with caution for treating arrhythmias from digitalis toxicity.

Advice to patient

- Do not double dose if one is missed but take the missed dose as soon as remembered (within 2 hours).
- Avoid driving and other activities requiring mental alertness or that are potentially dangerous until response to drug is known.
- Take OTC preparations only with approval from treating physician.

Adverse reactions

- Common: dizziness, diarrhea.
- Serious: **lupus-like syndrome**, ventricular fibrillation, bone marrow depression, AV block, widened QRS complex, QT prolongation, pericarditis, confusion, depression, hemolytic anemia, pleural effusion.

Clinically important drug interactions

- Drugs that increase effects/toxicity of procainamide: lidocaine, amiodarone, β blockers, antihypertensives, nitrates, antihistamines, antidepressants, atropine, phenothiazines, cimetidine, ranitidine, quinidine, trimethoprim, pimozide.
- Procainamide increases effects/toxicity of neuromuscular blocking agents, class IA or III antiarrthymics, phenothiazines, macrolide antibiotics, ketoconazoles, propulcid, lidocaine, quinidine.

Parameters to monitor

- CBC with differential and platelets every 2 weeks during the first 3 months of therapy. If leukopenia occurs, procainamide may have to be discontinued.
- Liver enyzmes.
- Cardiovascular status continuously during IV administration. Toxicity would be manifested by a widening of the QRS complex by 50% and a drop in BP >15 mm Hg.

- Antinuclear antibody periodically, particularly if administration is prolonged. If titer increases steadily, drug should be discontinued.
- Signs of lupus: fever, chills, pain when breathing, joint pain, skin rash.
- Serum procainamide level and level of *N*-acetylprocainamide, the major procainamide metabolite. Toxicity may occur if procainamide levels are in the range 8–16 µg/mL.
- Signs and symptoms of toxicity: confusion, drowsiness, tachyarrhythmias, dizziness.
- Signs of hypotension. Administer phenylephrine or norepinephrine.

Editorial comments

- Procainamide has a low therapeutic index. An acute dose of 5 g in an adult causes toxicity. Toxicity may be reversed by the following interventions: IV fluids, anticonvulsants, vasopressors, antiarrhythmics (lidocaine can be ideal for proarrhythmia because it shortens the action potential duration).
- Treat wide QRS intervals or hypotension by administering sodium bicarbonate and stopping or slowing the infusion.
- Procainamide can be administered and coadministered to patients in whom lidocaine has been unsuccessful or poorly tolerated for the treatment of ventricular tachycardia.
- Drugs levels of procainamide and *N*-acetylprocainamide, its active metabolite, should be monitored daily to prevent toxicity.
- Procainamide is an ideal IV drug to administer to patients with wide QRS complex tachycardia where diagnostic delineation of supraventricular versus ventricular tachycardia is not feasible and hemodynamically the patient is not in need of emergent cardioversion. Procainamide's usefulness is due to its blocking effect on sodium channels in atrial and ventricular fibers. In atrial fibrillation and flutter of less than 48 hours' duration, it has a 60% efficacy of pharmacologic conversion. Its proarrhythmic effects are 1–2%.
- Reduction of procainamide dosage should be done only after consulting a cardiologist or clinical electrophysiologist.

Procaine

Brand name: Novocaine.
Class of drug: Local and regional anesthetic.
Mechanism of action: Reversibly inhibits initiation and conduction of nerve impulses near site of injection.
Indications/dosage/route: Local injection only.
• Infiltration anesthesia
  – Adults: Total: 350–600 mg, with or without epinephrine 1:200,000.
  – Children: Maximum: 15/mg/kg using 0.5% solution.
• Peripheral nerve block
  – Adults: Total: 1000 mg, with or without epinephrine 1:200,000 or 1:1,000,000.
• Spinal anesthesia
  – Dilute stock solution (10% procaine) with sterile saline, sterile distilled water, or spinal fluid.
• Anesthesia of perineum
  – Adults: Total: 50 mg (0.5 mL 10% procaine plus 0.5 mL diluent).
• Anesthesia of perineum and lower extremities
  – Total: 100 mg (1 mL 10% procaine plus 1 mL diluent).
• Anesthesia up to costal margin
  – Total: 200 mg (2 mL 10% procaine plus 1 mL diluent).
Adjustment of dosage
• Kidney disease: No information available.
• Liver disease: No information available.
• Elderly: None.
• Pediatric: See above.
Food: No applicable.
Pregnancy: Category C.
Lactation: No data available. Use with caution.
Contraindications: Hypersensitivity for ester-type local anesthetic (eg, tetracaine).

Warnings/precautions
- Use local anethetics plus vasoconstrictor (eg, epinephrine, nor-epinephrine) with caution in patients with peripheral vascular disease, hypertension, administration of general anesthetics. Use local anesthetics with or without vasoconstrictor with caution in patients with severe liver disease. Use with extreme caution for lumbar and caudal epidural anesthesia, in patients with spinal deformities, pre-existing neurologic disease, severe uncontrolled hypotension, septicemia.
- Epidural anesthesia: A test dose of the local anesthetic should be given first before the full dose is administered to ensure that the catheter is not within a blood vessel. The test dose should include 10–15 µg epinephrine. Any increase in heart rate and systolic pressure within 45 seconds (the epinephrine response) would indicate that the injection is intravascular.
- Local anesthetics can trigger familial malignant hyperthermia. Symptoms of this condition include tachycardia, labile BP, tachypnea, muscle rigidity. The necessary means must be available to manage this condition (dantrolene, oxygen, supportive measures).
- A local anesthetic containing a vasoconstrictor should be injected with great caution into areas of the body supplied by end-organ arteries (nose, ears, penis, digits).

Editorial comments
- Procaine is not widely used as a local anesthetic today because of its short duration of action and tendency to cause contact dermatitis.
- This drug is not listed in the *Physicians' Desk Reference*, 54th edition, 2000.
- For additional information, see *bupivacaine*, p. 113.

Prochlorperazine

Brand name: Compazine.

Class of drug: Phenothiazine antipsychotic (neuroleptic), antiemetic.

Mechanism of action: Antagonizes dopamine at dopaminergic receptors in CNS neurons.

Indications/dosage/route: Oral, IV, IM, suppository.

• Severe nausea and vomiting
  – Adults: PO 5–40 mg t.i.d. or q.i.d.
  – Adults: Suppository 25 mg b.i.d.
  – Adults: IM 5–10 mg. Repeat q3–4h as needed.
  – Adults: IV 2.5–10 mg, slow injection or infusion. Maximum: 10 mg/dose, 40 mg/d.
  – Children, oral or rectal: 20–29 lb, 2.5 mg, 1 or 2 times/d; 36–39 lb, 2.5 mg b.i.d. or q.i.d.; 40–85 lb, 5 mg b.i.d.
  – Children 2–12 years: IM 0.06 mg/lb.

• Severe nausea and vomiting associated with surgery
  – Adults: IM 5–10 mg 1–2 hours before induction of anesthesia.
  – Adults: IV 5–10 mg, slow injection or infusion, 15–30 minutes before surgery. Maximum: 10 mg/dose, 5 mg/min.

• Anxiety disorder, severe
  – Adults: PO 5 mg t.i.d. or q.i.d.

• Psychotic disorders, mild
  – Adults: 5–10 mg t.i.d. or q.i.d.

• Psychotic disorders, moderate to severe
  – Adults: PO 10 mg t.i.d. or q.i.d. Maximum: 50–75 mg/d.
  – Adults: IM 10–20 mg as single injection. If needed, give 10–20 mg q4–6h.

• Psychotic disorders, children
  – Children 2–12 years: PO, rectal 2.5 mg b.i.d. or q.i.d. Maximum: 10 mg on first day.
  – Children 2–5 years: Maximum: 10 mg/d.
  – Children 6–12 years: Maximum: 25 mg/d.

Adjustment of dosage

• Kidney disease: Use with caution. Guidelines not available.
• Liver disease: Use with caution. Guidelines not available.
• Elderly: Use lower doses, increase dosage more gradually.
• Pediatric: See above. This drug should not be used in children <2 years.

Food: No data available.

Pregnancy: Category C.

Lactation: Probably appears in breast milk. Considered compatible with breastfeeding by American Academy of Pediatrics in 1983.

Contraindications: Hypersensitivity to phenothiazines, concurrent use of high-dose CNS depressants (alcohol, barbituates, benzodiazepines, narcotics), CNS depression, comatose state, pediatric surgery.

Warnings/precautions

• Use with caution in patients with cardiovascular, liver, kidney disease, glaucoma, chronic respiratory disorders, exposure to extreme heat, organophosphate insecticides or atropine-type drugs.

• Tardive dyskinesia is a syndrome associated with involuntary movements that occurs frequently after long-term administration of neuroleptic agents. Because this syndrome is potentially irreversible, close monitoring for drug-induced movement disorders is mandatory for all patients. Elderly women appear to be at highest risk. Medication must be discontinued if tardive dyskinesia develops.

• NMS is a potentially fatal symptom complex seen with administration of antipsychotic drugs. Symptoms include fever, muscular rigidity and autonomic instability, including arrhythmias and BP disturbances. Patients with suggestive symptoms must be evaluated immediately. Management includes drug discontinuation, close monitoring, and symptom-directed therapy including administration of dantrolene. Pharmacotherapy for NMS is not standardized at present.

• Make sure patient swallows drug and does not hoard tablets. Suicide attempts by drug overdose may occur even when patient's symptoms appear to be improving.

• Be aware of danger of aspiration of vomitus.

• Some preparations contain tartrazine (FD&C Yellow No. 5). This dye can cause a severe allergic reaction, even an asthmatic attack, in susceptible patients, particularly those who are allergic to aspirin. Prescribe a drug preparation that does not contain this dye for these individuals.

- Use lower doses initially in patients with prior insulin reactions and those receiving electroconvulsive therapy.
- Be aware that this drug, because of its antiemetic action, may obscure diagnosis and treatment of overdose of other drugs as well as diagnosis and treatment of such conditions as Reye's syndrome and intestinal obstruction.
- IM injections should be made slowly in upper quadrant of buttocks; avoid SC injection.

Advice to patient

- Avoid driving and other activities requiring mental alertness or that are potentially dangerous until response to drug is known.
- Patient and family members should avoid contact of the drug with skin or eyes as this can cause contact dermatitis or conjunctivitis.
- Discard if drug solution is any color other than yellow.
- Keep up compliance with dosing regimen and do not increase dose without approval of treating physician.
- Do not take any other medication including OTC products without approval from treating physician.
- Swallow enteric coated tablets whole; do not crush or chew.
- This drug may make you feel cold. If this occurs, use extra blankets only, not hot water bottle, heating pad, or electric blanket.
- Do not expose yourself to very high temperatures, ie, above 105°F (hot baths, sun lamps, sauna, whirlpool) as the drug may cause heat stroke. Symptoms of this condition include red, dry skin, dyspnea, strong pulse, body temperature above 105°F (40.6°C). Contact physician immediately.
- If you are experiencing dry mouth rinse with warm water frequently, chew sugarless gum, suck on ice cube, or use artificial saliva. Carry out meticulous oral hygiene (floss teeth daily).
- Do not stop taking drug abruptly as this may precipitate a withdrawal reaction, particularly extrapyramidal symptoms. Other symptoms of withdrawal include abdominal discomfort, dizziness, headache, tachycardia, insomnia. Reduce dosage gradually over a period of several weeks, eg, 10–25% q2wk.

- Be aware that your skin may turn yellow-brown to grayish-purple. This is a temporary condition.

Adverse reactions

- Common: Drowsiness.
- Serious: **hypotension, postural hypotension (IV injection), arrhythmias,** hepatitis, bone marrow depression, extrapyramidal reactions, dystonias, amenorrhea, galactorrhea, gynecomastia, tardive dyskinesia, NMS, hypersensitivity reaction, seizures, agranulocytosis, corneal and lens abnormalities, pigmentary retinopathy.

Clinically important drug interactions

- Drugs that increase effects/toxicity of phenothiazines: CNS depressants (barbiturates, opioids, general anesthetics, benzodiazepines, alcohol), quinidine, procainamide, anticholinergic agents, MAO inhibitors, antihistamines, nitrates, β blockers, tricyclic antidepressants, lithium, pimozide.
- Drugs that decrease effects/toxicity of phenothiazines: methyldopa, carbamazepine, barbiturates, aluminum- and magnesium-containing antacids, heavy smoking, amphetamines.
- Phenothiazines increase effects/toxicity of hydantoins.
- Phenothiazines decrease effects/toxicity of centrally acting antihypertensive drugs (guanethidine, clonidine, methyldopa), bromocriptine, levodopa.

Parameters to monitor

- CBC with differential and platelets, liver enzymes, serum BUN and creatinine.
- Observe patient receiving parenteral injection closely for hypotensive reaction. Patient should remain in recumbent position for at least 30 minutes following injection. If hypotensive reaction occurs, administer norepinephrine or phenylephrine; epinephrine is contraindicated under these conditions as it might cause a sudden drop in BP (vasomotor reversal). Recovery usually occurs spontaneously within 0.5 to 2 hours.
- Signs and symptoms of GI complications including fecal impaction and constipation. Urge patient to increase fluid intake and bulk-containing food.

- Signs and symptoms of fluid extravasation from IV injection.
- Signs and symptoms of bronchial pneumonia resulting from suppression of cough reflex. This may be a particular problem in the elderly and severely depressed patient.
- Signs and symptoms of tardive dyskinesia: Uncontrolled rhythmic movements of face, mouth, tongue, jaw, protrusion of tongue, uncontrolled rapid or wormlike movements of tongue, chewing movements. At first indication of tardive dyskinesia—vermicular movements of tongue—withdraw drug immediately. Tardive dyskinesia generally develops several months after treatment with a phenothiazine. Patient should be monitored every 6 months for possible development of tardive dyskinesia.
- Monitor blood and urine glucose in diabetic or prediabetic patients on high-dose drug for loss of diabetes control. If control is lost, it may be necessary to discontinue the drug and substitute another.
- Signs of agranulocytosis.
- Signs and symptoms of cholestatic jaundice: fever, flu-like symptoms, pruritus, jaundice. These effects may occur between the second and fourth weeks of treatment.
- Signs and symptoms of overdose: somnolence, coma. Treat by gastric lavage and patent airway. Do not induce vomiting.
- Ophthalmologic status, particularly in patients with glaucoma. Adverse ocular reactions include increased intraocular pressure, particle deposition in the cornea and lens, which may lead to venticular opacities, blurred vision, photophobia, ptosis.
- Signs of hypersensitivity reactions.
- Efficacy of treatment: improvement in mental status, including orientation, mood, general behavior, improved sleep, reduction in auditory and visual hallucinations, disorganized thinking, blunted affect, agitation.

Editorial comments: Phenothiazines have been a mainstay of treatment for psychosis. They have wide-ranging CNS effects and have complex effects on a variety of neurotransmitters. These properties cause frequent and often severe side effects. Because of prominent anticholinergic effects, extrapyramidal symptoms are less frequent than for high-potency dopaminergic blocking agents such as haloperidol.

Progesterone

Brand names: Prometrium, Crinone (gel).
Class of drug: Progestational hormone, contraceptive, increases endometrial receptivity for embryo implantation.
Mechanism of action: Inhibits secretion of pituitary gonadotropins (FSH, LH) by positive feedback.
Indications/dosage/route: Oral, IM, vaginal.
• Secondary amenorrhea
  – Adults: PO 400 mg as single daily dose, 10 days. Vaginal gel 4% every other day up to 6 doses; may increase to 8% if ineffective.
• Prevention of endometrial hyperplasia
  – Adults: PO 200 mg as single daily dose in p.m., 12 days.
• Assisted reproduction
  IM, vaginal gel 90 mg once or twice daily. If pregnancy develops, continue up to 10–12 weeks.
Adjustment of dosage
• Kidney disease: None.
• Liver disease: None.
• Elderly: None.
• Pediatric: Safety and efficacy have not been established.
Food: No restrictions.
Pregnancy: Category X (oral). Vaginal gel used for assisted pregnancy technology.
Lactation: Considered compatible by American Academy of Pediatrics.
Contraindications: Hypersensitivity to progestins, history of thrombophlebitis, active thromboembolic disease, cerebral hemorrhage, liver disease, missed abortion, use as diagnostic for pregnancy,

known or suspected pregnancy (first 4 months), undiagnosed vaginal bleeding, carcinoma of the breast, known or suspected genital malignancy.

Warnings/precautions

- Use with caution in patients with respiratory infection, history of depression, epilepsy, migraine, cardiac disease, renal disease, diabetes.
- Cigarette smoking significantly increases risk of cardiac complications and thrombotic events. At highest risk are women >35 years of age, smoking ≥15 cigarettes per day.

Advice to patient

- Weigh yourself twice a week and report to treating physician if there are any unusual changes in weight.
- If you observe a yellowing of skin or eyes, report to treating physician.
- If you experience changes in mental status suggestive of depression, report to treating physician.
- Discontinue medication if you experience sudden headaches or attack of migraine.
- Discontinue drug and notify physician if you miss a period or experience unusual bleeding.
- If you miss a dose, take the missed dose as soon as possible; do not double the next dose.
- If the drug is used as contraceptive and you miss a dose, stop taking and use an alternative method of contraception until period returns.
- Use good hygiene—flossing, gum massages, regular cleaning by dentist—to avoid gum problems.
- Keep an extra month supply of the drug on hand.
- Do not give this medication to anyone else.

Adverse reactions

- Common: irregular or unpredictable menstrual bleeding (spotting), amenorrhea, breakthrough bleeding, infertility for up to 18 months.
- Serious: thromboembolic events, depression, cholestatic jaundice.

Clinically important drug interactions: Drugs that decrease effects/toxicity of progestins: aminoglutethimide, phenytoin, rifampin.

Parameters to monitor
- Liver enzymes, cholesterol (total, LDL, HDL), triglycerides.
- Diabetic patient: Monitor blood glucose closely and adjust antidiabetic medication if necessary.
- Signs and symptoms of thromboembolic or thrombotic disorders: pain in leg, sudden chest pain, shortness of breath, migraine, sudden severe headache, vomiting. Discontinue drug.

Editorial comments
- Patient receiving a progesterone for contraceptive purposes should have a complete physical examination performed with special attention to breasts and pelvic organs as well as a Pap test before treatment and annually thereafter. If a patient experiences persistent or abnormal vaginal bleeding while on this drug, perform diagnostic tests including endometrial sampling, to determine cause.

Promazine

Brand name: Sparine.
Class of drug: Phenothiazine antipsychotic (neuroleptic).
Mechanism of action: Antagonizes dopamine at dopaminergic receptors in CNS neurons.
Indications/dosage/route: Oral, IV, IM (preferred).
- Psychotic disorders
  - Adults: PO 10–200 mg q4–6h. Maximum: 1000 mg/d.
  - Children >12 years: PO 10–25 mg q4–6h.
- Severely agitated patients
  - Adults: IM, continuous IV 50–100 mg. After 30 minutes, additional dose up to 300 mg may be given if needed. Maintenance: 10–200 mg q4–6h. Maximum: 1 g/d.
  - Children >12 years: IM, continuous IV 10–25 mg q4–6h.

Adjustment of dosage
- Kidney disease: Use with caution. Guidelines not available.

- Liver disease: Use with caution. Guidelines not available.
- Elderly: Use lower doses. Increase dosage more gradually.
- Pediatric: See above.

Food: No restrictions.

Pregnancy: Category C.

Lactation: No data available. Avoid breastfeeding.

Contraindications: Hypersensitivity to phenothiazines, concurrent use of high-dose CNS depressants (alcohol, barbituates, benzodiazepines, narcotics), CNS depression, comatose state.

Editorial comments

- Promazine should not be injected intraarterially.
- This drug is not listed in the *Physicians' Desk Reference*, 54th edition, 2000.
- For additional information, see *chlorpromazine*, p. 206.

Promethazine

Brand name: Phenergan.

Class of drug: Phenothiazine antipsychotic (neuroleptic).

Mechanism of action: Antagonizes dopamine at dopaminergic receptors in CNS neurons.

Indications/dosage/route: IM, IV.

- Allergic conditions
  - Adults: IM 25 mg. May be repeated in 2 hours if needed.
  - Children <12 years: IM 12.5 mg.
- Sedation, hospitalized patients
  - Adults: 25–50 mg
- Pre- or postoperative sedation
  - Adults: 25–50 mg along with analgesic or atropine-like drug.
- Nausea and vomiting
  - Adults: 12.5–25 mg; repeat q4h.
- Nausea and vomiting, postoperative

– Adults: IV, IM 12.5–25 mg.
• Obstetrics
  – Adults: IV, IM 50 mg. Repeat at reduced dose once or twice q4h.

Adjustment of dosage
• Kidney disease: Use with caution. Guidelines not available.
• Liver disease: Use at reduced dose in adults. Guidelines not available.
• Elderly: Use lower doses. Increase dosage more gradually.
• Pediatric: See above. Do not use in children showing signs and symptoms of Reye's syndrome or other hepatic disease.

Food: No restriction.
Pregnancy: Category C.
Lactation: Probably appears in breast milk. Potentially toxic to infant. Avoid breastfeeding.
Contraindications: Hypersensitivity to phenothiazines, concurrent use of high-dose CNS depressants (alcohol, barbituates, benzodiazepines, narcotics), CNS depression, comatose state.

Editorial comments
• Use of promethazine in children is limited to prolonged vomiting of known origin.
• For additional information, see *chlorpromazine,* p. 206.

Propafanone

Brand name: Rythmol.
Class of drug: Class Ic antiarrythmic.
Mechanism of action: Slows conduction in AV node, His-Purkinje system, and intraventricular conduction system.
Indications/dosage/route: Oral only.
• Life-threatening ventricular arrhythmia
  – Adults: PO 150 mg q8h. Increase after 3–4 days to 225 mg q8h. Maximum: 900 mg/d.

Adjustment of dosage: Oral only.
- Kidney disease: Consider dose reduction. Monitor carefully for signs of overdose.
- Liver disease: Reduce dose by 70–80%. Monitor carefully for signs of overdose.
- Elderly: Reduce dose. Monitor carefully for signs of overdose.
- Pediatric: Safety and effectiveness have not been established.

Onset of Action	Peak Effect	Duration
1 h	2–3 h	8–12 h

Food: May be taken with or without food.

Pregnancy: Category C.

Lactation: No data available. Potentially toxic to fetus. Avoid breastfeeding.

Contraindications: Hypersensitivity to propafanone, uncontrolled CHF; SA node, AV node, or intraventricular conduction disorders in absence of artificial pacemaker; marked hypotension, bronchospastic disease, electrolyte imbalance.

Warnings/precautions
- Use with caution in patients with kidney or liver disease, heart failure.
- If it is necessary to increase dosage, it should be done at intervals of at least 3–4 days because of the long half-life of the drug.
- Correct preexisting hypo- or hyperkalemia before drug administration.

Advice to patient
- Avoid driving and other activities requiring mental alertness or that are potentially dangerous until response to drug is known.
- Carry identification card at all times describing disease, treatment regimen, name, address, and telephone number of treating physician.

Adverse reactions
- Common: dizziness, altered taste, nausea, vomiting, constipation, headache, fatigue, visual disturbances.
- Serious: Arrhythmias, CHF, elevated antinuclear antibody titers and lupus-like syndrome, exacerbation of myasthenia gravis, agranulocytosis, seizures.

Clinically important drug interactions
- Propafanone increases effects/toxicity of digoxin, β blockers, local anesthetics, warfarin, cyclosporine.
- Drug that decreases effects/toxicity of propafanone: rifampin.

Parameters to monitor
- Cardiovascular status (BP, pulse) using ECG or Holter prior to and periodically.
- Symptoms of CHF.
- Signs and symptoms of toxicity.
- Signs and symptoms of anemia: shortness of breath, dizziness, angina, pale conjunctiva, skin, and nailbeds.
- Symptoms of agranulocytosis.

Editorial comments
- Because propafanone pharmacokintetics are very complex, it is necessary to individualize the dosage for each patient.
- It should be noted that propafanone has a very narrow therapeutic index and that if the serum level is only slightly above the therapeutic range, severe toxicity may occur. Major signs of toxicity may include the following changes in electrocardiogram: increases in PR, QRS, and QT intervals as well as amplitude of T wave. Treatment is supportive, ie, administration of fluids, anticonvulsants, and antiarrhythmics. Type IA agents should not be used to treat cardiotoxicity from propafanone. It may be necessary to institute ventricular pacing.
- Cardiac monitoring should be used during initiation of therapy or if it is necessary to increase doses.
- For acute cardiovascular collapse, the following should be used: atropine, isoprotenerol, pacemaker. Convulsions should be treated with IV diazepam.

- Propafanone, because of its class Ic pharmacokinetics and classification, is not actively used for ventricular arrhythmias following the CAST trial demonstrating poor results of Ic antiarrhythmics in patients with structural heart disease.
- It was originally felt that because of its concomitant β-blocker effect (weak), it might be a useful drug for atrial fibrillation/ atrial flutter suppression and prevention. However, large-scale clinical data are not available for this use. Clinically, propafanone is administered in certain cases of atrial fibrillation because treatment results in simultaneous lengthening of the effective refractory period in atrial tissue and AV nodal blockade.

Propantheline

Brand names: Norpanth, Pro-Banthine, Propanthel.
Class of drug: Cholinergic blocking agent.
Mechanism of action: Blocks acetylcholine effects at muscarinic receptors throughout the body.
Indications/dosage/route: Oral only.
- Hypermotility and spasms of GI tract
  - Adults: 15 mg 30 minutes before meals and 30 mg h.s.
  - Children: 0.375 mg/kg q.i.d.
- Urinary incontinence
  - Adults: 7.5–60 mg 3–5 times/d.
Adjustment of dosage
- Kidney disease: None.
- Liver disease: None.
- Elderly: None.
- Pediatric: See above.
Pregnancy: Category C.
Lactation: No data available. Potentially toxic to infant. Avoid breastfeeding.

Contraindications: Myasthenia gravis, narrow-angle glaucoma, GI obstruction, megacolon, colitis, ulcerative colitis, obstructive uropathy, hypersensitivity to atropine-type compounds (belladonna alkaloids).

Warnings/precautions

- Use with caution in patients with GI infections, chronic biliary disease, CHF, arrhythmias, pulmonary disease, BPH, hyperthyroidism, coronary artery disease, hypertension, seizures, psychosis, spastic paralysis.
- Anticholinergic psychosis can occur in sensitive individuals.
- Elderly may react with agitation and excitement even to small doses of anticholinergic drugs.

Clinically important drug interactions

- Drugs that increase effects/toxicity of systemic anticholinergics: phenothiazines and other antipsychotic agents, amantadine, thiazide diuretics, tricyclic antidepressants, MAO inhibitors, quinidine, procainamide.
- Drugs that decrease effects/toxicity of systemic anticholinergics: antacids, cholinergic agents.

Editorial comments

- This drug is rarely prescribed.
- This drug is listed without details in the *Physician's Desk Reference*, 54th edition, 2000.

Propoxyphene

Brand names: Darvon, Dolene, Wygesie.
Class of drug: Narcotic opioid analgesic, agonist.
Mechanism of action: Binds to opioid receptors and blocks ascending pain pathways. Reduces patient's perception of pain without altering cause of the pain.
Indications/dosage/route: Oral only.

- Mild to moderate pain
  - Adults: Capsules 65 mg q4h. Maximum: 390 mg/d.

– Adults: Tablets 100 mg q4h. Maximum: 600 mg/d.

Adjustment of dosage
• Kidney disease: Use with caution.
• Liver disease: Use with caution.
• Elderly: Use with caution.
• Pediatric: Not recommended for children.

Onset of Action	Peak Effect	Duration
30–60 min	2–2.5 h	4–6 h

Food: May be taken with food to lessen GI upset.

Pregnancy: Category C. Category D if prolonged use or if given in high doses at term.

Lactation: Appears in breast milk. Potentially toxic to infant. Considered compatible with breastfeeding by American Academy of Pediatrics.

Contraindications: Hypersensitivity to propoxyphene.

Warnings/precautions
• Use with caution in patients with head injury with increased intracranial pressure, serious alcoholism, prostatic hypertrophy, chronic pulmonary disease, severe liver or kidney disease, disorders of biliary tract, and in postoperative patients with pulmonary disease, suicidal or addiction-prone patients.
• Administer drug before patient experiences severe pain for fullest efficacy of the drug.
• Have the following available when treating patient with this drug: naloxone (Narcan) or other antagonist, means of administering oxygen, and support of respiration.
• Nausea, vomiting, and orthostatic hypotension occur most prominently in ambulatory patients. If nausea and vomiting persist, it may be necessary to administer an antiemetic, eg, droperidol or prochlorperazine.
• This drug can cause severe hypotension in a patient who is volume depleted or if given along with a phenothiazine or general anesthetic.

- Careful diagnosis must be made of acute abdominal condition before this drug is administered.

Editorial comments

- Proproxyphene increases plasma levels of the following drugs: carbamazepine, warfarin, tricyclic antidepressants. Dosages of these drugs should be reduced to avoid toxicity.
- This drug is generally available in combination with acetominophen, aspirin, and/or caffeine.
- For additional information, see *morphine*, p. 633.

Propranolol

Brand name: Inderal.
Class of drug: β-Adrenergic receptor blocker.
Mechanism of action: Competitive blocker of β-adrenergic receptors in heart and blood vessels.
Indications/dosage/route: Oral, IV.

- Hypertension
  - Adults: initial: PO 40 mg b.i.d. or 80 mg of sustained-release formulation once daily. Maintenance: PO, 120–240 mg/d in 2 to 3 divided doses or 120–160 mg of sustained-release formulation once daily. Maximum: 640 mg/d.
  - Pediatric: Initial: PO 0.5 mg/kg b.i.d. Increase to maximum of 8 mg/kg b.i.d. Usual dose: 2–4 mg/kg/d.
- Angina
  - Adults: Initial: PO 80–320 mg b.i.d., t.i.d., or q.i.d., or 80 mg of sustained-release preparation once daily. Maintenance: 160 mg/d. Maximum: 320 mg/d.
- Arrhythmias
  - Adults: 10–30 mg t.i.d. to q.i.d. given after meals and at bedtime.
- Hypertrophic subaortic stenosis
  - Adults: 20–40 mg t.i.d. to q.i.d. before meals and at bedtime or 80–160 mg of sustained-release preparation once daily.

- MI prophylaxis
  - Adults: 180–240 mg/d in 3 or 4 divided doses.
- Pheochromocytoma, preoperatively
  - Adults: 60 mg/d for 3 days before surgery.
- Migraine
  - Adults: Initial: PO 80 mg sustained-release preparation given once daily. Maintenance: 160–240 mg/d in divided doses.
- Life-threatening arrhythmias
  - Adults: IV 1–3 mg at 1 mg/min. Repeat after 2 min if needed. No further administration in <4 hours.

Adjustment of dosage
- Kidney disease: Use caution.
- Liver disease: Use caution.
- Elderly: Use caution. Increased risk for CNS and cardiovascular side effects.
- Pediatric: See above. Intravenous administration not recommended.

Food: No restriction.

Pregnancy: Category C.

Lactation: Appears in breast milk. Considered compatible by American Academy of Pediatrics.

Contraindications: Cardiogenic shock, asthma, CHF unless it is secondary to tachyarrhythmia treated with a β blocker, sinus bradycardia and AV block greater than first degree, severe COPD.

Warnings/precautions
- Use with caution in patients with diabetes, kidney disease, liver disease, COPD, peripheral vascular disease.
- Do not stop drug abruptly as this may precipitate arrhythmias, angina, MI or cause rebound hypertension. If necessary to discontinue, taper as follows: Reduce dose and reassess after 1–2 weeks. If status is unchanged, reduce by another 50% and reassess after 1–2 weeks.
- Drug may mask the symptoms of hyperthyroidism, mainly tachycardia.
- Drug may exacerbate symptoms of arterial insufficiency in patients with peripheral or mesenteric vascular disease.

Advice to patient
- Avoid driving and other activities requiring mental alertness or that are potentially dangerous until response to drug is known.
- Dress warmly in winter and avoid prolonged exposure to cold as drug may cause increased sensitivity to cold.
- Avoid drinks that contain xanthines (caffeine, theophylline, theobromine) including colas, tea, and chocolate because they may counteract the effect of drug.
- Restrict dietary sodium to avoid volume expansion.
- Drug may blunt response to usual rise in BP and chest pain under stressful conditions such as vigorous exercise and fever.

Adverse reactions
- Common: fatigue, headache, impotence.
- Serious: symptomatic bradycardia, decreased cardiac output, CHF, pulmonary edema, worsened AV block, depression, hallucinations, arterial thrombosis, bone marrow depression, lupus-like condition.

Clinically important drug interactions
- Drugs that increase effects/toxicity of β blockers: reserpine, bretylium, calcium channel blockers.
- Drugs that decrease effects/toxicity of β blockers: aluminum salts, calcium salts, cholestyramine, barbiturates, NSAIDs, rifampin.

Parameters to monitor
- Liver enzymes, serum BUN and creatinine, CBC with differential and platelets.
- Pulse rate near end of dosing interval or before the next dose is taken. A reasonable target is 60–80 beats/min for resting apical ventricular rate. If severe bradycardia develops, consider treatment with glucagon, isoproterenol, IV atropine (1–3 mg in divided doses). If hypotension occurs despite correction of bradycardia, administer vasopressor (norephinephrine, dopamine, or dobutamine).
- Symptoms of CHF. Digitalize patient and administer a diuretic or glucagon.
- Efficacy of treatment: decreased BP, decreased number and severity of anginal attacks, improvement in exercise tolerance.

Confirm control of arrhythmias by ECG, apical pulse, BP, circulation in extremities and respiration. Monitor closely when changing dose.

- CNS effects. If patient experiences mental depression reduce dosage by 50%. The elderly are particularly sensitive to adverse CNS effects.
- Signs of bronchospasm. Stop therapy and administer large doses of β-adrenergic bronchodilator, eg, albuterol, terbutaline, or aminophylline.
- Signs of cold extremities. If severe, stop drug. Consider β blocker with sympathomimetic properties.

Editorial comments

- Stopping a β blocker before surgery is controversial. Some advocate discontinuing the drug 48 hours before surgery; others recommend withdrawal for a considerably longer time. Notify anesthesiologist that patient has been on β blocker.
- β Blockers are first-line treatments for hypertension, particularly in patients with the following conditions: previous MI, ischemic heart disease, aneurysm, atrioventricular arrhythmias, migraine. These are drugs of first choice for chronic stable angina in conjunction with nitroglycerin.
- Many studies indicate benefit from administration of a β blocker following an MI.
- β Blockers are considered to be first-line drugs for prophylaxis of migraine headache in patients who have two or more attacks per month.

Propylthiouracil (PTU)

Brand name: Propyl-Thyracil.
Class of drug: Antihyperthyroid drug.
Mechanism of action: Inhibits synthesis of thyroid hormones; blocks thyroid gland oxidation of iodine.

Indications/dosage/route: Oral only.

• Hyperthyroidism
  – Adults: 300–900 mg/d divided t.i.d. Maintenance: 100–150 mg/d divided b.i.d. or t.i.d.
  – Neonates, children <6 years: 5–10 mg/kg/d divided doses q8h.
  – Children 6–10 years: 50–150 mg/d, divided doses q8h.
  – Children >10 years: 150–300 mg/d, divided doses q8h. Maintenance: 25 mg t.i.d. to 100 mg b.i.d. after 2 months.

• Thyroid toxic crisis
  – Adults: 200–400 mg q4h on first day.

Adjustment of dosage

• Kidney disease: Creatinine clearance 10–50 mL/min: 75% of normal dose; creatinine clearance <10 mL/min, 50% of normal dose.
• Liver disease: None recommended.
• Elderly: Reduce initial dose (150–300 mg/d).
• Pediatric: See above.

Onset of Action	Peak Effect	Duration
24–36 h	2–10 wk	—

Food: May be taken with food.

Pregnancy: Category D.

Lactation: Appears in breast milk. Considered compatible by American Academy of Pediatrics. Periodic check of infant's thyroid function advised.

Contraindications: Hypersensitivity to propylthiouracil.

Warnings/precautions: Use with extreme caution in patients receiving other drugs that are potentially able to cause agranulocytosis, kidney disease, elderly.

Advice to patient

• Avoid driving and other activities requiring mental alertness or that are potentially dangerous until response to drug is known.
• Avoid dietary sources of iodine, eg, iodized salt, shellfish.

• Carry identification card at all times describing disease, treatment regimen, name, address, and telephone number of treating physician.

Adverse reactions

• Common: nausea, vomiting, rash, fever.
• Serious: **leukopenia**, agranulocytosis, lupus-like syndrome, vasculitis, drug fever, hypersensitivity reactions, hepatotoxicity, neuritis, nephritis, coagulation disorders.

Clinically important drug interactions: Drugs that increase effects/toxicity of propylthiouracil: antineoplastic agents, lithium, potassium or sodium iodide, phenothiazines.

Parameters to monitor

• Signs and symptoms of hyperthyroidism or thyrotoxicosis: tachycardia, insomnia, diaphoresis, heat intolerance, weight loss, diarrhea.
• Signs and symptoms of hypothyroidism; intolerance to cold, constipation, dry skin. It may be necessary to adjust dosage.
• Signs of skin rash or swelling of cervical lymph nodes. It may be necessary to discontinue treatment if these occur.
• Thyroid function (TSH, T_3, T_4) before therapy, monthly during initiation of therapy, and every 2–3 months thereafter.
• Hematologic status, specifically for development of agranulocytosis.
• Weight 2–3 times/wk for signs of significant changes.
• Signs and symptoms of bone marrow depression.
• PT during therapy because PTU may cause hypoprothrombinemia and bleeding; it is necessary to do this before surgery.

Editorial comments

• Antithyroid drugs such as PTU are effective in elderly as well as younger adults. However, because of potential adverse effects, radioactive iodine is often preferable to PTU.
• If an antithyroid agent is needed during pregnancy, PTU is preferred over methimazole because it is less likely to cross the placental barrier and cause neonatal complications. Note, however, that PTU is considered to be teratogenic: pregnancy category D.

- Children should be checked every 6 months for appropriate development and growth when taking this drug.
- This drug is listed without details in the *Physician's Desk Reference*, 54th edition, 2000.

Protamine Sulfate

Class of drug: Treatment for heparin overdose.

Mechanism of action: Forms a complex with heparin that neutralizes the anticoagulant action.

Indications/dosage/route: IV only.

- Heparin overdose; neutralization of heparin during surgery or dialysis
  - Adults, children: 1 mg/90 units of heparin derived from lung tissue or 1 mg/155 units of heparin derived from intestinal mucosa. Administer as slow IV injection over 1–3 minutes. Maximum: 50 mg/10-minute period.

Onset of Action	Peak Effect	Duration
30–60 s	<5 min	2 h

Adjustment of dosage: None

Food: Not applicable.

Pregnancy: Category C.

Lactation: No data available. Best to avoid.

Contraindications: Hypersensitivity to protamine.

Warnings/precautions

- Use with caution in patients with postcardiac surgery, allergic reaction to fish, previous sensitization to protamine (present in protamine zinc insulin).
- Correct hypovolemia prior to protamine therapy. Otherwise, cardiovascular collapse may occur.

- Protamine is incompatible with several penicillins and cephalosporins.
- Protamine should not be administered rapidly as it may cause severe hypotension and anaphylaxis.

Advice to patient: Use caution in activities that may cause bleeding such as shaving with razor, brushing teeth, receiving injections. Such restrictions are necessary until the risk of hemorrhage is no longer present.

Adverse reactions
- Common: dyspnea.
- Serious: **hypotension, bradycardia**, pulmonary edema, acute pulmonary hypertension, hypersensitivity reactions.

Clinically important drug interactions: None.

Parameters to monitor
- Clotting factors: activated clotting time (ACT), activated partial thromboplastin time (aPTT), and thrombin time (TT). These values should be obtained 5–15 minutes after administration of protamine and repeated in 2–8 hours.
- Vital signs frequently. In particular, monitor BP as this may fall suddenly.
- Signs and symptoms of bleeding during administration. Be aware that bleeding may recur 8–9 hours after therapy due to rebound; rebound may occur even as late as 18 hours after administration of protamine.
- Signs of hypersensitivity reaction.

Protriptyline

Brand name: Vivactil.
Class of drug: Tricyclic antidepressant.
Mechanism of action: Inhibits reuptake of CNS neurotransmitters, primarily serotonin and norepinephrine.
Indications/dosage/route: Oral only.
- Depression

– Adults: 15–40 mg/d in 3 or 4 doses. Maximum: 60 mg/d.
– Elderly, adolescents: Initial: 15 mg/d in 3 doses.

Adjustment of dosage
- Kidney disease: None.
- Liver disease: None.
- Elderly: See above.
- Pediatric: Safety and efficacy have not been established.

Food: No restriction.

Pregnancy: Category C.

Lactation: Appears in breast milk. American Academy of Pediatrics expresses concern over use when breastfeeding.

Contraindications: Hypersensitivity to tricyclic antidepressants, acute recovery from acute MI, concomitant use of MAO inhibitor or SSRI, narrow-angle glaucoma, severe liver disease.

Editorial comments
- Use with caution in the elderly because of possibility of severe cardiovascular side effects.
- Protriptyline appears to be the most likely tricyclic antidepressant to cause tachycardia and postural hypotension.
- For additional information, see *amitriptyline*, p. 39.

Pyrazinamide

Brand names: Pyrazinamide, Rifater.
Class of drug: Antituberculosis drug.
Mechanism of action: Unknown.
Indications/dosage/route: Oral only.
- Adjunct for treatment of tuberculosis with primary and secondary antitubercular drugs when these are not successful
  – Adults: 15–30 mg/kg/d, 1–4 divided doses. Maximum: 3 g/d.

Adjustment of dosage
- Kidney disease: Use with caution. Some dose reduction may be required.

- Liver disease: Best to avoid.
- Elderly: Use lower dose and increase as tolerated.
- Pediatric: Not fully studied. Appears to be effective and well tolerated.

Food: May be taken with food.

Pregnancy: Category C.

Lactation: Appears in breast milk. Best to avoid.

Contraindications: Hypersensitivity to pyrazinamide, severe liver disease, acute gout.

Warnings/precautions

- Use with caution in patients with diabetes mellitus, renal failure, chronic gout.
- Advise diabetic patients that pyrazinamide may interfere with measurement of urinary ketones.

Advice to patient

- To minimize possible photosensitivity reaction, apply adequate sunscreen and use proper covering when exposed to strong sunlight.
- Notify treating physician if symptoms do not improve after several weeks on drug.
- Do not stop taking medication without consulting treating physician.

Adverse reactions

- Common: myalgia, nausea, vomiting, arthralgia, anorexia.
- Serious: thrombocytopenia, hepatotoxicity, nephritis, porphyria, gout, hypersensitivity reactions.

Clinically important drug interactions: Pyrazinamide decreases effects/toxicity of isoniazid.

Parameters to monitor

- Chest x-rays after initiation of treatment and at its completion.
- Signs and symptoms of hepatotoxicity.
- Uric acid levels. If there is a significant increase, probenecid or allopurinol administration may be instituted.
- Mycobacterial sensitivity before and periodically throughout therapy to detect possible resistance.
- Efficacy of treatment: Improvement should be noted after 2–3 weeks of therapy.

Editorial comments
- For HIV patients, physicians should consult the *Physicians' Desk Reference* for current CDC recommendations.
- Pyrazinamide is administered in combination regimens to prevent or delay development of resistant organisms.

Pyridostigmine Bromide

Brand Name: Mestinon.
Class of drug: Cholinesterase inhibitor.
Mechanism of action: Inhibits acetylcholinesterase, thereby increasing acetylcholine at cholinergic receptor sites.
Indications/dosage/route: Oral only.
- Myasthenia gravis
  – Adults: Syrup, tablets 60–120 mg q3–4h. Adjust dosage according to response. Maximum: 150 mg/d. Sustained-release tablets 180–450 mg, 1 or 2 times/d.
  – Children: 7 mg/kg/d in 5 or 6 divided doses.

Adjustment of dosage
- Kidney disease: None.
- Liver disease: None.
- Elderly: None.
- Pediatric: See above. Sustained-release tablets are not recommended for use in children.

	Onset of Action	Duration
Syrup, tablets	30–45 min	3–6 h
Sustained-release tablets	30–60 min	6–12 h

Food: Should be taken with food or milk to lessen GI side effects.
Pregnancy: Category C.

Lactation: Appears in breast milk. Considered compatible by American Academy of Pediatrics.

Contraindications: Hypersensitivity to the drug, peritonitis, mechanical obstruction of intestinal or urinary tract.

Editorial comments

• The parenteral form of pyridostigmine (Regonol) is listed without detail in the *Physicians' Desk Reference*, 54th edition, 2000.

• For additional information, see *neostigmine*, p. 652.

Pyrimethamine

Brand name: Daraprim.

Class of drug: Antimalarial.

Mechanism of action: Antagonizes folic acid, which is required for parasitic nucleic acid synthesis.

Indications/dosage/route: Oral only.

• Prophylaxis of malaria due to susceptible strains of plasmodia
  – Adults, children >10 years: 25 mg/wk.
  – Children 4–10 years: 12.5 mg/wk.
  – Children <4 years: 6.25 mg/wk.
  – Drug administration should be continued at least 10 weeks after leaving endemic areas.

• Acute malaria
  – Adults, children >15 years: 25–50 mg/d, 2 days.

• Toxoplasmosis
  – Adults: 50–75 mg/d, 3–4 weeks, together with 1–4 g of a sulfapyridine such as sulfadoxine, 3 or 4 divided doses. Continue for 1–3 weeks, depending on response. Then give half dose for 4–5 more weeks.

Adjustment of dosage

• Kidney disease: Use with caution. Consider dosage reduction.

• Liver disease: Use with caution. Consider dosage reduction.

• Elderly: None.
• Pediatric: See above.

Food: Administer with food or milk.

Pregnancy: Category C.

Lactation: Appears in breast milk. Considered compatible by American Academy of Pediatrics.

Contraindications: Megaloblastic anemia caused by a folic acid deficiency, hypersensitivity to pyrimethamine.

Warnings/precautions: Use with caution in patients with kidney and liver disease, bronchial asthma, severe allergies, seizure disorders, G6PD deficiency.

Adverse reactions

• Common: none.
• Serious: seizures, megaloblastic anemia (high doses), bone marrow depression, hematuria, arrhythmias, pulmonary eosinophilia, hypersensitivity reactions (including Stevens–Johnson syndrome, anaphylaxis, erythema multiforme, and toxic epidermal necrolysis).

Clinically important drug interactions: Drugs that increase effects/toxicity of pyrimethamine: antifolic agents (sulfonamides), antineoplastics, radiation therapy, methotrexate, lorazepam.

Parameters to monitor

• CBC with differential and platelets. May be required on a weekly basis in patients taking large doses of medication.
• Signs and symptoms of bone marrow depression.
• Signs of hypersensitivity reaction.
• Signs and symptoms of infection.
• Signs of folate deficiency (megaloblastic anemia). Under such conditions it may be necessary to decrease the dose or discontinue the drug. Alternatively, it may be necessary to give leucovorin to avoid complications when pyrimethamine is used >3–4 days. Leucovorin should be given at a dose of 3–9 mg/d for 3 days.

Editorial comments

• Pyrimethamine is no longer considered a first-line antimalarial agent. The following drugs are generally preferred: chloroquine, mefloquine, sulfadoxine.

- Pyrimethamine plus sulfadoxine should be used only when patients are exposed to malaria in areas where chloroquine-resistant malaria is present and only if it is anticipated that the traveler will remain in such an area >3 weeks.
- This drug should not be administered alone to nonimmune persons. In such individuals, pyrimethamine should be used with a drug such as chloroquine for 2 days. For chloroquinine-resistant strains, sulfonamides and possibly quinine should be administered with pyrimethamine.

Quinapril

Brand name: Accupril.
Class of drug: ACE inhibitor.
Mechanism of action: Inhibits ACE, thereby preventing conversion of angiotensin I to angiotensin II, resulting in decreased peripheral arterial resistance.
Indications/dosage/route: Oral only.
• Hypertension
– Initial: 10–20 mg, daily. Adjust dose q2wk. Maximum: 800 mg/d, single or divided doses. Initiate therapy at 3 mg/d in patients receiving diuretics.
• CHF
– Initial: 5 mg twice daily. Increase at weekly intervals to 10–20 mg b.i.d.
Adjustment of dosage
• Kidney disease: Creatinine clearance <40 mL/min: initial 3.75 mg/d, maximum 15 mg/d.
• Liver disease: Reduce dose.
• Elderly: None.
• Pediatric: Safety and efficacy have not been established.

Onset of Action	Peak Effect	Duration
Within 1 h	2–4 h	≤24 h

Food: Administer without regard to meals.
Pregnancy: Category C first trimester, Category D for second and third trimesters.
Lactation: No information available. Likely to be present in breast milk. Other similar agents considered safe.
Contraindications: Hypersensitivity to ACE inhibitors, hereditary or idieopathic angioedema, second and third trimesters of pregnancy.
Editorial comments: For additional information, see *enalapril*, p. 317.

Quinidine

Brand names: Quinaglute Duratabs, (quinidine gluconate), Cardioquin (quinidine polygalacturonate), Quinora (quinidine sulfate), Quinidex Extentabs (quinidine sulfate).

Class of drug: Antiarrythmic, class Ia.

Mechanism of action: Decreases myocardial conduction velocity and excitability. Depresses myocardial contractility. Suppresses automatically in His-Purkinje system.

Indications/dosage/route: Oral, IV, IM.

• Atrial flutter or fibrillation
  – Adults: PO 200 mg quinidine sulfate q2–3h. Increase dosage until sinus rhythm is restored or toxicity develops. Average maintenance dose: PO 200–400 mg t.i.d. or q.i.d.
• Paroxysmal supraventricular tachycardia
  – Adults: PO 400–600 mg quinidine sulfate q2–3h.
• Premature atrial contractions
  – Adults: Initial: PO 200–400 mg quinidine sulfate q2–4h; or IM 600 mg quinidine gluconate, then 400 mg q2h prn; or IV 800 mg quinidine gluconate, 16 mg/min.
  – Children: Initial: PO 30 mg/kg/d or 900 mg/m^2/d quinidine sulfate, 5 divided doses.

Note: Quinidine should be used only for life-threatening ventricular arrhythmias.

Adjustment of dosage

• Kidney disease: Creatinine clearance <10 mL/min: administer 75% of normal dose.
• Liver disease: No recommendations available, lower clearance in cirrhotics. Dose should be titrated on the basis of effectiveness and toxicity.
• Elderly: Safety and efficacy data not available. Caution advised.
• Pediatric: Safety and efficacy have not been established; however, children have been administered quinidine (see above).

Food: The following foods may alkalinize the urine and increase toxicity of quinidine: all fruits except prunes, cranberries, plums;

all vegetables. Administer with full glass of water on empty stomach 1 hour prior or 2 hours following meals.

Pregnancy: Category C.

Lactation: Appears in breast milk. Considered compatible by American Academy of Pediatrics.

Contraindications: Hypersensitivity to quinidine or related cinchona compounds, abnormal rhythms due to escape mechanisms (junctional or idioventricular pacemaker), history of quinidine-induced Torsade de pointes, myasthenia gravis, thrombocytopenia associated with previous quinidine administration.

Warnings/precautions

- Use with caution in patients with digitalis toxicity (AV conduction disorders), left bundle branch block or other intraventricular condition defects, thrombocytopenia purpura, kidney and liver disease, asthma, muscle weakness, infections, incomplete AV blocks, G6PD deficiency, arrthymic drug, sick sinus syndrome, and patients who have experienced transient Torsade de pointes when treated with a class Ia antiarrhythmic drug.
- It is best to avoid the IV route because of the possibility of producing severe hypotension.
- It is important to test the patient for quinidine intolerance before beginning administration on a regular basis. This is done by giving a test dose of 200 mg quinidine sulfate orally or 200 mg quinidine gluconate IM.

Advice to patient

- Do not use discolored quinidine solutions.
- Avoid driving and other activities requiring mental alertness or that are potentially dangerous until response to drug is known.
- Quinidine may cause light sensitivity and this can be minimized by wearing dark glasses.
- Take OTC medications only with approval of the treating physician.
- Carry identification card at all times describing disease, treatment regimen, name, address, and telephone number of treating physician.
- If you forget to take a dose, the following dose should not be doubled.

- Be aware of the fact that different quinidine preparations contain different amounts of quinidine. It is not advisable to change dosage or discontinue quinidine administration without consulting your treating physician.
- Do not chew or crush extended-release tablets.

Adverse reactions

- Common: diarrhea, nausea, vomiting, fever, rash, anorexia, lightheadedness.
- Serious: arrhythmias, hypotension, cinchonism (hearing loss, vertigo, confusion, delirium), inflammatory syndromes (bronchospasm, hemolytic anemia, vasculitis, thrombocytopenia, agranulocytosis, pneumonitis, lupus-like syndrome), hepatic injury, optic neuritis, respiratory depression.

Clinically important drug interactions

- Quinidine increases effects/toxicity of digoxin, verapamil, depolarizing and nondepolarizing muscle relaxants, β blockers, warfarin, procainamide, tricyclic antidepressants, phenothiazines, reserpine.
- Drugs that increase effects/toxicity of quinidine: amiodarone, cimetidine, alkalinizing agents, sodium bicarbonate, antihistamines, pimozide, succinylcholine, other neuromuscular blocking drugs.
- Drugs that decrease effects/toxicity of quinidine: phenobarbital, rifampin, phenytoin, cholinesterase inhibitors, neostigmine, pyridostigmine.

Parameters to monitor

- CBC with differential and platelets, liver enzymes.
- ECG, pulse, and BP continuously during IV administration. Discontinue if any of the following occurs: QRS complex widens by 50%; PR or QT intervals are prolonged. Switch to oral dosing when arrhythmia is treated successfully.
- Symptoms of arrhythmia: palpitations, shortness of breath, chest pain, syncope.
- Check liver enzymes during the first 4–8 weeks of quinidine administration and then every 6 months. If transaminases increase more than two or three times baseline values, it is best to discontinue quinidine and use a different drug.

- Symptoms of hemolysis. Use extreme caution in patients with G6PD deficiency.
- Signs and symptoms of hepatotoxicity.
- Serum quinidine levels. Therapeutic concentrations are 2–6 μg/mL. Toxicity usually is observed at concentrations >8 μg/mL.
- Symptoms of cinchonism: tinnitus, loss of hearing, headache, nausea, dizziness.

Editorial comments

- Quinidine (sulfate and gluconate) is one of the few antiarrhythmic drugs approved by the FDA for atrial fibrillation. In select patients it can be highly efficacious and tolerated; however, most patients have difficulty with GI side effects of nausea, diarrhea, and cramping.
- Blood dyscrasias are also prominent.
- The 2% incidence of Torsade de pointes also limits its usefulness and calls into question its use for non-life-threatening conditions such as atrial fibrillation.
- The proarrhythmic effects of quinidine can be seen anytime during its use when electrolyte and/or myocardial substrate changes occur. Usually proarrhythmia is seen within the first 48 hours of monitoring.
- Current clinical use of quinidine includes the treatment of ventricular tachycardia in conjunction with internal cardioverter defibrillators (ICDs). Where suppression is necessary, in certain cases of frequent shocks from ICDs, combinations of antiarrhythmics, including quinidine, may be helpful.
- Quinidine is considered to be the drug of first choice for the following conditions: new onset of atrial fibrillation or flutter (<1-year duration) when direct cardioversion is not considered to be desirable; maintenance of sinus rhythm after cardioversion in patients with paroxysmal atrial fibrillation or flutter; prevention of recurrent atrial fibrillation or flutter. Quinidine should not be used to treat atrial fibrillation or flutter if these are of longer than 1-year duration.

Ramipril

Brand name: Altace.
Class of drug: ACE inhibitor.
Mechanism of action: Inhibits ACE, thereby preventing conversion of angiotensin I to angiotensin II, resulting in decreased peripheral arterial resistance.
Indications/dosage/route: PO.
• Hypertension
 – Initial: 2.5 mg daily. May increase up to 20 mg/d in 1 or 2 divided doses (initiate therapy at 1.25 mg/d in patients receiving diuretics). Maintenance: 2.5–20 mg/d as single dose or 2 equally divided doses.
• CHF
 – Initial: 1.25–2.5 mg b.i.d. May be increased up to 5 mg b.i.d. Maintenance: 5 mg b.i.d.
Adjustment of dosage
• Kidney disease: Initial: 1.25 mg/d. Maximum: 5 mg/d.
• Liver disease: None.
• Elderly: None.
• Pediatric: Safety and efficacy have not been established.

Onset of Action	Peak Effect	Duration
Within 1–2 h	4–6.5 h	24 h

Food: Administer without regard to meals.
Pregnancy: Category C for first trimester. Category D for second and third trimesters.
Lactation: No information available. Likely to be present in breast milk. Other similar agents considered safe.
Contraindications: Hypersensitivity to ACE inhibitors, hereditary or idiopathic angioedema, second and third trimesters of pregnancy.
Editorial comments: For additional information, see *enalapril*, p. 317.

Ranitidine

Brand name: Zantac.
Class of drug: H_2 receptor blocker.
Mechanism of action: Competitively blocks H_2 receptors on parietal cells, thereby blocking gastric acid secretion.
Indications/dosage/route: Oral, IV, IM.
• Duodenal ulcer, short-term
  – Adults: PO 150 mg b.i.d. or 300 mg h.s. Maintenance: 150 mg h.s.
• Pathologic hypersecretory conditions
  – Adults: 150 mg b.i.d. Maximum: 6 g/d.
• Benign gastric ulcer
  – Adults: 150 mg b.i.d. Maintentance: 150 mg h.s.
• GERD
  – Adults: 150 mg b.i.d.
• Erosive esophagitis
  – Adults: 150 mg q.i.d. Maintenance of healing of erosive esophagitis
• Duodenal ulcer, hypersecretory conditions, GERD
  – Adults: IM 50 mg q6–8h. Intermittent IV injection or infusion: 50 mg q6–8h; maximum: 400 mg/d. Continuous IV infusion: 6.25 mg/h.
• Zollinger–Ellison syndrome
  – Continuous IV infusion: 1–2.5 mg/kg/h may be necessary
Adjustment of dosage
• Kidney disease: None.
• Liver disease: None.
• Elderly: None.
• Pediatric: Safety and efficacy have not been established.

	Onset of Action	Peak Effect	Duration
Oral	—	1–3 h	13 h

Food: Take with food.

Pregnancy: Category B.

Lactation: Appears in breast milk. Cimetidine (another H_2 blocker) is considered compatible by American Academy of Pediatrics.

Contraindications: Hypersensitivity to H_2 blockers.

Warnings/precautions

- Use with caution in the elderly, in patients with hepatic or liver disease, and in immunocompromised patients.
- Symptomatic relief does not mean absence of gastric malignancy.
- Adverse reactions are most likely to occur in elderly and in patients who have impaired renal function.
- Avoid driving and other activities requiring mental alertness or that are potentially dangerous until response to drug is known.
- Discontinue drug for 24–72 hours before performing skin test for allergens.
- Decreased gastric acidity may increase the possibility of intestinal parasites and bacterial overgrowth, particularly in immunocompromised patients.

Advice to patient

- Avoid alcohol and smoking.
- Avoid caffeine and foods that might cause GERD.
- Continue taking drug even after reduction in ulcer pain.
- Report ongoing use of OTC H_2 blockers to your physician.

Adverse reactions

- Common: none.
- Serious: arrythmias, jaundice, bone marrow suppression, aplastic anemia (rare), hypersensitivity reactions.

Clinically important drug interactions: None.

Parameters to monitor

- Efficacy of treatment: improved symptoms of gastroesophageal reflux or peptic ulcer disease.
- Presence of *Helicobacter pylori*: This is a standard approach in patients with peptic ulcer disease.
- Use endoscopy to prove healing of gastric ulcers. A nonhealing gastric ulcer may actually be due to gastric cancer.

- Symptoms of serious underlying disease requiring further testing (weight loss, worsening abdominal pain, early satiety, etc).

Editorial comments

- Current management of peptic ulcer disease uses diagnosis and treatment of *H. pylori* infection. Check if patients are receiving NSAIDs and discontinue when possible. Hypersecretory states are uncommon causes of peptic ulcer disease.
- H_2 blockers are the drugs of choice for the following conditions: dyspepsia not evaluated by endoscopy (empirical), mild to moderate GERD, peptic ulcer disease not due to *H. pylori* infection.
- Proton pump inhibitors are essentially replacing H_2 blockers for management of GERD.

Repaglinide

Brand name: Prandin.

Class of drug: Antidiabetic agent.

Mechanism of action: Closes ATP-dependent potassium channels in pancreatic beta cells, leading to opening of calcium channels. This results in the influx of calcium which increases insulin secretion.

Indications/dosage/route: Oral only.

- Type II diabetes mellitus
  - Adults: Initial, not previously treated with oral hypoglycemic drug: 0.5 mg before each meal.
  - Adults, previously treated with oral hypoglycemic agent: 1–2 mg before each meal. Maximum: 16 mg/d.

Adjustment of dosage

- Kidney disease: Use with caution.
- Liver disease: None.
- Elderly: None.
- Pediatric: Safety and efficacy have not been established.

Food: Should be taken before each meal.

Pregnancy: Category C.

Lactation: No data available. Potentially toxic to infant. Avoid breastfeeding.

Contraindications: Diabetic ketoacidosis, type I diabetes, hypersensitivity to repaglinide.

Clinically important drug interactions: None reported.

Editorial comments

- Repaglinide is a new oral hypoglycemic agent. It appears to have a good side effect profile. Adverse cardiovascular events in clinical trials were slightly higher (4%) compared with sulfonylureas (3%). The clinical significance of these results is presently unclear.
- Long-term safety of repaglinide has not been determined.
- For additional information, see *glipizide*, p. 404.

Rifampin

Brand names: Rifadin, Rifamate.

Class of drug: Treatment for tuberculosis. Adjunctive agent for staphylococcal and other infections.

Mechanism of action: Inhibits DNA-dependent RNA polymerase

Indications/dosage/route: Oral, IV.

- Pulmonary tuberculosis: used in conjunction with other agents (combination therapy)
  - Adults: PO or IV 600 mg as single daily dose.
  - Pediatric: PO or IV 10–20 mg/kg as single daily dose. Maximum: 500 mg daily. Treatment 6–10 months.
- Meningococcal prophylaxis
  - Adults: 600 mg b.i.d., 2 days.
  - Infants, children >1 month: PO 10 mg/kg b.i.d., 2 days.
  - Neonates <1 month: PO 5 mg/kg b.i.d., 2 days.
- Prophylaxis of *Hemophilius influenzae* type B infections
  - Adults, children: PO 2 mg/kg/d, 4 days.

Adjustment of dosage
- Kidney disease: None.
- Liver disease: Dosage reduction recommended. Specific guidelines not available.
- Elderly: Usual dose 10 mg/kg/d.
- Pediatric: Safety in children <5 years has not been established.

Food: Administer on empty stomach at least 1 hour prior or 2 hours following meals with a full glass of water.

Pregnancy: Category C. May cause vitamin K deficiency and hemorrhage during late pregnancy. Coadministration with vitamin K should be considered.

Lactation: Is excreted in breast milk. Considered compatible by American Academy of Pediatrics.

Contraindications: Hypersensitivity to rifampin or rifamycins.

Warnings/precautions
- Use with caution in patients with hepatic disease, porphyria.
- Inform patient that saliva, tears, sweat, and urine may become red-orange or red-brown. This is of little consequence in terms of the drug's effect.
- Rifampin may interfere with the dexamethasone suppression test. If such a test is needed, rifampin should be discontinued approximately 15 days before administration of dexamethasone.

Advice to patient
- Avoid driving or other activities requiring alertness until full response to rifampin is evaluated.
- Avoid alcohol.
- Rifampin may stain soft contact lenses permanently. Accordingly, soft contact lenses should not be worn during treatment with this drug.
- Do not discontinue taking rifampin without approval of treating physician.

Adverse reactions
- Common: diarrhea, red discoloration of urine and other body fluids.
- Serious: acute renal failure, confusion, bone marrow depression, hepatic injury.

Clinically important drug interactions
- Drugs that increase effects/toxicity of rifampin: alcohol, isoniazid, ketoconazole, miconazole.
- Rifampin decreases effects/toxicity of amiodarone, barbiturates, chloramphenicol, cisapride, corticosteroids, cyclosporine, digoxin, disopyramide, etoposide, halothane, indinavir, keto-conazole, opioids, oral contraceptives, oral hypoglycemics, phenytoin, quinidine, ritonivir, saquinavir, tacrolimus, tamox-ifen, teniposide, theophylline, verapamil, vinblastine, vincri-stine, warfarin.

Parameters to monitor
- In patients with pulmonary tuberculosis, respiratory status: lung sounds, character and amount of sputum. This should be done periodically throughout therapy.
- Renal function at least monthly during therapy.
- Liver function tests prior to therapy and then every 2–4 weeks thereafter.
- CBC with differential and platelets prior to and periodically after instituting therapy with rifampin.
- Signs and Symptoms of thrombocytopenia, bone marrow sup-pression, unusual bleeding or bruising.
- Culture and sensitivity testing before giving the first dose and repeatedly afterward to detect drug resistance.

Editorial comments
- Because resistance to rifampin by *Mycobacterium tuberculo-sis* develops rapidly, this drug is always given along with other antituberculosis agents.
- Rifampin is used during initial treatment of tuberculosis unless it is established that the organism is resistant or that rifampin is contraindicated.
- Hypersensitivity reactions and thrombocytopenia occur more frequently if intermittent therapy with rifampin is used.
- In general a four-drug regimen is used for the initial treatment of TB. The four drugs are as follows: isoniazid, rifampin, pyrazinamide, and streptomycin or ethambutol. This regimen may be altered once the susceptibility of the TB organism has been determined.

Rimantadine

Brand name: Flumadine.
Class of drug: Antiviral agent.
Mechanism of action: Inhibits uncoating of influenza virus A, thus interrupting early viral replication.
Indications/dosage/route: Oral only.
• Prophylaxis against influenza A virus
  – Adults, children >10 years: 100 mg b.i.d.
  – Children <10 years: 5 mg/kg/d, 1 or 2 divided doses. Maximum: 150 mg.
• Treatment of influenza A virus infections
  – Adults: 100 mg b.i.d., 7 days.
Adjustment of dosage
• Kidney disease: Creatinine clearance <10 mL/min: reduce dosage to 100 mg/d.
• Liver disease: Dosage reduction suggested. No specific guidelines available.
• Elderly: Reduce dose to 100 mg/d. At higher risk for side effects.
• Pediatric: Although rimantadine is recommended for the prophylaxis of influence A, its safety and effectiveness in children for treatment of symptomatic infection have not been established. Studies of prophylactic use of rimantadine in children <1 year have not been performed.
Food: May take with food.
Pregnancy: Category C.
Lactation: Probably appears in breast milk. Potentially toxic to infant. Avoid breastfeeding.
Contraindications: Hypersensitivity to rimantadine or amantadine.
Warnings/precautions
• Use with caution in patients with kidney or liver disease, seizure disorders.
• Begin therapy as soon as symptoms appear and continue for at least 7 days thereafter.
Advice to patient: Avoid crowds as well as persons who may have a contagious disease.

Adverse reactions
- Common: none.
- Serious: seizures, hallucinations, bronchospasm, CHF, snycope.

Clinically important drugs
- Drug that increases effects/toxicity of rimantadine: cimetidine.
- Drugs that decrease effects/toxicity of rimantadine: acetaminophen, aspirin.

Parameters to monitor: Respiratory status: rate, sputum, breath sounds, temperature. If symptoms occur, use supportive measures.

Editorial comments: The best way to prevent influenza is early annual vaccination.
- This drug is also available as a syrup.

Rimexolone

Brand name: Vexol.
Drug classification: Ocular antiinflammatory agent.
Mechanism of action: Inhibits migration of polymorphonuclear leukocytes; stabilizes lysosomal membranes; inhibits production of products of arachidonic cascade.
Indications/dosage/route: Topical (ophthalmic suspension).
- Postoperative ocular inflammation
  – Adults: 1–2 drops in conjunctival sac(s) q.i.d. 24 hours after surgery, continue for 2 weeks.
- Anterior uveitis
  – Adults: Initial: 1–2 drops in conjunctival sac(s) every hour, first week, 1 drop q2h, second week, until uveitis is resolved.

Adjustment of dosage
- Kidney disease: None.
- Liver disease: None.
- Elderly: None.
- Pediatric: Safety and efficacy have not been established.

Pregnancy: Category C.

Lactation: No data available. Best to avoid.

Contraindications: Superficial epithelial herpes simplex keratitis, other viral infections of cornea or conjunctiva, ocular tuberculosis, ocular fungal infections, acute untreated eye infection.

Warnings/precautions

- Steroid may mask acute untreated eye infections.
- Instruct patient regarding correct procedure for using ophthalmic solution or ointment.
- Children are particularly prone to develop posterior subcapsular cataract.
- Instruct patient regarding correct way to handle solutions to avoid contamination.
- When treating stromal keratitis or uveitis caused by herpes simplex, ocular steroid should be used only in conjunction with an antiviral drug.

Advice to patient: Do not touch any part of the container (cap or top) to eye.

Adverse reactions

- Common: elevated intraocular pressure, blurred vision, ocular pain, loss of visual acuity, blurred vision.
- Serious: secondary ocular infection, posterior subcapsular cataract.

Parameters to monitor

- Signs and symptoms of ocular toxicity: glaucoma, increased intraocular pressure, cataract, optic nerve damage, defects in visual acuity, appearance of fungal or viral exophthalmus infections (persistent corneal ulcerations). Ophthalmic examinations, in particular tonometry, should be carried out 2–3 weeks after beginning therapy and periodically afterward, particularly in elderly and those who have glaucoma.
- Efficacy of treatment: reduction of discomfort from local inflammation. If no improvement is noted after several days, drug should be discontinued and other therapy instituted. In such circumstances, dosage should be tapered to avoid exacerbation of the disease.

Editorial comment: If chronic topical ophthalmic steroid therapy is required, treatment must be undertaken under close supervision by an ophthalmologist.
• This drug is not listed in the *Physician's Desk Reference*, 54th edition, 2000.

Riseronate

Brand name: Actonel.
Class of drug: Bone growth regulator (biphosphonate).
Mechanism of action: Inhibits osteoblastic activity and decreases bone turnover and reabsorption.
Indications/dosage/route: Oral only.
• Paget's disease
  – Adults: 30 mg once daily with 6–8 oz of water. Duration of treatment: 2 months.
Adjustment of dosage
• Kidney disease: See contraindications.
• Liver disease: None.
• Elderly: None.
• Pediatric: Safety and efficacy have not been established.
Food: Should be taken at least 30 minutes before first food or drink of the day.
Pregnancy: Category C.
Lactation: No data available. Best to avoid.
Contraindications: Creatinine clearance <30 mL/min, hypocalcemia, hypersensitivity to riseronate.
Editorial comments
• It is now considered that riseronate, a new biphosphonate, is more effective than antidronate for treatment of Paget's disease of the bone. There is no information at this time as to how this drug compares with alendronate and tiludronate.
• For additional information, see *alendronate*, p. 15.

Risperidone

Brand name: Risperdal.
Class of drug: Antipsychotic.
Mechanism of action: Antagonist of serotonin receptors and dopamine-D_2 receptors in CNS.
Indications/dosage/route: Oral only.
- Management of psychotic symptoms in patients with schizophrenia
  - Adults: PO 1 mg b.i.d. Same dose on second and third days to target of 3 mg b.i.d. by third day. Usual maintenance dose: 4–8 mg/d. Maximum: 16 mg/d.

Adjustment of dosage
- Kidney disease: Starting dose: 0.5 mg b.i.d. Weekly incremental dosage increases of 0.5–1.0 mg/d.
- Liver disease: Starting dose: 0.5 mg b.i.d. Weekly incremental dosage increases of 0.5–1.0 mg/day.
- Elderly: Starting dose: 0.5 mg b.i.d. Weekly incremental dosage increases of 05–1.0 mg/d. Consider single daily doses.
- Pediatric: Safety and efficacy have not been established.

Food: May take with food.
Pregnancy: Category C.
Lactation: No data available. Best to avoid.
Contraindications: Hypersensitivity to resperidone.
Warnings/precautions
- Use with caution in patients with cardiovascular disease, cerebrovascular disease, hypovolemia, history of seizures, history of drug abuse or attempted suicide, kidney or liver disease, elderly.
- Efficacy of resperidone is established only for short-term use (6–8 weeks).
- Risperidone should be reserved for treatment of patients who are suffering from chronic illness that does not respond to other antipsychotic drugs.
- Resperidone should be prescribed at the smallest dose and for the shortest period for those who require chronic treatment.

Advice to patient
- Avoid exposure to extreme heat and cold.
- To minimize possible photosensitivity reaction, apply adequate sunscreen and use proper covering when exposed to strong sunlight.
- Change position slowly, in particular from recumbent to upright to minimize orthostatic hypotension. Sit at the edge of the bed for several minutes before standing, and lie down if feeling faint or dizzy. Avoid hot showers or baths and standing for long periods. Male patients may be safer urinating while seated on the toilet rather than standing.
- Avoid driving and other activities requiring mental alertness or that are potentially dangerous until response to drug is known.
- Avoid alcohol and other CNS depressants such as opioid analgesics and sedatives (eg, diazepam) when taking this drug.
- Use a nonhormonal form of contraception.
- Notify physician if you develop fever, particularly if associated with muscle rigidity.
- Report any visual disturbances to treating physician.

Adverse reactions
- Common: isomnia, agitation, anxiety, headache, constipation, dyspepsia.
- Serious: **extrapyrmidal reactions**, NMS, hypotension, orthostatic hypotension, arrhythmias, dystonia, tardive dyskinesia, seizures, paralytic ilius, cholestatic jaundice, leukopenia, decreased vision (irreversible).

Clinically important drug interactions
- Drugs that increase effects/toxicity of risperidone: alcohol, antihistamines, opioids, sedative–hyponotics, clozapine.
- Risperidone decreases effects/toxicity of levodopa, dopamine agonists.

Parameters to monitor
- CBC with differential and platelets, liver enzymes.
- Mental status before and periodically during therapy for signs of delusions, hallucinations.

- Possible suicidal tendencies. Prescribe a limited amount of drug to the patient at any given time.
- Efficacy of resperidone if used long-term (>6–8 weeks). Consider alternative therapy if efficacy is not demonstrated in this period.
- BP for orthostatic changes 3–5 days after initiating therapy or increasing the dose. It may be necessary to adjust the dose if significant hypotension occurs.
- Signs and symptoms of drug-induced extrapyramidal syndrome (pseudoparkinsonism): akinesia, tremors at rest, pill rolling, shuffling gait, masklike facies, drooling. If these occur while taking this medication drug discontinuation may be required. Alternatively, administration of diphenhydramine and benztropine may be indicated.
- Signs and symptoms of NMS: fever, tachycardia, convulsions, respiratory distress, irregular BP, severe muscle spasms. Use supportive measures and administer dantrolene.
- Signs and symptoms of bone marrow depression.
- Baseline and follow-up ophthalmologic examinations including visual acuity examinations required.

Editorial comments: This is a new antipsychotic agent. It appears to have fewer side effects than older drugs. In particular, it causes fewer extrapyramidal reactions. This could be a first-line drug in treating psychotic crises. When switching to risperidone from another antipsychotic drug, the previous drug may be stopped immediately. However, slow tapering of resperidone is generally better tolerated than abrupt withdrawal. Some overlapping of agents is acceptable; the duration of overlapping should be minimized.

Ritodrine

Brand name: Yutopar.
Class of drug: Inhibitor of uterine contractions, treatment for early labor.

Mechanism of action: Agonist at uterine β_2-adrenergic receptors. Causes relaxation of uterine muscle.

Indications/dosage/route: IV only.

• Adjunct for suppressing preterm labor after 34 weeks of gestation only
  – 50–100 µg/min. Increase by 50 µg/min q10–15 min Maximum: 350 µg/min. Use for 12 hours after contractions are over.

Adjustment of dosage

• Kidney disease: None.
• Liver disease: None.
• Elderly: Not applicable.
• Pediatric: Not used in infants and children.

Onset of Action	Duration
5 min	—

Food: Not applicable.

Pregnancy: Category B.

Lactation: Not applicable.

Contraindications: Hypersensitivity to ritodrine, gestation <20 weeks, conditions in which continuing pregnancy would be hazardous to mother or fetus (eclampsia, preeclampsia, antipartum hemorrhage, intrauterine death, placenta previa), maternal hyperthyroidism, hypovolemia, pulmonary hypertension, cardiac arrhythmias, cardiac disease, uncontrolled hypertension, diabetes mellitus, bronchial asthma treated with corticosteroids or β-adrenergic agonists.

Warning/precautions

• Use with caution in patients with moderate preeclampsia, diabetes.
• Use in advanced labor (cervical dilation >4 cm) has not been established.
• Perform ultrasound and amniocentesis to determine fetal maturity.
• Avoid concurrent use of β blockers.

Adverse reactions

Common: dry mouth, urinary retention, constipation, blurred vision, orthostatic hypotension, sedation.

Serious: arrhythmias (ventricular tachycardia), myocardial ischemia, pulmonary edema (maternal).

Clinically important drug interactions

• Drugs that increase effects/toxicity of ritodrine: anticholinergics, corticosteroids.

• Drugs that decrease effects/toxicity of ritodrine: β blockers.

• Ritodrine increases effects/toxicity of sympathomimetics.

Parameters to monitor

• BP, heart rate.

• Strength, frequency of uterine contractions.

• Fetal heart rate.

• Respiratory status: lung sounds to determine fluid status and signs of pulmonary edema (dyspnea, rales, frothy sputum).

• Signs and symptoms of electrolyte imbalance: acidosis, hypokalemia.

• Status of neonate: Monitor for hypotension, hypocalcemia, hypo- or hyperglycemia.

Editorial comments

• This drug is used in selected patients to prolong gestation when prolongation of interim life would be a benefit to the fetus, ie, to reduce the incidence of neonatal respiratory distress and death from premature birth.

• This drug is not listed in the *Physician's Desk Reference*, 54th edition, 2000.

Rocuronium

Brand name: Zemuron.

Class of drug: Nondepolarizing neuromuscular blocker.

Mechanism of action: Blocks nicotinic acetylcholine receptors at neuromuscular junction, resulting in skeletal muscle relaxation and paralysis.

Indications/dosage/route: IV only.
- Tracheal intubation
  - Adults: Initial: 0.6 mg/kg. Maintenance: 0.1–0.2 mg/kg.
  - Children: Initial: 0.6 mg/kg. Maintenance: 0.075–0.125 mg/kg.
  - Elderly (>65 years): Initial: 0.6 mg/kg. Maintenance: 0.1–0.15 mg/kg.
- Continuous infusion
  - Initial: 0.01–0.02 mg/kg/min. Maintenance: 0.004–0.016 mg/kg/min.

Adjustment of dosage
- Kidney disease: None.
- Liver disease: Prolonged duration of action, higher volume of distribution. Higher initial dose may be required for rapid sequence induction.
- Elderly: None.
- Pediatric: See above.

Food: Not applicable.

Pregnancy: Category B.

Lactation: No data available. Best to avoid.

Contraindications: Hypersensitivity to rocuronium and chemically related drugs.

Warnings/precautions
- Use with caution in patients with liver disease, kidney disease, impaired pulmonary function, respiratory depression, myasthenia gravis, dehydration, porphyria, muscle spasms, hypokalemia, hypermagnesemia, dehydration, underlying cardiovascular disease, fractures, hyperthermia, shock, thyroid disorders, familial periodic paralysis.
- Neuromuscular blocking agents do not produce analgesia. The patient is fully aware of sensory input when such drugs are used. Accordingly, an antianxiety agent (benzodiazepine) or analgesic (narcotic) is administered along with these drugs.
- Long-term use in the ICU setting has not been studied.
- Therapeutic index (margin of safety between the dose required and respiratory paralysis) is very small. Accordingly, appropriate measures must be on hand to provide respiratory support should this be necessary.

- Not recommended for rapid sequence induction for cesarean section.
- Patient who is to required to have prolonged ventilation must be adequately sedated.
- To protect the cornea, apply eyedrops and eye patches to patient.
- Drug should not be administered until patient is unconscious. As consciousness is not affected by the drug, use caution in conversation near patient.
- Prolonged duration of action and slower recovery time are anticipated in patients with cardiac dysfunction and liver disease and in the elderly.
- Burn patients may exhibit resistance to the actions of the drug.
- Imbalance of potassium (hypokalemia) and magnesium (hypermagnesemia) can potentiate the neuromuscular blocking potency of the drug and should be corrected before drug administration.
- Direct medical supervision is required when this drug is administered.
- Atropine and a cholinersterase inhibitor such as neostigmine must be readily available when drug is administered.
- Rapid IV administration may predispose the patient to respiratory paralysis and/or bronchospasm.

Adverse reactions

- Common: none.
- Serious: arrythmia, cardiovascular collapse, bronchospasm, hypersensitivity reactions.

Clinically important drug interactions: Drugs that increase effects/toxicity of neuromuscular blockers: inhalation anesthetics, aminoglycosides, quinidine, lincomycin, tetracycline, lithium, magnesium sulfate, polymyxin D, vancomycin, bacitracin, colistin.

Parameters to monitor

- Respiratory status continuously. Maintain patent airway and ventilation until normal respiration is recovered. If respiratory depression persists, administer a cholinesterase inhibitor, eg, neostigmine or pyridostigmine. Coadminister atropine to counteract excessive muscarinic stimulation.

- Postoperative respiratory distress and muscle weakness.
- Neuromuscular status: Use peripheral nerve stimulator every 4 hours during surgery and afterward to evaluate recovery and effectiveness of muscle relaxation.
- Pulmonary status at frequent intervals: respiratory rate, frequency, breath sounds.
- Signs of excessive vagal stimulation using ECG: bradycardia, hypotension, arrhythmias.
- Recovery from the drug: Evaluate by grip strength and 5-second head lift.
- Signs of hypotension (ganglionic blockade) prior to and during use.
- Symptoms of histamine release: bronchospasm, salivation.
- Evidence of pain during surgery. Administer analgesic drug to control pain adequately.

Editorial comment: Neuromuscular blocking drugs should be administered by or under supervision of experienced clinicians who are thoroughly familiar with these drugs and know how to treat potential complications that might arise from their use. Administration of these drugs should be made in a setting where there are facilities available for the following: tracheal intubation, administration of oxygen, drugs for reversing drug effects, and administration of artificial respiration.

Rofecoxib

Brand name: Vioxx.
Class of drug: Antiinflammatory, analgesic, COX-2 inhibitor.
Mechanism of action: Selective inhibitor of COX-2, the enzyme required for synthesis of prostaglandins and other products of the arachidonic acid cascade.
Indications/dosage/route: Oral only.
- Osteoarthritis
  – Adults: 12.5–25 mg/d.

- Analgesia
  – Adults: 25–50 mg/d. Maximum: 5 days.

Adjustment of dosage

- Kidney disease: None. Potentially toxic to kidney.
- Liver disease: Reduce dosage. Monitor carefully.
- Elderly: Use lowest recommended dose.
- Pediatric: Safety and efficacy have not been determined in children <18 years.

Food: May be taken with or without food.

Pregnancy: Category C. Category D in third trimester and near delivery.

Lactation: No data available. Best to avoid.

Contraindications: Severe liver disease, history of allergic reaction to aspirin or other NSAIDs, hypersensitivity to rofecoxib.

Warnings/precautions

- Use with caution in patients with active gastric ulcer, history of ulcer disease or GI bleeding, active asthma, hypertension, fluid retention, chronic kidney or liver disease.
- Rofecoxib can cause significant GI bleeding despite being a specific COX-2 inhibitor.
- Potentially toxic to kidneys, particularly when prostaglandins maintain renal blood flow (renal and heptatic insufficiency, CHF).

Advice to patient: Report to treating physician if you experience dyspepsia, changes in stool, abdominal pain, or swelling of ankles.

Adverse reactions

- Common: none.
- Severe: GI bleeding, arrhythmias, allergic reactions.

Clinically important drug interactions

- Drugs that increase effects/toxicity of rofecoxib: rifampin, other P450 inhibitors, aspirin.
- Drugs that decrease effects/toxicity of rofecoxib: antacids.
- Rofecoxib increases effects/toxicity of methotrexate, warfarin, lithium.
- Rofecoxib decreases effects/toxicity of furosemide, thiazide diuretics.

Parameters to monitor
- Improvement in pain and inflammation.
- Signs and symptoms of salt and water retention.
- Signs and symptoms of GI toxicity.
- Signs and symptoms of renal toxicity.

Editorial comments: In limited studies, rofecoxib is as effective as other NSAIDs in osteoarthritis and has a lower incidence of GI toxicity than the older drugs. However, the incidence of long-term GI effects has not been determined as compared with NSAIDs or other COX-2 inhibitors. Future uses of Cox-2 inhibitors may include chemoprevention of colonic neoplasms.

Rosiglitazone

Brand name: Avandia.
Class of drug: Oral hypoglycemic agent.
Mechanism of action: Increases sensitivity to insulin in type II diabetics.
Indications/dosage/route: Oral only.
- Type II diabetes
  - 2 mg b.i.d. or 4 mg once/d. Increase dose to 4 mg b.i.d or 8 mg/d if inadequate.

Note: This drug may be used alone or in combination with a sulfonylurea or insulin.

Adjustment of dosage
- Kidney disease: None.
- Liver disease: None.
- Elderly: None.
- Pediatric: Safety and efficacy have not been established.

Food: Should be taken with or between meals.
Pregnancy: Category C.
Lactation: No data available. Potentially toxic to infant. Avoid breastfeeding.
Contraindications: Type I diabetics, treatment of diabetic ketoacidosis, hypersensitivity to rosiglitazone.

Warnings/precautions: Use with caution in patients with CHF.
Advice to patient
- Do not undereat because skipping meals may result in loss of glucose control.
- Avoid even moderate amounts of alcohol, eg, >2 oz 100-proof whiskey. The combination with the drug you are taking may result in a disulfiram reaction: flushing, sweating, palpitation, nausea, vomiting, abdominal cramps.
- To minimize possible photosensitivity reactions, apply adequate sunscreen and use proper covering when exposed to strong sunlight.
- Carry identification card at all times describing disease, treatment regimen, name, address, and telephone number of treating physician.
- Carry hard candy or candy bar at all times.

Adverse reactions
- Common: none.
- Serious: hypoglycemia.

Clinically important drug interactions: None.

Parameters to monitor
- Serum glucose.
- Serum alanine aminotransferase level before beginning treatment, every 2 months afterward for 1 year, and periodically thereafter. If ALT is more than 2.5 times upper normal limit, drug administration should not be undertaken. If the value is more than 3 times higher than normal upper limit, drug administration should be stopped.

Editorial comments
- At this time, FDA has approved use of rosiglitazone, a newer hypoglycemic agent, only as monotherapy for type II diabetes. Long-term benefits of treatment with this drug have not yet been determined.
- Unlike troglitazone, significant hepatotoxic effects and liver failure have not been described to occur with rosiglitazone.

Salmeterol

Brand name: Serevent.
Class of drug: β-Adrenergic agonist, bronchodilator.
Mechanism of action: Relaxes smooth muscles of the bronchioles by stimulating β_2-adrenergic receptors.
Indications/dosage/route: Inhalation only.
• Bronchodilation, asthma
  – Adults, children >12 years: 2 inhalations b.i.d.
• Prevention of exercise-induced bronchospasm
  – Adults, children >12 years: 2 inhalations 30–60 minutes before exercise.
• Asthma or bronchospasm
  – Inhalation powder for adults, children >12 years: 1 inhalation b.i.d.
Adjustment of dosage
• Kidney disease: None.
• Liver disease: None.
• Elderly: None.
• Pediatric: See above.

Onset of Action	Peak Effect	Duration
<20 min	—	12 h

Food: Not applicable.
Pregnancy: Category C.
Lactation: No data available. Best to avoid.
Contraindications: Hypersensitivity to adrenergic compounds, tachycardia (idiopathic or from digitalis).
Editorial comments
• This drug is indicated for maintenance therapy. It is not initiated for acute, deteriorating asthma. Not to be used more than twice a day.
• Immediate hypersensitivity reactions have been reported with salmeterol.
• For additional information, see *metaproterenol*, p. 575.

Scopolamine

Brand names: Transderm-Scōp, Isopto Hyoscine (ophthalmic), Hyoscine.

Class of drug: Anticholinergic, antiemetic, ophthalmic (mydriatic).

Mechanism of action: Scopolamine blocks acetylcholine effects at muscarinic receptors throughout the body.

Indications/dosage/route: IV, IM, SC, ophthalmic, transdermal.

• Preoperative or antiemetic
  – Adults: IM, IV, SC 0.3–0.65 mg. Repeat q4–6h or 3 times per day as needed.
  – Children: IM, IV, SC 6 μg/kg/dose. Repeat q6–8h as needed.

• Ophthalmic: refraction
  – Adults: 1–2 drops 0.25% solution in eyes 1 hour before procedure.

• Ophthalmic: iridocyclitis
  – Adults: 1–2 drops, 0.25% in eyes maximum q.i.d.
  – Children: 1 drop 0.25% in eye, maximum t.i.d.

• Ophthalmic: cycloplegic refraction
  – Adults: 2 drops 0.25% solution in eye 1 hour before refraction.
  – Children: 1 drop 0.25% solution in eye b.i.d. for 2 days before refraction.

• Ophthalmic: iritis, uveitis
  – Adults: 1–2 drops 0.25% solution/d, maximum t.i.d.
  – Children: 1 drop 0.25% solution, maximum t.i.d.

• Prevention of motion sickness: transdermal
  – Adults: 1.5 mg Transderm-Scōp, applied 4 hours prior to travel.

Adjustment of dosage

• Kidney disease: None recommended.
• Liver disease: None recommended.
• Elderly: Reduce dosage: higher likelihood of side effects.
• Pediatric: Higher rate of side effects. Avoid use in children.

	Onset of Action	Peak Effect	Duration
Mydriatic action	10–30 min	30–45 min	72
Motion sickness effect (transdermal)	4 h	—	72 h
Antiemetic action (PO, IM, SC)	30 min	1h	4–6 h

Food: Not applicable.

Pregnancy: Category C.

Lactation: No data available. Best to avoid.

Contraindications: Hypersensitivity to scopolamine, bromide (solutions for ophthalmic and injection purposes only), narrow-angle glaucoma, tachycardia, thyrotoxicosis, acute GI hemorrhage, obstructive uropathy, asthma, myasthenia gravis, intestinal atony.

Warnings/precautions

- Use with caution in patients with intestinal obstruction, chronic liver, pulmonary, kidney, or cardiac disease, BPH, hyperthyroidism, cornary artery disease, heart failure, hypertension, ulcerative colitis, seizures, psychosis.

Advice to patient

- Take medication exactly as directed. If dose is missed, patient should not double subsequent dose when it is remembered.
- Avoid tasks that require mental alertness until full effects of drug have been evaluated.
- Use caution when exercising in hot weather.
- Avoid alcohol.
- Chew sugarless gum or candy to minimize dry mouth.
- If administered ophthalmic preparations, use dark glasses to minimize sensitivity of eyes to light.

Adverse reactions

- Common: dry mouth, blurred vision, (decreased accommodation), drowsiness, tachycardia, urinary hesitancy.
- Serious: disorientation, hallucinations, acute narrow-angle glaucoma.

Clinically important drug interactions

- Drugs that increase effects/toxicity of scopolamine: antihistamines, antidepressants, disopyramide, quinidine, alcohol, opioids, sedative-hypnotics.
- Scopolamine increases effects/toxicity of oral potassium chloride preparations in wax matrix.
- Scopolamine decreases effects of Ketoconazole.

Parameters to monitor

- Heart rate, periodically.
- Signs of urinary retention, periodically.

Editorial comments: A withdrawal syndrome including disequilibrium, nausea, headaches, and dizziness can occur on withdrawal of transdermal scopolamine. Patients should wash hands carefully after patch application.

Selegiline

Brand names: Elderpryl, Carbex.
Class of drug: Anti-Parkinson MAO inhibitor.
Mechanism of action: Selective, irreversible, inhibitor of MAO type B activity. Increases level of dopamine in CNS.
Indication/dosage/route: Oral only.
• Adjunct to levodopa–carbidopa in the symptomatic treatment of Parkinson's disease
  – Adults: 10 mg/d: 5 mg at breakfast, 5 mg at lunch. Gradually decrease carbidopa–levodopa dosage (10–30%) 2–3 days after initiating selegiline.
Adjustment of dosage
• Kidney disease: None.
• Liver disease: None.
• Elderly: None.
• Pediatric: Safety and efficacy have not been established.

Onset of Therapeutic Action	Duration
<1 h	24–72 h

Food: Patients should avoid foods that contain tyramine (aged cheese, Chianti wine, pickled herring, chopped liver, broad beans).
Pregnancy: Category C.
Lactation: No data available. Best to avoid.
Contraindications: Hypersensitivity to selegiline and those who are taking opioid-type drugs, especially meperidine.

Warnings/precautions
- Warn patients regarding signs and symptoms of MAO toxicity, in particular hypertensive crisis, when selegiline is taken along with tyramine-containing foods. Symptoms include: severe headache, vomiting, chest pain, enlarged pupils. Limit dose to 10 mg, thereby greatly minimizing the tyramine reaction.
- This drug is not to be used at dose above 10 mg/d.
- It may be necessary to reduce the dose of L-dopa after initiating therapy with selegiline.

Advice to patient
- Avoid tryamine containing foods as listed by physician.
- Avoid alcohol.
- Selegiline may cause dizziness, particularly at the beginning of therapy, and this may cause you to fall.

Adverse reactions
- Common: nausea (20%), dizziness, abdominal pain (8%), dry mouth (66%).
- Serious: arrhythmias, confusion, hallucinations, sleep disturbances, orthostatic hypotension.

Clinically important drug interactions: Selegiline increases effects/toxicity of opioids, fluoxetine, and other SSRIs, amitriptyline, protriptyline, other tricyclic antidepressants.

Parameters to monitor
- Improvement in Parkinsonism.
- Improvement in symptoms of depression.

Editorial comments: Selegiline must be discontinued for at least 14 days prior to initiation of antidepressant therapy with a tricyclic or SSRI.

Sertraline

Brand name: Zoloft.
Class of drug: SSRI
Mechanism of action: Inhibits serotonin reuptake into CNS neurons.

Indications/dosage/route: Oral only.
- Depression
  - Adults: Initial: 50–200 mg/d in either the morning or evening.
- Obsessive–compulsive disorder
  - Adults: 50–200 mg/d.
  - Children 6–12 years: 25 mg/d.
  - Adolescents 13–17 years: 50 mg/d.
- Panic attacks
  - Adults: Initial: 25 mg/d. Maintenance: 50–200 mg/d.

Adjustment of dosage
- Kidney disease: Use with caution.
- Liver disease: Decrease dose and/or frequency.
- Elderly: None.
- Pediatric: See above.

Food: May be taken with meals.

Pregnancy: Category B.

Lactation: Appears in breast milk. Best to avoid. American Academy of Pediatrics expresses concern with use during breastfeeding.

Contraindications: MAO inhibitor taken within 14 days, hypersensitivity to sertraline.

Warnings/precautions
- Use with caution in patients with diabetes mellitus, seizures, liver, kidney disease.
- Advise patient that effectiveness of the drug may not be apparent until 4 weeks of treatment.
- A withdrawal syndrome has been described after abrupt withdrawal of this drug. Symptoms include blurred vision, diaphoresis, agitation, and hypomania.
- Mania or hypomania may be unmasked by SSRIs.
- Patients should wear a bracelet identifying their condition and possibility of developing hypoglycemia.

Advice to patient
- Avoid driving and other activities requiring mental alertness or that are potentially dangerous until response to drug is known.
- Avoid alcohol and other CNS depressants such as opiate analgesics and sedatives (eg, diazepam) when taking this drug.

- Report excessive weight loss to treating physician.
- Take this drug in the morning as it may cause insomnia.

Adverse reactions

- Common: insomnia, drowsiness, nausea, diarrhea, dry mouth, male sexual dysfunction.
- Serious: urticaria, suicidal tendency, hepatitis, bronchospasm, psychosis.

Clinically important drug interactions

- Drugs that increase effects/toxicity of sertraline: MAO inhibitors (combination contraindicated), clarithromycin, tryptophan, cimetidine.
- Sertraline increases effects/toxicity of tricyclic antidepressants, dextromethorphan, encainide, haloperidol, perphenazine, propafenone, thioridizine, trazadone, warfarin, carbamazepine, lithium.

Parameters to monitor

- Signs of progressive weight loss. Recommend dietary management to maintain weight. This may be particularly important in underweight patients.
- Signs of hypersensitivity reactions.

Editorial comments

- SSRIs are recommended for patients who are at risk for medication overdose because they are safer than tricyclic antidepressants.
- SSRIs may be a better choice than tricyclic antidepressants for those who cannot tolerate the anticholinergic effects or excessive daytime sedation of tricyclic antidepressants, and those who experience psychomotor retardation or weight gain. They are generally well tolerated.
- If coadministered with tricyclic antidepressant, dosage of the latter may need to be reduced and blood monitored.
- Do not administer for at least 14 days after discontinuing a MAO inhibitor. Do not initiate MAO inhibitor until at least 5 weeks after discontinuing this agent.
- SSRIs have generally replaced other antidepressants (tricyclics, MAO inhibitors) as drugs of choice for depression.
- Nausea and loose stools are common GI side effects of sertraline.

Sildenafil

Brand name: Viagra.
Class of drug: Drug for erectile dysfunction.
Mechanism of action: Enhances effect of nitric oxide by inhibiting phosphodiesterase in corpus cavernosum.
Indications/dosage/route: Oral only.
• Erectile dysfunction.
 – 25–100 mg once/d, 0.5–4 hours before sexual activity.
Adjustment of dosage
• Kidney disease: Begin with 25 mg.
• Liver disease: Begin with 25 mg.
• Elderly: Begin with 25 mg.
• Pediatric: Not indicated.

Onset of Action	Peak Effect	Duration
30 min	60–120 min	4 h

Food: Take on empty stomach. High-fat meal delays absorption.
Pregnancy: Not applicable.
Lactation: Not applicable.
Contraindications: Concomitant use of nitrates, including patch; hypersensitivity to sildenafil.
Warnings/precautions
• Use with caution in patients with cardiovascular disease, hypotension, bleeding disorder, active peptic ulcer, sickle cell anemia, multiple myeloma, leukemia, retinitis pigmentosa, anatomical deformation of the penis; MI, cardiovascular accident, or arrhythmia in prior 6 months, kidney or liver disease, elderly.
• Provide patient with list of drugs that potentiate sildenfil action (see Clinically Important Drug Interactions).
• Determine cause of erectile dysfunction: psychologic, organic, drug-induced.
• Priapism has occurred with this agent.
Advice to patient
• Practice safe sex as drug has no effect on disease transmission.

- Additional sexual stimulation is often required after drug is taken to enhance erectile response.
- If erection is present longer than 6 hours, seek medical attention.

Adverse reactions
- Common: headache, dyspepsia, flushing, visual disturbances.
- Serious: severe hypotension when taken along with nitrates, angina, MI, arrhythmias, CVA, depression, neuropathy, hearing loss, ocular toxicity.

Clinically important drug interactions
- Drugs that increase effects/toxicity of sildenafil: cimetidine, erythromycin, itraconazole, ketoconazole.
- Drug that decreases effects/toxicity of sildenafil: rifampin.

Parameters to monitor
- BP, pulse, ECG.
- Ophthalmologic status.
- Efficacy of treatment: success in acquiring and maintaining penile erection during sexual intercourse.

Editorial comments
- Sildenafil, an extremely popular drug, has proven to provide beneficial responses in patients with impotence associated with diabetes, cardiovascular disease, spinal cord injury, radical prostatectomy and in patients taking drugs for hypertension, depression, or psychosis. Cardiovascular events described with the drug's use have generally occurred in the setting of preexisting disease. These may represent effects of sexual activity in a high-risk population.
- Long-term effects of the drug have not been determined.
- This drug is not listed in the *Physician's Desk Reference,* 54th edition, 2000.

Silver Sulfadiazine

Brand name: Silvadene Cream.
Class of drug: Topical antiinfective agent.

Mechanism of action: Disrupts bacterial cell architecture, including cell walls and membranes.

Indications/dosage/route: Oral only.

• Prevention and treatment of wound infections (second- and third-degree burns)

   – Adults, children: 1/16-inch thickness of ointment applied to cleaned and debrided wound, once or twice a day.

Adjustment of dosage

• Kidney disease: None.

• Liver disease: None.

• Elderly: None.

• Pediatric: Silver sulfadizine is contraindicated in premature infants or infants <2 months.

Food: Not applicable.

Pregnancy: Category B, use with caution at term.

Lactation: Avoid during treatment and for several days afterward.

Contraindications: neonates <2 months, hypersensitivity to drug, pregnant women at or near term, G6PD deficiency.

Warnings/precautions

• Use with caution in patients with hypersensitivity to silver sulfadizine, kidney and liver disease. May have cross-sensitivity with thiaziades, sulfonylaurate, sulfonylureal anhydrase inhibitors.

• Continue drug adminsitration until burn is healed or a skin graft is performed.

• Inform patient that if cream becomes dark, it should be discarded.

Advice to patient: Cover entire wound with thin layer cream. If cream has rubbed off a portion of the affected area, it may be reapplied. Your physician may recommend coverings over the area being treated with silver sulfadiazine.

• Notify treating physician if condition persists or becomes worse.

Adverse reactions

• Common: pain, itching.

• Serious: bone marrow suppression, hemolytic anemia, hepatic injury.

Clinically important drug interactions: Silver sulfadiazine reduces effects of fibrinolysin, deoxyribonuclease, collagenase, sutilains, papain.

Parameters to monitor
- Burn tissue for signs of infection: purulent discharge, excessive odor and moisture. Patient may require coadministration of local/systemic anesthetic.
- Signs of sepsis: fever, shock, increased WBC count.
- Hypersensitivity to silver sulfadizine: rash, burning sensation, itching at sites of application and surrounding tissue.
- Signs of fungal superinfection.
- Urine for crystalluria and formation of renal calculi.
- Serum electrolytes.

Editorial comments: It should be noted that appreciable amounts of silver sulfadiazine may be absorbed and produce systemic adverse reactions.

Simvastatin

Brand name: Zocor.
Class of drug: Antilipidemic agent.
Mechanism of action: Inhibits HMG-CoA reductase. Reduces total LDL cholesterol, serum triglyceride levels. There is little if any effect on serum HDL levels.
Indications/dosage/route: Oral only.
- Hypercholesterolemia (types IIA and IIB)
  – Adults: Initial: 20 mg in the evening. Maintenance: 5–80 mg/d in the evening.
  – Elderly: Initial: 5 mg/d. Maintenance:10 mg/d.
- Homozygous familial hypercholesterolemia
  – Adults: 40 mg/d in the evening or 80 mg/d in 3 divided doses (20 mg, 20 mg, 40 mg in the evening).

Adjustment of dosage
- Kidney disease (severe): Initial: 5 mg/d.
- Liver disease: None.
- Elderly: See above.
- Pediatric: Safety and efficacy have not been established.

Food: Take with meals.

Pregnancy: Category X. Contraindicated.

Lactation: Appears in breast milk. Contraindicated.

Contraindications: Hypersensitivity to statins, active liver disease or unexplained persistent elevations of serum transaminase, pregnancy, lactation.

Warnings/precautions

- Use with caution in patients with renal insufficiency, history of liver disease and in alcohol abusers.
- Discontinue if drug-induced myopathy develops. This is characterized by myalgia, creatinine kinase levels >10 times normal. May cause acute renal failure from rhabdomyolysis. This may occur more frequently when drug is combined with gemfibrozil or niacin.
- Discontinue drug if patient experiences severe trauma, surgery, or serious illness.

Advice to patient

- Avoid alcohol.
- Exercise regularly, reduce fat and alcohol intake, and stop smoking.

Adverse reactions

- Common: none.
- Serious: myopathy, rhabdomyolysis, neuropathy, cranial nerve abnormalities, hypersensitivity reactions, pancreatitis, hepatic injury including hepatic necrosis and cirrhosis, lens opacities.

Clinically important drug interactions

- Drugs that increase effects/toxicity of HMG-CoA reductase inhibitors: gemfibrozil, clofibrate, erthyromycin, cyclosporine, niacin, clarithromycin, itraconazole, protease inhibitors.
- HMG-CoA reductase inhibitors increase effects/toxicity of oral anticoagulants.

Parameters to monitor

- Total cholesterol, LDL and HDL cholesterol, triglycerides. Values should be obtained prior to and periodically after treatment begins to ascertain drug efficacy.
- Serum BUN and creatinine.

- Liver enzymes before beginning therapy, at 3, 6, and 12 months thereafter, and semiannually afterward.
- Signs and symptoms of myopathy: unexplained skeletal muscle pain, muscle tenderness or weakness particularly when accompanied by fever or fatigue. Check creatinine kinase levels. If these are markedly elevated or patient is symptomatic, discontinue drug.
- Discontinue drug if transaminase level exceeds 3 times normal values. It may be advisable to take a liver biopsy if transaminase elevation persists after drug is discontinued.
- Ophthalmic state should be evaluated once a year following treatment. If lens opacity occurs, consider discontinuing drug.

Editorial comments: Current literature suggests that the most effective reduction of total and LDL cholesterol occurs with a combination of exercise, weight reduction, low-fat diet, and lipid-lowering agents.

Sodium Polysterene Sulfonate

Brand name: Kayexalate.
Class of drug: Potassium cation-exchange resin.
Mechanism of action: Binds potassium ions in intestine and prevents absorption.
Indications/dosage/route: Oral, rectal.
- Treatment of mild to moderate hyperkalemia
  - Adults: PO 15 g 1–4 times/d in water or sorbitol. Rectal 30–50 g q6h (as rention enema).
  - Children: PO 1 g/kg/dose.

Adjustment of dosage:
- Kidney disease: None.
- Liver disease: None.
- Elderly: Use with caution (at higher risk for fecal impaction).

- Pediatric: Smaller children, infants: Dosage is based on the following calculation: 1 mEq of potassium is bound for each 1 g of resin.

	Onset of Action in Serum Potassium	Duration
Oral	2–12 h	6–24 h
Rectal	2–12 h	No data

Food: Administer sodium polystyrene sulfonate with water or sorbitol, not with orange juice. Suspension may be chilled to improve taste.

Pregnancy: Category C.

Lactation: No data available. Best to avoid.

Contraindications: Hypersensitivity to sodium polysterene sulfonate or components, hypokalemia.

Warnings/precautions

- Use with caution in patients with sodium intake restriction (severe heart failure, marked edema, hypertension), constipation.
- Large oral dose may cause fecal impaction, particularly in elderly. Advise patients experiencing constipation to increase intake of fluids and to consume high-fiber foods (bran, wholegrain bread, raw vegetables and fruits).
- An osmotic laxative, eg, sorbitol, should be administered along with sodium polystyrene to minimize constipation.

Advice to patient

- Retain enema for several hours for best results.

Adverse reactions

- Common: constipation, diarrhea, nausea, vomiting.
- Serious: sodium retention, intestinal obstruction, colonic necrosis (when combined with aluminum hydroxide) alkalosis, pulmonary edema.

Clinically important drug interactions

- Drugs that increase effects/toxicity of sodium polysterene sulfonate: magnesium hydroxide, aluminum carbonate, other aluminum- and magnesium-containing antacids and laxatives.

- Drugs that decrease effects/toxicity of sodium polysterene sulfonate: nonabsorbing cation-donating antacids.
- Sodium polystyrene sulfonate increases effects/toxicity of digitalis glycosides (due to hypokalemia).

Parameters to monitor

- Serum potassium, calcium, BUN, and creatinine.
- Symptoms of potassium abnormalities, ie, hyper- or hypokalemia. Serum potassium should be monitored at least once daily. Potassium levels should be maintained at 4–5 mEq/L. Symptoms of hyperkalemia include muscle weakness, paresthesias, ECG abnormalities. Symptoms of hypokalemia include cardiac arrhythmias, ECG changes (flat or inverted T waves, prominent U waves), confusion, muscle weakness, diarrhea.
- Serum calcium, particularly for patients receiving sodium polystyrene sulfonate >3 days.
- Intake of fluids and urinary and other fluid output to minimize renal toxicity. Closely monitor electrolyte levels.
- Symptoms of digitalis toxicity for patients on cardiac glycosides: visual disturbances, anorexia, nausea, diarrhea, arrhythmias.

Editorial comments: When administering sodium polystyrene sulfonate it may be necessary to discontinue or modify the dosage of drugs that increase serum potassium: potassium-sparing diuretics, ACE inhibitors, potassium substitutes.

Somatropin

Brand names: Genotropin, Humatrope, Nutropin, Saizem, Norditropin.
Class of drug: Recombinant human growth hormone.
Mechanism of action: Stimulates linear growth in children with growth hormone deficiency. Improves metabolism of proteins, carbohydrates, lipids in these patients.
Indications/dosage/route: IM, SC.

- Treatment of children with inadequate levels of endogenous growth hormone

– Humatrope: IM, SC 0.18 mg/kg/wk, daily, 3 alternate days, or 6 times/wk. Maximum: 0.3 mg/kg/wk.

– Nutropin: SC 0.3 mg/kg/wk, divided doses.

• Turner syndrome
  – 0.375 mg/kg/wk, divided doses.

• Adults with childhood- or adult-onset growth hormone deficiency
  – 0.006 mg/kg/d. Increase gradually to maximum 0.0125 mg/kg/d.

Adjustment of dosage
• Kidney disease: No data available.
• Liver disease: No data available.
• Elderly: No data available for patients >60 years.
• Pediatrics: See above.

Food: Not applicable.

Pregnancy: Category C.

Lactation: No data available. Best to avoid.

Contraindications: Growth promotion in children with closed epiphyses (if used for growth stimulation [girls 14–15, boys 15–16]), intracranial lesion with ongoing neoplastic activity, hypersensitivity to *m*-cresol or glycerin (present in somatropin), critically ill patients.

Warnings/precautions
• Use with caution in patients with hypothyroidism, coexisting ACTH deficiency, dysfunctional thyroid gland, intracranial lesions.
• Constitute only with supplied diluent; however, do not use diluent that is supplied if patient is sensitive to *m*-cresol or glycerin. Reconstitute with sterile water.
• Do not use in critically ill patients who are postoperative from myocardial or abdominal surgery or patients with recent trauma or respiratory failure.

Advice to patients
• Use only if solution is clear.
• Change injection sites to prevent lipodystrophy.

Adverse reactions
• Common: edema, arthralgia, myalgia, headache.
• Serious: intracranial hypertension (pediatric patients), antigrowth hormone antibodies, insulin resistance, diabetes, leukemia.

Clinically important drug interactions

- Drugs that decrease effects/toxicity of somatropin: glucocorticoids.
- Somatropin may decrease effects/toxicity of glucocorticoids, anticonvulsants, cyclosporine.

Parameters to monitor

- Serum glucose.
- Development: bone age (annually), growth rate, height, weight, the latter every 3–6 months. Treatment should be continued only if growth is at the rate of 2 cm/y.
- Thyroid function. If hypothyroidism develops, it may be necessary to use thyroid replacement therapy.
- Monitor patient's insulin requirements. These may change in patients with diabetes receiving human growth hormone.
- Symptoms of intracranial hypertension: headache, pupilledema, visual problems.
- Symptoms of slipped capital epiphysis: knee or hip pain, limp.
- Possible development of neutralizing antibodies to somatostatin, particularly if growth rate does not exceed 2.5 cm/half-year.

Editorial comments

- Administration of growth hormone should be undertaken only by a physician who is experienced in diagnosis and treatment of pituitary disorders.
- Patients should be strongly advised not to use growth hormone to increase athletic performance.
- Off-label indications include HIV-infected patients with AIDS-wasting syndrome.

Sotalol

Brand name: Betapace.
Class of drug: β-Adrenergic receptor blocker.
Mechanism of action: Competitive blocker of β-adrenergic receptors in heart and blood vessels.

Indications/dosage/route: Oral only.
• Ventricular arrhythmias
   – Adults: Initial: 80 mg b.i.d. Maintenance: 240 or 640 mg/d.
Adjustment of dosage
• Kidney disease: Creatinine clearance >60 mL/min: dosing interval 12 hours; creatinine clearance 30–59 mL/min: dosing interval 24 hours; creatinine clearance 10–29 mL/min: dosing interval 36–48 hours; creatinine clearance <10 mL/min: individualize dose.
• Liver disease: None.
• Elderly: None.
• Pediatric: Safety and efficacy have not been established.
Food: No restriction.
Pregnancy: Category B.
Lactation: Appears in breast milk. Considered compatible by American Academy of Pediatrics. Observe infant for bradycardia and hypotension.
Contraindications: Cardiogenic shock, asthma, CHF unless it is secondary to tachyarrhythmia treated with a β blocker, sinus bradycardia and AV block greater than first degree, severe COPD.
Editorial comments
• Note that this drug is pregnancy category B (most β blockers are category C).
• For additional information, see *propranolol*, p. 790.

Sparfloxacin

Brand name: Zagam.
Class of drug: Broad-spectrum quinolone antibiotic.
Mechanism of action: Inhibits DNA gyrase, thereby blocking bacterial DNA replication.
Susceptible organisms *in vivo*: *Staphylococcus aureus, Streptococcus pneumoniae* (penicillin sensitive), *Enterobacter cloacae, Hemophilus influenzae, Hemophilus parainfluenzae, Klebsiella pneumoniae, Moraxella catarrhalis, Chlamydia pneumoniae, Mycoplasma pneumoniae.*

Indications/dosage/route: Oral only.
- Community-acquired pneumonia, acute bacterial exacerbation of chronic bronchitis
  - Adults, children >18 years: 100 mg on the first day, as a loading dose. Then 100–200 mg q24h for a total of 10 days.

Adjustment of dosage
- Kidney disease: Creatinine clearance >50 mL/min: loading dose 400 mg on day 1; then 200 mg q48h for ≥8 days.
- Liver disease: None.
- Elderly: None.
- Pediatric: Safety and efficacy have not been established in children <18 years.

Food: Take 1 hour before or 2 hours after meals with a glass of water.

Editorial comments
- Sparfloxacin has advantage over levofloxacin of improved *Bacteroides fragilis* activity.
- Important toxic effects include increased QT interval and phototoxicity which occur more commonly than with other quinolones.
- For additional information, see *ciprofloxacin,* p. 218.

Spironolactone

Brand name: Aldactone.
Class of drug: Potassium-sparing diuretic.
Mechanism of action: Competitively inhibits aldesterone action on distal renal tubules, resulting in excretion of sodium and water and retention of potassium.
Indications/dosage/route: Oral only.
- Edema, ascites
  - Adults: Initial: 25–200 mg/d in 2–4 divided doses, at least 5 days. Maintenance: 75–400 mg/d in 2–4 divided doses.
  - Children: 3.3 mg/kg/d as a single dose or 2–4 divided doses.

- Hypertension alone or with other diuretics or antihypertensive drugs
  - Adults: Initial: 50–100 mg/d, single dose or 2–4 divided doses for at least 2 weeks. Maintenance: adjust to individual response.
  - Children: 1–2 mg/kg in a single dose or 2–4 divided doses.
- Hypokalemia
  - Adults: 25–100 mg/d as single dose or 2–4 divided doses.
- Diagnosis of primary hyperaldosteronism
  - Adults: 400 mg/d, 4 days (short test) or 3–4 weeks (long test)
- Hyperaldosteronism, prior to surgery
  - Adults: 100–400 mg/d in 2–4 doses prior to surgery.

Adjustment of dosage
- Kidney disease: Creatinine clearance 10–50 mL/min: dose q12–24h; creatinine clearance <10 mL/min: do not use.
- Liver disease: None.
- Elderly: None.
- Pediatric: Safety and efficacy have not been established.

Onset of Action	Peak Effect	Duration
—	1–3 h	>24 h

Food: Take with food or milk.
Pregnancy: Category B.
Lactation: Metabolite appears in breast milk. Considered compatible by American Academy of Pediatrics.
Contraindications: Anuria, hyperkalemia, severe renal insufficiency, serum potassium level >5 mEq/L, patients receiving other potassium-sparing diuretics or potassium supplements, hypersensitivity to spironolactone.

Warnings/precautions
- Use caution in patients with dehydration, acute and chronic liver disease, hyponatremia, kidney disease, concurrent use of ACE inhibitors (danger of hyperkalemia).

- May cause severe and life-threatening hyperkalemia.
- Initiation of antihypertensive therapy with a fixed combination of diuretics, eg, potassium-sparing diuretics plus thiazide is generally not recommended. Each drug should be titrated separately and the combination used if appropriate.

Advice to patient

- Change position slowly, in particular from recumbent to upright, to minimize orthostatic hypotension. Sit at the edge of the bed for several minutes before standing, and lie down if feeling faint or dizzy. Avoid hot showers or baths and standing for long periods. Male patients should sit on the toilet while urinating rather than stand.
- Avoid excessive intake of high-potassium foods (bananas, citrus fruits, peaches, dates) and potassium-containing salt substitutes.
- Do not take OTC drugs unless approved by treating physician. In particular, avoid those containing significant amounts of sodium or potassium (eg, Alka-Seltzer).

Adverse reactions

- Common: none.
- Serious: hypotension, bradycardia, heart failure, hyperkalemia, hyponatremia, acidosis, dehydration, male sexual dysfunction, hepatorenal syndrome (cirrhosis).

Clinically important drug interactions

- Drugs that increase effects/toxicity of potassium-sparing diuretics: ACE inhibitors, cimetidine.
- Drugs that decrease effects/toxicity of potassium-sparing diuretics: NSAIDs.
- Potassium-sparing diuretics increase effects/toxicity of digoxin, lithium.
- Potassium-sparing diuretics decrease effects/toxicity of oral hypoglycemics.

Parameters to monitor

- Serum electrolytes including sodium, potassium, bicarbonate, chloride, serum BUN and creatinine. Serum potassium should be determined every 3–4 days at beginning of therapy. If the level reaches 5–5.9 mEq/L, withhold drug, then decrease dosage by 50% or use alternative drug.

- Evaluate patient for orthostasis before and after initiating therapy.
- Signs and symptoms of fluid and electrolyte imbalance: thirst, abdominal cramps, lethargy, paresthesias, weakness, confusion.
- Signs and symptoms of hyperkalemia: muscle weakness, paresthesias, flaccid paralysis of extremities, bradycardia, life-threatening arrthymias, ECG changes in T wave, R wave, S wave, QRS complex.
- Signs and symptoms of severe hyponatremia: seizures, hyperreflexia.
- Signs and symptoms of hypokalemia: weakness, fatigue, Q wave on ECG, polyuria, arrthymias.
- Monitor acid–base balance frequently for possible acidosis (metabolic or respiratory), headache, abdominal pain, nausea, vomiting, severe weakness.
- Intake of fluids and urinary and other fluid output.
- For patients with preexisting severe liver disease, monitor for possible hepatic encephalopathy: confusion, tremors, coma, jaundice.
- ECG. If significant changes develop, drug should be stopped regardless of serum potassium.
- Therapeutic efficacy by weighing patient before breakfast and immediately before voiding. This should be done on the same scale at the same time each day and with the same clothing.
- Mental confusion or lethargy. Reduce dose if these occur.
- For those with hepatic disease, monitor for changes in mental status: stupor, lethargy.

Editorial comments

- For the treatment of essential hypertension, potassium-sparing diuretics are usually combined with other diuretics or antihypertensive drugs.
- This drug has been shown to be carcinogenic in laboratory animals.

Stavudine

Brand name: Zerit. Also known as d4T.
Class of drug: Antiviral, thymidine nucleoside.
Mechanism of action: Inhibits HIV reverse transcriptase, decreases viral DNA synthesis and replication.
Indications/dosage/route: Oral.
• Treatment of HIV infections in patients who do not respond to or cannot tolerate other therapy
  – Adults ≥132 lb: 40 mg q12h.
  – Adults <132 lb: 30 mg q12h.
  – Children <30 kg: 1 mg/kg q12h.
  – Children >30 kg: adult dose.

Adjustment of dosage
• Kidney disease: Creatinine clearance >50 mL/min: usual dose; creatinine clearance 26–50 mL/min: reduce dose by 50% and administer q12h; creatinine clearance 10–25 mL/min: reduce dose by 50% and administer q24h.
• Liver disease: None recommended.
• Elderly: No data available.
• Pediatric: See above.
Food: May be taken with food.
Pregnancy: Category C.
Lactation: Contraindicated. CDC recommends that HIV-infected mothers not breastfeed due to chance of maternal–fetal virus transmission.
Contraindications: Hypersensitivity to stavudine.

Warnings/precautions
• Use with caution in patients with kidney disease, peripheral neuropathy, preexisting bone marrow suppression, folic acid or vitamin B_{12} deficiency.

Adverse reactions
• Common: headache, insomnia, depression, nervousness, abdominal pain, nausea, vomiting, diaphoresis, rash, myalgia, chills, fever, dyspnea.

- Serious: **peripheral neuropathy (20%)**, bone marrow depression, hepatic injury, lactic acidosis with severe hepatic steatosis, pancreatitis.

Clinically important drug interactions: Drugs that increase effects/toxicity of stavudine: chloramphenicol, cisplatin, ethambutol, hydra- lazine, lithium, metronidazole, phenytoin, vincristine.

Parameters to monitor

- Liver enzymes.
- Signs and symptoms of hepatotoxicity. Discontinue if present.
- Symptoms of opportunistic infection.
- Signs of peripheral neuropathy: numbness, pain in hands or feet, tingling sensation. Discontinue if symptoms of neuropathy develop. Drug may be cautiously reintroduced at 50% of prior maintenance dose if symptoms resolve.
- Signs of pancreatitis: nausea, vomiting, abdominal pain. Confirm diagnosis with serum amylase and lipase levels.

Editorial comments

- Stavudine is used in combination therapy with zidovudine or other nucleoside antiviral drugs.

Streptokinase

Brand names: Kibikase, Streptase.

Class of drug: Thrombolytic enzyme.

Mechanism of action: Activates plasminogen conversion to plasmin. This stimulates the formation of anticoagulant proteins, resulting in dissolution of clot.

Indications/dosage/route: IV only.

- Management of acute coronary thrombosis
  - Adults: 500,000 IU infused over 60 minutes. Loading dose of 20,000 IU via coronary catheter. Maintenance: 2000 IU/min, 60-minute IV infusion.
- Pulmonary embolus, other emboli (deep vein, arterial), thrombosis

- Adults: 150,000-IU loading dose followed by 100,000 IU/h, 24 hours for pulmonary embolus, 72 hours for recurrent pulmonary embolus or deep vein thrombosis.
- Adults: Loading dose: 250,000 IU, 30-minute infusion. Sustaining dose:100,000 IU/h, IV infusion, 72 hours for deep vein thrombosis, 100,000 IU/h over 24 hours for pulmonary embolism.
- Cannula occlusion injection
  - Adults: 100,000–250,000 IU. Clamp cannula for 2 hours, then aspirate.
- Acute transmural MI (intracoronary and intravenous infusion)
  - Adults: 20,000-IU bolus, then 2000 IU/min, 60 minutes.

Adjustment of dosage
- Kidney disease: None.
- Liver disease: Contraindicated.
- Elderly: May be a greater risk for bleeding after streptokinase.
- Pediatric: Safety and effectiveness have not been established. Arterial occlusions have been treated IV with 1000 IU/kg loading doses, with IV infusions of 1000 IU/kg/h for ≤12 hours.

Onset of Action	Duration
Rapid	12 h

Food: Not applicable.

Pregnancy: Category C. Avoid during first 18 weeks and use only when there is no safe alternative.

Lactation: Not recommended.

Contraindications: Active internal bleeding, recent CVA, ulcerative colitis, severe hypertension, acute left heart arterial embolus, acute or chronic liver disease, recent cerebral embolism or hemorrhage, recent liver or kidney biopsy or other surgical procedure, streptococcal infections within the last 6 months, tuberculosis, brain cancer, uncontrolled hypertension (systolic >180 mm Hg, diastolic >110 mm Hg), ophthalmic hemorrhage, history of allergic reaction to any thrombolytic agents.

Warnings/precautions

- Use with caution in patients with arterial embolus that originates from left side of the heart, obstetric delivery, major surgery within 10 days, internal organ biopsy, arterial puncture; in patients having had prior streptokinase; and in patients receiving anticoagulants or antiplatelet drugs.
- Venipuncture or arterial puncture should be conducted with care.
- If minor allergic reaction occurs, this can be treated with an antihistamine as well as parenteral corticosteroid. If fever occurs, this may be treated with acetaminophen but not aspirin.

Advice to patient: Avoid taking NSAIDs together with this drug.

Adverse reactions

- Common: superficial bleeding
- Serious: angioneuritic edema, bronchospasm, severe internal hemorrhage, Guillain–Barré syndrome, hypersensitivity reaction.

Clinically important drug interactions

- Drugs that increase effects/toxicity of streptokinase: anticoagulants, aspirin, NSAIDs, antiplatelet drugs.
- Drugs that decrease effects/toxicity of streptokinase: antifibrinolytics (aminocaproic acid).

Parameters to monitor

- Signs of bleeding.
- Signs of allergic reaction.

Editorial comments

- Streptokinase is probably the most widely used fibrinolytic therapy in the world. Huge populations of acute MI patients (transmural) have undergone enrollment in randomized trials investigating dosing and combination therapies. These trials have determined that large single bolus doses ($\approx 1.5 \times 10^6$ IU) with concomitant treatments with aspirin, β blockers and, after 12 hours, heparin (half-life of streptokinase is short and reinfarctions are not uncommon if heparin is not added) are effective. Tissue plasmonogen activator has the ability to prevent reinfarction without the use of heparin IV.
- The advent of direct angioplasty and stenting has decreased the use of fibrinolytic therapy in acute MI. In many communities, however, thrombolysis is the only aggressive therapy

available. The addition of better antiplatelet therapy is a burgeoning area of research in acute coronary syndromes.
- Thrombolysis is also used as therapy of acute brain thrombus/stroke and for pulmonary embolus and some types of acute arterial occlusions.

Streptomycin

Brand name: Streptomycin.
Class of drug: Antibiotic, aminoglycoside.
Mechanism of action: Binds to ribosomal units in bacteria, inhibits protein synthesis.
Susceptible organisms *in vivo*: *Mycobacterium tuberculosis, Yersinia pestis, Francisella tularensis, Brucella*; synergism against enterocococi and streptococcoi.
Indications/dosage/route: IM only.
- Inguinal granuloma, chancroid; respiratory, endocardial, meningeal infections (*Hemophilus influenzae*), pneumonia, UTIs, bacteremia (gram-negative bacillary)
  – Adults: 15 mg/kg/d. Maximum: 1 g/d.
  – Children: 20–40 mg/kg/d. Maximum: 1 g/d.
- Tuberculosis
  – Adults: 1 g or 15 mg/kg/d, 2–3 months, then 1 g 2–3 times/wk. Maximum: 1 g/d.
  – Children: IM 20–40 mg/kg/d. Maximum: 1 g/d.
- Tularemia
  – Adults: 1–2 g/d in divided doses, 7–14 days.
- Plague
  – Adults: 2 g/d in 2 divided doses, minimum 10 days.
- Streptococal endocarditis (for synergism with a β-lactam)
  – Initial: 1 g b.i.d. (first week), then 500 mg b.i.d. second week.
- Enterococcal endocarditis (with penicillin) (for synergism with ampicillin or vancomycin)
  – Initial: 1 g b.i.d. (2 weeks), then 5 mg b.i.d. next 4 weeks.

Adjustment of dosage
- Kidney disease: Creatinine clearance 10–50 mL/min: administration interval 24–72 hours; creatinine clearance <10 mL/min: administration interval 72–96 hours.
- Liver disease: None.
- Elderly: None.
- Pediatric: See above.

Food: No restrictions.

Pregnancy: Category D.

Lactation: Appears in breast milk. Considered compatible by American Academy of Pediatrics.

Contraindications: Hypersensitivity to aminoglycoside antibiotics.

Warnings/precautions
- Use with caution in patients with renal disease, neuromuscular disorders (eg, myasthenia gravis, parkinsonism), hearing disorders.
- Do not combine this drug with any other drug in the same IV bag.

Adverse reactions:
- Common: none.
- Serious: renal toxicity, ototoxicity, neuromuscular paralysis, respiratory depression (infants), superinfection.

Clinically important drug interactions
- Drugs that increase effects/toxicity of aminoglycosides: loop diuretics, amphotericin B, enflurane, vancomycin, NSAIDs.
- Drugs that decrease effects/toxicity of aminoglycosides: penicillins (high dose), cephalosporins.

Parameters to monitor
- Peak and trough serum levels 48 hours after beginning therapy and every 3–4 days thereafter as well as after changing doses. Peak (therapeutic): = 15–40 µg/mL; trough: <4 µg/mL.
- Signs of ototoxicity: tinnitus, vertigo, hearing loss. The drug should be stopped if tinnitus or vertigo occurs. Limit administration to 7–10 days to decrease the risk of ototoxicity.
- Renal function periodically. If serum creatinine increases by more than 50% over baseline value, it may be advisable to

discontinue drug treatment and use a less nephrotoxic agent, eg, a quinolone or cephalosporin.
- Efficacy of drug action. If there is no response in 3–7 days, reculture and consider another drug.
- Neuromuscular function when administering the drug IV. Too rapid administration may cause paralysis and apnea. Have calcium gluconate or pyridostigmine available to reverse such an effect.
- Neurologic status if the drug is given for hepatic encephalopathy.
- Signs and symptoms of allergic reaction.

Editorial comments
- Streptomycin has the greatest activity of all the aminoglycosides against *M. tuberculosis*. It is a first-line drug for tuberculosis though not as effective as isoniazid and rifampin.
- Streptomycin is the drug of choice to treat plague and brucellosis.
- Streptomycin and gentamicin are the drugs of choice to treat tularemia.

Succinylcholine (Suxamethonium)

Brand names: Anectine, Sucostrin, Quelicin.
Class of drug: Skeletal muscle relaxant (depolarizing).
Mechanism of action: Depolarizes motor endplate at myoneural junction, preventing stimulation by endogenous acetylcholine.
Indications/dosage/route: IV, IM.
- Skeletal muscle paralysis after induction of anesthesia for surgical procedures
  - Adults: Short procedures: IV or IM 0.3–1.1 mg/kg over 10–30 seconds. Maintenance: 0.04–0.07 mg/kg q5–10min. Maximum: 150 mg.
  - Infants: IV 1–2 mg/kg. Maintenance: 0.3–0.6 mg/kg q5–10 min.

– Older children, adolescents: 1 mg/kg IV or 3-4 mg/kg IM. Maximum 150 mg.

Note: Succinylcholine should be reserved for use in children who require emergency intubation, who do not have an accessible vein, and for whom an airway can be readily secured.

Adjustment of dosage

- Kidney disease: Use with caution; may precipitate hyperkalemia in renal failure patients.
- Liver disease: Use cautiously, high risk for side effects; reduce dose.
- Elderly: Use with caution.
- Pediatric: See above.

	Onset of Action	Peak Effect	Duration
IV	0.5–1 min	1–2 min	14–20 min
IM	2–3 min	No data	10–30 min

Pregnancy: Category C.

Lactation: No data available; best to avoid.

Contraindications: Hypersensitivity to succinylcholine, low plasma pseudocholinesterase (hepatocellular disease), atypical plasma cholinesterase, malnutrition, severe anemia, severe burns, cancer, dehydration, collagen diseases, family or personal history of acute malignant hyperthermia, acute narrow-angle glaucoma, myopathies (high serum creatinine phosphokinase), penetrating eye injuries, multiple traumas, denervation of skeletal muscle (due to CNS injury).

Warnings/precautions

- Use with caution in patients undergoing cesarean section; in patients with kidney and severe liver disease, respiratory depression, severe anemia, severe burns, hyperkalemia, cerebrovascular accident, myasthenia gravis, thyroid disorders, porphyria, eye surgery, pheochromocytoma, chronic abdominal infection, subarachnoid hemorrhage, degenerative neuromuscular disease, patients receiving cardiac glycosides, fractures, dislocations; and in patients recovering from severe trauma.

- Patient should be premedicated with atropine or scopolamine to prevent excessive salivation.
- Neostigmine or pyridostigmine should be available to counteract neuromuscular blockade after drug is stopped.
- Patient is fully conscious and thus aware of surroundings, including conversations.
- Tachyphylaxis may occur with continuous infusion or repeated administration. It is preferable to administer the drug by continuous infusion rather than fractional doses to minimize tachyphylaxis.
- A test dose of succinylcholine may be administered initially to determine the degree of sensitivity of the patient as well as recovery time. This test dose should consist of 5–10 mg or 0.1 mg/kg.
- Patient with fracture or muscle spasm may experience additional trauma because of muscle fasciculations. Administer tubocurarine to prevent this.

Adverse reactions
- Common: muscle fasciculations, postoperative muscle pain, increased intraocular pressure, hypertension, salivation.
- Serious: malignant hyperthermia, bradycardia, hypotension, tachycardia, arrthymias, cardiac arrest, hyperkalemia, severe prolonged neuromuscular blockade, severe prolonged respiratory depression or apnea.

Clinically important drug interactions: Drugs that increase effects/toxicity of succinylcholine: cholinesterase inhibitors, oral contraceptives, cyclophosphamide, thiotepa, inhalation anesthetics, aminoglycosides, tetracyclines, vancomycin, cyclosporine, isofluorophate, echothiophate, aminoglycosides, clindamycin, quinidine, procainamide, β blockers, lithium, non-potassium-sparing diuretics, opioids, digitalis glycosides.

Parameters to monitor
- Signs and symptoms of toxicity, particularly in those with low plasma pseudocholinesterase activity.
- Respiratory status continuously. If respirations do not return in a few seconds after discontinuing administration, use of oxygen is necessary.

- Neuromuscular response using a peripheral nerve stimulator. Responses should be determined during and after surgery to monitor efficacy and recovery.
- Cardiovascular status throughout. Monitor for bradycardia, arrhythmias, hypotension.
- Signs of malignant hyperthermia: muscle spasm, particularly of the jaw, loss of laryngeal relaxation, hyperthermia, unstable BP, tachyarrthymias, hypercarbia. Hyperthermia is a late manifestation. Stop infusion if these symptoms are noted.
- Electrolytes: calcium and in particular potassium for hyperkalemia. This is especially necessary for patients with severe trauma or burns.
- Signs and symptoms of increased intraocular pressure. This is usually transient; if it persists this could be dangerous to the eyes.

Editorial comments

- Succinylcholine should be used only by individuals who are well versed and experienced in endotracheal intubation. Equipment for intubation should be available immediately if needed.
- Succinylcholine has no effect on pain threshold. If a painful or long procedure is anticipated, an analgesic must be administered along with succinylcholine. A benzodiazepine or conventional analgesic should be used.

Sufentanil

Brand name: Sufenta.
Class of drug: Narcotic analgesic, agonist.
Mechanism of action: Binds to opiate receptors and blocks ascending pain pathways. Reduces patient's perception of pain without altering cause of the pain.
Indications/dosage/route: IV only.
- Analgesia

- Adults: Initial: 1–2 µg/kg with oxygen and nitrous oxide. Maintenance: 10–25 µg as required.
- Complicated surgery
  - Adults: 2–8 µg/kg with oxygen and nitrous oxide. Maintenance: 10–50 µg.
- General anesthesia
  - Adults: 8–30 µg/kg with 100% oxygen and a muscle relaxant. Maintenance: 25–50 µg.
  - Children <12 years: 10–25 µg/kg with 100% oxygen. Maintenance: 25–50 µg.
- General anesthesia in children <12 years undergoing cardiovascular surgery
  - Initial: 10–25 µg/kg with 100% oxygen. Maintenance: 25–50 µg.

Adjustment of dosage
- Kidney disease: None.
- Liver disease: None.
- Elderly: None.
- Pediatric: See above.

Onset of Action	Peak Effect	Duration
1.5–3 min	No data	No data

Food: Not applicable.

Pregnancy: Category C. Category D if prolonged use or if given in high doses at term.

Lactation: No information available. Avoid breastfeeding.

Contraindications: Hypersensitivity to opiates of the same chemical class, bronchial asthma, severe respiratory depression, abdominal pain of undetermined origin.

Warnings/precautions
- Use with caution in patients with head injury with increased intracranial pressure, serious alcoholism, prostatic hypertrophy, chronic pulmonary disease, severe liver or kidney disease, post disorders of biliary tract, and in postoperative patients with pulmonary disease.

- Administer drug before patient experiences severe pain for fullest efficacy.
- Nausea, vomiting, and orthostatic hypotension occur most prominently in ambulatory patients. If nausea and vomiting persist, it may be necessary to administer an antiemetic, eg, droperidol or prochlorperazine.
- This drug can cause severe hypotension in a patient who is volume depleted or if given along with a phenothiazine or general anesthetic.
- Careful diagnosis must be made of acute abdominal condition before this drug is administered.

Editorial comments
- This drug should be administered only by personnel who have experience in the use of IV and general anesthetics as well as how to manage possible respiratory depression by narcotic drugs. The following must be immediately available should the need arise: resuscitative and intubation equipment, oxygen, narcotic antagonist. Patient should be continuously monitored for oxygen saturation, vital signs, and signs of upper airway obstruction and hypotension.
- This drug is listed without details in the *Physician's Desk Reference,* 54th edition, 2000.
- For additional information, see *morphine*, p. 633.

Sulfasalazine

Brand name: Azulfidine.
Class of drug: Antiinflammatory agent/immunomodulator.
Mechanism of action: Metabolite (5-aminosalicyclic acid) is believed to act as antiinflammatory agent.
Indications/dosage/route: Oral only.
- Ulcerative colitis
  – Adults: Initial: 1–2 g daily. Increase to 3–4 g daily if needed. Maintenance: 2 g/d.

– Children >2 years: 40–60 mg/kg/d in 3–6 divided doses. Maintenance: 30 mg/kg/day in 4 divided doses.
• Rheumatoid arthritis
 – Adults: Initial: 0.5–1 g daily. Increase to 2–3 g/d in evenly divided doses as needed.

Adjustment of dosage
• Kidney disease: Use with caution only after careful appraisal.
• Liver disease: Use with caution only after careful appraisal.
• Elderly: None.
• Pediatric: See above. Contraindicated in children <2 years.

Food: Should be taken with food to minimize GI upset.

Pregnancy: Category B

Lactation: Appears in breast milk. Potentially toxic to infant. American Academy of Pediatrics recommends caution with administration during breastfeeding.

Contraindications: Hypersensitivity to sulfasalazine, sulfonamides (sulfa drugs, thiazides, oral hypoglycemic drugs), salicylates; intestinal or urinary obstruction, porphyria.

Warnings/precautions: Use with caution in patients with mild to moderate liver or kidney disease, bronchial asthma, blood dyscrasia, G6PD deficiency, severe allergies.

Advice to patient
• Drink large amounts of fluid (2.5–3 L) per day and maintain adequate fluid intake after discontinuing the drug.
• To minimize possible photosensitivity reaction, apply adequate sunscreen and use proper covering when exposed to strong sunlight.
• Report to treating physician if you experience the following symptoms: sore throat, fever, jaundice.
• To prevent relapse, continue to take sulfasalazine even if your ulcerative colitis or rheumatoid arthritis shows improvement.
• Do not take antacids with sulfasalazine.
• Be aware that your urine and skin may turn orange-yellow and that soft contact lenses may be permanently stained.

Adverse reactions
• Common: skin rash, anorexia, headache, nausea, vomiting, gastric distress, fever, oligospermia (reversible).

- Serious: Stevens–Johnson syndrome, Lyell's syndrome, granulocytopenia, leukopenia, thrombocytopenia, aplastic anemia, hepatitis, interstitial nephritis, serum sickness.

Clinically important drug interactions
- Sulfasalazine decreases effects/toxicity of digoxin, folic acid.
- Ferrous sulfate decreases absorption of sulfasalazine.

Parameters to monitor
- CBC with differential, liver function tests. These should be carried out before starting therapy and periodically during the first 3 months. These tests are recommended monthly during the next 3 months and afterward every 3 months.
- Periodic serum BUN and creatinine, urinalysis with microscopic examination.
- Signs and symptoms of skin rash.
- Signs of hemolytic anemia in patients with G6PD deficiency.
- Serum sulfapyridine levels. Level of this metabolite >50 µg/mL are associated with an increase in adverse reactions.
- Efficacy in treating ulcerative colitis: reduction of stool frequency, rectal bleeding, abdominal pain, increase in energy level.

Editorial comments: In general, new forms of 5-aninosalicylate preparations (which do not contain sulfapyridine) are preferred for the treatment of inflammatory bowel disease because of their better side effect profiles. However, sulfasalazine may be somewhat more potent and is much less costly than the newer alternatives.

Sulindac

Brand name: Clinoril.
Class of drug: NSAID.
Mechanism of action: Inhibits cyclooxygenase, resulting in inhibition of synthesis of prostaglandins and other inflammatory mediators.
Indications/dosage/route: Oral only.

- Osteoarthritis, rheumatoid arthritis, ankylosing spondylitis
  – Adults: 150 mg b.i.d.
- Acute painful shoulder, acute gouty arthritis
  – Adults: 200 mg b.i.d., 7–14 days.
- Gout
  – Adults: 200 mg b.i.d., 7 days.

Adjustment of dosage
- Kidney disease: None.
- Liver disease: None.
- Elderly: May be necessary to reduce dose for >65 years.
- Pediatric: Safety and efficacy have not been established.

Food: Take with food or large quantities of water or milk.

Pregnancy: Category B. Category D in third trimester or near delivery.

Lactation: Not data available. Best to avoid.

Contraindications: Hypersensitivity to sulindac and cross-sensitivity with other NSAIDs and aspirin.

Editorial comments
- Sulindac has been shown to be efficacious as a chemoprophylactic agent for limiting growth of adenomatous polyps in patients with familial adenomatous polyposis.
- For additional information, see *ibuprofen*, p. 445.

Sumatriptan

Brand name: Imitrex.

Class of drug: Antimigraine.

Mechanism of action: Activates selective serotonin 5-HT$_1$ receptors in cerebral artery vessels. As a result, vasoconstriction occurs and reduction in inflammation.

Indications/dosage/route: Oral, SC.
- Acute migraine headache with or without aura
  – Adults: SC 5–20 mg total dose, 2 divided doses/d. Nasal spray: administer as 5 or 10 mg both nostrils or 20 mg one nostril.

– Adults: Initial: PO 25–100 mg. Second dose of 25–100 mg after 1–2 hours if no response; another dose after 2 hours of 25–100 mg may be given. Maximum daily dose: 300 mg.

Adjustment of dosage

• Kidney disease: None.
• Liver disease: Use with caution; higher blood levels expected.
• Elderly: Use with caution.
• Pediatric: Safety and efficacy have not been established.

	Onset of Action	Peak Effect	Duration
Oral	<30 min	2–4 h	24 h
SC	30 min	12 min	24 h

Food: Unknown.

Pregnancy: Category C.

Lactation: Excreted in breast milk. Best to avoid.

Contraindications: Hypersensitivity to sumatriptan, uncontrolled hypertension, ischemic heart disease, hemiplegic or basilar migraine, Prinzmetal's angina, GI lesions (history or active), use within 14 days of MAO inhibitor therapy, concurrent ergotamine, IV route, peripheral vascular disease, ischemic bowel, severe liver disease.

Warnings/precautions: Use with caution in postmenopausal women, in male patients >40 years who may be at risk for coronary artery disease, and in patients with family history of heart disease, hypertension, obesity, diabetes, liver disease.

Advice to patient

• Do not administer IV, only SC. Sumatriptan should be used only during a migraine attack and is best taken at the first sign of attack. It is not to be used to prevent or reduce the number of attacks.
• Lie down in darkened room following administration of sumatriptan.
• Avoid driving and other activities requiring mental alertness or that are potentially dangerous until response to drug is known.

- Avoid alcohol and other CNS depressants such as sedatives (eg, diazepam) when taking this drug.

Adverse reactions
- Common: taste disturbances, nausea and vomiting.
- Serious: coronary vasospasm, myocardial ischemia, ventricular tachycardia, ventricular fibrillation, MI, GI bleeding, syncope.

Clinically important drug interactions
- Drugs that increase effects/toxicity of sumatriptan: lithium, SSRIs, ergot-containing drugs, MAO inhibitors.
- Sumatriptan increases effects/toxicity of ergot containing drugs.

Parameters to monitor
- Signs of hypersensitivity reaction: wheezing, tightness in chest, pain, swelling of eyelids or face, rash, hives. If these occur, discontinue administration of sumatriptan.
- Following symptoms: tingling in extremities, flushing, drowsiness, dizziness.
- BP before and at least 1 hour after initial injection.
- ECG for ischemic changes including angina.

Editorial comments
- Physician should provide patient with information pamphlet and perhaps the instructional video available from manufacturer when administering sumatriptan.
- Sumatriptan is indicated only for patients who have a clear diagnosis of migraine.
- It is suggested that the first dose of sumatriptan should be taken in the physician's office because of the rare possibility of occurrence of severe cardiac events.

Tacrine

Brand name: Cognex.

Class of drug: Cholinesterase inhibitor, symptomatic treatment for dementia.

Mechanism of action: Tacrine is a reversible cholinesterase inhibitor that decreases the breakdown of acetycholine in the brain. Increased CNS acetylcholine theoretically will maintain function in nondegenerated neurons in the cerebral cortex and forebrain.

Indication/dosage/route: Oral only.

• Mild to moderate Alzheimer's disease

 – Adults: Initial: 10 mg q.i.d. Continue for 4 weeks and check ALT level. If patient tolerates this dose level and transaminases are stable, increase dosage up to 20 mg q.i.d. Further increases up to every 4 weeks may be instititued if drug is tolerated and no changes occur in liver enzymes.

Adjustment of dosage

• Monitor transaminase levels every other week for 16 weeks, then every 6 months. Adjust doses based on the following recommendations for patients in whom elevations occur: ALT 2 times upper normal limits: continue; ALT >2 to <3 times upper limit of normal: continue treatment, monitor transaminase weekly; ALT >3 to <5 times upper limit of normal: reduce dose by 40 mg/d, monitor ALT weekly, resume normal dosing/ titration when ALT normalizes; ALT >5 times upper limit of normal; stop drug. If jaundice develops consult specialist.

• Pediatric: No studies have been performed to document efficacy of tacrine in children with dementia.

Food: Should be taken between meals on an empty stomach. May be taken with food if GI upset occurs.

Pregnancy: Category C.

Lactation: No data available. Potentially toxic to infant.

Contraindications: Hypersensitivity to tacrine or acridine derivatives, patients who have developed tacrine-related jaundice from previous treatment with this drug.

Warnings/precautions

- Use with caution in patients with sick sinus syndrome, bradycardia, liver disease, kidney disease, asthma, prostatic hypertrophy, Parkinson's disease, active peptic ulcer.
- If jaundice occurs or bilirubin is ≥3 mg/dL, discontinue tacrine permanently.

Advice to patient

- Do not double dose if a single dose is missed.
- Do not increase dose without consulting treating physician.
- Do not discontinue tacrine without consulting treating physician. If tacrine 80 mg/d is discontinued, it may result in a severe decline in cognitive function as well as behavioral disturbances.
- If nausea and vomiting become persistent and troublesome, notify treating physician.

Adverse reactions

- Common: elevation of transaminase levels, headache, dizziness, nausea, vomiting, diarrhea.
- Serious: liver injury, seizures, heat exhaustion, cholinergic crises, bone marrow suppression, parkinsonism, hypotension, arrhythmias, bradycardia, bone marrow depression.

Drug interactions

- Drugs that increase effects/toxicity of tacrine: cimetidine, other inhibitors of cytochrome P450, fluvoxamine.
- Tacrine increases effects/toxicity of theophylline, succinycholine, other cholinesterase inhibitors, cholinergic agonists (eg, bethanechol).
- Tacrine decreases effects/toxicity of anticholinergic agents.

Parameters to monitor

- Liver enzymes, CBC with differential and platelets.
- Pulse and BP periodically for evidence of bradycardia, hypotension.

- Signs of symptoms of gastric ulcer development.
- Signs and symptoms of toxicity: severe nausea, sweating, bradycardia, hypotension, seizures, muscle weakness. If these symptoms occur, administer atropine IV, initial dose 1–2 mg. Give subsequent doses on the basis of clinical response.
- Signs of hypersensitivity reactions: urticaria, rash, wheezing, pruritis, hypotension. Discontinue drug.

Editorial comments: Tacrine therapy probably does not stop the neurologic degenerative processes associated with Alzheimer's disease. The full effect of tacrine on the natural history of this condition is not known.

Tacrolimus

Brand name: Prograf.
Class of drug: Immunosuppressant, antirejection agent in patients with organ transplantation.
Mechanism of action: Inhibits T-lymphocyte activation and suppresses cell-mediated immunity.
Indication/dosage/route: Oral, IV.

- Prophylaxis for organ rejection in patients with kidney or liver transplantation
  - Adults: IV: Initial: 0.03–0.05 mg/kg/d, given no sooner than 6 hours after transplant. Continuous IV infusion maintained until patient can tolerate oral administration. Generally, given with concomitant parenteral corticosteroid therapy.
  - Adults: Oral (liver transplantation): 0.1–0.15 mg/kg/d, 2 divided doses q12h. Start 8–12 hours after discontinuing infusion.
  - Adults: Oral (kidney transplantation): 0.2 mg/kg/d, 2 divided doses, q12h. Initial dose within 24 hours of transplantation; may be delayed until serum creatinine <4.0 mL/min.
  - Children: IV 0.1 mg/kg/day, no sooner than 6 hours after transplantation. Maintain IV route until patient can tolerate oral administration. Then give 0.3 mg/kg/d PO, 2 divided

doses q12h. Begin 8–12 hours after discontinuation of IV infusion.

Adjustment of dosage
• Kidney disease: Lower doses should be used.
• Liver disease: Use with caution. Give lowest possible dose.
• Elderly: None.
• Pediatric: See above.

Food: Administer oral tacrolimus on empty stomach.

Pregnancy: Category C.

Lactation: Appears in breast milk. Contraindicated.

Contraindications: Hypersensitivity to castor oil derivative (present in IV form).

Warnings/precautions
• Use with caution in patients with kidney or liver disease.
• Do not administer potassium-sparing diuretics to patients taking tacrolimus.
• Replace IV administration with oral therapy as soon as possible.
• Cyclosporine should not be administered with tacrolimus. Either agent should be discontinued at least 24 hours before beginning the other.

Advice to patient: Avoid grapefruit juice.

Adverse reactions
• Common: tremor, headache, diarrhea, hypertension, nausea, vomiting, hyperglycemia, paresthesias, insomnia, chest pain.
• Serious: **nephrotoxicity, hyperglycemia, hyperkalemia, hypomagnesemia**, hypokalemia, hepatitis, bone marrow depression, paresthesias, neuropathy, anaphylaxis, dyspnea, myocardiol, hypertrophy, pulmonary edema, pleural effusion.

Clinically important drug interactions
• Drugs that increase effect/toxicity of tacrolimus: aminoglycosides, cisplatin, cyclosporine, potassium-sparing diuretics, ACE inhibitors, antifungal agents (clotrimazole, fluconazole, itraconazole, ketoconazole), bromocriptine, calcium channel blockers, cimetidine, clarithromycin, erythromycin, metoclopramide, cisapride, methylprednisolone, danazol, protease inhibitors.

- Drugs that decrease effects/toxicity of tacrolimus: phenobarbital, phenytoin, carbamazepine, rifampin, rifabutin.

Parameters to monitor

- BP closely during therapy. If hypertension occurs, it should be treated.
- Hypersensitivity reaction: rash, edema of face, eyelids, nasal membranes, and/or larynx, hypotension, wheezing, pruritis, cardiovascular irregularity. The following should be immediately available to counteract these effects: IV epinephrine (1:1000), IV antihistamines (best Benadryl), or IV corticosteroids, equipment for artificial ventilation.
- Monitor tacrolimus blood levels as an aid to determine efficacy and toxicity and to assess compliance.
- Signs and symptoms of infection.
- Frequent monitoring of the following is suggested: serum potassium, magnesium, triglycerides, cholesterol, calcium, phosphate, CBC.

Editorial comments: There is a possibility of increased risk for developing lymphomas or other malignancies particularly of the skin in patients who receive tacrolimus.

Tamoxifen

Brand name: Nolvadex.
Class of drug: Antiestrogen agent.
Mechanism of action: Inhibits DNA synthesis by binding to estrogen receptors on tumor cells.
Indications/dosage/route: Oral only.

- Adjuvant or palliative therapy for breast cancer
  – 10–20 mg b.i.d.

Adjustment of dosage

- Kidney disease: None.
- Liver disease: None.
- Elderly: None.
- Pediatric: Not applicable.

Food: Administer with food or fluids.

Pregnancy: Category D.

Lactation: Inhibits lactation and is potentially toxic to newborn. Contraindicated.

Contraindications: Hypersensitivity to tamoxifen, pregnancy, history of DVT, requirement for coumadin.

Warnings/precautions

- Use with caution in patients with leukopenia, thrombocytopenia, retinopathy, decreased visual activity.
- Perform estrogen receptor assay before initiating therapy to make certain that tamoxifen is indicated.
- Perform regular gynecologic examination including PAP and vaginal smears.
- Tamoxifen increases risk of developing hepatocellular carcinoma.

Advice to patient: This drug may cause bone pain and hot flashes when starting therapy. These effects usually disappear after a short time while on continuous treatment. Notify physician if vaginal bleeding occurs.

Adverse reactions

- Common: nausea, vomiting, irregular menses, flushing, bone and tumor pain (transient, subsides rapidly with continuing administration), hot flashes (transient), skin rash, vaginal bleeding.
- Serious: Thromboembolic occurrences, hypersensitivity reactions, thrombocytopenia, thromboembolic occurrences, hypercalcemia, endometrial carcinoma, confusion.

Clinically important drug interactions

- Drugs that increase effects/toxicity of tamoxifen: Cytotoxic agents, ritonavir.
- Drugs that decrease effects/toxicity of tamoxifen: estrogens.
- Tamoxifen increases effects/toxicity of coumadin, cyclosporine.

Parameters to monitor

- Serum cholesterol and triglycerides.
- Thyroid function, in particular T_4, periodically.
- Hematologic status including CBC periodically.
- Weight on a weekly basis. If there is significant weight gain, therapy should be evaluated. This may indicate edema.

- Increase in pain in bone or tumor. Advise patient that this pain will subside despite continued treatment. If pain is severe, administer appropriate analgesics.
- Efficacy of treatment by determining the decrease in size or spread of the breast cancer. Effectiveness may not be observed until 4–10 weeks after beginning drug administration.

Editorial comments

- An increase in bone pain is often associated with a good response of the tumor. This generally occurs shortly after beginning therapy.
- Best results in using tamoxifen occur when the patient exhibits positive estrogen receptors in the tumor.

Tamsulosin

Brand name: Flomax.

Class of drug: α_1-Adrenergic antagonist.

Mechanism of action: Blocks α_1-adrenergic receptors in prostate, resulting in relaxation of bladder neck and prostatic smooth muscle.

Indications/dosage/route: Oral only.

- BPH
  – Adults: 0.4 mg/d, administered 30 minutes after the same meal each day. If there is no response after 2–4 weeks, increase dose to 0.8 mg/d.

Adjustment of dosage

- Kidney disease: Creatinine clearance <10 mL/min: has not been studied.
- Liver disease: None in moderate dysfunction.
- Elderly: Consider reduced dose.
- Pediatric: Contraindicated.

Food: Patient should be advised to take tamsulosin 30 minutes after the same meal each day.

Pregnancy: Category B.

Lactation: Not applicable.

Contraindications: Hypersensitivity to tamsulosin, treatment of hypertension with α blockers, children.

Warnings/precautions: May cause orthostatic hypotension and syncope.

• Use with caution in patient receiving warfarin concurrently.

Advice to patient

• Change position slowly, in particular from recumbent to upright, to minimize orthostatic hypotension. Sit at the edge of the bed for several minutes before standing, and lie down if feeling faint or dizzy. Avoid hot showers or baths and standing for long periods. Patients with orthostatic hypotension may be safer urinating while seated on the toilet rather than standing.

• Avoid driving and other activities requiring mental alertness or that are potentially dangerous until response to drug is known.

Adverse reactions

• Common: dizziness, rhinitis, fatigue.

• Serious: orthostatic hypotension, syncope, ejaculation abnormalities.

Clinically important drug interactions: Drugs that increase effects/toxicity of tamsulosin: α-adrenergic blockers, warfarin, cimetidine.

Parameters to monitor: BP to check if significantly lowered.

Editorial comments: Because the symptoms of BPH and carcinoma of the prostate are quite similar, prostatic carcinoma should be ruled out before initiating therapy.

Temazepam

Brand name: Restoril.

Class of drug: Benzodiazepine.

Mechanism of action: Potentiates effects of GABA in limbic system and reticular formation.

Indications/dosage/route: Oral only.

• Insomnia

 – Adults: 7.5–30 mg h.s.
 – Elderly: Initial: 15 mg h.s. Adjust dosage according to response.

Adjustment of dosage
• Kidney disease: None.
• Liver disease: None.
• Elderly: See above.
• Pediatric: Safety and efficacy have not been established in children <18 years.

Food: No restrictions.

Pregnancy: Category D.

Lactation: Appears in breast milk. Potentially toxic to infant. American Academy of Pediatrics expresses concern about breast-feeding while taking benzodiazepines. Avoid breastfeeding.

Contraindications: Hypersensitivity to benzodiazepines, pregnancy.

Editorial comments
• Use with caution in patients who are severely depressed.
• Do not use for more than 2 weeks.
• This drug is listed without details in the *Physician's Desk Reference*, 54th edition, 2000.
• For additional information, see *diazepam*, p. 273.

Terazosin

Brand name: Hytrin.

Class of drug: α-Adrenergic blocker antihypertensive agent.

Mechanism of action: Hypotensive effect: Blocks α_1-adrenergic receptors, resulting in decreased BP. Also blocks adrenergic receptors in neck of bladder and in prostate, resulting in smooth muscle relaxation and improved urine flow.

Indications/dosage/route: Oral only.
• Hypertension
 – Adults: Initial: 1 mg h.s. Maintenance: 1–5 mg/d. Maximum: 20 mg/d.

- BPH
  - Adults: Initial: 1 mg/d. Maintenance: 10 mg/d. Maximum: 20 mg/d.
- Concomitant therapy with a diuretic or other antihypertensive drug
  - Reduce dose initially and titrate up until desired effect is produced.

Adjustment of dosage
- Kidney disease: None.
- Liver disease: Reduce dose, use with caution.
- Elderly: None.
- Pediatric: Safety and efficacy have not been established in children <18 years.

	Onset of Action	Peak Effect	Duration
Hypertension	15 min	1–2 h	12–24 h

Food: Take with meals or milk to minimize GI upset.
Pregnancy: Category C.
Lactation: Present in breast milk. Best to avoid.
Contraindications: Hypersensitivity to terazosin and other quinazoline drugs (prazosin and doxazosin).

Warnings/precautions
- Use with caution in patients with pulmonary embolism, aortic and mitral valve stenosis, liver disease.
- Syncope may occur with first dose due to orthostatic hypotension.
- Use with caution when adding another antihypertensive agent to this drug or adding this drug to another antihypertensive regimen, to avoid rapid fall in BP.

Advice to patient
- Avoid driving and other activities requiring mental alertness or that are potentially dangerous until response to drug is known.
- Limit alcohol intake.
- Avoid standing for long periods, especially during hot weather.
- Take first dose at bedtime; lie down shortly after first dose.

- Use caution when going from lying down or seated position to standing, especially when dosage is being adjusted.
- Avoid excessive intake of caffeine (regular coffee), theobromine (cocoa, chocolates), and theophylline (regular tea).
- Report significant weight gain or ankle edema to treating physician.
- Notify physician if prolonged penile erection occurs.

Adverse reactions
- Common: dizziness, headache, edema.
- Serious: hypotension, orthostatic hypotension, depression, priapism.

Clinically important drug interactions
- Drugs that increase effects/toxicity of α blockers: β blockers, diuretics, verapamil.
- Drugs that decrease effects/toxicity of α blockers: NSAIDs.
- α Blockers decrease effects of clonidine.

Parameters to monitor
- BP for possible first-dose orthostatic hypotension and syncope, particularly when increasing dose.
- Intake of fluids and urinary and other fluid output to minimize renal toxicity. Increase fluid intake if inadequate. Closely monitor electrolyte levels.
- Efficacy of treatment for patient with BPH: decreased nocturia, urgency, and frequency of urination.

Editorial comments: This drug appears to cause dizziness less frequently than doxazosin.

Terbutaline

Brand name: Brethine.
Class of drug: β-Adrenergic agonist, bronchodilator.
Mechanism of action: Relaxes smooth muscles of the bronchioles by stimulating β_2-adrenergic receptors.
Indications/dosage/route: Oral, IV, SC, inhalation.

- Bronchodilation
  - Adults, children >15 years: Initial: PO 5 mg t.i.d. q6h. Maximum: 15 mg q24h.
  - Children 12–15 years: PO 2.5 mg t.i.d. not to exceed 7.5 mg q24h.
- Bronchodilation
  - Adults: Initial: SC 0.25 mg. Repeat after 15–30 minutes. Maximum: 0.5 mg q4h.
- Premature labor
  - Initial: IV infusion 10 µg/min. Increase rate by 0.005 mg/min q10min. Continue 4–8 hours after contractions cease.
- Bronchodilation: metered dose inhaler
  - Adults, children >12 years: 1–2 inhalations q4–6h, separated by 60-second intervals. Repeat q4–6h if needed.

Adjustment of dosage

- Kidney disease: None.
- Liver disease: None.
- Elderly: Lower doses may be required.
- Pediatric: Safety and efficacy have not been established in children <12 years.

	Onset of Action	Peak Effect	Duration
PO	30 min	—	4—8 h
SC	5–15 min	—	1.5—4 h
Inhalation	5–30 min	—	3—6 h

Food: Not applicable.

Pregnancy: Category B. Tocolytic agent in second and third trimesters.

Lactation: Excreted in breast milk. Considered compatible by American Academy of Pediatrics.

Contraindications: Hypersensitivity to adrenergic compounds, tachycardia (idiopathic or from digitalis).

Editorial comments: Seizures, liver enzyme elevations, and hypersensitivity reactions have rarely been reported with terbutaline use.

- For additional information, see *metaproterenol*, p. 575.

Testosterone

Brand name: Delatestryl, Virilon IM.

Class of drug: Androgenic hormone.

Mechanism of action: Stimulates receptors in androgen-responsive organs, thereby promoting growth and development of male sex organs. Maintains secondary male characteristics in deficit states.

Indications/dosage/route: Only IM.

- Androgen replacement therapy
  – 25–50 mg 2–3 times weekly.
- Delayed puberty
  – 40–50 mg/m^2 monthly for 6 months. IM 50–200 mg q2–4wk.
- Male hypogonadism
  – 40–50 mg/m^2 monthly. IM 50–400 mg q2–4wk.
- Palliation of mammary cancer
  – 50–100 mg 3 times/wk. IM 200–400 mg q2–4wk.
- Postpartum breast engorgement
  – 25–50 mg for 3–4 days, starting at delivery.

Adjustment of dosage

- Kidney disease: None.
- Liver disease: None.
- Elderly: Use with caution because of possibility of developing prostatic hypertrophy.
- Pediatric: Use with great caution. Drug should be administered only by physician who is aware of possible adverse effects of drug on bone maturation. Head and wrist should be examined radiologically every 6 months.

Food: Information not available.

Pregnancy: Category X. Contraindicated.

Lactation: No data available. Best to avoid.

Contraindications: Hypersensitivity, males with carcinoma of the breast, known or suspected carcinoma of the prostate, serious cardiac, renal or hepatic decompensation.

Editorial comments: For additional information, see *methyl-testosterone*, p. 596. This drug is listed without detail in *Physician's Desk Reference,* 54th edition, 2000.

Testosterone Transdermal System

Brand names: Testoderm, Androderm.
Class of drug: Androgenic hormone.
Mechanism of action: Stimulates receptors in androgen-respon-sive organs, thereby promoting growth and development of male sex organs. Maintains secondary male characteristics in deficit states.
Indications/dosage/route: Transdermal.
• Primary hypogonadism, hypogonadotropic hypogonadism.
• Testoderm
 – Initial: 6-mg/d system applied to scrotum. Wear 22–24 hours.
• Androderm
 – Initial: 5-mg or 2.5-mg system. Applied nightly for 24 hours to back, abdomen, upper arms, or thighs.
Adjustment of dosage
• Kidney disease: No experience with use in renal insufficiency.
• Liver disease: No experience with use in hepatic insufficiency.
• Elderly: Use with caution because of possibility of developing prostatic hyperplasia or prostatic carcinoma.
• Pediatric: Safety and efficacy have not been established.
Food: Information not available.
Pregnancy: Not for use in women.
Lactation: Not for use in women.
Contraindications: Hypersensitivity to testosterone, males with carcinoma of the breast, known or suspected carcinoma of the prostate, serious cardiac, renal or hepatic decompensation.
Editorial comments
• If desired results are not achieved in 6–8 weeks, another form of testosterone replacement should be considered.
• For additional information, see *methyltestosterone*, p. 596.

Tetracaine

Brand name: Pontocaine.
Class of drug: Spinal anesthetic.
Mechanism of action: Reversibly inhibits initiation and conduction of nerve impulses near site of injection.
Indications/dosage/route: Local injection only.
• Spinal anesthesia
  – Dilute 1% solution with equal volume of CSF immediately before use or dissolve 5 mg of powder in 1 mL CSF.
• Anesthesia of perineum and lower extremities
  – Adults: 10 mg.
• Spinal anesthesia up to costal margin
  – Adults: 15–20 mg.
• Saddle block anesthesia for vaginal delivery
  – Adults: 2–5 mg.
Adjustment of dosage
• Kidney disease: No information available.
• Liver disease: No information available.
• Elderly: None.
• Pediatric: Safety and efficacy have not been established.
Food: Not applicable.
Pregnancy: Category C.
Lactation: No data available. Use with caution.
Contraindications: Hypersensitivity for ester-type local anesthetic (eg, procaine).
Warnings/precautions: Use with caution in patients with severe liver disease, spinal deformities, existing neurologic disease, severe uncontrolled hypotension, septicemia, infection at site of injection, abnormal or reduced levels of serum cholinesterase.
Editorial comments: If an oxytocic drug has been administered along with tetracaine, extreme care must be used when a vasopressor agent is used to treat the hypotension that frequently accompanies spinal anesthesia. Such vasopressors may cause

severe and persistent hypertension and/or rupture of cerebral blood vessels.

• This drug is listed in the *Physician's Desk Reference*, 54th edition, 2000 only for topical application.

• For additional information, see *bupivacaine*, p. 113.

Tetracycline

Brand names: Achromycin, Tetracycline.

Class of drug: Tetracycline antibiotic.

Mechanism of action: Inhibits bacterial protein synthesis after specific ribosomal binding.

Susceptible organisms *in vivo*: *Borrelia burgdorferi, Borrelia recurrentis, Brucella* sp, *Calymmatobacterium granulomatis, Chlamydia pneumoniae, Chlamydia psittaci, Chlamydia trachomatis, Ehrlichia* sp, *Helicobacter pylori, Rickettsia* (Q fever), *Rickettsia* sp, *Vibrio* sp.

Indications/dosage/route: Oral, IV, IM.

• Usual dose
  – Adults: PO 1–2 g/d in 2 or 4 equal doses.
  – Children >8 years: Daily dose is 10–20 mg/lb (25–50 mg/kg in 4 equal doses).

• Brucellosis
  – PO 500 mg 4 times/d for 3 weeks, accompanied by 1 g streptomycin IM 2 times/d the first week and once daily the second week.

• Syphilis
  – PO 30–40 g in equally divided doses over 10–15 days. Perform close follow-up and laboratory tests.

• Uncomplicated urethral, endocervical, or rectal infections caused by *C. trachomatis.*
  – PO 500 mg 4 times/d for at least 7 days.

• Severe acne
  – PO: Initial: 1 g/d in divided doses. Maintenance: 125–500 mg/d.

- Lymphogranuloma venereum: genital, inguinal or anorectal
  - PO 500 mg 4 times/d for at least 2 weeks.
- Nongonococcal urethritis
  - PO 500 mg 4 times/d for 7 days.
- Acute pelvic inflammatory disease, ambulatory treatment
  - Adults: 2 g IM cefoxitin, 3 g oral amoxicillin, 3.5 g oral ampicillin, 4.8×10^6 units IM aqueous procaine penicillin G at 2 sites or 250 mg IM ceftriaxone. Each (except ceftriaxone) should be accompanied by 1 g oral probenecid. Follow with 500 mg tetracycline 4 times/d.
  - Children >8 years: 150 mg/kg/d IV cefuroxime or 100 mg/kg/d IV ceftriaxone followed by 30 mg/kg/d IV tetracycline in 3 doses, continued for at least 4 days. Thereafter, continue tetracycline orally to complete at least 14 days of therapy.

Adjustment of dosage
- Kidney disease: None.
- Liver disease: None.
- Elderly: None.
- Pediatric: Not to be used in children <8 years unless all other drugs are either ineffective or contraindicated.

Food: Take 1 hour before or 2 hours after meals. Dairy products interfere with tetracycline absorption.

Pregnancy: Category D.

Lactation: Appears in breast milk. Considered compatible by American Academy of Pediatrics.

Contraindications: Hypersensitivity to any tetracycline, patients with esophageal obstruction, children ≤8 years.

Warnings/precautions
- Use with caution in patients with impaired kidney function.
- Administer IM by deep injection into large muscle. If injected inadvertently SC or into fat layer, severe pain may result. This can be relieved by means of an ice pack. IM solution should be used within 24 hours of preparation.
- The drug may permanently discolor (yellow brown to gray) deciduous or permanent teeth or cause enamel hypoplasia. Premature infants may experience decreased fibula growth.

- Do not administer antacids that contain calcium, aluminum, or magnesium.

Advice to patient

- Discard drug if it is beyond expiration date. Outdated drug can cause severe kidney toxicity (Fanconi-like syndrome).
- To minimize possible photosensitivity reaction, apply adequate sunscreen and use proper covering when exposed to strong sunlight.
- Store drug away from light, heat, and high humidity.
- Use two forms of birth control including hormonal and barrier methods.
- Do not take drug at bedtime.

Adverse reactions

- Common: nausea, vomiting, diarrhea, anorexia.
- Serious: renal toxicity, hypersensitivity reactions, benign intracranial hypertension (pseudotumor cerebri), pericardits, diabetes insipidus, pseudomembranous colitis, hepatitis, anaphylaxis.

Clinically important drug interactions

- Drugs that decrease effects/toxicity of tetracyclines: aluminum antacids, iron preparations, calcium salts, magnesium salts, sodium bicarbonate, zinc salts, bismuth salts, cimetidine.
- Tetracyclines increase effects/toxicity of oral anticoagulants, bumetanide, digoxin, thiazide diuretics, ethacrynic acid, furosemide, insulin, methoxyflurane.
- Tetracyclines decrease effects/toxicity of penicillins.

Parameters to monitor

- Serum BUN and creatinine, liver enzymes.
- Signs of possible oliguria, which may result in accumulation of the drug.
- Signs and symptoms of pseudotumor cerebri in adults: headaches, diplopia.
- Signs and symptoms of pseudomembraneous colitis: Discontinue drug if possible. If necessary, treat with vancomycin, metronidazole, and cholestyramine.
- Signs and symptoms of phlebitis from IV injections.

- Renal function in patients with preexisting renal impairment. If indicated, monitor serum drug levels. Maintain level below 15 µg/mL.
- Serum enzymes in patients with preexisting kidney or liver disease or those receiving concomitant hepatotoxic drug.

Editorial comments
- Uses for tetracyclines include treatment of early Lyme disease, *Vibrio* infections such as cholera, and rickettsial infections including typhus, Q fever, and Rocky Mountain spotted fever. They are also used to treat genital infections (granuloma inguinale, nongonococcal urethritis, pelvic inflammatory disease, and other infections caused by *C. trachomatis*).

Theophylline

Brand names: Aerolate, Aminophyllin, Marax, Respbid, Slo-Phyllin, Theo-Dur, Theolair (also many other name brands).
Class of drug: Bronchodilator.
Mechanism of action: Inhibits phosphodiesterase, resulting in increased levels of cAMP. This results in release of epinephrine, bronchodilation, cardiac and CNS stimulation.
Indications/dosage/route: Oral, IV.
- Bronchodilator for reversible airway obstruction due to asthma or COPD
  - Adults, children <16 years, PO: 5 mg/kg. Maintenance: 300 mg/d in divided doses of 6–8 hours. Increase dose to 400 mg/d after 3 days and again up to 600 mg/d after 3 more days.
  - Full-term infants to 1 year, PO: Maintenance: 0.2 mg/kg.
  - Full-term infants <6 months, PO: 0.2 mg/kg in divided doses q6h.
  - Premature infants >24 weeks postnatal, PO: Maintenance: 1.5 mg/kg q12h.
  - Premature infants <24 weeks postnatal, PO: 1 mg/kg q12h.

- Adults, IV: Loading dose: 5 mg/kg. Maintenance: 0.55 mg/kg/h (nonsmoker). Reduce to 0.39 mg/kg/h after 12 hours or 0.47 mg/kg/h (elderly, right heart failure), then 0.24 mg/kg/h after 12 hours.
- Children 1–16 years, IV: Loading dose: 5 mg/kg. Maintenance: 0.7 mg/kg/h.
- Full-term infants ≤1 year, IV: Maintenance dose 0.2 mg/kg/day.
- Premature infants >24 weeks postnatal, IV: Maintenance: 1.5 mg/kg q12h.
- Premature infants <24 weeks postnatal, IV: Maintenance: 1 mg/kg q12h.

Adjustment of dosage
- Kidney disease: None.
- Liver disease: Reduce dose; monitor theophylline levels frequently.
- Elderly: Lower initial doses should be administered and such patients should be monitored closely for adverse reactions (see IV dosage).
- Pediatric: See above.

Food: Patient should take limited amounts of xanthine-containing foods or beverages (caffeine-containing coffees, colas, chocolates, teas). Patient should also be advised to avoid charcoal-broiled foods. Theophylline may be taken with food if GI upset occurs; however, it is felt that most consistent blood levels occur when the drug is administered in the fasting state.

Pregnancy: Category C. It should be noted that theophylline appears in significant amounts in the fetus.

Lactation: Appears in breast milk. May cause irritability to infant. Considered compatible with breastfeeding by American Academy of Pediatrics.

Contraindications: Hypersensitivity to xanthine compounds (caffeine, theobromine), uncontrolled seizures, uncontrolled arrhythmias.

Warnings/precautions: Use with caution in patients with CHF, cor pulmonale, kidney or liver disease, peptic ulcer, diabetes, glaucoma, hypertension, angina, acute MI, elderly, chronic alco-holism.

Advice to patient

- Drink sufficient liquids, at least 2000 mL/d.
- Limit intake of protein and carbohydrates.
- Avoid OTC products for cough and cold since these may contain sympathomimetic drugs.
- Do not smoke.
- Do not change theophylline brand or dosage form without first consulting with the treating physician.
- If a dose is missed, the next dose should be taken as soon as possible. Doses should not be doubled if missed.
- Read written guidelines provided by your physician that identify early signs and symptoms of overdosage as well as the most important adverse effects of the drug.

Adverse reactions

- Common: nervousness, nausea, vomiting, tachycardia.
- Serious: arrhythmias, seizures.

Clinically important drug interactions

- Drugs that increase effects/toxicity of theophylline: sympathomimetic drugs, erythromycin and other macrolide antibiotics, cimetidine, glucocorticoids, interferon, oral contraceptives, β blockers, tetracycline, mexiletine, ciprofloxacin and other quinolones, allopurinol, thyroid hormone, halothane, troleandomycin, calcium channel blockers, disulfiram, thiabendazole.
- Drugs that decrease effects/toxicity of theophylline: aminoglutethimide, isoniazid, carbamazepine, isoproteranol, moricizine, phenobarbitol, phenytoin, rifampin, loop diuretics, sulfinpyrazone, smoking.
- Theophylline decreases effects/toxicity of adenosine, lithium, phenytoin, diazepam, flurazepam, lorazepam, midazolam, pancuronium.

Parameters to monitor

- Oxygen therapy during an acute asthma attack. Make sure oxygen intake is correct.
- Therapeutic efficacy in patients with chronic bronchitis on the basis of pulmonary function tests.

- Fluid overload: intake and output ratios.
- ECG for the following changes: PVCs, supraventricular tachycardia, ventricular tachycardia. Make sure that resuscitative equipment is close at hand if needed.
- Monitor serum theophylline levels on a regular basis particularly if high doses are required or if there is a need for prolonged therapy. Samples should be obtained at peak and trough 15 and 30 minutes after IV loading dose, 4 and 12 hours after admin-istration of extended-release form. Therapeutic plasma level is in the range 5–15 µg/mL. Levels above 20 µg/mL are frequently associated with toxicity.
- Symptoms of drug toxicity: nausea, vomiting, headache, increased urination, insomnia, arrhythmias.

Editorial comments

- Status asthmaticus is not rapidly responsive to usual doses of conventional bronchodilators. This medical emergency requires close monitoring and the use of parenteral drugs. Treatment is preferably carried out in an intensive care setting. An oral preparation of theophylline is not used for treating status asthmaticus.
- It is advisable to calculate dosage on the basis of lean body weight.
- It is advisable to have the following available to treat an overdose of theophylline if the patient is conscious without seizures: ipecac syrup, cathartics, equipment for gastric lavage.
- If the patient is unconscious or having seizures, the following should be available for treatment: mechanical ventilator, diazepam, oxygen, IV fluids.

Thiabendazole

Brand name: Mintezole.
Class of drug: Anthelmintic.

Mechanism of action: May act by inhibiting helminth-specific fumarate reductase.

Indications/dosage/route: Oral only.

• Pinworm, roundworm, whipworm, threadworm infestation
  – Adults, children: 30–150 lb: 4.5 mg/kg q12h, 2 days.
  – Adults, children >150 lb: 1.5 g q12h, 2 days. Maximum dose: 3 g/d.
• Trichinosis infections
  – 4.5 mg/kg b.i.d., 2–4 successive days.
• Cutaneous larva migrans
  – 4.5 mg/kg/d, 7 successive days.

Adjustment of dosage

• Kidney disease: None.
• Liver disease: None.
• Elderly: None.
• Pediatric: Limited data in children <30 lb.

Food: Should be taken after meals. Advise patient to drink fruit juice which aids in expelling worms.

Pregnancy: Category C.

Lactation: No data available. Best to avoid.

Contraindications: Hypersensitivity to thiabendazole, use for pinworm infestation.

Warnings/precautions: Use with caution in patients with kidney or liver disease, anemia, severe malnutrition, vomiting.

Advice to patient

• Avoid driving and other activities requiring mental alertness or that are potentially dangerous until response to drug is known.
• Wash perianal area daily and change bedclothes on daily basis.
• Have other family members tested and treated if necessary.

Adverse reactions

• Common: drowsiness, headache, hypotension, anorexia, nausea, vomiting, rash.
• Serious: jaundice, Stevens–Johnson syndrome, angioedema, anaphylaxis, seizures, hypotension, hallucinations, leukopenia, liver damage.

Clinically important drug interactions: Thiabendazole increases effects/toxicity of aminophylline, theophylline.

Parameters to monitor
- Signs and symptoms of anemia.
- Symptoms of dehydration: thirst, weakness, fatigue, dry mucous membranes.
- Signs and symptoms of malnutrition.
- Signs and symptoms of CNS toxicity: loss of mental alterness, muscular weakness.

Editorial comments: This drug is not to be used as a prophylactic therapy for pinworm infestation.

Thioridazine

Brand name: Mellaril.
Class of drug: Phenothiazine antipsychotic (neuroleptic).
Mechanism of action: Antagonizes dopamine at dopaminergic receptors in CNS neurons.
Indications/dosage/route: Oral only.
- Psychotic disorders
  - Adults: Initial: 25–100 mg t.i.d. Maintenance: 200–800 mg/d in 2–4 doses.
- Psychoneurotic symptoms (depression plus anxiety in adults, agitation, tension, sleep disturbance in geriatric patients)
  - Adults, elderly: Initial: 25 mg t.i.d. Maintenance: 20–200 mg/d.
- Behavioral disorders
  - Children 2–12 years: 0.5–3 mg/kg/d. Maximum: 3 mg/kg/d.
- Hospitalized, severely disturbed or psychotic patients
  - Adults: Initial: 50–100 mg t.i.d. Increase to 200 mg q.i.d. if necessary. Increase gradually as needed.
  - Children: Initial: 25 mg b.i.d. or t.i.d.

Adjustment of dosage
- Kidney disease: Use with caution. Guidelines not available.
- Liver disease: Use with caution. Guidelines not available.
- Elderly: For other than psychoneurotic symptoms, see above.
- Pediatric: This drug is not recommended for children <2 years.

Food: No restriction.

Pregnancy: Category C.
Lactation: No data available. Potentially toxic to infant. Avoid breastfeeding.
Contraindications: Hypersensitivity to phenothiazines, concurrent use of high-dose CNS depressants (alcohol, barbituates, benzodiazepines, narcotics), CNS depression, comatose state.

Editorial comments
- This drug is not listed in the *Physicians' Desk Reference*, 54th edition, 2000.
- For additional information, see *chlorpromazine*, p. 206.

Thiotepa

Brand name: Thioplex.
Class of drug: Alkylating antineoplastic.
Mechanism of action: Inhibits protein synthesis by disrupting crosslinking of strands in DNA and RNA.
Indications/dosage/route: IV, local injections.

- Carcinoma of the breast, ovary; intracavitary effusions in advanced neoplasms; papillary carcinoma of the bladder; lymphoma, Hodgkin's disease
  - Dosage must be carefully individualized. Generally, initial treatment is followed by maintenance doses every 1–4 weeks. Maintenance doses are adjusted according to hematologic parameters.
  - Adults, children >12 years: IV initial: 0.3–0.5 mg/kg/d. Repeat q4wk.
- Bladder tumors (intravesicular)
  - Adults, children >12 years: 60 mg in 30–60 mL sodium chloride, retained in bladder for 2 hours. Usually weekly for 4 weeks. May repeat (use extreme caution due to bone marrow depression).
- Neoplastic effusions (intracavity or intratumor)
  - Adults, children: Initial: 0.6–0.8 mg/kg. Repeat q1–4wk.

Adjustment of dosage
• Kidney disease: Use with extreme caution. Best to avoid.
• Liver disease: Use with extreme caution. Best to avoid.
• Elderly: Consider lower doses.
• Pediatric: See above.

Food: Not applicable.

Pregnancy: Category D.

Lactation: No data available. Potentially toxic to infant. Avoid breastfeeding.

Contraindications: Hypersensitivity, severe bone marrow depression, liver disease (relative contraindicated), kidney disease (relative contraindicated).

Warnings/precautions
• Use with caution in patients with kidney or liver disease, bone marrow suppression.
• Caregivers should screen visitors for infection before they enter the patient's room; visitation should be limited.
• IM injection should not be made if platelet count is <100,000/mm^3.
• Withhold fluids 8–10 hours prior to instilling thiotepa into the bladder.

Advice to patient
• Use two forms of birth control including hormonal and barrier methods.
• Avoid alcohol.
• Do not receive any vaccinations (particularly live attenuated viruses) unless permitted by treating physician.
• Drink large amounts of fluids to facilitate excretion of uric acid.

Adverse reactions
• Common: nausea, vomiting, febrile reaction, dermatitis.
• Serious: **bone marrow depression**, anaphylactic reactions, hemorrhagic cystitis (intravesicular), hyperuricemia, secondary carcinogenesis.

Clinically important drug interactions
• Drugs that increase effects/toxicity of thiotepa: antineoplastic agents, radiation therapy.

- Drugs that decrease effects/toxicity of thiotepa: clofibrate, phenobarbital.
- Thiotepa increases effects/toxicity of succinylcholine (may cause prolonged apnea).
- Thiotepa decreases antibody response to live virus vaccines.

Parameters to monitor
- CBC and differential prior to administration and weekly during therapy. Discontinue therapy or reduce dose at the first sign of a sudden large decrease in leukocyte or platelet count. Therapy should be resumed when leukocyte count and thrombocyte count increase to >2000 mm^3 and 50,000 mm^3, respectively.
- Signs and symptoms of infection: fever, sore throat, backache.
- Determine whether patient is showing excessive bleeding or bruising.
- Intake of fluids and urinary and other fluid output to minimize renal toxicity. Increase fluid intake if inadequate. Closely monitor electrolyte levels.
- Signs and symptoms of GI upset, eg, nausea, vomiting, anorexia. Administer antiemetic drug if necessary.
- Signs and symptoms of anemia: shortness of breath, dizziness, angina, pale conjunctivae, skin and nailbeds.
- Signs of hyperuricemia: gouty arthritis, uric acid kidney stones.

Editorial comments
- Following bladder installation, patient should retain the drug for 2 hours. Patient should not receive anything by mouth for 6 hours following instillation. Patient should be repositioned every 15 minutes to obtain maximum bladder area contact.
- This drug's major use currently is as a part of conditioning regimens for autologous stem cell transplants (ie, it is part of the high-dose chemotherapy preparative regimen).

Thiothixene

Brand name: Navane.
Class of drug: Phenothiazine antipsychotic (neuroleptic).

Mechanism of action: Antagonizes dopamine at dopaminergic receptors in CNS neurons.

Indications/dosage/route: Oral, IM.

• Psychotic disorders, milder conditions
  – Adults, children over 12: PO 2 mg t.i.d. Increase to 15 mg/d as needed.
• Psychotic disorders, severe
  – Adults, children over 12: PO 5 mg b.i.d. Maintenance: 20–30 mg/d. Maximum: 60 mg/d.
  – Adults: IM 4 mg 2–4 times/d. Maintenance: 16–20 mg/d.

Adjustment of dosage

• Kidney disease: Use with caution. Guidelines not available.
• Liver disease: Use with caution. Guidelines not available.
• Elderly: Use lower doses. Increase dosage more gradually.
• Pediatric: Safety and efficacy have not been established in children <12 years.

Food: No restriction.

Pregnancy: Category C.

Lactation: No data available. Potentially toxic to infant. Avoid breastfeeding.

Contraindications: Hypersensitivity to phenothiazines, concurrent use of high-dose CNS depressants (alcohol, barbituates, benzodiazepines, narcotics), CNS depression, comatose state, blood dyscrasias.

Editorial comments: For additional information, see *chlorpromazine*, p. 206.

Ticarcillin

Brand name: Ticar.

Class of drug: Antibiotic, penicillin family.

Mechanism of action: Inhibits bacterial cell wall synthesis.

Susceptible organisms *in vivo*: Staphylococci, *Staphylococcus aureus, Streptococcus pneumoniae*, beta-hemolytic streptococci,

Enterococcus faecalis, Escherichia coli, Hemophilus influenzae, Neisseria gonorrhoeae, Proteus mirabilis, Salmonella sp, *Morganella morganii, Proteus vulgaris, Providencia rettgeri, Pseudomonas aeruginosa, Serratia* sp, *Clostridium* sp, *Peptococcus* sp, *Peptostreptococcus* sp, *Bacteroides* sp, *Fuso-bacterium* sp, *Eubacterium* sp, *Veillonella* sp.

Indications/dosage/route: IV, IV infusion, IM.

• Bacterial septicemia, intraabdominal infections, skin and soft tissue infections, infections of the female genital system and pelvis, respiratory infections
  – Adults: 200–300 mg/kg/d by IV infusion in divided doses q4–6h.
  – Children <40 kg: 200–300 mg/kg/d by IV infusion every 4 or 6 hours.
• UTIs, uncomplicated
  – Adults: 1 g IM or direct IV q6h.
  – Children <40 kg: 50–100 mg/kg/d IM or direct IV in divided doses every 6 or 8 hours.
• Neonates with sepsis due to *pseudomonas, Proteus,* or *E. coli*
  – <7 days and <2 kg: 75 mg/kg q12h.
  – >7 days and <2 kg: 75 mg/kg q8h.
  – <7 days and >2 kg: 75 mg/kg q8h.
  – >7 days and >2 kg: 100 mg/kg q8h, IM or IV infusion over 10–20 minutes.

Adjustment of dosage

• Kidney disease: Creatinine clearance >60 mL/min: 3 g q4h; creatinine clearance 30–60 mL/min: 2gq8h; creatinine clearance 10–30 mL/min: 2 g q12h; creatinine clearance <10 mL/min: 2 g q24h. All doses given IV after loading dose of 3 g ticarcillin IV.
• Liver disease: None.
• Elderly: None.
• Pediatric: See above.

Food: Not applicable.

Pregnancy: Category B.

Lactation: Appears in breast milk. Considered compatible by American Academy of Pediatrics.

Contraindications: Hypersensitivity to penicillin or cephalosporins.
Editorial comments: Ticarcillin has poor efficacy against *Enterococcus faecalis* (which is susceptible to piperacillin and mezlocillin).
• Ticarcillin is effective against *Pseudomonas aeruginosa*, although piperacillin is more effective.
• Ticarcillin/clavulanate (Timentin) also covers penicillinase-producing Staphylococcus aureus (MSSA, not MRSA), anaerobic organisms (*Bacteroides fragilis*), *Hemophilus influenzae*, and *Branhamella catarrhalis.*
• For additional information, see *penicillin G*, p. 708.

Ticlopidine

Brand name: Ticlid.
Class of drug: Antithrombotic.
Mechanism of action: Inhibits platelet function, resulting in increased bleeding time. The exact mechanism of this effect is undetermined.
Indications/dosage/route: Oral only.
• Prevention of stroke in patients with history of stroke or stroke precursor; antithrombotic agent in patients who are unable to tolerate aspirin or other anticoagulants
– Adults: 250 mg b.i.d. Increase to 750 mg/d depending on response.
Adjustment of dosage
• Kidney disease: Consider dosage reduction.
• Liver disease: Avoid in severe hepatic dysfunction; otherwise use with extreme caution.
• Elderly: None.
• Pediatric: Safety and efficacy in children under 18 has not been established.

Onset of Action	Time for Maximum Platelet Inhibition	Duration of Platelet Inhibition
1–2 days	3–6 days	4–10 days

Food: Take with food or immediately after eating.

Pregnancy: Category B. Avoid breastfeeding.

Lactation: No data available. Best to avoid.

Contraindications: Hypersensitivity to ticlopidine, neutropenia, history of thrombocytopenia, active bleeding from peptic ulcer, active intracranial bleeding, other active bleeding diatheses, severe liver disease.

Warnings/precautions

- Use with caution in patients with risk of bleeding (surgery, history of ulcer disease), kidney or severe liver disease, gout, asthma, angina, hemodynamic instability, biliary obstruction.
- Discontinue ticlopidine 10–14 days before surgery.
- If ticlopidine is substituted for another anticoagulant drug, the previous drug should be discontinued before ticlopidine is administered.
- Neutropenia is a serious side effect seen in 2.4% of patients treated with ticlopidine. Severe neutropenia (ANC <450 neutrophils/mm^3) occurs in 0.8% of patients. This side effect may occur 3 weeks to ≥3 months after treatment.
- CBC and white cell differential count must be performed every 2 weeks beginning with the second week through the end of the third month of therapy. If a patient's neutrophil count declines consistently and is only 30% less than baseline count, more frequent monitoring is necessary.

Advice to patient

- Avoid aspirin and aspirin-containing products, in particular those obtained OTC. Such medications should not be used without first consulting the treating physician.
- Use an electric razor and soft bristle toothbrush to minimize bleeding.

Adverse reactions

- Common: rash, diarrhea, nausea, vomiting.
- Serious: intracerebral bleeding, nephrotic syndrome, neutropenia, bone marrow depression, allergic pneumonitis, serum sickness, neuropathy, angioedema, elevated liver enzymes.

Clinically important drug interactions
- Drugs that increase effects/toxicity of ticlopidine: cimetidine, anticoagulants, theophylline, phenytoin.
- Drugs that decrease effects/toxicity of ticlopidine: antacids, corticosteroids.
- Tipclopidine increases effects/toxicity of theophylline, anticoagulants, NSAIDs.

Parameters to monitor
- Signs and symptoms of bone marrow depression.
- Coagulation status. If bleeding time is excessively prolonged, IV methylprednisolone or a transfusion of platelets may be needed to normalize bleeding time.
- Signs and symptoms of hepatotoxicity.
- Signs of hypersensitivity reactions.
- Signs of diarrhea (incidence approximately 20%). Reduce dose or advise patient to take drug with food.
- Avoid aspirin and aspirin-containing products, in particular those obtained OTC. Such medications should not be used without first consulting the treating physician.

Editorial comments
- The drug of choice for male patients after a completed stroke is aspirin. There are some studies suggesting that ticlopidine may be slightly more effective in female patients.
- In general ticlopidine is reserved as a first-line agent only for patients intolerant to aspirin because of the risk of neutropenia or agranulocytosis.

Timolol

Brand names: Blocadren, Timoptic.
Class of drug: β-Adrenergic receptor blocker.
Mechanism of action: Competitive blocker of β-adrenergic receptors in heart, blood vessels, and eyes.

Indications/dosage/route: Oral, topical (ophthalmic).
- Hypertension
  - Initial: PO 10 mg b.i.d. alone or with a diuretic. Maintenance: 20–40 mg/d. Maximum: 80 mg/d.
- MI prophylaxis for patients who have survived the acute phase
  - PO 10 mg b.i.d.
- Migraine prophylaxis
  - Initial: PO 10 mg b.i.d. Maintenance: 20 mg/d given as single dose. Total daily dose may be increased to 30 mg in divided doses.
- Ophthalmic preparation
  - 1 drop of 0.25–0.50% in each eye b.i.d. Maintenance: 1 drop once a day.

Adjustment of dosage
- Kidney disease: None.
- Liver disease: None.
- Elderly: None.
- Pediatric: Safety and efficacy have not been established.

Food: No restriction.

Pregnancy: Category C.

Lactation: Appears in breast milk. Considered compatible by American Academy of Pediatrics. Observe infant for bradycardia and hypotension.

Contraindications: Cardiogenic shock, asthma, CHF unless it is secondary to tachyarrhythmia treated with a β blocker, sinus bradycardia and AV block greater than first degree, severe COPD.

Editorial comments: For additional information, see *betaxolol*, p. 95.

Tobramycin

Brand name: Nebcin.
Class of drug: Antibiotic, aminoglycoside.

Mechanism of action: Binds to ribosomal units in bacteria, inhibits protein synthesis.

Susceptible organisms *in vivo*: Staphylococci (penicillinase and nonpenicillinase), *Staphylococcus epidermidis, Acinetobacter* sp, *Citrobacter* sp, *Enterobacter* sp, *Escherichia coli, Klebsiella* sp, *Proteus* sp, *Providencia* sp, *Pseudomonas* sp, *Serratia* sp.

Indications/dosage/route: IV, IM.

- Septicemia, lower respiratory tract infections, CNS infections (meningitis), intraabdominal infections (peritonitis), skin, bone, and skin structure infections, complicated and recurrent UTIs.
- Serious infections
  – Adults: 3 mg/kg/d in 3 equal doses q8h.
  – Children: 6–7.5 mg/kg/d in 3 or 4 equally divided doses.
  – Premature or neonates ≤1 week: ≤4 mg/kg/d in 2 equal doses q12h.
- Life-threatening infections
  – Adults: 5 mg/kg/d in 3 or 4 equal doses.

Adjustment of dosage: None.

Food: No restrictions.

Pregnancy: Category D.

Lactation: Appears in breast milk in small amounts. Potentially toxic to infant. Best to avoid.

Contraindications: Hypersensitivity to aminoglycoside antibiotics.

Warnings/precautions

- Use with caution in patients with renal disease, neuromuscular disorders (eg, myasthenia gravis, parkinsonism), hearing disorders.
- Do not combine this drug with any other drug in the same IV bag.

Adverse reactions

- Common: none.
- Serious: renal toxicity, ototoxicity, neuromuscular paralysis, respiratory depression (infants), superinfection.

Clinically important drug interactions

- Drugs that decrease effects/toxicity of aminoglycosides: penicillins (high dose), cephalosporins.

• Drugs that increase effects/toxicity of aminoglycosides: loop diuretics, amphotericin B, enflurane, vancomycin, NSAIDs.

Parameters to monitor

• Monitor peak and trough serum levels 48 hours after beginning therapy and every 3–4 days thereafter as well as after changing doses.

• Ototoxicity: tinnitus, vertigo, hearing loss. The drug should be stopped if tinnitus occurs. Limit administration to 7–10 days to decrease the risk of ototoxicity.

• Renal function periodically. If serum creatinine increases by more than 50% over baseline value, it may be advisable to discontinue drug treatment and use a less nephrotoxic agent, eg, a quinolone or cephalosporin.

• If there is no response in 3–7 days, reculture and consider another drug.

• Neuromuscular function when administering the drug IV. Too rapid administration may cause paralysis and apnea. Have calcium gluconate or pyridostigmine available to reverse such an effect.

• Neurologic status if the drug is given for hepatic encephalopathy.

• Signs and symptoms of allergic reaction.

Editorial comments

• Tobramycin is superior to gentamicin for the treatment of *P. aeruginosa* (in combination with an antipseudomonal β-lactam antibiotic for serious infections).

• Gentamicin is the preferred aminoglycoside used in the combination treatment of enterococcal endocarditis (with ampicillin or vancomycin).

Tocainide

Brand name: Tonocard.
Class of drug: Antiarrthymic, class Ib.

Mechanism of action: Reduces or suppresses automaticity of conducting tissue and spontaneous dipolarization of ventricle during diastole. Blocks myocardial excitability by reducing membrane conductance of sodium and potassium ions.

Indications/dosage/route: Oral only.

• Suppression and prevention of symptomatic life-threatening ventricular arrthymias
  – Adults: Initial: 400 mg q8h. Maintenance: 1200–1800 mg/d, divided into 3 doses.

Adjustment of dosage

• Kidney disease: Creatinine clearance <30 mL/min: 50% of normal dose should be administered.
• Liver disease: Maximum daily dose: 1200 mg.
• Elderly: None.
• Pediatric: Safety and efficacy in children have not been established.

Food: Should be taken with food.

Pregnancy: Pregnancy category C.

Lactation: No data available. Potentially toxic to fetus.

Contraindications: Second- or third-degree AV block in absence of artificial pacemaker; advanced heart block, hypersensitivity to tocainide, lidocaine, or other amide-type local anesthetics.

Warnings/precautions

• Use with caution in patients with heart failure, kidney or liver disease.
• Correct preexisting hypokalemia before instituting tocainide therapy.

Advice to patient

• Take missed drug as soon as remembered if within 4 hours of previous drug. Do not double dose.
• Avoid driving and other activities requiring mental alertness or that are potentially dangerous until response to drug is known.
• Carry identification card at all times describing disease, treatment regimen, name, address, and telephone number of treating physician.

Adverse reactions
- Common: anorexia, diarrhea, nervousness, rash, mood alteration, tremor, dizziness, nausea.
- Serious: **ventricular arrhythmia**, pulmonary fibrosis, interstitial pneumonitis, fibrosis alveolitis, pulmonary edema, pneumonia, agranulocytosis, bone marrow depression, septic shock.

Clinically important drug interactions: Drugs that increase effects/toxicity of tocainide: lidocaine, metoprolol, rifampin.

Parameters to monitor
- ECG, pulse, BP prior to and periodically when administering tocainide.
- Monitor pulmonary status periodically for the following symptoms: cough, wheezing, shortness of breath. Perform chest x-rays if there are signs or symptoms of pulmonary complications.
- Hematologic status including WBC with differential and platelet counts.
- Signs of infection: fever, chills, sore throat.
- Signs and symptoms of bone marrow depression.
- Signs of tremor. This is the first indication that the maximum dose has been reached. Tocainide blood levels should be in the range of 4–10 μg/mL.

Editorial comments
- Tocainide is not often used because its side effects overshadow its efficacy as an antiarrhythmic.
- Tocainide may be used as a means of switching from IV lidocaine to an oral antiarrhythmic agent.
- Because of the possibility of agranulocytosis, CBC, white blood cell count, differential, and platelet counts should be carried out at weekly intervals for the first 3 months of tocainide administration and frequently thereafter. Such measurements should be carried out frequently afterward. If the patient develops any signs of infection or excessive bruising or bleeding, complete blood counts should be performed promptly. If a hematologic disorder has been identified as being responsible, tocainide should be discontinued.
- Tocainide has a narrow therapeutic index and if the blood level

is even slightly above the therapeutic range, severe toxicity may occur.

Tolazamide

Brand name: Tolinase.
Class of drug: Oral hypoglycemic agent, first generation.
Mechanism of action: Stimulates release of insulin from pancreatic beta cells; decreases glucose production in liver; increases sensitivity of receptors for insulin, thereby enhancing effectiveness of insulin.
Indications/dosage/route: Oral only.
• Diabetes, type II (non-insulin-dependent diabetes mellitus)
  – Adults: Initial: 100 mg/d if fasting blood sugar is < 200 mg/100 mL, 250 mg/d if fasting blood sugar is >200 mg/100 mL.
  – Elderly: 100 mg/d with breakfast. Adjust dose by increments of 50 mg/d every week. Maximum: 1 g/d.
Adjustment of dosage
• Kidney disease: None.
• Liver disease: None.
• Elderly: See above.
• Pediatric: Not recommended.

Onset of Action	Duration
4–6 h	12–24 h

Food: No restriction. Patient should be told to eat regularly and not skip meals. Sugar supply should be kept handy at all times. If stomach is upset Tums should be taken with meal. Dose is best administered before breakfast or, if taken twice a day, before the evening meal.
Pregnancy: Category C.

Lactation: Probably appears in breast milk. Potentially toxic to infant. Avoid breastfeeding.

Contraindications: Hypersensitivity to the drug, diabetes complicated by ketoacidosis.

Editorial comments

- This drug is listed without details in the *Physician's Desk Reference*, 54th edition, 2000.
- For additional information, see *glyburide*, p. 409.

Tolbutamide

Brand name: Orinase.

Class of drug: Oral hypoglycemic agent.

Mechanism of action: Stimulates release of insulin from pancreatic beta cells; decreases glucose production in liver; increases sensitivity of receptors for insulin, thereby enhancing effectiveness of insulin.

Indications/dosage/route: Oral only.

- Diabetes, type II (non-insulin-dependent diabetes mellitus)
  - Adults: Initial: 1–2 g/d. Maintenance: 0.25–3 g/d.

Adjustment of dosage

- Kidney disease: None.
- Liver disease: None.
- Elderly: See above.
- Pediatric: Not recommended.

Onset of Action	Duration
1 h	6–12 h

Food: No restriction. Patient should be told to eat regularly and not to skip meals. Sugar supply should be kept handy at all times. If stomach is upset, Tums should be taken with meal. Dose is best administered before breakfast or, if taken twice a day, before the evening meal.

Pregnancy: Category C.
Lactation: Appears in breast milk. Potentially toxic to infant. Considered compatible by American Academy of Pediatrics.
Contraindications: Hypersensitivity to the drug, diabetes complicated by ketoacidosis.
Editorial comments
• This drug is listed without details in the *Physician's Desk Reference*, 54th edition, 2000.
• For additional information, see *glyburide*, p. 409.

Tolmetin Sodium

Brand name: Tolectin.
Class of drug: NSAID.
Mechanism of action: Inhibits cyclooxygenase, resulting in inhibition of synthesis of prostaglandins and other inflammatory mediators.
Indications/dosage/route
• Rheumatoid arthritis, osteoarthritis
  – Adults: 400 mg t.i.d. Maintenance: 600–1800 mg/d in 3 to 4 divided doses. Maximum: 1800 mg/d.
• Juvenile rheumatoid arthritis
  – Children ≥2 years: Initial: 20 mg/kg/d in 3 to 4 divided doses. Maintenance: 15–30 mg/kg/d. Maximum: 30 mg/kg/d.
Adjustment of dosage
• Kidney disease: None.
• Liver disease: None.
• Elderly: May be necessary to reduce dose for patients >65 years.
• Pediatric: Safety and efficacy have not been established in children <2 years.
Food: Take with food or large quantities of water or milk.
Pregnancy: Category C. Category D in third trimester or near delivery.

Lactation: Appears in breast milk. Considered compatible with breastfeeding by American Academy of Pediatrics.
Contraindications: Hypersensitivity to tolmetin and cross-sensitivity with other NSAIDs and aspirin.
Editorial comments: For additional information, see *ibuprofen*, p. 445.

Torsemide

Brand name: Demadex.
Class of drug: Loop diuretic.
Mechanism of action: Inhibits sodium and chloride reabsorption in proximal part of ascending loop of Henle.
Indications/dosage/route: Oral, IV.
• CHF
  – Adults, initial: PO, IV 10 or 20 mg once daily.
• Chronic renal failure.
  – Adults: Initial: PO, IV 20 mg once daily.
• Hepatic cirrhosis
  – Adults: Initial: PO, IV 5 or 10 mg once daily along with aldosterone antagonist or a potassium-sparing diuretic.
• Hypertension
  – Adults: Initial: PO 5 mg once daily. Increase to 10 mg once daily if needed.
Adjustment of dosage
• Kidney disease: None.
• Liver disease: Use with caution.
• Elderly: Use with caution. At higher risk for toxicity.
• Pediatric: Safety and efficacy in children has not been established.

	Onset of Action	Peak Effect	Duration
Oral	Within 60 min	60–120 min	6–8 h
IV	Within 10 min	Within 60 min	6–8 h

Food: Take with food or milk.
Pregnancy: Category B.
Lactation: No data available. Use with caution.
Contraindications: Hypersensitivity to sulfonamides, anuria, hepatic coma, severe electrolyte depletion.

Editorial comments

• Torsemide has the advantage of a safer pregnancy category than other loop diuretics.
• For additional information, see *furosemide*, p. 394.

Tramadol

Brand name: Ultram.
Class of drug: Narcotic (opioid) analgesic.
Mechanism of action: Most likely produces analgesia by binding to opioid receptors. Also inhibits reuptake of norepinephrine and serotonin.
Indications/dosage/route: Oral only.

• Moderate to moderately severe pain
  – Adults: 50–100 mg q4–6h prn. Maximum: 400 mg/d.

Adjustment of dosage

• Kidney disease: Creatinine clearance <30 mL/min: 50–100 mg q12h. Maximum: 200 mg/d.
• Liver disease (cirrhosis): 50 mg q12h.
• Elderly: Maximum daily dose of 300 mg in patients >75 years.
• Pediatric: Safety and efficacy of tramadol have not been established in children <16 years.

Onset of Action	Peak Effect	Duration
1 h	2–3 h	4–6 h

Food: May take with food.
Pregnancy: Category C.

Lactation: Appears in breast milk. Best to avoid.

Contraindications: Hypersensitivity to tramadol or opioids; acute intoxication with alcohol; other analgesics, opioids, hypnotics, or psychotropic agents.

Warnings/precautions

- Use with caution in patients with increased cranial pressure, head injury, alcohol and drug withdrawal, respiratory depression, acute abdominal conditions, history of physical dependence on opioids, and in those concomitantly using (SSRIs), tricyclic antidepressants, neuroleptics, drugs decreasing seizure threshold, kidney or liver disease, elderly.
- Tramadol has been associated with seizures. There is an increased risk in patients with conditions that predispose to seizures, eg, head injury.
- Tramadol is not recommended for patients who have exhibited dependence on opioids or have received opioids previously for more than 1 week.
- Prolonged use of tramadol may result in physical or psychologic dependence although this is not as intense as with opioids.
- Do not give tramadol to patients with abdominal pain without adequate evaluation to rule out structural or pathophysiologic causes.
- Tramadol should be discontinued gradually after long-term use to avoid withdrawal symptoms.
- Patients who have exhibited a previous allergic reaction to opioids may experience seizures if given tramadol.
- It is recommended that tramadol be given on a regular basis rather than prn.

Advice to patient

- Avoid driving and other activities requiring mental alertness or that are potentially dangerous until response to drug is known.
- Change position slowly, in particular from recumbent to upright, to minimize orthostatic hypotension. Sit at the edge of the bed for several minutes before standing, and lie down if feeling faint or dizzy. Avoid hot showers or baths and standing for long periods. Male patients with orthostatic hypotension

may be safer urinating while seated on the toilet rather than standing.
- Avoid alcohol.
- If experiencing constipation, increase intake of fluids and consume high-fiber foods (bran, whole-grain bread, raw vegetables and fruits).

Adverse reactions
- Common: dizziness, vertigo, headache, nausea, constipation, somnolence.
- Serious: CNS stimulation, seizures, anaphylaxis.

Clinically important drug interactions
- Drugs that increase effects/toxicity of tramadol: alcohol, antihistamines, opioids, sedatives, hypnotics, other psychotropic drugs, MAO inhibitors, tricyclic antidepressants, SSRIs, carbamazepine, quinidine.
- Tramadol increases effects/toxicity of digoxin, warafarin, MAO inhibitors.

Parameters to monitor: BP and respiratory rate before and periodically after drug administration.

Editorial comments
- This agent has proven to be highly beneficial for patients with chronic pain in whom other opioids and/or NSAIDs are to be avoided. It produces less respiratory depression than narcotic agents. In some clinical trials, tramadol was comparable or superior to adult dosages of codeine with/without acetaminophen.
- Abuse and dependence on tramadol have been reported; avoid overuse. Use caution if administering to individuals with a prior history of opioid dependence or abuse of other drugs.

Trazodone

Brand name: Desyrel.
Class of drug: Antidepressant.

Mechanism of action: Inhibits reuptake of norepinephrine and serotonin into CNS neurons in animals. Mechanism in humans is not fully understood.

Indications/dosage/route: Oral only.

• Depression
  – Adults: Initial: 150 mg/d, divided doses. Maintenance: 150–600 mg/d. Maximum: 600 mg/d. Chronic dosage should be at lowest effective dose; downward titration is suggested.

Adjustment of dosage

• Kidney disease: None.
• Liver disease: None.
• Elderly: Initial 25 mg/d; increase as needed q3–4d.
• Pediatric: Safety and efficacy have not been established in children <18 years.

Food: Take on an empty stomach or at least 2 hours after last meal.

Pregnancy: Category C.

Lactation: Appears in breast milk. Best to avoid. American Academy of Pediatrics expresses concern regarding use of trazodone while breastfeeding.

Contraindications: Recovery from MI, hypersensitivity to trazodone, concurrent electroconvulsive therapy.

Warnings/precautions: Use with caution in patients with cardiac disease, risk of suicide.

Advice to patient

• May cause priapism. Discontinue if inappropriate or prolonged erections occur.
• Avoid driving and other activities requiring mental alertness or that are potentially dangerous until response to drug is known.
• Avoid alcohol and other CNS depressants such as opiate analgesics and sedatives (eg, diazepam) when taking this drug.
• If you are experiencing dry mouth rinse with warm water frequently, chew sugarless gum, suck on ice cube, or use artificial saliva. Carry out meticulous oral hygiene (floss teeth daily).

Adverse reactions

• Common: dry mouth, dizziness, drowsiness, fatigue, insomnia, anxiety, nausea.

• Serious: hypotension, orthostatic hypotension, arrthymias, priapism, leukopenia.

Clinically important drug interactions: Trazodone increases effects/toxicity of digoxin, phenytoin.

Parameters to monitor: Evidence of improvement in depression, anxiety.

Editorial comments

• For chronic treatment, keep use at lowest effective dose. No formal studies have demonstrated effect beyond 6 weeks.

• It may require 2–4 weeks before full effects of this drug are realized.

• This drug is not listed in detail in the *Physician's Desk Reference*, 54th edition, 2000.

Triamterene

Brand name: Dyrenium.

Class of drug: Potassium-sparing diuretic.

Mechanism of action: Acts on distal renal tubules to inhibit sodium–potassium exchange.

Indications/dosage/route: Oral only.

• Diuretic

– Adults: Initial: 100 mg b.i.d. after meals. Maximum: 300 mg/d.

Adjustment of dosage

• Kidney disease: Contraindicated in patients with anuria, acute and chronic renal insufficiency, or significant renal dysfunction.

• Liver disease: None.

• Elderly: None.

• Pediatric: Safety and efficacy have not been established.

Onset of Action	Peak Effect	Duration
2–4 h	6–8 h	12–16 h

Food: Take with food or milk.

Pregnancy: Category B.

Lactation: No data available. Best to avoid.

Contraindications: Anuria, hyperkalemia, severe renal insufficiency, serum potassium level >5 mEq/L, patients receiving other potassium-sparing diuretics or potassium supplements, hypersensitivity to triamterine, significant renal dysfunction.

Editorial comments

• Use with caution in diabetics with those preparations combined with a thiazide diuretic, as they may worsen hyperglycemia. Use with caution in patients with history of kidney stones (triamterene may incorporate into stones).

• Generally combined in lower doses (37.5 mg or 50 mg) with thiazide diuretic for potassium-sparing effect.

• For additional information, see *spironolactone*, p. 849.

Trifluoperazine

Brand name: Stelazine.

Class of drug: Phenothiazine antipsychotic (neuroleptic).

Mechanism of action: Antagonizes dopamine at dopaminergic receptors in CNS neurons.

Indications/dosage/route: Oral, IM.

• Psychotic disorders
  – Adults, adolescents: Initial: PO 2–5 mg b.i.d. Maintenance: 15–20 mg/d, 2 or 3 divided doses.
  – Adults: IM 1–2 mg q4–6h. Maximum: 10 mg/d.
  – Children 6–12 years: PO 1 mg 1–2 times/d.
  – Children, severe symptoms only: PO 1 mg 1–2 times/d.

• Anxiety, nonpsychotic
  – Adults, adolescents: PO 1–2 mg b.i.d. Maximum: 6 mg/d, no longer than 12 weeks.

Adjustment of dosage

• Kidney disease: None.

• Liver disease: None.

- Elderly: Use dosage in lower range.
- Pediatric: There is little experience with this drug in children. For emergency purposes, 1 mg may be administered IM once or twice a day.

Food: No restriction.

Pregnancy: Category C.

Lactation: No data available. Potentially toxic to infant. Avoid breastfeeding.

Contraindications: Hypersensitivity to phenothiazines, concurrent use of high-dose CNS depressants (alcohol, barbituates, benzodiazepines, narcotics), CNS depression, comatose state.

Editorial comments: For additional information, see *chlorpromazine*, p. 206.

Trihexyphenidyl

Brand name: Artane.

Class of drug: Anticholinergic.

Mechanism of action: Blocks acetylcholine effects at muscarinic receptors throughout the body.

Indications/dosage/route: Oral only

- Parkinsonism
  - Adults: Initial, 1 mg on day 1. Increase by 2 mg q 3–5 days until daily dose is 6–10 mg/day in divided doses. Maximum 12–15 mg/day.
- Adjunct L-DOPA therapy for Parkinsonism
  - Adults: 3-6 mg/day in divided doses.
- Drug-induced extrapyramidal symptoms
  - Adults: Initial, 1 mg/day. Increase to daily dose of 5-15 mg as needed.

Adjustment of dosage

- Kidney Disease: None.
- Liver Disease: None.
- Elderly:None.
- Pediatric: Safety and efficacy have not been established in children.

Pregnancy: Category C.
Lactation: No data available. Potentially toxic to infant. Avoid breastfeeding.
Contraindications: Myasthenia gravis, narrow angle glaucoma, GI obstruction, megacolon, active ulcerative colitis, obstructive uropathy, hypersensitivity to atropine-type compounds (belladonna alkaloids).

For additional information, see *atropine*, p. 67.

Trimethobenzamide

Brand name: Tigan.
Class of drug: Antiemetic.
Mechanism of action: Depresses chemoreceptor trigger zone in the medulla.
Indications/dosage/route: Oral, IM, suppositories.
• Nausea and vomiting
  – Adults, capsules: 250 mg t.i.d. or q.i.d.
  – Adults, suppositories: 200 mg t.i.d. or q.i.d.
  – Adults: IM 200 mg t.i.d. or q.i.d.
  – Children, capsules: 100–200 mg t.i.d. or q.i.d.
  – Children <30 lb, suppositories: 100 mg t.i.d. or q.i.d.
  – Children 30–90 lb, suppositories: 100–200 mg t.i.d. or q.i.d.
Adjustment of dosage
• Kidney disease: None.
• Liver disease: None.
• Elderly: None.
• Pediatric: See above.

	Onset of Action	Duration
PO, IM	10–40 min	3–4 h

Food: Not applicable.
Pregnancy: Category C.

Lactation: No data available. Best to avoid.

Contraindications: Injectable form in children, suppositories in premature and newborn infants, hypersensitivity to trimethobenzamide, sensitivity to benzocaine (suppository).

Warnings/precautions: Use with caution in uncomplicated vomiting in children and in patients with febrile illness, encephalitides, gastroenteritis, dehydration, electrolyte imbalance.

Advice to patient

• Notify physician if worsening nausea develops, particularly if associated with fever, abdominal pain and/or distention, dizziness, or headache.

• Use minimal dosage required to control symptoms.

Adverse reactions

• Common: drowsiness, hypotension, dizziness, headache, diarrhea, muscle cramps.

• Serious: skin reactions (allergic type), seizures, coma.

Clinically important drug interactions

• Trimethobenzamide decreases effects/toxicity of oral anticoagulants.

• Drugs that increase effects/toxicity of trimethobenzamide: atropine-type drugs, alcohol and other CNS depressants (phenothiazines, barbiturates).

Parameters to monitor

• Signs and symptoms of allergic skin reactions.

• Signs and symptoms of extrapyramidal reactions and other CNS toxic effects (convulsions, coma), particularly in the elderly and debilitated patients.

Editorial comments: The antiemetic action of trimethobenzamide may obscure and render difficult the diagnosis of such conditions as appendicitis and evidence of toxicity due to overdose of other drugs.

Trimethoprim–Sulfamethoxazole (TMP–SMZ)

Brand names: Bactrim, Co-Trimoxazole, Septra.

Class of drug: Folic acid antagonist antiinfective.

Mechanism of action: Blocks folic acid synthesis, thus inhibiting biosynthesis of nucleic acids and proteins in susceptible organisms.

Susceptible organisms *in vivo*
- Gram positive: *Streptococcus pneumoniae*, *Staphylococcus aureus*, streptococci, *Listeria*.
- Gram negative: *Escherichia* coli (including enterotoxigenic strains), *Hemophilus influenzae*, Enterobactericeae, *Citrobacter*, *Salmonella, Shigella*, Typhoid.
- Unusual organisms: mycobacteria other than tubercle—*Mycobacterium cheloneae, Mycobacterium fortunotum, Pneumocystis carinii, Cyclospora cayetanensis, Isospora belli, Nocardia*.

Indications/dosage/route: Oral, IV.
- Severe UTIs, shigellosis
  - Adults, children: IV 8–10 mg/kg (based on trimethoprim component), in 3 or 4 equal doses every 6, 8, or 12 hours, up to 14 days for UTI, 5 days for Shigellosis. Maximum: 48 g/d.
  - Adults: PO 160 mg trimethoprim plus 800 mg sulfamethoxazole (1 double-strength tablet or 2 ordinary tablets) q12h, 10–14 days for UTI, 5 days for shigellosis.
- UTIs, shigellosis, acute otitis media in pediatric patients
  - PO 8 mg/kg trimethoprim plus 40 mg/kg sulfamethoxazole q12h, 10 days for UTI, 5 days for shigellosis.
- Acute exacerbation of chronic bronchitis
  - Adults: PO 160 mg trimethoprim plus 800 mg sulfamethoxazole q12h, 14 days.
- Treatment of *P. carinii* pneumonia
  - Adults, children: PO 15–20 mg/kg trimethorpim plus 75–100 mg/kg sulfamethoxazole per day in divided doses q6h, 14–21 days.
- Prophylaxis of P. carinii pneumonia
  - Adults: PO 160 mg trimethoprim plus 800 mg sulfamethoxazole per day.
  - Children: PO, 150 mg/m^2 trimethoprim plus 750 mg/m^2 sulfamethoxazole in equal doses for 3 consecutive days/week.

- Traveler's diarrhea
  - Adults: PO 160 mg trimethoprim plus 800 mg sulfamethoxazole q12h, 5 days.

Adjustment of dosage

- Kidney disease: Creatinine clearance >30 mL/min: usual dose; creatinine clearance 15–30 mL/min: 50% of usual dose; creatinine clearance <15 mL/min: not recommended.
- Liver disease: None.
- Elderly: Use with caution, particularly in those with liver or kidney disease.
- Pediatric: See above. This drug is contraindicated for use in infants <2 months.

Food: Oral medication should be taken with 8 oz of water 1 hour before or 2 hours after eating.

Pregnancy: Contraindicated.

Lactation: Contraindicated.

Contraindications: Hypersensitivity to trimethoprim or sulfonamides, thiazide diuretics, oral hypoglycemics, megaloblastic anemia due to folate deficiency, pregnancy, lactation, treatment of streptococcal pharyngitis.

Warnings/precautions

- Use with caution in patients with possible folate deficiency (chronic alcoholics, elderly), concurrent anticonvulsant therapy, blood dyscrasias, G6PD deficiency, severe allergies, bronchial asthma, AIDS.
- Administer folinic acid if bone marrow depression occurs.

Advice to patient

- Drink large amounts of fluids (2.5–3 L) per day and maintain adequate fluid intake after discontinuing the drug.
- To minimize possible photosensitivity reaction, apply adequate sunscreen and use proper covering when exposed to strong sunlight.

Adverse reactions

- Common: anorexia, nausea, vomiting, glossitis, rash.
- Serious: Stevens–Johnson syndrome (rare), pseudomembranous colitis, agranulocytosis, aplastic anemia, megaloblastic anemia, hyperkalemia, hemolysis (patients with G6PD deficiency).

Clinically important drug interactions
- Drugs that increase effects/toxicity of trimethoprim–sulfamethoxazole: salicylates and other NSAIDs.
- Trimethoprim–sulfamethoxazole increases effects/toxicity of warfarin, phenytoin, methotrexate, cyclosporine, digoxin, oral hypoglycemic drugs.

Parameters to monitor
- Early signs and symptoms of Stevens–Johnson syndrome.
- CBC and differential, liver enzymes, kidney function. Discontinue drug if there is significant reduction in any formed element.
- Signs and symptoms of renal toxicity. Perform urinalysis with microscopic examination as well as kidney function tests.

Editorial comments: Uses for trimethoprim–sulfamethoxazole include the treatment of UTIs acquired in the community (superior to amoxicillin). Other important uses include treatment of *Listeria* meningitis (in patients allergic to penicillin), *Pneumocystis* pneumonia in AIDS, *Enterobacter* infections, and Whipple's disease.

Trimipramine

Brand name: Surmontil.
Class of drug: Tricyclic antidepressant.
Mechanism of action: Inhibits reuptake of CNS neurotransmitters, primarily serotonin and norepinephrine.
Indications/dosage/route: Oral only.
- Depression
  - Adults: Initial: 75 mg/d in divided doses. Maintenance: 100–150 mg/d. Maximum: 200 mg/d.
  - Elderly, adolescents: 50 mg/d. Maintenance: 100 mg/d.

Adjustment of dosage
- Kidney disease: None.
- Liver disease: None.
- Elderly: See above.
- Pediatric: Safety and efficacy in children <12 have not been established.

Food: No restriction.
Pregnancy: Category C.
Lactation: Appears in breast milk. American Academy of Pediatrics expresses concern over use when breastfeeding.
Contraindications: Hypersensitivity to tricyclic antidepressants, acute recovery from MI, concomitant use of MAO inhibitor.
Editorial comments: For additional information, see *amitriptyline*, p. 39.

Troleandomycin

Brand name: TAO.
Class of drug: Antibiotic, macrolide.
Mechanism of action: Inhibits RNA-dependent protein synthesis at the level of the 50S ribosome.
Susceptible organisms *in vivo*: *Staphylococcus pyogenes, Staphylococcus pneumoniae*.
Indications/dosage/route: Oral only.
• Pneumonia or respiratory tract infection caused by sensitive pneumoccoci or group A beta-hemolytic streptococci
  – Adults: PO 250–500 mg q6h.
  – Children: PO 125–250 mg q6h.
Adjustment of dosage: None.
Food: Take on empty stomach.
Pregnancy: Safety has not been established.
Lactation: No data available. Best to avoid.
Contraindications: Hypersensitivity to macrolide antibiotics.
Editorial comments
• For additional information, see *erythromycin*, p. 329.

Tubocurarine

Brand name: Tubocurarine.

Class of drug: Nondepolarizing neuromuscular blocker.

Mechanism of action: Blocks nicotinic acetylcholine receptors at neuromuscular junction, resulting in skeletal muscle relaxation and paralysis.

Indications/dosage/route: IV, IM.

• Adjunct to surgical anesthesia
  – Adults: Initial: IM, IV 6–9 mg, then 3–4.5 mg in 3–5 min if needed.
  – Pediatric ≤4 weeks: Initial: IV 0.3 mg/kg, then increments of one-fifth to one-sixth the initial dose.
  – Infants, children: IV 0.6 mg/kg.
• Electroshock therapy
  – Adults: IV 0.1–0.2 mg/kg.
• Diagnosis of myasthenia gravis
  – Adults: IV 0.004–0.033 mg/kg. Terminate test by injecting 2 mg neostigmine IV 2 or 3 minutes after tubocurarine.

Adjustment of dosage

• Kidney disease: None.
• Liver disease: Prolonged duration of action, higher volume of distribution. Higher initial dose may be required for rapid induction.
• Elderly: None.
• Pediatric: See above.

Food: Not applicable.

Pregnancy: Category C.

Lactation: No data available. Best to avoid.

Contraindications: Hypersensitivity to tubocurarine and chemically related drugs.

Warnings/precautions

• Use with caution in patients with liver disease, kidney disease, impaired pulmonary function, respiratory depression, myasthenia gravis, dehydration, porphyria, muscle spasms, hypokalemia, hypermagnesemia, dehydration, underlying cardiovascular disease, fractures, hyperthermia, shock, thyroid disorders, familial periodic paralysis.
• Neuromuscular blocking agents do not produce analgesia. The patient is fully aware of sensory input when such drugs are

used. Accordingly, an antianxiety agent (benzodiazepine) or analgesic (narcotic) is administered along with these drugs.

- Long-term use in the ICU setting has not been studied.
- Therapeutic index (margin of safety between the dose required and respiratory paralysis) is very small. Accordingly, appropriate measures must be on hand to provide respiratory support should this be necessary.
- Not recommended for rapid sequence induction for cesarean section.
- Patient who is to required to have prolonged ventilation must be adequately sedated.
- To protect the cornea, apply eyedrops and eye patches to patient.
- Drug should not be administered until patient is unconscious. As consciousness is not affected by the drug, use caution in conversation near patient.
- Prolonged duration of action and slower recovery time are anticipated in patients with cardiac dysfunction and liver disease and in the elderly.
- Burn patients may exhibit resistance to the actions of the drug.
- Imbalance of potassium (hypokalemia) and magnesium (hypermagnesemia) can potentiate the neuromuscular blocking potency of the drug and should be corrected before drug administration.
- Direct medical supervision is required when this drug is administered.
- Atropine and a cholinersterase inhibitor such as neostigmine must be readily available when drug is administered.
- Rapid IV administration may predispose the patient to respiratory paralysis and/or bronchospasm.

Adverse reactions
- Common: none.
- Serious: arrythmias, cardiovascular collapse, bronchospasm, hypersensitivity reaction.

Clinically important drug interactions: Drugs that increase effects/ toxicity of neuromuscular blockers: inhalation anesthetics, aminoglycosides, quinidine, lincomycin, tetracycline, lithium, magnesium sulfate, polymyxin D, vancomycin, bacitracin, colistin.

Parameters to monitor

- Respiratory status continuously: Maintain patent airway and ventilation until normal respiration is recovered. If respiratory depression persists, administer a cholinesterase inhibitor, eg, neostigmine or pyridostigmine. Coadminister atropine to counteract excessive muscarinic stimulation.
- Monitor patient for postoperative respiratory distress and muscle weakness.
- Neuromuscular status: Use peripheral nerve stimulator every 4 hours during surgery and afterward to evaluate recovery and effectiveness of muscle relaxation.
- Pulmonary status at frequent intervals: respiratory rate, frequency, breath sounds.
- Signs of excessive vagal stimulation using ECG: bradycardia, hypotension, arrhythmias.
- Recovery from the drug. Evaluate by grip strength and 5-second head lift.
- Signs of hypotension (ganglionic blockade) prior to and during use.
- Symptoms of histamine release: bronchospasm, salivation.
- Evidence of pain during surgery. Administer analgesic drug to control pain adequately.

Editorial comments

- Neuromuscular blocking drugs should be administered by or under supervision of experienced clinicians who are thoroughly familiar with these drugs and know how to treat potential complications that might arise from their use. Administration of these drugs should be made in a setting where there are facilities available for the following: tracheal intubation, administration of oxygen, drugs for reversing drug effects, and administration of artificial respiration.
- This drug is not listed in the *Physician's Desk Reference,* 54th edition, 2000.

Valacyclovir

Brand name: Valtrex.
Class of drug: Antiviral purine nucleoside.
Mechanism of action: Inhibits viral DNA polymerase.
Indications/dosage/route: Oral only.
• Herpes zoster in immunocompetent patients
  – Adults: 1 g t.i.d., 7 days.
• Recurrent genital herpes in immunocompetent patients
  – Adults: 500 mg b.i.d., 5 days.
Adjustment of dosage
• Kidney disease: Creatinine clearance 30–49 mL/min: 1 g every 12 hours; creatinine clearance 10–29 mL/min: 1 g every 24 hours; creatinine clearance <10 mL/min: 500 mg every 24 hours.
• Elderly: Adjustment may be necessary depending on renal status.
• Pediatric: Safety and effectiveness in children have not been established.
Food: No restriction.
Pregnancy: Category B.
Lactation: No data available. Best to avoid.
Contraindications: Hypersensitivity to valacyclovir, acyclovir, immunocompromised patients.
Warnings/precautions: Use with caution in patients with renal disease, hemolytic anemia, and in patients receiving other nephrotoxic drugs.
Advice to patient
• Male patients should use condoms if engaging in sexual intercourse while using this medication.
• Do not receive any vaccinations (particularly live attenuated viruses) without permission from treating physician.
Adverse reactions
• Common: headache, dizziness, nausea, vomiting.
• Serious: none.
Clinically important drug interactions: Drugs that increase effects/toxicity of valacyclovir: probenecid, cimetidine.

Parameters to monitor
• Signs and symptoms of renal toxicity.
• Signs and symptoms of infection.

Editorial comments
• It is most important to institute valacyclovir therapy as soon as possible following signs or symptoms of herpes zoster infection. The drug is most effective if started within 48 hours of the onset of rash. It is unknown how effective treatment would be more than 72 hours after onset of rash.
• Advise patient to report if there is any recurrence of herpes zoster infection. Such recurrences are rare and may indicate an underlying malignancy or dysfunction of the immune system.

Valproic Acid

Brand names: Depacon (valproate sodium injection), Depakote (tablets), Depakene (capsules, syrup).
Class of drug: Anticonvulsant.
Mechanism of action: Increases brain levels of GABA.
Indications/dosage/route: Oral, IV.
• Complex partial seizures, monotherapy
  – Adults, children >10 years: Initial: PO, IV 10–15 mg/kg/d. Increase by 5–10 mg/kg/d as needed. Maximum: 60 mg/d.
• Complex partial seizures, adjunct to anticonvulsant therapy
  – Adults: Initial: PO, IV 10–15 mg/kg/d. Increase by 10–15 mg/kg/d as needed. Maximum: 60 mg/kg/d.
• Simple and complex absence seizures
  – Adults, children >10 years: Initial: IV 15 mg/kg/d. Increase at 1-week intervals by 10–15 mg/kg. Maximum: 60 mg/kg/d.
• Mania
  – Adults: PO 750 mg/d in divided doses. Increase rapidly until desired therapeutic effect is achieved. Maximum: 60 mg/kg/d.

- Migraine
  - Adults: Initial: PO 250 mg b.i.d. Maximum: 1000 mg/d.

Adjustment of dosage

- Kidney disease: None.
- Liver disease: Contraindicated.
- Elderly: No specific data available for use in elderly. Adjustment of dose not considered necessary.
- Pediatric: See above. Not recommended for treatment of mania in children <18 years or of migraine in children <16 years.

Food: Capsules or tablets should be swallowed whole to avoid irritation of oral mucosa. Should be taken with food but carbonated beverages should be avoided.

Pregnancy: Category D.

Lactation: Appears in breast milk. Considered compatible with breastfeeding by the American Academy of Pediatrics.

Contraindications: Liver disease or hepatic dysfunction, hypersensitivity to valproic acid.

Warnings/precautions

- Use with caution in patients with previous history of liver disease, patients on multiple anticonvulsants (see drug interactions below), congenital metabolic disorders, organic brain disease, severe seizures accompanied by mental retardation.
- This drug may cause thrombocytopenia and severe bleeding disorders.
- Children under 2 years old are at considerable risk for hepatotoxicity.
- Drug should be discontinued at first sign of hepatic dysfunction.

Advice to patient

- Do not drive or perform other activities requiring alertness until effects of the drug are known.
- Avoid alcohol and other central nervous system depressants (sedatives, narcotics).
- Report the following adverse effects to treating physician immediately: yellowing of skin, unusual bruising or bleeding, unexplained fever, sore throat.

- Do not discontinue drug suddenly as this may precipitate status epilepticus. Do not alter dosage without approval from treating physician.
- Carry identification card listing drug as well as type of seizure disorder, name, address and telephone number of treating physician.

Adverse reactions

- Common: Nausea, vomiting, abdominal cramping, dyspepsia, diarrhea, anorexia.
- Serious: Hepatotoxicity, thrombocytopenia, erythema multiforme, confusion, pancreatitis.

Clinically important drug interactions

- Drugs that increase effects/toxicity of valproic acid: aspirin, alcohol, felbamate, rifampin, diazepam.
- Drug that decreases effects/toxicity of valproic acid: clonazepam (avoid combination).
- Valproic acid increases effects/toxicity of the following drugs: diazepam, ethosuximide, lamotrigine, phenobarbital, primidione, phentoin, warfarin.
- Valproic acid decreases effects/toxicity of carbamazepine.

Parameters to monitor

- CBC with differential and platelet count, liver enzymes, thyroid function tests.
- Serum valproic acid levels.
- Liver function for signs and symptoms of hepatotoxicity. Discontinue drug immediately at first signs of hepatic dysfunction.
- Check serum levels of valproic acid when adding another anticonvulsant (see drug interactions).
- Monitor patient for signs and symptoms of thrombocytopenia. Perform platelet counts and coagulation tests before initiating therapy and periodically thereafter.

Editorial comments

- Therapeutic serum levels are 50–100 microgram/mL. Toxicity is seen with serum levels >100 mcg/mL.
- Overdoses are characterized by hallucinations, deep sleep, followed by coma.

Valsartan

Brand name: Diovan.
Class of drug: Angiotensin II receptor antagonist, antihypertensive.
Mechanism of action: Blocks binding of angiotensin II to vascular smooth muscle receptors. This results in inhibition of vasoconstriction. Also diminishes aldosterone activity.
Indications/dosage/route: Oral only.
• Hypertension
 – Adults: Initial: 80 mg/d, once a day. Increase to 160–320 mg/d or diuretic may be added (eg, hydrochlorothiazide.)
Adjustment of dosage
• Kidney disease: Mild to moderate: none; severe: use with caution.
• Liver disease: Mild to moderate: none; severe: use with caution.
• Elderly: None.
• Pediatric: Safety and efficacy have not been established.
Food: Advise patients to limit foods containing potassium: salt substitutes, orange juice, bananas.
Pregnancy: Category C. Category D in second and third trimesters. Discontinue valsartan as soon as possible when pregnancy is detected.
Lactation: No data available. Potentially toxic to infant. Avoid breastfeeding.
Contraindications: Hypersensitivity to valsartan, anuria, hypersensitivity to sulfonamides (thiazide diuretics, oral hypoglycemic drugs).
Editorial comments: For additional information, see *losartan*, p. 541.

Vancomycin

Brand names: Vancocin, Vancoled, Lyphocin.
Class of drug: Antibiotic.

Mechanism of action: Inhibits bacterial cell wall synthesis.
Indications/dosage/route: Oral, IV.
- Severe infections caused by methicillin-resistant staphylococcus (documented or suspected), also streptococcal infections, *Corynebacterium* sp, *Streptococcus pneumoniae, Listeria, Bacillus anthrancis*, and *Enterococcus* sp.
  – Adults: IV 500 mg q6h or 1 g q12h.
  – Children, infants >1 month: IV 40 mg/kg/d, divided q6h.
  – Neonates: Initial: IV 15 mg/kg. Increase to 10–15 mg/kg IV q6–8h up to age 1 month.
  – Neonates ≤7 days: Depending on body weight, IV q12h to q24h.
- Pseudomembranous colitis
  – Adults: PO 125–500 mg q6h, 7–14 days.
  – Children: PO 40 mg/kg/d q6–8h, 7–10 days. Maximum: 2 g/d.
  – Neonates: PO 10 mg/kg/d q6–8h.
- Prophylaxis of endocarditis
  – Adults: IV 1 g starting 1 hour before procedure.
  – Children <27 kg: IV 20 mg/kg.
  – Children >27 kg: adult dose.

Adjustment of dosage
- Kidney disease: Creatinine clearance 40–90 mL/min: administer q24h; creatinine clearance 10–20 mL/min: administer q96h; creatinine clearance <10 mL/min: administer 5–7 days.
- Liver disease: Reduce dose by 60%.
- Elderly: Patients are at greater risk for developing ototoxicity.
- Pediatric: See above.

Food: Take oral vancomycin with food.
Pregnancy: Category C.
Lactation: Appears in breast milk. Best to avoid.
Contraindications: Hypersensitivity to vancomycin.
Warnings/precautions
- Use with caution in patients with: hearing impairment, intestinal obstruction, and in patients receiving other potentially nephrotoxic or ototoxic drugs, kidney disease, elderly.
- Vancomycin may not be administered by the IM route.

Advice to patient
- If diarrhea is experienced, an antidiarrheal agent should not be taken except following physician approval.
- If you have artificial heart valves, notify physician prior to invasive dental or medical procedures.

Adverse reactions
- Common: nausea, vomiting, taste disturbances, rash on face and upper body (parenteral administration).
- Serious: anaphylaxis, ototoxicity, thrombocytopenia, renal failure, interstitial nephritis, hypotension, vasculitis.

Clinically important drug interactions: Vancomycin increases effects/toxicity of aspirin, aminoglycosides, cyclosporine, loop diuretics, nondepolarizing neuromuscular blockers, general anesthetics.

Parameters to monitor
- Serum BUN and creatinine.
- Sensitivity prior to and throughout therapy.
- Patency of IV catheter, infiltration associated with discomfort at IV site, skin erythema along venous distribution. If extravasation is suspected, remove catheter and discontinue administration.
- Signs and symptoms of Red Man syndrome: erythema, maculopaplar rash of neck and back, chills, paresthesias, hypotension. Treat with antihistamine or slow down infusion rate.
- Signs and symptoms of ototoxicity: tinnitus, vertigo, hearing loss, initially in range 4000–8000 Hz.
- Serum vancomycin level throughout course of therapy. Draw peak 30–60 minutes after conclusion of infusion (1-hour duration). Draw trough prior to preceding dose. Therapeutic levels of vancomycin: peak, 25–40 µg/mL; trough, 5–12 µg/mL.
- Signs and symptoms of renal toxicity.
- Intake of fluids and output of urinary and other fluids. Increase fluid intake if inadequate in order to minimize renal toxicity. Closely monitor serum electrolyte levels.
- Signs and symptoms of antibiotic-induced bacterial or fungal superinfection.

Editorial comments: Vancomycin is used for a variety of infections including methicillin-resistant *Staphylococcus aureus* and *Staphylococcus epidermidis* infections. It is used to treat enterococcal infections resistant to ampicillin, preferable in combination with an aminoglycoside. In oral form, it is used to treat *Clostridium difficile* colitis.

Vasopressin (Antidiuretic Hormone)

Brand name: Pitressin.

Class of drug: Antidiuretic hormone, vasoconstrictor, prokinetic drug.

Mechanism of action: Antidiuretic action: increases cAMP at renal tubule and collecting duct, resulting in increased urine osmolality and decreased rate of urinary flow. Peristaltic stimulant action: stimulates contraction of GI tract smooth muscle. Hemostatic action: constricts capillaries and small arterioles in GI tract.

Indications/dosage/route: IV, IM, SC.

• Diabetes insipidus
  – Adults: IM or SC 5–10 units b.i.d. or q.i.d. as needed.
  – Children: IM or SC 2.5–10 units b.i.d. or q.i.d. as needed.
• Postoperative abdominal distention
  – Adults: Initial: IM 5 units, then same dose q3–4h. Maximum: 10 units.
  – Children: 2.5–5 units.
• Upper GI tract hemorrhage
  – Adults: IV 0.1–0.4 unit/min. Increase dose until bleeding stops. At this point decrease dose and discontinue within 24–48 hours.

Adjustment of dosage

• Kidney disease: None.
• Liver disease: May require decreased dose.
• Elderly: May have a decreased effect.
• Pediatric: See above.

Onset of Action	Duration
Rapid	2–8 h

Pregnancy: Category C.

Lactation: No data available. Best to avoid.

Contraindications: Chronic nephritis (until controlled), hypersensitivity to beef/pork proteins, hypersensitivity to vasopressin, coronary artery disease, angina pectoris.

Warnings/precautions

• Use with caution in patients with seizures, asthma, migraine, heart failure, goiter, atherosclerosis.

• Do not inject vasopressin during the first stage of labor.

• May cause gangrene or ischemic bowel during infusion.

Advice to patient

• Avoid alcohol and other CNS depressants such as opioid analgesics and sedatives (eg, diazepam) when taking this drug.

• Carry identification card at all times describing disease, treatment regimen, name, address, and telephone number of treating physician.

Adverse reactions

• Common: hypertension, headache, fever, skin pallor, tremor, abdominal cramps, nausea, diaphoresis.

• Serious: MI, arrhythmias, bradycardia, water intoxication, seizures, bronchoconstriction, venous thrombosis, anaphylaxis.

Clinically important drug interactions

• Drugs that increase effects/toxicity of vasopressin: carbamazepine, clofibrate, chlorpropamide, ganglionic blockers, fludrocortisone, phenformin, urea.

• Drugs that decrease effects/toxicity of vasporessin: alcohol, lithium, heparin, epinephrine, norepinephrine.

Parameters to monitor

• Intake of fluids and urinary and other fluid output to minimize renal toxicity. Closely monitor electrolyte levels.

• Signs and symptoms of fluid extravasation from IV injection.

• When treating diabetes insipidus, monitor patient for the following: urine volume, specific gravity and osmolality, serum and urine sodium, fluid intake, symptoms of dehydration (excessive thirst, tachycardia, dry skin), edema. Weigh patient daily and monitor intake and output.

• Signs of water intoxication: confusion, headache, difficulty urinating, seizures, weight gain. Discontinue vasopressin if these symptoms occur. Administer mannitol or furosemide if symptoms are severe.

• BP twice daily. If BP is elevated, this may signify that the drug is not working properly.

• When treating abdominal distension, monitor characteristics of bowel sounds, passage of stool or flatus.

Editorial comments

• Physician should be advised that dosage for treating diabetes insipidus is highly variable. Titrate administered dose based on serum and urine osmolality and sodium.

• Elderly patients should be cautioned about increasing water or fluid intake beyond that needed to satisfy their thirst.

• This drug is not listed in the *Physician's Desk Reference*, 54th edition, 2000.

Venlafaxine

Brand name: Effexor.

Class of drug: SSRI.

Mechanism of action: Inhibits reuptake of serotonin into CNS neurons.

Indications/dosage/route: Oral.

• Depression
  – Adults: Initial: 75 mg/d in 2 or 3 divided doses. Maintenance: 150–225 mg/d in divided doses.

Adjustment of dosage

• Kidney disease: Mild to moderate: reduce dose by 25%; severe: reduce dose by 50%.

• Liver disease: Reduce dose by 50% or more.

• Elderly: Use with caution.

• Pediatric: Safety and efficacy have not been established in children <18 years.

Food: May be taken with meals.

Pregnancy: Category C.

Lactation: Appears in breast milk. Best to avoid. American Academy of Pediatrics expresses concern with use during breastfeeding.

Contraindications: MAO inhibitor taken within 14 days, hypersensitivity to venflaxine.

Editorial comments

• Male sexual dysfunction and diarrhea appear to be less common than with some other SSRIs.

• For additional information, see *fluoxetine*, p. 378.

Verapamil

Brand names: Calan, Covera, Verelan, Isoptin.

Class of drug: Calcium channel blocker.

Mechanism of action: Inhibits calcium movement across cell membranes.

Indications/dosage/route: Oral, IV.

• Angina
  – Adults: Initial: PO 40–120 mg t.i.d. Maintenance: PO 240–480 mg/d.

• Arrhythmias
  – Digitalized patients with chronic atrial fibrillation: 240–320 mg/d in divided doses t.i.d. to q.i.d.

• Hypertension
  – Initial: PO 80–120 mg t.i.d.
  – Elderly: initial: PO 40 mg t.i.d.

Extended–release forms

• Hypertension
  – Initial: 240 mg/d in morning.

– Elderly: 120 mg/d. Increase to 240 mg in morning and 120 mg in evening and then 240 mg q12h if needed.

- Supraventricular tachyarrhythmias
  – Adults: Initial: IV 5–10 mg given over 2 min, then 10 mg 30 min later if needed.
  – Infants ≤1 year: IV 0.1–0.2 mg/kg as IV bolus over 2 minutes.
  – Children 1–15 years: 0.1–0.3 mg/kg over 2 minutes. It may be repeated after 30 minutes if needed.

Adjustment of dosage

- Kidney disease: Administer with caution. Monitor P-R interval.
- Liver disease: Reduce dose by 70% in severe liver disease.
- Elderly: None.
- Pediatric: Safety and efficacy have not been established.

Onset of Action	Peak Effect	Duration
1–2 h 1–5 min IV	1–2 h 5 h extended-release form	8–10 h 24 h extended-release form

Food: No restriction.

Pregnancy: Category C.

Lactation: Appears in breast milk in small amounts. Considered compatible by American Academy of Pediatrics. Manufacturer recommends discontinuing breastfeeding.

Contraindications: Hypersensitivity to calcium channel blockers.

Warnings/precautions

- Use with caution in patients with CHF, severe left ventricular dysfunction, and in those concomitantly using β blockers or digoxin, kidney or liver disease.
- Do not withdraw drug abruptly, as this may result in increased frequency and intensity of angina.
- For the diabetic patient, the drug may interfere with insulin release and therefore produce hyperglycemia.
- Patient should be tapered off β blocker before beginning calcium channel blocker to avoid exacerbation of angina due to abrupt withdrawal of the β blocker.

Advice to patient
- Use two forms of birth control including hormonal and barrier methods.
- Change position slowly, in particular from recumbent to upright, to minimize orthostatic hypotension. Sit at the edge of the bed for several minutes before standing, and lie down if feeling faint or dizzy. Avoid hot showers or baths and standing for long periods. Male patients should sit on the toilet while urinating rather than standing.
- Avoid driving and other activities requiring mental alertness or that are potentially dangerous until response to drug is known.
- Use OTC medications only after first informing the treating physician.
- Determine BP and heart rate aproximately at the same time each day and at least twice a week, particularly at the beginning of therapy.
- Be aware of the fact that this drug may also block or reduce anginal pain, thereby giving a false sense of security on severe exertion.
- Include high-fiber foods to minimize constipation.
- Limit consumption of xanthine-containing drinks: regular coffee (more than 5 cups/d), tea, cocoa.

Adverse reactions
- Common: cough, headache, edema, constipation.
- Serious: CHF, bradycardia, first-, second-, and third-degree AV block, galacorrhea.

Clinically important drug interactions
- Drugs that increase effects/toxicity of calcium blockers: cimetidine, β blockers, cyclosporine.
- Drugs that decrease effects of calcium blockers: barbiturates.

Parameters to monitor
- BP during initial administration and frequently thereafter. Ideally, check BP close to the end of dosage interval or before next administration.
- Status of liver and kidney function. Impaired renal function prolongs duration of action and increases tendency for toxicity.

- Intake of fluids and urinary and other fluid output to minimize renal toxicity. Increase fluid intake if inadequate. Closely monitor electrolyte levels.
- Efficacy of treatment for angina: decrease in frequency of angina attacks, need for nitroglycerin, episodes of ST segment elevation, anginal pain. If anginal pain is not reduced at rest or during effort, reassess patient as to medication.
- GI side effects: use alternative.
- ECG for development of heart block.
- Symptoms of CHF.

Vidarabine

Brand name: Vira-A.
Class of drug: Antiviral agent.
Mechanism of action: Inhibits DNA polymerase, is incorporated into viral DNA interfering with DNA synthesis.
Indications/dosage/route: IV, topical (ophthalmic).
- Acute conjunctivitis and recurrent epithelial keratitis caused by herpes simplex virus types I and II
  – Administered as 3% ophthalmic ointment. Apply 1/2 inch into lower conjunctival sac 5 times/d at 3-hour intervals. Continue treatment for 7 days after reepithelialization is complete. If reepithelialization has not occurred in 21 days, other therapy should be considered.
- Herpes simplex viral encephalitis, neonatal herpes simplex viral infections
  – IV 15 mg/kg/d, 10 days.
- Herpes zoster
  – IV 10 mg/kg/d, 5 days.
Adjustment of dosage: None.
Pregnancy: Category C.
Lactation: No data available. Best to avoid.
Contraindications: Hypersensitivity to vidarabine.

Warnings/precautions: Do not administer for bacterial infection or other viral conjunctivitis not cited above.

Adverse reactions

• Common: lacrimation, irritation, infection of the conjunctiva.

• Serious: none.

Clinically important drug interactions: None.

Parameters to monitor: Monitor conjunctive for efficacy of treatment. There should be improvement within 7 days and reepithelialization in 21 days. After reepithelialization, reduce frequency to b.i.d. for 7 days.

Editorial comments

• May be administered together with topical gentamicin, erythromycin, and chloramphenicol.

• This drug is not listed in the *Physician's Desk Reference*, 54th edition, 2000.

Vinblastine

Brand name: Velban.

Class of drug: Antineoplastic agent, vinca alkaloid.

Mechanism of action: Disrupts cell division in metaphase by inhibition of microtubule formation.

Indications/dosage/route: IV only.

• Hodgkin's and non-Hodgkin's lymphoma; testicular, lung, breast, head, and neck carcinoma; Kaposi's sarcoma; idiopathic thrombocytopenic purpura, mycosis fungoides, histiocytosis, choriocarcinoma

 – Adults: 0.1 mg/kg weekly q7–14d. Alternative dose: 4–10 mg/m^2. Increase in increments of 50 µg/kg to maximum of 0.5 mg/kg/wk. Five-day infusion: 1.5–2 mg/m^2/d.

 – Children: 2.5 mg/m^2, single dose every week. Increase to maximum of 7.5 mg/m^2.

Adjustment of dosage

• Kidney disease: None.

- Liver disease: Serum bilirubin 1.5–3.0 mg/dL: 50% of normal dose; serum bilirubin 3.0–5.0 mg/dL: 25% of dose; serum bilirubin >5.0 mg/dL: avoid administration.
- Elderly: None.
- Pediatric: See above.

Pregnancy: Category D.

Lactation: No data available. Potentially toxic to infant. Avoid breastfeeding.

Contraindications: Significant granulocytopenia, active bacterial infection.

Warnings/precautions

- Use with caution in patients with decreased bone marrow reserve, liver disease.
- Dosage must be individualized based on hematologic parameters. Administer only when WBC >4000/mm^3. Decrease doses in patients receiving other chemotherapy or with recent radiation therapy.
- For intravenous use only; do not use as intrathecal injection (will cause fatality).
- Do not confuse vinblastine with vincristine when administering.
- Administer an antiemetic before vinblastine.
- If used as intermittent dosage, vinblastine should not be administered more often than weekly. Leukocyte count should be checked prior to each administered dose.

Advice to patient

- Use two forms of birth control including hormonal and barrier methods. Practice contraception for at least 2 months following conclusion of therapy.
- Drink at least 2 quarts of fluid/d.
- Avoid taking NSAIDs together with this drug.
- Avoid alcohol.
- Receive vaccinations (particularly live attenuated viruses) only if approved by treating physician.
- Eat a high-fiber diet to prevent constipation.
- To minimize possible photosensitivity reaction, apply adequate sunscreen and use proper covering when exposed to strong sunlight.

Adverse reactions

- Common: alopecia, nausea, vomiting, stomatitis, constipation, taste disturbances, hypertension, urinary retention, muscle pain, hyperuricemia, photosensitivity.
- Serious: **bone marrow depression**, Raynaud's phenomenon, bronchospasm, tissue necrosis (extravasation), peripheral neuropathy, seizures, autonomic neuropathy, hemorrhagic colitis, depression, orthostatic hypotension, paralytic ileus.

Clinically important drug interaction

- Drugs that increase effects/toxicity of vinblastine: antineoplastic agents (cause bone marrow suppression), mitomycin (bronchospasm), erythromycin, ritonavir.
- Vinblastine decreases effects/toxicity of phenytoin.

Parameters to monitor

- CBC with differential and platelet count.
- BP, pulse.
- Respiratory status; evaluate for bronchospasm.
- Signs of infection.
- Signs and symptoms of neuropathy: burning, tingling, numbness in hands or feet; loss of peripheral sensation, motor weakness, discoordination, ataxia, diminished deep tendon reflexes, foot or wrist drop, paralytic ileus. If a medication-induced neuropathy is suspected, discontinue treatment immediately.
- Signs and symptoms of fluid extravasation from IV injection. Observe for patency of IV catheter, infiltration associated with discomfort at IV site, skin erythema along with venous distribution. If extravasation is suspected, remove catheter and discontinue administration. Hyaluronidase is a specific antidote for vinca alkaloid extravasation.
- Signs and symptoms of bone marrow depression.
- Signs and symptoms of anemia.
- Signs of hyperuricemia.
- Hematologic status prior to and frequently during course of therapy. If WBC falls to <4000/µL, withhold treatment until recovery occurs.
- Signs and symptoms of stomatitis. Treat with peroxide, tea, topical anesthetics such as benzocaine or lidocaine, or antifungal drug.

Editorial comments

- Do not administer by the following routes: SC, IM, or intrathecal. It is to be used only by the IV route.
- Combining vinblastine with mitomycin C may result in severe bronchospasm. This toxic effect may occur within a few minutes of mitomycin C administration or may occur up to 2 weeks following administration of a single dose of mitomycin.
- Following radiation therapy or chemotherapy, the dose of vinblastine should be reduced; single maximum doses should not exceed 5.5 mg/m^2.
- Although rare, a neurotoxic syndrome resembling that seen with vincristine can occur with high-dose vinblastine therapy. Signs and symptoms include peripheral neuropathy, headache, confusion, urinary retention, and seizures.

Warfarin

Brand name: Coumadin.
Class of drug: Oral anticoagulant.
Mechanism of action: Inhibits synthesis of hepatic vitamin K-dependent clotting factors.
Indications/dosage/route: Oral, IV.
• Anticoagulation
  – Adults: Initial: PO, IV 5–10 mg/d for 2–4 days, then adjust dose based on prothrombin or INR determinations. Maintenance: 2–10 mg/d based on prothrombin or INR.
• Prophylaxis, prosthetic heart valve replacement
  – PO 2–5 mg/d.
Adjustment of dosage
• Kidney disease: None.
• Liver disease: None.
• Elderly: May need to have reduced dosage.
• Pediatric: Safety and efficacy have not been established in children <18 years.
Pregnancy: Category X.
Lactation: Not detected in breast milk. Considered compatible by American Academy of Pediatrics.
Contraindications: Pregnancy, hemorrhagic disorders, hemophilia, blood dyscrasias, thrombocytopenia purpura, malignant hypertension, recent surgery (eg, brain, eye), head injury, threatened abortion, spinal puncture, hypersensitivity to warfarin.
Warnings/precautions
• Use with caution in patients with CHF, kidney and liver disease, heparin-induced thrombocytopenia, and in menstruating women.
• Heparin is generally started prior to warfarin to decrease time required for anticoagulation. Heparin should be withdrawn when steady-state anticoagulation is achieved.
• Stop this drug 3 days before anticipated surgery. Oral

anticoagulation should be reinstituted 3 days after surgery and INR should be checked 5–7 days after restarting anticoagulation.

- Before beginning therapy test patient for occult blood in stool or urine.
- Begin oral anticoagulant therapy in progressing stroke only if a CAT scan shows there is no brain hemorrhage.
- Many drugs interact in an unfavorable way with oral anticoagulants.
- Treat overdose from oral anticoagulant as follows: (1) stop one or two doses; (2) consider administration of phytonadione (vitamin K) 1–10 mg orally or 20–40 mg IV, 1 mg/min; (3) if bleeding is severe or persistent, it may be necessary to administer parenteral vitamin K, plasma (fresh or frozen), or whole blood.
- Only administer warfarin when there is no need for arterial puncture.

Advice to patient

- Carry identification card at all times describing disease, treatment regimen, name, address, and telephone number of treating physician.
- Avoid alcohol.
- Do not take OTC products containing aspirin or related drugs, eg, ibuprofen.
- Do not change brands unless approved by treating physician.
- Use soft toothbrush and electric razor.
- Do not change diet extensively without consulting physician.
- Notify physician immediately if you sustain a serious injury. Avoid situations that could result in falls, bumps, cuts (eg, contact sports).
- Notify physician if you experience nosebleeds, excessive bleeding from a cut, etc.
- Notify physician if you observe red or tarry-black stools or red or dark brown urine.
- Avoid vitamin supplements or foods high in vitamin K (eg, spinach, broccoli, cabbage, turnips, milk, yogurt, cheeses).

- Use two forms of birth control including hormonal and barrier methods.

Adverse reactions

- Common: none.
- Serious: hemorrhage, warfarin-induced necrosis, cholesterol microembolism.

Clinically important drug interactions

- Drugs that increase effects/toxicity of warfarin: NSAIDs, aspirin, cimetidine.
- Drugs that decrease effects/toxicity of warfarin: barbiturates, rifampin.

Parameters to monitor

- PT, INR, and other suitable coagulation tests. Therapeutic PT should be 1.5–2.5 times control. Therapeutic INR = 2–3. Adjust dosage to achieve these parameters.
- INR or PT at least once a month in menstruating female.
- Efficacy of treatment: prevention of deep vein thrombosis or pulmonary embolism.
- Signs of "purple toes syndrome": local pain, purple-black skin surrounded by red area.
- Signs of skin necrosis or local pain in elderly and obese patients.
- Signs and symptoms of local thrombosis or vasculitis, which may occur 2–10 days after starting therapy. Give vitamin K if this occurs and stop drug administration.
- Signs of internal bleeding: hematuria (red, dark brown, or cloudy urine), hematemesis (dark brown or red vomitus), bleeding gums, petechiae, blood in sputum, abdominal pain or swelling, chest pain, severe headache, dizziness or fainting (intracranial bleeding), excessive bleeding from minor injury.

Editorial comments: All patients receiving an oral anticoagulant must be under close medical supervision. Laboratory facilities must be available to monitor therapy; personnel must know how to treat the hemorrhagic patient.

Zafirlukast

Brand name: Accolate.
Class of drug: Antiasthmatic, leukotriene receptor antagonist.
Mechanism of action: Blocks leukotriene D_4 and E_4, reducing bronchospasm and inflammation.
Indications/dosage/route: Oral only.
• Chronic treatment of asthma
  – Adults, children >12 years: 20 mg b.i.d.
Adjustment of dosage
• Kidney disease: None.
• Liver disease: Reduce dosage.
• Elderly: Use with caution.
• Pediatric: Safety and efficacy have not been established in children <12 years.
Food: Should be taken 1 hour before or 2 hours after meals.
Pregnancy: Category B.
Lactation: Appears in breast milk. Best to avoid.
Contraindications: Hypersensitivity to zafirlukast, acute attack of asthma, status asthmaticus.
Warnings/precautions
• Use with caution in patients with liver disease.
• Patient should continue all other antiasthma medications as prescribed.
Advice to patient: If a dose is missed, do not double the next dose.
Adverse reactions
• Common: headache.
• Serious: hepatitis, eosinophilia, vasculitis, urticaria.
Clinically important drug interactions
• Drugs that decrease effects/toxicity of zafirlukast: erythromycin, theophylline, aspirin, magnesium or aluminum-containing antacids.
• Zafirlukast increases effects/toxicity of warfarin, theophylline.
Parameters to monitor: Signs and symptoms of asthma: Monitor respiratory rate, pulmonary function and oxygen saturation.
Editorial comments: Rare cases of Churg–Strauss syndrome with eosinophilia, vasculitic rashes, worsening lung status, cardiac

disease, and peripheral neuropathy have been seen with zafirlukast therapy, usually after decreased steroid dosage. If this syndrome is suspected, zafirlukast must be immediately discontinued.

Zalcitabine

Brand name: Hivid.
Class of drug: Antiretroviral agent.
Mechanism of action: Converted to active metabolite that inhibits HIV replication by blocking reverse transcriptase.
Indications/dosage/route: Oral only.
• Treatment of advanced HIV infection
  – Adults ≥ 66 lb: 0.75 mg zalcitabine plus 200 mg ziduvidine, q8h.
Adjustment of dosage
• Kidney disease: Creatinine clearance >40 mL/min: normal dose; creatinine clearance 10–40 mL/min: 0.75 mg q12h; creatinine clearance <10 mL/min: 0.75 mg q24h.
• Liver disease: None.
• Elderly: Safety and efficacy have not been established in HIV patients >65 years.
• Pediatric: Safety and efficacy have not been established in HIV-infected children <13 years.
Food: Take on empty stomach.
Pregnancy: Category C.
Lactation: Data not available. CDC suggests that HIV-infected mothers should not breastfeed due to potential for HIV transmission to infant.
Contraindications: Hypersensitivity to zalcitabine, coadministration with other pancreatoxic agents (eg, pentamidine).
Warnings/precautions
• Use with caution in patients with peripheral neuropathy, kidney disease, heart failure, history of pancreatitis.
• Zalcitabine is used with extreme caution in patients with CD4 cell counts <50/mm^3.

Advice to patient

- Do not discontinue this drug without consulting treating physician.
- If a dose is missed, do not double the next dose.
- Avoid alcohol.
- Male patients should use condoms if engaging in sexual intercourse while using this medication.

Adverse reactions

- Common: See Serious.
- Serious: **peripheral neuropathy**, seizures, pancreatitis, cardiomyopathy, CHF, hepatitis, liver failure.

Clinically important drug interactions: Drugs that increase effects/toxicity of zalcitabine: other potentially neurotoxic drugs including cisplatin, chloramphenicol, dapsone, disulfiram, ethionamide, glutethimide, gold, hydralazone, iodoquinol, isoniazid, metronidazole, nitrofurantoin, ribavirin, phenytoin, vincristine, alcohol, azathioprine, pentamidine, tetracyclines, thiazides, valproic acid, aminoglycosides, foscarnet.

Parameters to monitor

- Signs and symptoms of anemia: shortness of breath, dizziness, angina, pale conjunctiva, skin, and nailbeds.
- Signs and symptoms of infection.
- Signs and symptoms of neuropathy. If these symptoms last more than 3 days, drug should be discontinued. If peripheral neuropathy improves, zalcitabine may be readministered at 50% of the initial dose.
- CD4 levels prior to and at frequent intervals after therapy is instituted.
- Signs and symptoms of pancreatitis: nausea, vomiting, abdominal pain.
- Levels of serum amylase and triglycerides. If serum amalyase increases by 1.5–2 times normal or symptoms of pancreatitis occur, zalcitabine should be discontinued.
- Signs and symptoms of bone marrow depression.
- Signs and symptoms of hepatotoxicity.

Editorial comments

- Zalcitabine is approved for use in adult patients with advanced HIV infection who have experienced clinical and/or immunologic deterioration in their condition. For this purpose it is often used only in combination with zidovudine.

• It is recommended that treatment with zalcitabine be made in consultation with a physician experienced in treating HIV infection.

• Zalcitabine has the potential to produce serious and life-threatening toxic effects. The prescribing physician should be cognizant of these toxic effects and should advise the patient to discontinue the drug should they occur. Toxic effects include peripheral neuropathy (potentially reversible), pancreatitis (1.1% potentially fatal), and liver failure.

Zidovudine (Azidothymidine, AZT)

Brand names: Retrovir, Combivir.
Class of drug: Antiretroviral agent.
Mechanism of action: Active metabolite inhibits HIV replication by blocking reverse transcriptase.
Indication/dosage/route: Oral, IV.

• Symptomatic HIV infection, asymptomatic HIV infection, CD4 count <500/mm^3
  – Adults, children >12 years: PO 100 mg q4h. Alternative dosing: IV 1 mg/kg q4h.
  – Children 3 months–12 years: 180 mg/m^2 q6h. Maximum: 200 mg q6h.

• Prevention of transmission of HIV from mother to fetus (after week 14 of pregnancy)
  – Maternal dosage: 100 mg q5h until start of delivery.
  – During labor and delivery: IV 2 mg/kg over 1 hour. Then continuous infusion of 2 mg/kg/h.
  – Infant dosing: PO 2 mg/kg q6h, within 12 hours of birth. Continue through 6 weeks of age.
  – Maternal dosing: IV 1–2 mg/kg q4h until PO therapy can be administered.

Adjustment of dosage

- Kidney disease: Creatinine clearance < 10 mL/min: 100 mg q6–8h.
- Liver disease: Dose reduced by 50% or double the dosing interval in cirrhotic patients.
- Elderly: No information available.
- Pediatric: See above.

Food: Should be taken 30 minutes before or 1 hour after meal with a glass of water.

Pregnancy: Category C.

Lactation: HIV-infected mothers should avoid breastfeeding.

Contraindications: Hypersensitivity to zidovudine.

Warnings/precautions

- Use with caution in patients with advanced HIV, severe bone marrow depression, renal insufficiency, liver disease, myopathy, neuropathy, anemia.
- Administer around the clock to maintain constant serum levels.
- When given long-term, zidovudine may cause a myopathy that resembles HIV-induced myopathy.

Advice to patients

- Take only prescribed dose and do not discontinue without consulting the treating physician. If a dose is missed, do not double the subsequent dose.
- Male patients should use condoms if engaging in sexual intercourse while using this medication.
- Avoid crowds as well as persons who may have a contagious disease.
- Consume 2–3 L of fluid/d.
- Avoid using acetaminophen.

Adverse reactions

- Common: nausea, headache, malaise, diarrhea, anorexia.
- Serious: **neuropathy**, anemia, neutropenia, leukopenia, thrombocytopenia, myopathy, hepatitis.

Clinically important drug interactions

- Zidovudine increases effects/toxicity of dapsone, gancyclovir, vincristine, vinblastine, flucytosine, adriamycin, doxorubicin.
- Drugs that increase effects/toxicity of zidovudine: probenecid, fluconazole, acetaminophen, cimetidine, indomethacin, lorazepam,

aspirin, clarithromycin, valproic acid, α interferon, phenytoin, trimethoprim, acyclovir, gancyclovir, pentamidine, indinavir.

Parameters to monitor

- CBC with differential count every 2 weeks during the first 8 weeks of therapy in patients with advanced HIV disease. Beyond this time, monitoring should be carried out on a chronic basis.
- Hematologic status. Reduce dose under the following conditions: hemoglobin <7.5 m/dL, or granulocyte count <750 mm^3 or >50% decrease from baseline.
- Signs and symptoms of infection.
- Symptoms of myopathy. If this occurs, it may be necessary to reduce the dosage or stop drug administration.

Zolmitriptan

Brand name: Zomig.

Class of drug: Antimigraine drug.

Mechanism of action: Selective angonist for 5-HT$_1$ receptors on basilar and cranial arteries. Produces cranial vasoconstriction and decreased release of inflammatory neuropeptides.

Indications/dosage/route: Oral only.

- Acute migraine headache
  - Adults: Initial: 2.5–5 mg. Repeat in 2 hours if necessary.

Adjustment of dosage

- Kidney disease: None.
- Liver disease: None.
- Elderly: Use with caution in patients >40 years.
- Pediatric: None

Food: No restriction.

Pregnancy: Category C.

Lactation: No data available. Best to avoid.

Contraindications: Ischemic heart disease, uncontrolled hypertension, *prophylaxis* of migraine, angina, history of MI, concurrent use of MAO inhibitor or within 2 weeks of stopping one.

Warnings/precautions: Use with caution in postmenopausal women and in patients with diabetes, obesity, cigarette smoking, hypercholestremia, family history of coronary artery disease.

Clinically important drug interactions: Drugs that increase effects/toxicity of zomitriptan: MAO inhibitors, oral contraceptives, cimetidine, SSRIs, ergotamine-containing or ergot-type medications (dihydroergotamine, methysergide).

Editorial comments

• Zolmitriptan, a new agent for acute treatment of migraine headaches, is very similar to sumatriptan. Some patients who do not respond to sumatriptan may respond to zolmitriptan.

• This drug is not listed in the *Physicians' Desk Reference*, 54th edition, 2000.

• For additional information, see *sumatriptan*, p. 867.

Zolpidem

Brand name: Ambien.

Class of drugs: Nonbarbiturate, nonbenzodiazepine hypnotic.

Mechanism of action: Binds to and modulates GABA–benzodiazepine receptor complex in CNS neurons.

Indications/dosage/route: Oral only.

• Short-term management of insomnia
  – Adults: 10 mg h.s. Do not exceed nightly dose of 10 mg.

Adjustment of dosage

• Kidney disease: None.

• Liver disease: Initial dose: 5 mg h.s. Monitor for daytime sleepiness.

• Elderly: Initial dose: 5 mg h.s.

• Pediatric: Safety and effectiveness have not been established in children <18 years.

Food: Should be taken on an empty stomach.

Pregnancy: Category B. Should be used only if needed.

Lactation: Appears in breast milk. Considered compatible by American Academy of Pediatrics.

Contraindications: None.
Warnings/precautions
- Use with caution in patients with decreased respiratory drive (eg, COPD), history of alcohol or drug abuse, depression, suicide attempts, history of psychiatric illness, liver and kidney disease.
- There is the possibility of a withdrawal reaction if abruptly withdrawn after ≥2 weeks. This consists of insomnia, muscle cramps, vomiting, panic attacks, seizures.
- Do not prescribe more than a 1-month supply.

Advice to patient
- Avoid alcohol.
- Avoid driving and other activities requiring mental alertness or that are potentially dangerous until response to drug is known.
- Use only as directed by your physician: how and when to take the drug and for how long. Do not use this drug longer than directed by your physician. Do not increase the dose prescribed by your physician.

Adverse reactions
- Common: headache, drowsiness, dizziness, diarrhea, drugged sensation, dry mouth.
- Serious: anaphylaxis, depression, cardiac toxicity, bone marrow depression.

Clinically important drug interactions
- Drugs that increase effects/toxicity of zolpidem: CNS depressants, imipramine, chlorpromazine.
- Flumazenil reverses the effects of zolpidem.

Parameters to monitor
- Pain status in those with acute or chronic pain. Consider addition of an analgesic. Untreated pain decreases sedative action of this drug.
- Evidence of dependence, depression, alcoholism, or addiction.

Editorial comments
- Patient should be reevaluated if zolpidem is taken longer than 2–3 weeks. Limit use to 7–10 days.
- In the event of overdose, flumazenil may be used to reverse CNS depression from zolipidem.

APPENDICES

TABLE 1

Food and Drug Administration Pregnancy Categories

A. Controlled studies performed in pregnant women do not demonstrate a risk to the fetus during the first trimester of pregnancy with no evidence of risk in the second or third trimesters. The possibility of fetal harm appears highly unlikely.

B. Either studies in reproducing animals do not demonstrate a fetal risk but there are no controlled studies in pregnant women, or animal reproduction studies have shown adverse effects (other than a decrease in fertility) that were not confirmed in controlled studies in pregnant women in the first trimester and there is no evidence of a risk in later trimesters.

C. Either study in animals has demonstrated adverse effects on the fetus (teratogenic, embryocidal, or other effects) and there are no controlled studies in women, or studies in women and animals are not available. These drugs should be given only if the potential benefits of the drug justify the potential or unknown risk to the fetus.

D. There is positive evidence of human fetal risk, but the benefits from administration in pregnant women may be acceptable despite the risk. For example, if the drug is needed in a life-threatening situation or for a serious disease for which safer drugs cannot be used or are ineffective, administration may be indicated.

X. Animals or human studies have demonstrated fetal abnormalities or there is evidence of risk to the fetus based on human experience, or both. The risk of the use of the drug in pregnant women clearly outweighs any possible benefit. The drug is therefore contraindicated in women who are or may become pregnant.

TABLE 2

Common Aminoglycosides: General Information

Group A	Dosage (adult) once daily	Maintenance Loading	Maintenance Daily	Peak (µg/mL)	Trough (µg/mL)	Comments
Gentamicin	7.5 mg/kg	2 mg/kg	1.7 mg/kg	4–10	1–2	Preferred for enterococcal infections (synergistic)
Tobramycin	7.5 mg/kg	2 mg/kg	1.7 mg/kg q8h	4–10	1–2	Preferred for pseudomonal infections (synergistic)
Amikacin	15 mg/kg	7.5 mg/kg	7.5 mg/kg q12h	15–30	5–10	Still effective for gram-negative infections resistant to gentamicin and tobramycin
Streptomycin	15 mg/kg 2 or 3 times weekly; 25–30 mg (tuberculosis)		(*Yersinia pestis*) 7.5 mg/kg q12h (plague)			Synergistic with ampicillin and vancomycin for enterococcal endocarditis unless highly resistant to streptomycin

(continued)

TABLE 2 (CONTINUED)

Common Aminoglycosides: General Information (continued)

Aminoglycoside spectrum

1. As single agents: gram-negative aerobic bacilli (*Acinetobacter*, *Enterobacter*, most Enterobacteriaceae)
2. Synergistic for *Pseudomonas aeruginosa* (tobramycin, amikacin superior to gentamicin). Should be combined with β-lactam (piperacillin, mezlocillin, ticarcillin, ceftazidime, cefepime, imipenem, aztreonam)
3. Synergistic for enterococcus (gentamicin only). Combined with either ampicillian or vancomycin if organisms highly resistant to gentamicin
4. Synergistic for streptococcal endocarditis
5. Synergistic for staphylococcal endocarditis

TABLE 3

First-Generation Cephalosporins

Generic name	Brand name	Route	Spectrum
Cefadroxil	Duricef	Oral	All first-generation cephalosporins have excellent activity against various gram-positive cocci including (1) *Staphylococcus aureus* but not MRSA, and (2) streptococci (group A, group B, and viridans). Not effective against *Enterococcus* sp (like all cephalosporins). Moderately effective against *Streptococcus pneumoniae* Poor gram-negative activity, except for community-acquired *Escherichia coli, Proteus mirabilis* (indole positive), *Klebsiella* sp, *Branhamella catarrhalis*. Poor activity against *Hemophilus influenzae*. Not effective against *Bracillus fragilis*.
Cefazolin First-choice parenteral agent	Ancef	IM/IV	
Cephalexin First-choice oral agent	Keflex	Oral	
Cephalothin	Keflex	IM, IV	
Cephapyrim	Cefadyl	IM, IV	
Cephradine	Velosef	PO IM/IV	

TABLE 4

Second-Generation Cephalosporins

Generic name	Brand name	Route	Spectrum
			Cefuroxime subgroup
Cefuroxime	Zinacef	IV, IM	• *S. aureus*: good, but less than first-generation
Cefamandole	Mandol	IV, IM	• *S. pneumoniae*: more active than first-generation for beta-hemolytic streptococci
Cefonicid	Monocid	IV, IM	• More active against gram-negative bacteria including: *Hemophilus influenzae*, *Neisseria gonorrhoeae*, *Moraxella catarrhalis*, *E. coli*, *P. mirabilis*, *Klebsiella* sp, *Citrobacter* sp, *Morganella* sp
			• Cefuroxime good for meningitis, but ceftriaxone superior
			• Cefamandole better for *S. aureus*, not as good for gram-negative especially *H. influenzae*
			Cephamycin subgroup
Cefoxitin	Mefoxin	IV, IM	• Cefoxitin best anaerobic activity in second-generation cephalosporins: covers *Bacteroides* sp
Cefotetan	Cefotan	IV, IM	• Less active against gram-positive than first- and second-generation cephalosporins
Cefmetazole	Zefazone	IV, IM	

962

TABLE 4 (CONTINUED)

- More active against gram-negative than first-generation, but less active than cefuroxime against *H. influenzae*
- Cefotetan less active against *Bacteroides* DOT group, more active against gram-negative

Oral second-generation

- Treat mild to moderate community-acquired infections (ie, skin, soft tissue, UTI [other agents better])
- Respiratory infections, sinusitis, otitis media, strep throat; preferred agent—cefuroxime axetil

Cefaclor	Ceclor	PO
Cefprozil	Cefzil	PO
Ceftibuten	Cedax	PO
Loracarbef (Carbacephem)	Lorabid	PO
Cefuroxime axetil	Ceftin	PO

Note: MTT chain: Inhibits activation of vitamin K. → bleeding   cefamandole
Disulfiram-like reaction with alcohol   cefotetan
    cefmetazole
    cefoperazone (third-generation)

TABLE 5

Third-Generation Cephalosporins

Generic name	Brand name	Route	Spectrum
Ceftriaxone (good CSF, biliary sludge)	Rocephin	IV, IM	• Superior efficacy against *S. pneumoniae* and good CSF levels; also, covers *Neisseria meningitidis* and *H. influenzae*, therefore good for meningitis
Cefotaxime (good CSF)	Claforan	IV, IM	• Superior activity against streptococci • Poor activity against *S. aureus* • Good activity against gram-negative, *E. coli, P. mirabilis, Klebsiella* sp. not *P. aeruginosa*
Ceftizoxime	Cefizox	IV, IM	• Not as effective as ceftriaxone or cefotaxime against *S. pneumoniae* • Good anaerobic activity including many *B. fragilis* strains (66–80%)
Cefoperazone (MTT chain, poor CSF)	Cefobid	IV, IM	• Modest *P. aeruginosa* efficacy (50%) • Less effective against gram-positive

TABLE 5 (CONTINUED)

Drug	Brand names	Route	Comments
Ceftazidime (good CSF)	Fortaz, Tazicef, Tazidime	IV, IM	• Low activity for many inducible β-lactamase producers • Excellent gram-negative coverage (including *P. aeruginosa*) • Poor anaerobe and *S. aureus* coverage
Cefixime	Suprax	PO	• Antimicrobial activity against penicillin-resistant *S. pneumoniae* is low
Cefpodoxime	Vantin	PO	
Ceftibuten	Cedax	PO	
Cefdinir	Omnicef	PO	

TABLE 6

Fourth-Generation Cephalosporin

Generic name	Trade name	Route	Spectrum
Cefepime	Maxipime	IV, IM	Compared with ceftazidime, improved gram-positive activity (including *S. pneumoniae*, MSSA, streptococci); good *P. aeruginosa* activity

TABLE 7

Macrolides: Susceptible Organisms

	Gram-positive	Gram-negative	Others
Erythromycin	Group A streptococcus (increased resistance outside United States)	*Neisseria gonorrhoeae*	Lung
	Streptococcus pneumoniae (increased resistance outside United States)	*Neisseria meningitides*	*M. pneumoniae*
	S. aureus (moderately effective)	*Helicobacter pylori*	*C. pneumoniae*
	Viridans streptococci	*C. jejuni*	*Legionella* sp
	C. diphtheriae	*M. catarrhalis*	Genital
	Whooping cough (*Hemophilus influenzae*)		*Chlamydia trachomatis*
	Listeria (nonmeningeal)		*Ureaplasma*
	P. acne		*M. hominis*
	Clostridium perfringens		

(*continued*)

TABLE 7 (CONTINUED)

Macrolides: Susceptible Organisms (continued)

	Gram-postive	Gram-negative	Others
Azithromycin	Less active	More active, especially *M. catarrhalis*, *Shigella* sp *Campylobacter* sp	Nongonococcal urethritis (1 g single dose effective) Prophylaxis for MAI in AIDS Early Lyme disease
Clarithromycin	Active especially against *S. pneumoniae* and *S. aureus*	Same as erythromycin but not active against *H. influenzae* and *H. pylori*	Treatments: MAI in AIDS, other mycobacterial infections, early Lyme disease

MAI, *Mycobacterium avium–intracellulare*.

TABLE 8

Quinolones: General Information

Generic name	Brand name	Route	Important adverse effects	Spectrum and use
First Generation: not fluorinated				
Nalidixic Acid	Neg Gram	PO	—	• Only aerobic gram-negative; not *Pseudomonas aeruginosa* covers Enterobacteriaceae, *Hemophilus influenzae*, *Neisseria gonorrhoeae*, and *catarrhalis*
Second Generation: fluorinated ⇒ fluoroquinolones				
Ciprofloxacin	Cipro	PO, IV	—	• Excellent gram-negative activity, the quinolone of choice for *P. aeruginosa*; covers all Enterobacteriaceae
				• Good activity against *S. aureus* including MRSA; Second-line agent used for osteomyelitis
				• Excellent for atypical pneumonia, (ie, *Legionella, Mycoplasma, C. pneumoniae*)
				• Not used for *S. pneumoniae*, as single agent for community-acquired pneumonia, acute or chronic sinusitis, otitis media, or skin infections

(continued)

TABLE 8 (CONTINUED)

Quinolones: General Information (continued)

Generic name	Brand name	Route	Important adverse effects	Spectrum and use
Norfloxacin	Noroxin	PO	—	• Excellent for genital infections (including prostatitis), ie, *N. gonorrhoeae* (single dose), *Chlamydia trachomatis, M. hominis, Ureaplasma* • Poor coverage for anaerobic and streptococci
Enoxacin	Penetrex	PO	—	• Narrower spectrum; used for UTI, prostatitis, *N. gonorrhoeae* • Not for *P. aeruginosa, S. aureus,* or *Chlamydia* sp • Similar to ofloxacin
Ofloxacin	Floxin	PO, IV	—	• Similar to ciprofloxacin, but less effective against *P. aeruginosa*
Lomefloxacin	Maxaquin	PO	Phototoxicity	• Similar to ofloxacin

TABLE 8 (CONTINUED)

Quinolones with improved gram-positive coverage

Levofloxacin	Levoquin	PO, IV	—	• Levo isomer of ofloxacin with activity against *Streptococcus pneumoniae* and streptococci; some anaerobic activity (not *Bacillus fragilis*)
Sparfloxacin	Zagam	PO	Increased QT, interval, phototoxicity	• Like levofloxacin, but improved activity against *B. fragilis*
Grepafloxacin	Raxar	PO	Increased QT interval	• Excellent *Pseudomonas aeruginosa* activity, good gram-positive activity, excellent anaerobic coverage including *B. fragilis*
Trovafloxacin	Trovan	PO, IV	Liver failure, used only for severe infections	• Good *P. aeruginosa* activity, excellent gram-positive and anaerobic coverage.
Gatifloxacin	Tequin	PO	—	• Excellent anaerobic and gram-positive coverage

TABLE 9

Antifungal Agents

Spectrum and Uses

Agent	Brand name	Route	CNS	Candida	Cryptococcus	Fungi	Molds	Others
Ketoconazole	Nizoral	PO	No	Good	Avoid especially in CNS infections	Blastomycosis, histoplasmosis, coccidioidomycosis	No	*Leishmania major*
Fluconazole	Diflucan	PO, IV	Yes	Excellent activity but not *C. glabrata* *C. krusei*	Excellent even for CNS infections	Coccidioidomycosis, meningitis (do not use for blastomycosis, histoplasmosis, ringworm, sporotrichosis)	No	No

TABLE 9 (CONTINUED)

Itraconazole	Sporanox	PO	Yes	Excellent activity even in resistant organisms	No	Blastomycosis, histoplasmosis, coccidioidomycosis, sporotrichosis	Aspergillosis	Tinea versicolor, onychomycosis, ringworm
Voriconazole	Investigational	PO, IV	?	Excellent	?	?	Aspergillosis (even severe?)	—
Miconazole	Monistat	Topical, No IV		Good, topical	—	—	*Pseudallescheria boydii*	—
Terbinafine	Lamisil	PO		—	—	—	—	Onychomycosis, tinea versicolor, tinea pedis, tinea cruris

TABLE 9 (CONTINUED)

Antifungal Agents (continued)

Agent	Brand Name	Route	Spectrum and Uses					
			CNS	Candida	Cryptococcus	Fungi	Molds	Others
Griseofulvin	Fulvicin	PO	—	—	—	—	—	Second-line agent except possibly in children with tinea capitis
Flucytosine	Ancobon	PO	—	Synergism with amphotericin B	Synergism with amphotericin B	Chromomycosis (drug of choice)	—	—

TABLE 10

Oral Contraceptives

Combination Estrogen/Progestin Preparations: Schedules and Dosages

Brand Name	Estrogen	Progestin
Monophasic		
Brevicon 21-Day and 28-Day	Ethinyl estradiol (35 µg)	Norethindrone (0.5 mg)
Demulen 1/35-21 and 1/35-28	Ethinyl estradiol (35 µg)	Ethynodiol diacetate (1 mg)
Demulen 1/50-21 and 1/50-28	Ethinyl estradiol (50 µg)	Ethynodiol diacetate (1 mg)
Desogen (28-day)	Ethinyl estradiol (30 µg)	Desogestrel (0.15 mg)
Genora 0.5/35 21 Day and 28 Day	Ethinyl estradiol (35 µg)	Norethindrone (0.5 mg)
Genova 1/35 21 Day and 28 Day	Ethinyl estradiol (35 µg)	Norethindrone (1 mg)
Genova 1/50 21 Day and 28 Day	Mestranol (50 µg)	Norethindrone (1 mg)
Levlen 21 and 28	Ethinyl estradiol (30 µg)	Levonorgestrel (0.15 mg)
Levora 0.15/30-21 and -28	Ethinyl estradiol (30 µg)	Levonorgestrel (0.15 mg)
Loestrin 21 1/20	Ethinyl estradiol (20 µg)	Norethindrone acetate (1 mg)
Loestrin 21 1.5/30	Ethinyl estradiol (30 µg)	Norethindrone acetate (1.5 mg)

(continued)

TABLE 10 (CONTINUED)

Oral Contraceptives

Combination Estrogen/Progestin Preparations: Scheduled and Dosages (continued)

Brand Name	Estrogen	Progestin
Loestrin Fe 1/20 (28 day)	Ethinyl estradiol (20 μg)	Norethindrone acetate (1 mg)
Loestrin Fe 1.5/30 (28 day)	Ethinyl estradiol (30 μg)	Norethindrone acetate (1.5 mg)
Lo/Ovral-21 and -28	Ethinyl estradiol (30 μg)	Norgestrel (0.3 mg)
Modicon 21 and 28	Ethinyl estradiol (35 μg)	Norethindrone (0.5 mg)
Necon 0.5/35-21 Day and 28 Day	Ethinyl estradiol (35 μg)	Norethindrone (0.5 mg)
Necon 1/35-21 Day and 28 Day	Ethinyl estradiol (35 μg)	Norethindrone (1 mg)
Necon 1/50-21 Day and 28 Day	Mestranol (50 μg)	Norethindrone (1 mg)
Necon 1/50-21 Day and -28 Day	Ethinyl estradiol (50 μg)	Norethindrone (1 mg)
N.E.E. 1/35 21 Day and 28 Day	Ethinyl estradiol (35 μg)	Norethindrone (1 mg)
Nelova 0.5/35E 21 Day and 28 Day	Ethinyl estradiol (35 μg)	Norethindrone (0.5 mg)
Nelova 1/35E 21 Day and 28 Day	Ethinyl estradiol (35 μg)	Norethindrone (1 mg)
Nelova 1/50M 21 Day and 28 Day	Mestranol (50 μg)	Norethindrone (1 mg)

TABLE 10 (CONTINUED)

Nordette-21 and -28	Ethinyl estradiol (35 μg)	Levonorgestrel (0.15 mg)
Norethin 1/35E 21 Day and 28 Day	Ethinyl estradiol (35 μg)	Norethindrone (1 mg)
Norethin 1/50M 21 Day and 28 day	Mestranol (50 μg)	Norethindrone (1 mg)
Norinyl 1 + 35 21-Day and 28-Day	Ethinyl estradiol (35 μg)	Norethindrone (1 mg)
Norinyl 1 + 50 21-Day and 28-Day	Mestranol (50 μg)	Norethindrone (1 mg)
Ortho-Cept 21 Day and 28 Day	Ethinyl estradiol (30 μg)	Desogestrel (0.15 mg)
Ortho-Cyclen-21 and -28	Ethinyl estradiol (35 μg)	Norgestimate (0.25 mg)
Ortho Novum 1/35-21 and -28	Ethinyl estradiol (35 μg)	Norethindrone (1 mg)
Ortho Novum 1/50-21 and -28	Mestranol (50 μg)	Norethindrone (1 mg)
Ovcon-35 21 Day and 28 Day	Ethinyl estradiol (35 μg)	Norethindrone (0.4 mg)
Ovcon-50 21 Day and 28 Day	Ethinyl estradiol (50 μg)	Norethindrone (1 mg)
Ovral 21 Day and 28 Day	Ethinyl estradiol (50 μg)	Norgestrel (0.5 mg)
Zovia 1/35E-21 and -28	Ethinyl estradiol (35 μg)	Ethynodiol diacetate (1 mg)
Zovia 1/50E-21 and -28	Ethinyl estradiol (50 μg)	Ethynodiol diacetate (1 mg)

(continued)

977

TABLE 10 (CONTINUED)

Oral Contraceptives

Combination Estrogen/Progestin Preparations: Scheduled and Dosages (continued)

brand Name	Estrogen	Progestin
Biphasic		
Jenest-28	Ethinyl estradiol (35 µg)	Norethindrone (10 tabs of 0.5 mg followed by 11 tabs of 1 mg)
Necon 10/11 21 Day and 28 Day	Ethinyl estradiol (35 µg)	Norethindrone (10 tabs of 0.5 mg followed by 11 tabs of 1 mg)
Nelova 10/11-21 and -28	Ethinyl estradiol (35 µg)	Norethindrone (10 tabs of 0.5 mg followed by 11 tabs of 1 mg)
Ortho-Novum 10/11-21 and -28	Ethinyl estradiol (35 µg)	Norethindrone (10 tabs of 0.5 mg followed by 11 tabs of 1 mg)
Triphasic		
Ortho-Novum 7/7/7 (21 or 28 days)	Ethinyl estradiol (35 µg)	Norethindrone (0.5 mg for 7 days, 0.75 next 7 days, 1 mg last 7 days)

TABLE 10 (CONTINUED)

Ortho-Tri-Cyclen (21 or 28 days)	Ethinyl estradiol (35 µg)	Norgestimate (0.18 mg first 7 days, 0.125 mg next 7 days, 0.25 mg last 7 days)
Tri-Levlen 21 Day and Tri-Levlen 28 Days	First 6 days: ethinyl estradiol (30 µg); next 5 days: ethinyl estradiol (40 µg); last 10 days: ethinyl estradiol (30 µg)	Levonorgestrel (0.05 mg) Levonorgestrel (0.075 mg) Levonorgestrel (0.125 mg)
Tri-Norinyl (21 or 28 day)	Ethinyl estradiol (35 µg)	Norethindrone (0.5 mg first 7 days, 1 mg next 9 days, 0.5 mg last 5 days)
Triphasil (21 or 28 day)	First 6 days: ethinyl estradiol (30 µg); next 5 days: ethinyl estradiol (40 µg); last 10 days: ethinyl estradiol (30 µg)	Levonorgestrel (0.05 mg) Levonorgestrel (0.075 mg) Levonorgestrel (0.125 mg)

Reprinted from "PDR nurse's Handbook," 1998 by permission from Medical Economics Company, Montvale, New Jersey.